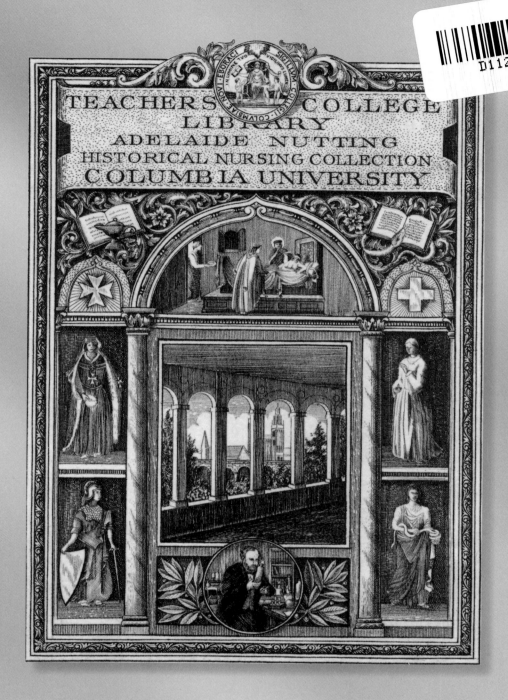

NURSING
THE FINEST ART

Third Edition

An Illustrated History

NURSING
THE FINEST ART

Third Edition

An Illustrated History

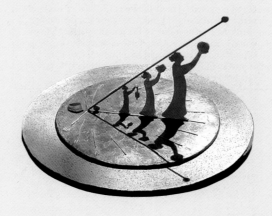

M. Patricia Donahue, PhD, RN, FAAN
Professor Emerita
College of Nursing
The University of Iowa
Iowa City, Iowa

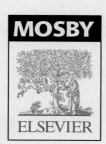

MOSBY
ELSEVIER

MOSBY
ELSEVIER

3251 Riverport Lane
Maryland Heights, Missouri 63043

Notice

Knowledge and best practice in this field are constantly changing. As new research and experience broaden
our knowledge, changes in practice, treatment and drug therapy may become necessary or appropriate.
Readers are advised to check the most current information provided (i) on procedures featured or (ii) by the
manufacturer of each product to be administered, to verify the recommended dose or formula, the method
and duration of administration, and contraindications. It is the responsibility of the practitioner, relying on
their own experience and knowledge of the patient, to make diagnoses, to determine dosages and the best
treatment for each individual patient, and to take all appropriate safety precautions. To the fullest extent of
the law, neither the Publisher nor the Authors assumes any liability for any injury and/or damage to persons
or property arising out of or related to any use of the material contained in this book.

Previous editions copyrighted 1996 and 1985.

Library of Congress Cataloging-in-Publication Data
Donahue, M. Patricia.
    Nursing, the finest art : an illustrated history / M. Patricia Donahue. — 3rd ed.
        p. ; cm.
    Inclues bibliographical references and index.
        ISBN 978-0-323-05305-1 (hardcover : alk. paper)   1. Nursing—History. 2. Nursing—United
States—History. 3. Nursing in art.   I.   Title.
    [DNLM: 1. History of Nursing. 2. Art. WY 11.1 D674n 2010]
    RT31.D66 2010
    610.73—dc22   2009047276

Senior Editor: Yvonne Alexopoulos
Senior Developmental Editor: Lisa P. Newton
Publishing Services Manager: Jeff Patterson
Senior Project Manager: Clay Broeker
Designer: Charles Seibel

Printed in China
Last digit is the print number: 9 8 7 6 5 4 3 2 1

THIS BOOK IS DEDICATED TO NURSES WORLDWIDE
—PAST, PRESENT, AND FUTURE—
WHO REMAIN DEDICATED TO PROFESSIONAL,
COMPETENT, AND COMPASSIONATE CARE AND DRAMATICALLY
INTERPRET THE JOY AND PAIN OF THEIR WORK.

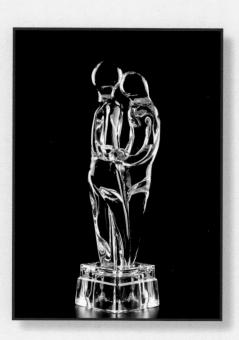

Foreword

We celebrate the appearance of this third edition of *Nursing: The Finest Art: An Illustrated History*. It is an amazing assemblage of visual representations of nursing from earliest times to the present and continues to surpass all other works. Patricia Donahue offers us paintings from renowned artists, sculptures, drawings, photographs, and every imaginable art form to stimulate, inform, and broaden our concept of nursing and its meaning to humankind.

The works range from inspiring and cautionary to satirical and charming. The text and timelines orient and clarify the history of nursing care in all its forms and locations. We readily absorb the intensity of the care-giving and care-receiving relationship through these images, and we find the multiple and varied roles played by nurses over time and in societies around the world.

Read and enjoy this beautiful book. Start anywhere; you will find images you have never seen. Furthermore, I know that every time you open this book, you will thank the creative and tireless scholar who is providing you with knowledge and with the joy of art.

JOAN E. LYNAUGH, RN, PhD, FAAN
Professor Emerita, School of Nursing
University of Pennsylvania
Director Emerita, Barbara Bates Center for the Study
of the History of Nursing
Philadelphia, Pennsylvania

Preface

Approximately 2 weeks before my retirement from The University of Iowa College of Nursing, my secretary asked whether I planned to write the third edition of *Nursing: The Finest Art: An Illustrated History.* I looked at her in utter amazement and replied that the thought had never crossed my mind and that it was highly unlikely that I would contemplate doing this. I was looking forward to retirement and the reduction of job-related pressure and stress. Three days later, I received a phone call from an editor at Elsevier informing me that a discussion was being held regarding the possibility of doing the third edition. Would I be interested? It was an extremely difficult decision to make as I vividly recalled the amount of time and effort required to produce the past editions. On the other hand, I also remembered the rich rewards I have received from nursing over the past 50 years that are so intangible and almost indescribable. Part of my motivation for the previous editions of the book included the possibility of being able to articulate these rewards as well as facilitate an understanding of nursing as it has progressed through time by incorporating artwork with text. This third edition would present me with the opportunity to once again express my deep sentiments about these nursing rewards that I acknowledged in *Nursing: The Finest Art: Master Prints:* "In truth, no one had ever adequately prepared me for the wonders of nursing: the emotional ups and downs; the physical dimensions that demand strength and exertion that may be stretched to the very limits of one's being; the spiritual element that can tax one's faith, can shake it to its very foundation; the observation of miracles; and the growth and development that occur beyond one's wildest imagination. In the final analysis, nursing puts us in touch with being human." Hopefully, I would again be able to provide some insight into that which is truly nursing, into that which is truly a nurse. As some would say, "The rest is history!"

It is almost inconceivable that over 24 years have passed since the first edition was published and 14 years since the second edition. *Nursing: The Finest Art* was the first nursing book of its kind that incorporated artwork of all types with the written words of nursing's history. Although the publishing company was rather nervous about whether this type of book would be accepted by the nursing community, it proved to be a successful undertaking. In a sense, the publication acted as a trailblazer for other publications of this type as numerous nursing publications have emerged that are enhanced with artwork. This combination of visual representation and the written word has proven to be a significant and valuable means to facilitate an understanding of all types of knowledge and phenomena.

It is difficult to capture the totality of nursing in a book of this type, which attempts to portray not only nursing's history but also its eloquent beauty and vitality as represented by the written word and a variety of art forms. As in the first and second editions, art has been used to facilitate the depiction of the particular shifts and changes in the roles and functions of the nurse and the effects of major social, political, and historical forces in society. The majority of the artwork in this third edition is new, and a decided effort was made to incorporate art that would represent nursing as a global community. Every attempt was made to more closely align appropriate artwork with the text, although this presents a challenge in a book of this type. The previous content has been reorganized and new content has been added to address the current status of the nursing profession, with particular emphasis on the global scene. Some might argue that there is too much information on hospitals and medicine, but the fact remains that nursing and its history do not exist in a vacuum and are affected by the historical happenings related to both hospitals and medicine. As with any publication, this text represents a much larger body of information available about nursing's history. It can, however, be used to augment both nursing and art courses and its esthetic value appreciated by all lovers of art.

The illustrated history is not entirely chronological but more representative of a thematic representation; for example, the Nurses in Wars unit incorporates all wars rather than having them discussed in the units that correspond to their specific dates. Numerous resources were used to update the timelines that appear in each unit. The intent of these timelines is to provide the reader with an overview of significant global and nursing events that have occurred; they represent only a fraction of the material that could have been included. Unfortunately, a discussion of nursing evolution in all countries is not feasible in a book of this type, but hopefully the shifting realities of nursing's education and practice are evident as a global reality.

It is true that some significant events, persons, and places were omitted from the text. This is not atypical when writing a book such as this that depicts the history of nursing from primitive times to the present. Any author must be selective with material that is so broad in scope. Indeed, I have chosen specific occurrences in an attempt to balance the artwork with the text and yet render a fair appraisal of nursing's journey through time. Selected events, topics, and individuals important to the development of nursing have been highlighted. These represent a larger body of information that could be used to demonstrate nursing's struggles, growth, challenges, dilemmas, humanitarianism, and beauty. All would reinforce the recurring themes evident in the text and reaffirm the need to effectively communicate the true essence of nursing.

There continues to be discussion about whether nursing is an art as well as a science. Perhaps the difficulty in this discussion is how art is defined and the fact that much of contemporary nursing is focused on the sciences; most nursing educational programs are science based. Far less consideration has been given to nursing's state as an art due to the inability to truly explain the nursing art. There is no doubt that it is difficult to articulate the synthesis of art and science that takes place in nursing practice or to express why and how nursing is an art. Yet, nursing as an art is a form of qualitative inquiry that draws its substance from the aesthetic insight. It is not merely a technique but a process that incorporates the soul, mind, and creative imagination. It is that which inserts the humanistic aspects into the practice of nursing and provides a variety of mechanisms beneficial to effective nurse-patient relationships. Although the discussions may continue, I believe that nursing is an art that defies expression and is equally significant to an understanding of the true essence of nursing.

Many individuals have been involved with this project in different ways, particularly my family and friends. To all of them I extend my sincere appreciation. Those persons who are not identified know of their invaluable assistance and unique contributions. My deepest gratitude is extended to my research assistant, Coralie Pederson, MSN, RN, WHNP, who performed innumerable tasks with persistent enthusiasm for the project. Her determination, organization, and precision were a primary factor in the completion of this work. Always bubbly and cheerful, Coralie inserted a ray of sunshine whenever difficulties occurred. It was so enjoyable to observe her emerging interest in the history of nursing and to be challenged by her insightful questions. Many individuals at Elsevier were instrumental in moving this project forward. Yvonne Alexopoulos, Senior Editor, and Lisa Newton, Senior Developmental Editor, provided sustained support, encouragement, and understanding, particularly during some difficult aspects of the project. They were flexible when I needed them to be and provided sensitive guidance as we progressed. They afforded me the opportunity to participate in every aspect of the publication and permitted me a great deal of autonomy related to the artwork. I will be forever grateful for their genuine trust in my abilities even when I was behind in the anticipated deadlines. Last, but certainly not least, I am deeply indebted to Heather Rippetoe, Editorial Assistant, who inherited the project and handled the artwork permissions. Heather actually became the hub of the wheel that moved artwork production along its journey to completion of the book. Heather was never too busy to answer my questions, return my calls, and research artwork locations I could not find. I have been truly blessed to work with all of them, including the production staff of the company.

M. Patricia Donahue, PhD, RN, FAAN
Golden Valley, Minnesota
August 2009

Contents

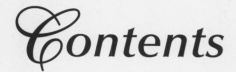

UNIT One

CONTENTS

UNIT Two

Nursing in a Christian World, 38

CONTENTS

UNIT Three

Nursing in Transition, 82

UNIT Four

The Development of Nursing in America, 126

CONTENTS

CONTENTS

UNIT Five

Nurses During War, 178

UNIT Six

Nursing in an Era of Change and Challenge, 216

CONTENTS

UNIT Seven

The Nursing Transformation, 252

CONTENTS

UNIT Eight

The Healing Spirit of Nursing, 288

UNIT Nine

A Global View of Nursing and Healthcare, 316

CONTENTS

UNIT Ten

NURSING
THE FINEST ART
Third Edition

An Illustrated History

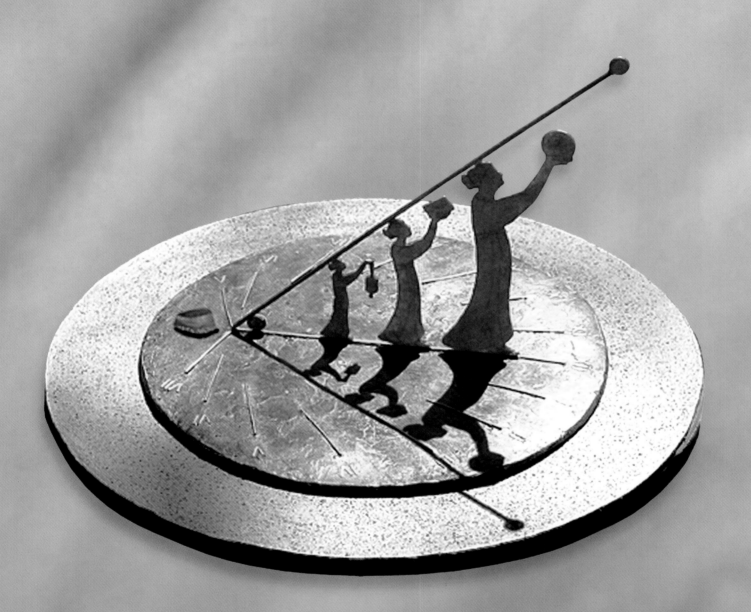

UNIT One

The Origin of Nursing

oman is an instinctive nurse, taught by Mother Nature. The nurse has always been a necessity, thus lacking in social status. In primitive times she was a slave, and in the civilized era a domestic. Overlooked in the plans of legislators and forgotten in the curricula of pedagogues, she was left without protection and remained without education. She was not an artisan who could obtain the help of a hereditary guild; there was no Hanseatic League for nurses. Drawn from the nameless and numberless army of poverty, the nurse worked as a menial and obeyed as a servant. Denied the dignity of a trade and devoid of professional ethics, she could not rise above the degradation of her environment. It never occurred to the Aristotles of the past that it would be safer for the public welfare if nurses were educated, instead of lawyers. The untrained nurse is as old as the human race; the trained nurse is a recent discovery. The distinction between the two is a sharp commentary on the follies and prejudices of mankind.

– VICTOR ROBINSON

The figures of the MGH Nursing Sundial sculpture depict the profession's past (holding a lantern, charting the course for the profession), present (holding a book, representing the scientific knowledge base for the profession), and future (holding a globe, representing the far reaching, global impact of nursing and its universal and multicultural dimensions). Quotes by Nightingale ("Nursing is an Art; the finest of the Fine Arts") and Sleeper ("Always, always more to see, more to learn, more to do…to improve both care and cure") and an exact replica of the MGH nurses' cap complete the sculpture's important nursing message.

Nancy Schon, *Nursing Sundial*, sculpture; base is Chelmsford Granite, 10' in diameter and 18" high; bronze dial is 7' in diameter, and the bronze gnomon is 14' high at the top; gift from the MGH Nurses' Alumnae Association to the Massachusetts General Hospital; September 24, 2004; functioning sundial on lawn by Bulfinch Building of Massachusetts General Hospital, Boston, MA.

The Origin of Nursing

	45,000 BC	30,000 BC	20,000 BC	10,000 BC	5000 BC
Nursing	Nursing as a separate occupation is not well documented during this period. The following is generally known: • Midwives accepted as specialists to women in childbirth • Children's nurses given some distinction in some cultures • Priestesses believed to have performed functions that are now recognized as nursing functions • Men as well as women function as caregivers • Details of nursing principles and practices given in ancient writings • Nurse, pharmacist, and physician recorded in ancient Greek mythology				
Medicine and Health Care					**2900-2800 BC** Imhotep identified as greatest priest physician of Egypt
Science and Technology		**37,000 BC** Rudimentary counting devices used in Africa	**18,550 BC** Bone needles from wallaby shin bone used in Australia		**4241 BC** Egyptians produce 12-month calendar **4000 BC** Writing developed in Mesopotamia **3300 BC** Syrian clay tablets part of earliest phase of writing
The Visual Arts	**45,000 BC** Rock engravings in South Australia	**24,000 BC** First rock paintings in Africa			**3000 BC** First known pottery in the Americas
Daily Life			**17,000 BC** Wild grain harvesting in Middle East **13,000 BC** Earliest evidence of colonization in North America	**6500 BC** Human populations raise sheep, goats, and cattle	**5000 BC** Rice cultivation established in China **4000 BC** Babylonian civilization flourishes **3761 BC** The first year of the Jewish calendar that begins with Rosh Hashana **3500-3001 BC** Linen produced in Middle East

			250 BC World's first nursing school founded in India, but only men are considered "pure" enough to become nurses	
2500-2001 BC Sumerian medicine discovers healing qualities of mineral springs	**2000-1500 BC** Contraceptives used in Egypt **1900 BC** Code of Hammurabi inscribed on shaft of black stone **1800 BC** Mosaic health code developed	**1134 BC** Asklepios is worshipped in temples in Greece	**500 BC** Acupuncture and moxibustion performed in China halls of healing **460-370 BC** Hippocrates credited with establishment of scientific medicine **400 BC** Trephination performed to treat head injuries, migraine headaches, and seizures **300 BC** Medical schools connected with temples of Asklepios in Greece **200 BC** Greek physicians are made slaves and forced to practice throughout Rome	**90 BC** Asclepiades, Greek physician, practices nature healing in Rome
2500-2001 BC Egyptians discover use of papyrus	**2000 BC** Bronze used in tools in China and Europe **2000 BC** Iron tools and weapons developed **1876 BC** First eclipse recorded in China **1800 BC** Bronze weapons used in Europe **1600 BC** Glass molded to form objects and vessels	**1400 BC** Phonetic alphabet widely used in the Levant **800 BC** Use of alphabet adopted in Greece **600 BC** Earliest coins issued by kings of Lydia (modern Turkey)		**80 BC** Greek astronomical calculator computes changing positions of heavenly bodies
2650 BC Stepped pyramid of King Zoser of Egypt built **2650-2150 BC** Most famous Egyptian pyramids built at Giza, Saqqara, and Dahshur **2500 BC** Burial urns painted in western China	**2100 BC** Stonehenge reaches final form in Great Britain **2000 BC** Temples and ritual centers flourish in the Huanaco Valley of Central Peru	**1000-900 BC** Brush-and-ink painting in China **800 BC** Egyptian coffin lids decorated with painted scenes	**500 BC** Terra-cotta sculptures made in Northern Nigeria **500-200 BC** Celtic art style becomes prominent	
2800-2400 BC Flint widely traded **2500-2000 BC** Earliest Egyptian mummies		**1500 BC** Vedas, historical documents of India, written **1280 BC** Hypostyle hall at Karnak uses 134 columns for support **776 BC** First recorded Olympic Games held in Greece **550-331 BC** System of roads established in Persia	**469-399 BC** Socrates pioneers the philosophy of Classical Greece **450-400 BC** Plague in Athens **400-300 BC** Open-air theaters such as Epidauros built **400-300 BC** Use of chopsticks becomes common in China **250-200 BC** Oil lamps introduced in Greece **200 BC** Woven sandals worn by Anasazi people	

Adequate identification and descriptions of the exact origins of nursing are difficult because nothing is known about the actual work of the nurse in prehistory. Everything that has been written about nursing during this period is merely inference based on the discoveries of prehistorians, archaeologists, and anthropologists. Yet early records do provide information about the legacy left to civilized humans by primitive societies. From the dawn of civilization, evidence supports the premise that *nurturing* has been essential to the preservation of life. Survival of the human race, therefore, is inextricably intertwined with the development of nursing.

NURSING AND HUMAN CARING

It is difficult at times to distinguish nursing from medicine in this evolutionary process because the early stages of each are so closely interwoven. Historically, Florence Nightingale is recognized as the founder of nursing as a profession in which individuals were trained and educated but not associated with a religious order. Yet nursing is as old as and actually predates medicine. The interdependence of the two is evident throughout history and has produced a unique and curious relationship. At some periods, such as the Hippocratic era, rational medicine functioned without nursing, whereas at other times, for example, during the Middle Ages, nursing was practiced without rational medicine. According to Davison (1943), who identified four main cycles of medicine (primitive, Renaissance, pharmacy, and modern), nursing approached adequacy in three of those cycles (not pharmacy), and only in these did medicine progress. Davison believes that nursing merits recognition as the "cornerstone of [medicine's] foundation." Certainly the mother-nurse must have preceded the magician-priest or the medicine man or woman. It is even possible that these two types of service were at first united but eventually divided to produce two practitioners of the healing arts—the medicine giver and the caretaker (Stewart and Austin, 1962). Indeed, the modern doctor has the aura of the medicine man, but the seeds of medical knowledge were sown by the natural remedies of the mother.

Nursing has been called the oldest of the arts and the youngest of the professions. As such, it has gone through many stages and has been an integral part of societal movements. Nursing has been involved in the existing culture—shaped by it and yet helping to develop it. The history of nursing has been one of frustration, ignorance, and misunderstanding. It is a great epic involving trials and triumph, romance and adventure. Most important, it is the story of an occupational group whose status has always been affected by the prevalent standards of humanity. The great turning points in world progress have also been important turning points in nursing. Events that give rise to "higher degrees of consideration for those who are helpless or oppressed, kindliness and sympathy for the unfortunate and for those who suffer, tolerance for those of differing religion, race, color, etc.—all tend to promote activities like nursing which are primarily humanitarian" (Dock and Stewart, 1925, p. 3).

In any text concerning the genesis of nursing, there is considerable content that refers to the history of nursing as an episode in the history of woman. In fact, one historian described this phenomenon with a clear and emphatic statement: "The nurse is the mirror in which is reflected the position of woman through the ages" (Robinson, 1946, p. vii). During the periods when women were closely restricted to the home by social convention, and their energies were limited to family life, nursing must have had the character of a household art. The duties of women, their degree of economic independence, the freedom of women outside the family, and other factors have seriously influenced the progress of nursing. The fullest development of nursing was not possible without emancipation from the conditions of subjection endured by women. Ultimately, the full demands of nursing could not be realized without education and knowledge of the social conditions and needs of the day.

Confusion exists regarding the proper role or function of the nurse because the connotations of the word *nurse* have changed over the course of human history. Even now, the words *nurse* and *nursing* have many meanings, a condition that causes varying interpretations of the appropriate work and functions of the nurse. Throughout history the development of nursing has been closely related to the evolution of the word *nurse,* specific definitions of which are dependent upon the major social forces of the day. It is apparent that the meaning of the word has progressed from indicating a woman who performs the basic, unlearned human activity of suckling an infant to describing a person who is highly learned and part of a sophisticated profession. These shifts in meaning are clearly reflected in changes in the nursing role.

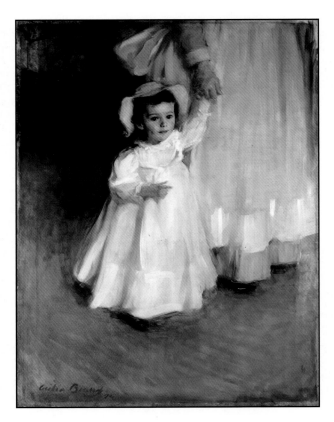

Ernesta Drinker, the artist's niece, looks out as she grasps the hand of her nurse, Mattie. The painter cropped the nurse at the waist, giving the observer the child's view of a starched apron. The child holds hands with her nurse, symbolizing trust, protection, caring, and touch.

Cecilia Beaux, *Child with Nurse*, 1894, painting, 128.3 × 96.5 cm, Metropolitan Museum of Art, NY, Maria DeWitt Jesup Fund, 1965 (65.49). Copyright The Metropolitan Museum of Art.

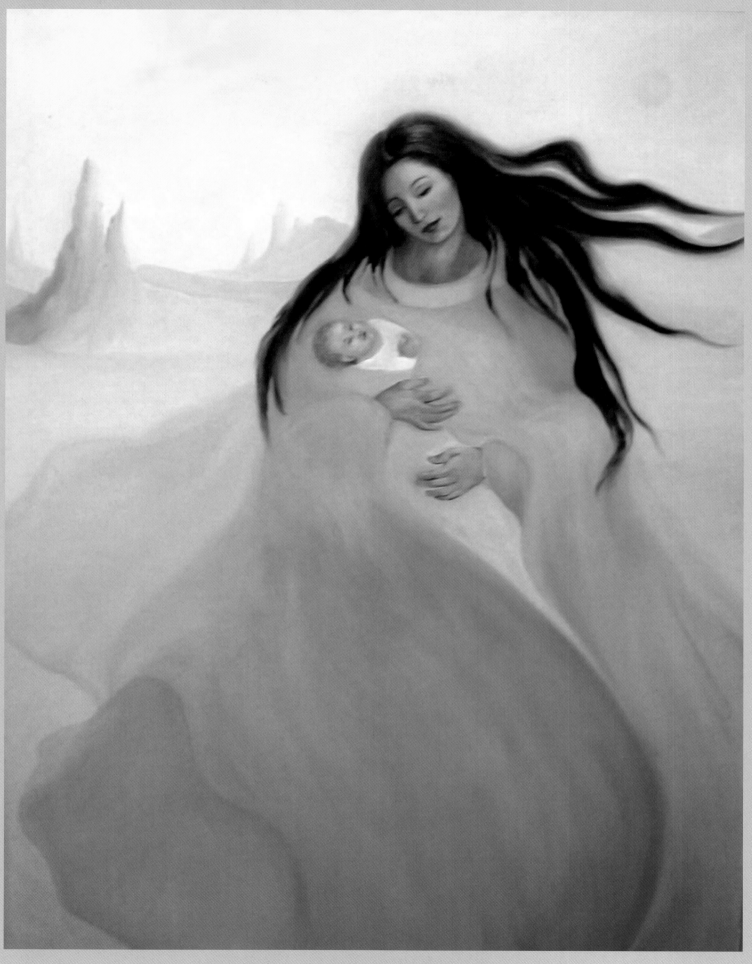

Margo Mandette, *Desert Mother & Child*, 1994, oil, 24″ × 36″, Anderson Mandette Art Gallery, Jerome, AZ.

Nursing has its origin in the mother-care of helpless infants and must have coexisted with this type of care from earliest times. The term *nurse* has been used to indicate a nursing mother, and it commonly referred to a woman who suckled a child who was not her own—that is, a wet nurse. The term stemmed from Latin and French roots and was first used in English in the 13th century. Through this evolution of the word, another dimension was added to its meaning: a woman who cares for and tends young children. The meaning of the word *nurse* continued to broaden to encompass more and more functions related to the care of all humanity. By the 16th century, meanings of the noun included "a person, but usually a woman, who waits upon or tends the sick." It was not until the 18th century that the meaning stopped specifying *woman* and said simply "to wait upon or tend a person who is sick." During the 19th century two more components were added: the training of those who tend the sick and the carrying out of such duties under the supervision of a physician.

Although the aspect of nurturing has long been identified with nursing, it has been even more closely associated with education, particularly with respect to the rearing, training, and general upbringing of the young. "This accounts for the two kinds of helpers who appeared quite early in some households—child-nurses and sick-nurses. Sick-nurses became more closely associated with the healing arts and child-nurses with the teaching and training of children. Often, the two functions were combined" (Stewart and Austin, 1962, p. 4). The words *nursemaid, nanny,* and *governess* thus emerged and became titles for the girls or young women who functioned in the role of child-nurse.

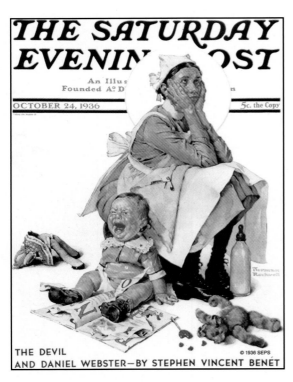

THE DEVIL AND DANIEL WEBSTER—BY STEPHEN VINCENT BENÉT

The nurse was portrayed in a variety of ways while functioning in different roles. The child nurse, nursemaid, or nanny fulfilled an important role throughout history.

The origin of the nurse as mother perpetuated the idea that nursing could be done only by women. The maternal instinct provided that strong impulse or motive necessary to care for those who were suffering or helpless. Women, because of their maternal instinct, were considered "born nurses." Consequently, the nurse as a loving mother who intuitively comforts and renders care continues to be a popular image. The term *parental instinct* more accurately describes this strong motive and is present in both sexes of all races and occurs in all age-groups. It is, however, generally thought that women possess a greater degree of this instinct because of their traditional role in the family, a position that has provided greater experiences in parental activities. Yet the timeless spirit of nursing contains no sexual boundaries. Human beings of both sexes have a natural tendency to respond to helplessness or to a threat to life resulting from disease or injury. Men as well as women have functioned as nurses throughout various periods in history.

The role of the nurse gradually expanded to include a much broader scope. Care of the sick, the aged, the helpless, the infirm, and the handicapped and promotion of health became vital components of the whole of nursing. In addition, care eventually encompassed affection, concern, and solicitude as well as responsibility for individuals in need. In the ancient periods the woman cared for her own kin. As the nursing concept broadened, she also took care of the members of her own tribe. With the development of early civilizations, slaves and servants of households and estates also received care, and nursing began to be performed outside the home. As nursing care became more complex, it became apparent that factors other than a strong motive were necessary to do the work of a nurse. Yet this motivation continued to be a vital component of nursing's development and prompted the motivation to care for the suffering and the helpless. In its fullest development it produced altruism, or humanitarianism, the noblest forms of love and kindness. Compelling societal forces such as religious fervor reinforced this motive at various historical eras and paved the way for people to lead lives of service and self-sacrifice for the sake of others.

As time progressed, it became apparent that love and caring alone were not sufficient to nurture health or overcome disease. The development of nursing depended on two additional essential ingredients—skill and expertise plus knowledge. Great manual dexterity in the carrying out of specific procedures was evident even among primitive tribes and continued to be perfected through experience. As more and more information about illness and disease became available, emphasis on the necessity of knowledge began to emerge. Knowledge of facts and principles would provide the initiating force for nursing to become both an art and a science (Dock and Stewart, 1925). The head, the heart, and the hands became truly united to provide the strong foundation for modern-day nursing. These three essentials were also referred to as the science, spirit, and skill of nursing and, at still another point, became synonymous with the theoretical, practical, and moral and ethical aspects of nursing (Stewart, 1918, 1921). The neglect or overemphasis of any one of these would cause an imbalance in care.

The concept of nursing that has been evolving throughout the ages has not yet reached its fullest maturity. The question of whether it ever will is compounded by the fact that it continues to grow and develop to include widening spheres of nursing service and practice and expanding func-

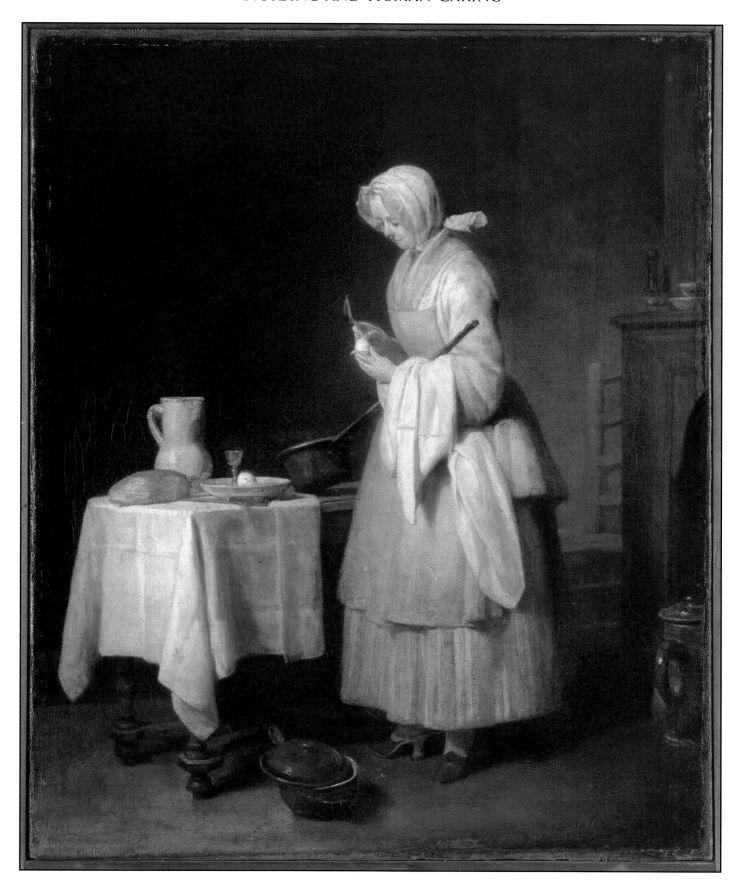

tions that reflect nursing in a global context. It can no longer be viewed as functioning in a particular state, region, or country because it now must embrace the entire world. In addition, it can never "rise higher than the human instruments by which it is administered and the resources they are able to draw upon in the culture of their age and their group" (Stewart and Austin, 1962, p. 10).

The attentive nurse gives special consideration to the needs, desires, and comfort of patients. The nurse is mindful, observant, and receptive in the process of caring.

Jean-Baptiste-Simeon Chardin, *The Attentive Nurse*, 1738, painting, 18³/₁₆″ × 14⁹/₁₆″, Samuel H. Kress Collection. Image courtesy of the Board of Trustees, National Gallery of Art, Washington, DC.

NURSING: THE SEED OF EARLY COMMUNITY SERVICE

Nursing can be distinguished as a form of community service early in its history. This service was originally related to a strong instinct for the preservation and protection of the tribe and its members. Love and concern for family and tribe extended to neighbors and strangers. One rudimentary way to assist in this effort was through the nursing of individuals who became ill. As more sophisticated civilizations developed, the care of the sick expanded to include concern for other human conditions. Methods of dealing with problems such as poverty, prevention of disease, and any type of helplessness added a social dimension to nursing work. The functions commonly associated with present-day social workers were incorporated into the role of the nurse. Historically, the nurse and social worker were one. This phenomenon continued until another group of workers was trained to handle the problems associated with the social ills of society. Even then, as now, nurses were in a sense true social workers, constantly battling adverse social conditions that directly affected the health and welfare of society. Dock and Stewart (1925, pp. 374-375) regarded this as a very important aspect of nursing: "When we consider the whole movement of social progress—the breaking down of the spirit of hatred and prejudice, the promotion of kindlier and more humane relations between human beings, the organization of practical and effective measures for reducing human suffering and distress—it would be hard to find any group of workers, who have contributed more to the sum total of social effort."

During specific periods this sense of community was influenced by waves of religious awakening, ideas of chivalry, patriotism and democracy, and social and humanitarian efforts. In these instances, nursing combined with other available branches of charitable aid and kindness. The religious influence, however, was probably the strongest. For long periods nursing was regarded as a calling that could be done only by those who renounced the world. This intensely religious motive, combined with the element of self-sacrifice, provided an excellent qualification for assuming the nursing role.

Concern for the health of the public or the community was evident in antiquity and continued as civilizations developed. Nearly all primitive tribes fostered some type of sanitary practices so the environment would not be tainted. These elementary practices became more sophisticated as technological advances occurred and provided improvements such as water-drainage systems. Eventually, concern broadened to include disease and its communicability and an overall emphasis on health.

From its inception, nursing was involved in this social movement, even during the periods when nursing care was integrated into the practice of medicine men, priests, wise women, and midwives. Service to the community as well as to the individuals within it was readily incorporated into a basic conception of nursing that included both health and illness. These early roots of public health became a prominent aspect of the nursing role and ultimately provided a variety of community services to achieve this goal. Branches of public service evolved as extensions of nursing and extended into the innermost structures of society. Visiting nurses, school nurses, public health nurses (an older term for community health nurses), nursing settlements, and other facets of community service emerged to become forever a vital and necessary component of nursing.

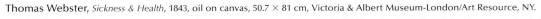

Thomas Webster, *Sickness & Health*, 1843, oil on canvas, 50.7 × 81 cm, Victoria & Albert Museum-London/Art Resource, NY.

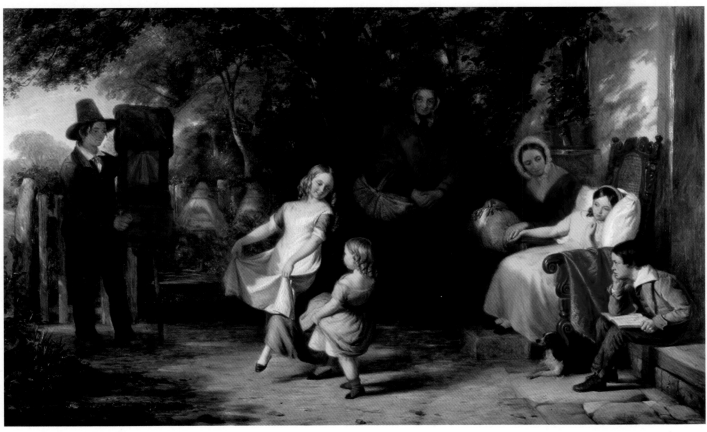

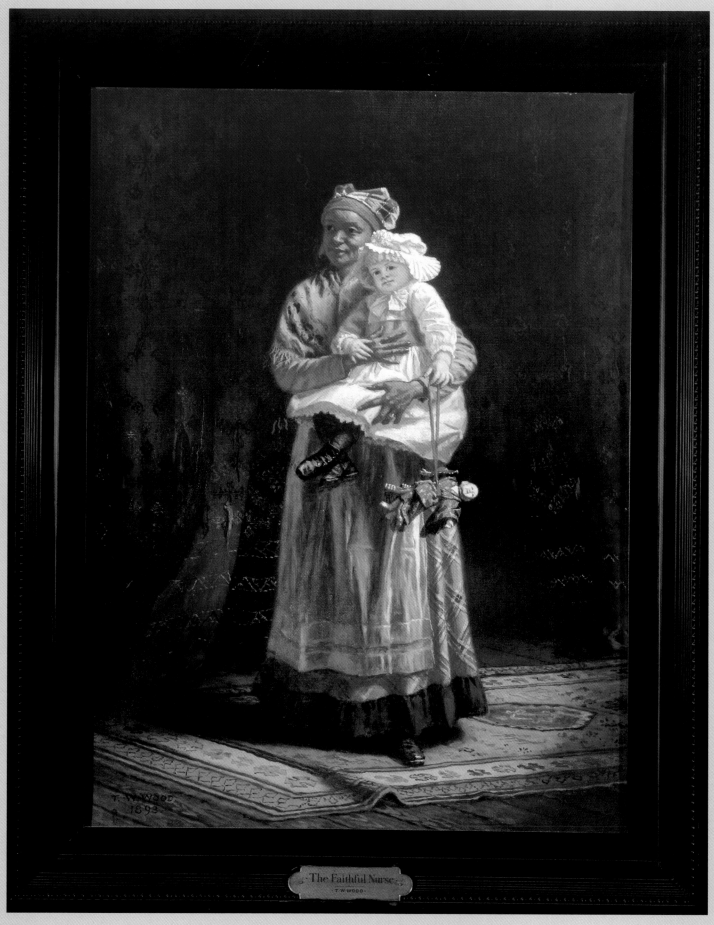

The Faithful Nurse
T. W. WOOD

Blacks have been typically shown as slaves, nursemaids, and "nannies" who are ever-faithful to their charges. However, a minority group of nurses has dealt admirably with impediments from both society and nursing itself. They have worked constantly for the acceptance of Blacks in nursing, and for the promotion of equal opportunities for all minority persons. Numerous Black nurses have emerged as significant nursing leaders, made valuable contributions to nursing, and brought the concerns of Blacks to the attention of nurses and the general public.

Thomas Waterman Wood, *The Faithful Nurse,* 1893, painting, 71.12 × 50.8 cm, T.W. Wood Gallery & Arts Center.

CARE OF THE SICK AMONG PRIMITIVE PEOPLE

It is possible that some of the first ideas related to medical treatment and nursing care were acquired through the observation of animals. Although it may be difficult for some to consider that simple medical and nursing procedures were prehuman in origin, support for this premise exists in natural history. The first traces of parental love, kindness, and mutual aid were exhibited by birds and other animals. The lower animals, in particular, subjected themselves to appropriate medical and surgical treatment when necessary, treated themselves when injured or ill, and assisted one another (Berdoe, 1893).

Primitive people, to escape the ravages of illness and disease, needed to learn how to protect themselves and find means of treatment and cure. During that period of history, people were much closer to nature and moved throughout the animal kingdom with minimal fear. They were readily able to observe and learn the animal practices associated with ailments. Even animals attempted to relieve pain and to remove the causes of infection. Animals cleansed their wounds by licking; ate grasses, leaves, and other plant life, which acted as emetics and purgatives; submerged inflamed wounds in water; and engaged in other practices that had significant effects on their well-being.

It was not possible for primitive people to find treatments for every illness through this observational process. Nor were they able to detect more than the most obvious natural circumstances leading to illness by using such a system. Yet, instinctively aware that other causal factors of diseases existed, people turned to searching for additional explanations. Close intimacy with nature, however, colored their ideas about myriad forms of life, of which they had no scientific knowledge. People ascribed to all such forms the qualities they identified within themselves. All natural objects—rocks, rivers, trees, mountains, the wind—were alive, or animate, and possessed a spirit or soul (psyche, anima). Natural phenomena, including those causing disaster or disease, could thus be explained. This basic belief in animism unlocked the door to a still greater world in the minds of humans, that of imagination.

The introduction of a belief in spirits, good and evil, profoundly affected the development of practices related to treatments and remedies. Ideals of an occult nature, superstitions, became tightly linked to the causes of diseases because supernatural origins of most happenings, including illness, were accepted by primitive people. Humans lived in two worlds—the visible and the invisible—so a combination of occult practices and empirical practices occurred and provided the necessary climate for the use of magic. The supernatural world could and did affect primitive humans.

The cause of illness and disease was attributed to evil spirits, so cures were attempted through intervention with these spirits. Consequently, a great body of tribal lore arose, and they included incantations, rites, rituals, and spells. In time, certain types of symptoms were ascribed to the work of particular spirits, and means of driving them away were devised. The primary goal was to make the patient's body an unpleasant dwelling place for the spirit. Repeated pummeling and pounding of the inhabited area of the body were meant to dislodge the evil spirit. (It is possible that the practice of massage originated from these techniques.) Plants that had unpleasant effects were used to make concoctions that would be disagreeable to the spirits. Expulsion could occur in two ways: through the intestinal tract or through the mouth, so appropriate herbs, which acted as purgatives or emetics, were chosen and administered. Evil spirits lodged in the head were to be released through holes in the skull. Trephined skulls of primitive peoples give evidence of this extreme measure. Fire, hot instruments, and blistering appliances were used as counterirritants to burn out the spirits. Cold baths, sweating, starvation, bad smells, and hideous noises were all used in the attempt to expel demons from the suffering body.

The magical lore that accumulated became too complex to be understood by the ordinary tribal people. Chosen individuals who supposedly had special insight or intimate contact with the spirits devoted their time to mastering and interpreting this lore for the benefit of the tribe. These men, and sometimes women, usually went through a long and arduous training period. In addition, they might have lived through some mystical experience, spent weeks alone in fellowship with the spirits, or recovered from a critical illness or injury. In time, these medicine men, witch doctors, or shamans became the guardians and disseminators of the esoteric knowledge and skills. More important, their possession of life-giving powers granted them a place of prestige, and they were set apart from and above the rest of the tribe. "Here was the beginning of specialization in the art of healing" (Shryock, 1959).

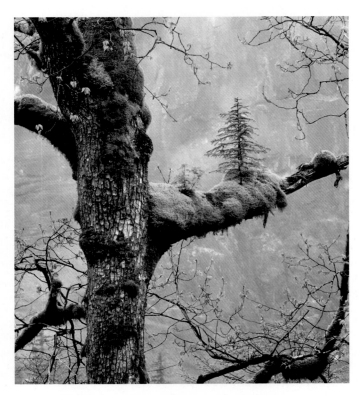

A coniferous seedling grows on a moss-covered branch of a nursing tree. "All new and sustained life is nurtured by the dying past" (E. Clark White, 2009).

Gunter Marx, *A Coniferous Tree Growing on a Moss Covered Deciduous Tree Branch,* photograph, photo taken at Pacific West Coast Rainforest, near Bella Coola. Gunter Marx Studios, British Columbia, Canada.

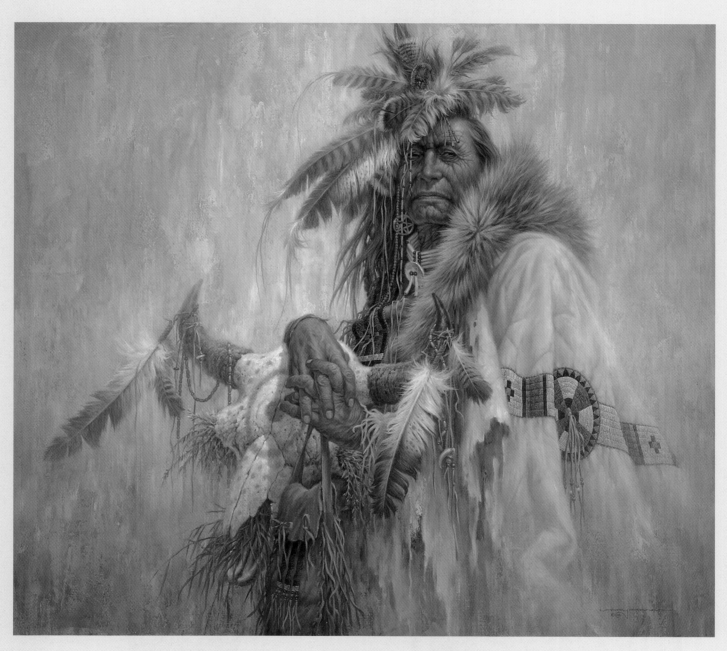

Larry Fanning, *Medicine Skull—Blackfoot Shaman*, 2006, painting, 36" × 40", Larry Fanning Studios, LLC, Evergreen, CO.

Healers were concerned primarily with occult lore and procedures, although they undoubtedly became authorities on tribal folk medicine. In most instances the challenge was not to give the illness a name but to find a cure. Consequently, a magical cause had to be identified in order to overcome the malady. Healers were also faced with another aspect of the occult related to the cure of disease or the dispelling of misfortune. They had to develop the ability to use their magic in an evil or a good way. The use of these two separate functions gave rise to a system of black magic and white magic. White magic invoked the help of good spirits to drive off evil ones and was practiced for benevolent purposes. Black magic, hostile and destructive in its aims, was used to bring disaster or disease upon enemies. This was accomplished with the aid of evil spirits, poisons, and malice.

These practices were organized into ritualistic ceremonies that eventually assumed a religious tone. The result of this union was the labeling of the medicine man as a holy person. Primitive medicine became a mixture of magic, religion, and natural remedies. According to some sources, the medicine man became the priest-physician (Dolan, Fitzpatrick, and Hermann, 1983; Jamieson and Sewall, 1950). Other authors subscribe to belief in the development of higher and lower ranks among healers, with the priest-physician being the highest (Dock and Stewart, 1925; Stewart and Austin, 1962), or to the idea that it is unclear whether primitives made distinctions between priests and medicine men (Shryock, 1959). What is clear, however, is that both types of healers dealt with problems of life and death and were authorities on traditional lore.

The omnipotence of these early healers was supported by the use of strange disguises, elaborate ceremonies, mystical signs, charms (amulets and talismans), and fetishes. Skins, hooves, and horns of animals as well as feathers, grasses, and other objects adorned the ceremonial garb. Extreme drama and mystery kept the observers in awe of the medicine man. The ceremonies might last for hours or days and often included dancing, singing, and the playing of instruments. The medicine man's ability to frighten off evil spirits was demonstrated by these props.

As the caste of medicine men developed, a class of practitioners became associated with them. These individuals, most often the women of the tribe, applied the treatments, ascertained the qualities of drugs, became skillful in dressing wounds, and learned to reduce fevers. Theirs was a practical knowledge of appliances and drugs. These tribal women were the discoverers of medical herbs; they were the first empirical physicians, and they learned to prepare potions to be used as remedies (Mason, 1894). Some of these women, particularly the elderly, must have been the earliest prototypes of the so-called witch. These wise women, who were extremely knowledgeable about medicinal secrets and who went out early and late to gather herbs, became prominent as caretakers for the sick through the prehistoric ages (Alexander, 1782). In time, as a result of superstitious feelings, wise women, or witches, were credited with uncanny powers that were both good and evil, particularly the ability to cause illness and wasting diseases. Eventually, this belief led to the persecution of perhaps the first rivals of the

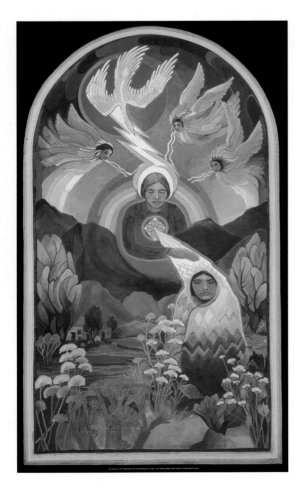

Cynthia West, *The Healer*, 1977-1987, painting.

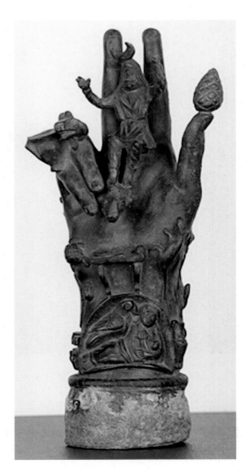

Sabazius is a god of vegetation or reproduction. On the wrist, a woman nurses a baby, a reference to the god's protection of women in labor and of mothers and babies.

Hand of Sabazius, sculpture, Napoli, Italy. With permission from the Ministero per i Beni e le Attivita Culturali-Soprintendenza archaeologica de Pompei.

medicine men (Dock and Stewart, 1925). Many similar superstitions still exist today in isolated communities.

The exact relationship between the practical attendants (nurses) and the medicine men or priest-physicians is not clearly understood. If the attendant received orders for the treatment of the patient from the medicine man, the relationship was probably that of physician and nurse. If the attendant prescribed the simple treatments and herbs and the medicine man limited his work to incantations, the relationship could have been the symbolic representation of the combination of the theory and practice of medicine. The latter would be indicative of the yet unspecialized category called nursing (Nutting and Dock, 1937). It is also possible that some rivalry began to occur as the struggle for a monopoly of power emerged or the differentiation of roles and functions became necessary.

The individuals who provided rudimentary nursing probably varied with the customs of each group or tribe. These practical tasks were first, however, the work of mothers and wives. This naturally occurred as a result of the division of labor: men hunted for the food and provided the defense for the tribe; women cared for the children and eventually for those individuals afflicted by disease, age, injury, or other incapacitating conditions. As knowledge increased, others became specialized in particular areas of medical work.

Primitive societies sowed the seeds of hygiene, sanitation, and public health as well as medicine, surgery, psychiatry, midwifery, nursing, and other branches of the healing arts. Within this structure, nursing's heritage was derived. The role of the nurse as mother, the concept of nursing as a feminine occupation, and the expansion of nursing to include people who were not related emerged and became a vital part of society. The interrelationship and the separation between the medical practitioner and the nursing practitioner were established.

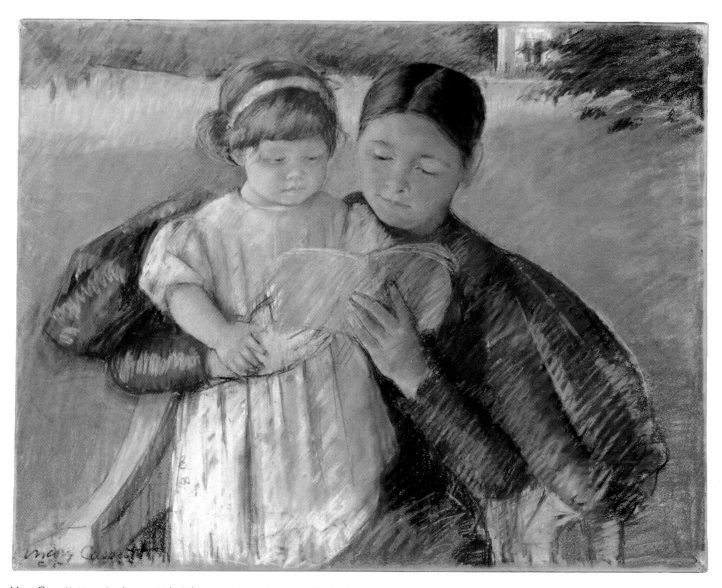

Mary Cassatt, *Nurse Reading to a Little Girl*, 1895, painting, 23⅝″ × 28¾″ (60 × 73 cm), the Metropolitan Museum of Art, gift of Mrs. Hope Williams Read, 1962. Copyright The Metropolitan Museum of Art.

ANCIENT CIVILIZATIONS

To fully understand the origin of nursing, one must also understand the intimate and universal connection between religion and medicine that permeated the majority of ancient civilizations. This potentially impacted the rendering of care and the identification of the caregiver; a search throughout ancient history reveals little about attendants to the sick—nurses. The lack of history may have occurred because it is unusual or striking events rather than ordinary ones that are generally recorded in history. People have always nursed their sick as a matter of course. It was not until cities became large and problems became acute that the matter of care in illness warranted specific mention. Yet one can be reasonably sure that nurses, male or female, functioned in early civilizations to a greater or lesser extent, depending on the particular civilization. From earliest times the midwife has been accepted in her role during childbirth, as has the child's nurse. Slaves, attendants, and women of good character probably cared for those with curable conditions. Priestesses are believed to have performed many functions now recognized as those of the nurse. Indeed, the beliefs, mores, and culture of each civilization directly influenced the way in which nursing care was given. In addition, who rendered nursing care and what constituted nursing care were reflections of the prevailing society.

Nature worship became the basic principle upon which the mythologies and religions of the ancient civilizations were founded. The belief in evil spirits as causes of disease progressed to the belief that disease was caused by the failure to do things that the gods wished or by some moral transgression (Goodnow, 1942). Thus, illness was a curse, a punishment set forth by the gods and directed at individuals, at families and their descendants, and at sinners. The many gods of ancient times "were all originally nature gods, or simply external forces of nature or attributes of the physical and intellectual man symbolised and personified" (Nutting and Dock, 1937, p. 26). Legends and myths about deities who watched over health and had powers over life and death were composed and cultivated by nations. This served to bring some order out of the old confusion about innumerable demons associated with the earlier magical medicine. Fewer beings now needed to be appeased. Furthermore, traditions of worship and methods of requesting divine aid for the sick were established. Many temples were built to these gods, and they became temples for healing and, ultimately, sanctuaries for the sick.

The lifestyles of primitive tribes led to constant changes in their locations. These nomadic people naturally followed the presence of food, tending to migrate toward the south, where warmth, rich soil, and vegetative growth made it possible to live with less effort and a greater degree of comfort. Evolutionary improvements such as the development of tools (during the Stone Age) followed by the incorporation of the use of several metals (during the Iron Age) occurred along with the domestication of plants and animals. These advances paved the way for tribal people to settle down as herders and farmers and to supplant the roving life with village life. Slowly, in certain fertile areas, civilization began to develop.

It is generally believed that the movement of these tribes radiated from the interior of Europe and Asia toward the warm shores of the Mediterranean Sea, India, and China. Migration of a much lesser degree evolved in the direction of western Europe and the British Isles. In most instances, movement followed the shores of great rivers. Although early civilizations also appeared in China and Japan, they exerted little influence on the Western world because of limited contact.

Regions bordering the Mediterranean Sea came to form the greater part of the known world. This body of water was believed to occupy the center of the earth, as its name implies. Consequently, all areas to the east of the Mediterranean Sea became known as "eastern"; those to the west became known as "western."

The cultural patterns in these early centers of civilization exhibited interdependence of religion, government, social welfare, and health care. As in primitive tribal societies, magic, superstition, and early forms of religion were used to control the forces of nature when other measures were ineffectual. Through the use of magic and superstition, government authority was enforced, property disputes were settled, woman's place was determined, social welfare was secured, and disease and injury were cured. Justice and charity toward the poor, the weak, and the sick were taught in some cultures. Human sacrifices might be demanded, and mutilation of the body was not encouraged.

Religious beliefs and myths were the foundations of medical practice in early civilizations, so religious leaders were originally given the responsibility for curing and treating the sick and the injured. As time progressed, two ideas regarding the cause of illness became accepted: illness was caused by the displeasure of the gods, and all illnesses were the result of natural causes. Dualism, the first step medicine needed to make the transition from the magical to the rational, was thus exhibited. Rational observations and treatments were preceded and followed by religious chants and rites to ensure cure. With the development of empirical knowledge, health care was delegated to priest-physicians and eventually to secular physicians. The latter development occurred primarily in Greek and Roman civilizations. This evolution resulted in the development of significant medical contributions (special procedures, biological sciences, diagnostic measures, classification of diseases, and observation recording) that began to transform medicine from magic into a science.

THE NEAR EAST

EGYPT

One of the first civilizations to emerge clearly from barbarism was that of Egypt. The very long, narrow valley on either side of the Nile River composed its boundaries. The people who settled on this fertile strip built a civilization that far exceeded that of other groups who settled elsewhere. Signs of prosperity became increasingly evident in Egypt: systems of irrigation were devised, roads and ships were built, trade was established, practical arts were developed, architecture became dignified, family and other social relationships were maintained through the use of accepted moral codes, and the entire society was held together by an absolute monarchy headed by the pharaoh, or king. Egypt is well remembered; impressive and enduring monuments still exist to herald its glory. Pyramids, tombs, temples, and other edifices are among the wonders of the contemporary world.

More is known about Egypt than about any other ancient culture. Surviving Egyptian records are related to periods as distant as 3000 BC. A system of writing was introduced, at first in the form of pictures and later as signs, or hieroglyphics. Formal records were carved in stone or written in inks on paper scrolls called papyri (writing materials made from the pith of the tall sedge plant). In the dry sands of Egypt these papyri, which contained the most complete examples of ancient medical literature, were preserved. They were named after their discoverers or owners—for example, the Brugsch, Ebers, Smith, Hearst, Berlin, and London scrolls (Frank, 1953). The Ebers papyrus is known as the oldest complete medical book in the world.

> No less than five medical papyri have come down to our time, the finest being the celebrated Ebers papyrus, bought at Thebes by Dr. Ebers in 1874. The papyrus contains one hundred and ten pages, each page consisting of about twenty-two lines of bold hieratic writing. It may be described as an Encyclopedia of Medicine as known and practised by the Egyptians of the eighteenth dynasty, and it contains prescriptions for all kinds of diseases—some borrowed from Syrian medical lore, and some of such great antiquity that they are ascribed to the mythological ages, when the gods yet reigned personally upon earth.
>
> — *EDWARDS, 1892, P. 219*

The Smith papyrus reveals a high level of Egyptian surgical practice arranged according to the general parts of the body (only the section relating to the upper parts survives).

The Hearst, London, and Berlin papyri, which focus almost entirely on the treatment of the diseases of the anus, may have been practical handbooks. The Ebers papyrus outlines many of the diseases known to modern science and mi-

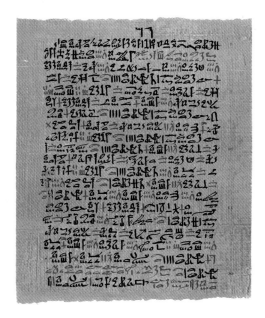

Papyrus Ebers, University of Leipzig Library. Photo courtesy of the National Library of Medicine, Bethesda, MD.

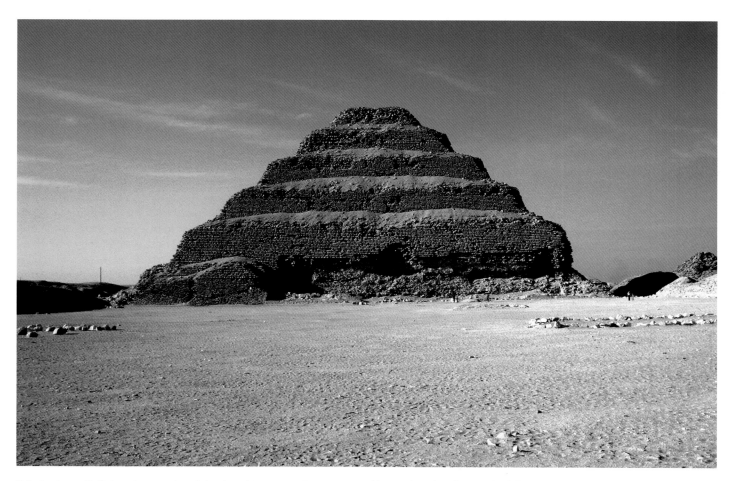

This structure with its temples, complex of chambered terraces, and great courtyard is now thought to be a medical shrine built under the direction of Imhotep.

Saqqara Djoser (Zoser) Step Pyramid, Egypt. Copyright Art Resource.

nutely describes their symptoms. In addition, more than seven hundred substances from the vegetable, mineral, and animal kingdom are given as drugs, along with descriptions of their preparation. The complexity of these prescriptions suggests the need for specialists to compound them. The Ebers papyrus also, however, contains incantations and verbal charms.

Three essential elements are present in these manuscripts: religion, magic, and accounts of illness and treatments. This is consistent with Berdoe's (1893, p. 61) description: "The art of medicine in ancient Egypt consisted of two branches, the higher, which was the theurgic part, and the lower, which was the art of the physician proper. The theurgic class devoted themselves to magic, counteracting charms by prayers, and to the interpretation of the dreams of the sick who had sought aid in the temples. The inferior class were practitioners who simply used natural means in their profession." It is possible, however, that the word *magic* did not convey the true medical state, because the Egyptians practiced hypnotism and were aware of how to control the mind and imagination. It is not clear who gave the orders for the practical treatment of the patient, the priest-magician (priest) or the priest-physician (doctor). What is clear is that the two professions dealt with the sick at the same time but in different ways. In some instances the two combined to become one, commonly known as the priest-physician.

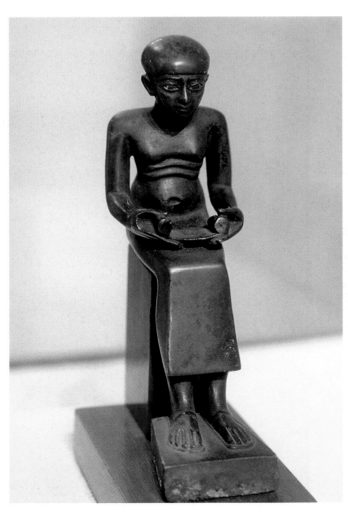

Imhotep, sculpture. Image from Ancient Art and Architecture Collection Ltd.

Out of this structure emerged the first physician known to history. Sometime during the Third Dynasty (c. 2900-2800 BC) Imhotep is identified as the greatest priest-physician of Egypt. His stature as a historical personage grew according to his deeds. He was recognized as a surgeon and architect to one of the pharaohs and as a temple priest, a learned scribe, and a successful magician (priest-physician). Imhotep was noted for his great wisdom and learning in the fields of health, magic, and religion. He was so successful in healing the sick that statues and temples were erected in his honor. After Imhotep's death the Egyptian people elevated him to the rank of Egyptian God of Medicine, the god of healing.

The philosophy of the Egyptians was a form of nature worship that included some aspects of animism. Diseases were believed to have partly natural, partly supernatural causes. The development of astrology also led to the belief that disease, as well as destiny, was influenced by changes in celestial phenomena, such as the movement of sun and stars and the passage of seasons. Astrological medicine arose and functioned harmoniously with mythical premises.

A spirit world inhabited by many gods developed in the Nile valley. Ultimately a trinity assumed control of bodily and spiritual welfare: Isis, Osiris, and Horus, their son. Isis (Mother Earth) and Osiris (Day or Light or Sun God) were regarded as the creators of agriculture and the medical arts. Isis gave her help to the sick most often through the medium of dreams. From his mother, Horus learned medicine as well as the gift of prophecy. Osiris sat in judgment of the souls of those who died, and immortality became an established belief. Magnificent temples emerged and became significant as molding influences in the civilization. Originally built as meager shelters to protect the gods, the temples became centers of community and national life. Priest-physicians functioned in those temples, which were frequented by individuals in search of better health.

Concern for the question of life after death was especially prevalent in Egyptian society. The people hoped for personal survival beyond the grave. Therefore, symbols of immortality, the pyramids, were erected. Bodies were skillfully embalmed so that souls could remain within them or return to them once the afterlife had begun. Aromatics, resins, and other preservatives were employed in this process. The custom of embalming enabled the Egyptians to become familiar with the organs of the human body. More than two hundred fifty different diseases were identified on the basis of clinical observations. Treatments were developed that incorporated the use of drugs and procedures, including surgery. Specialization became a reality, perhaps because of the large quantity of writings that may have necessitated concentration on a limited area of knowledge. Herodotus, the Greek historian, explained, "Medicine is practiced among them on a plan of separation; each physician treats a single disorder and no more: thus the country swarms with medical practitioners, some undertaking to cure diseases of the eye, others of the teeth, others of the head, others of the intestines, and some of those which are invisible." Splendid examples of the art of bandaging emerged as thousands of yards of linen of various widths and patterns were used on one mummy. These bandages were hardened with a gluey substance to form an impenetrable case for an aseptically cleansed body. Safe repositories in the form of elaborate tombs were constructed to ensure the preservation of body and soul for all time.

The ancient Egyptians also established public hygiene and sanitation at a relatively high level. They appear to have had a corps of sanitary inspectors or health officers (Nutting and Dock, 1937). The Egyptians recognized the importance of an adequate drainage system, a good water supply, and the inspection of slaughter houses. They were very particular about the cleanliness of their bodies and their dress, which was always of linen. They practiced circumcision from earliest times. Strict rules were developed to regulate such matters as cleanliness, food, drink, exercise, and sexual relations. Some sources indicate that the rigid hygienic regulations of the Jews originated from these Egyptian practices. Others believe they came from the writings of the Old Testament and were given as laws from God, not developed from captivity in Egypt.

Modern researchers have yet to disclose evidence regarding the existence of any building identifiable as a hospital. However, according to Caton, "There is reason to believe that institutions closely related to infirmaries or hospitals existed in Egypt many centuries earlier than the Hieron of Epidauros, but no structural trace of such building has been discovered" (Nutting and Dock, 1937, p. 54). Whether there were or were not hospitals, the temples had some type of housing for the sick. In the temples frequented by individuals in search of good health, priest-physicians engaged in medical practice. The existence of priestesses or "temple women" is also certain; what their duties were is not clear, although it is assumed that they performed some type of nursing functions.

The position of women in ancient Egypt was higher than that in other Eastern countries. In general, women enjoyed considerable freedom and dignity. Within their own households they held a position of authority and importance. It is probable that nursing care was the chief responsibility of the mother or the daughters in the home. In addition, physicians in ancient Egypt did not practice obstetrics; this field was left entirely to midwives. Wet nurses were engaged on contract to breast-feed infants for approximately six months.

In a nation as sophisticated in medicine, pharmacy, and sanitation as ancient Egypt, it is almost impossible to believe that there were no persons, male or female, who engaged specifically in the work of nurses and nursing. History, however, fails to make this point clear.

PERSIA (IRAN)

Persia is currently called Iran, a form of the word *Arya,* which indicates that the Persians spoke an Aryan, or so-called Indo-European, language. The Plateau of Iran was positioned to the east of the Fertile Crescent and between the Persian Gulf and the Caspian Sea. In ancient times the land was occupied by the Medes and the Persians. However, by 500 BC the Persians had conquered the Medes, moved their borders eastward to the Indus River in India, and conquered all of the Fertile Crescent and Egypt. The energies of Persia were directed toward war, tyranny, and the acquisition of wealth and power. The result of these efforts was the founding of the most extensive empire that had appeared in the Near East. Fortunately, this empire, which exerted an almost totally destructive influence, existed for only about two hundred years.

The religion of the Persians, Zoroastrianism, revolved around Zoroaster, who lived about 600 BC. This prophet wrote the sacred books of Persia, the *Zendavesta,* which introduced a world ruled by two creators, one producing light and good, the other darkness and evil. Although good and evil were constantly at war, good always triumphed. In addition, sacred elements were identified: fire, earth, and water, with fire being described as the purest. According to the sacred books, immortality was a mental rather than a physical state. The principal virtues of veracity, virility, and hard work would enable people to achieve happiness. So happiness or unhappiness depended on the righteousness or evil of people on Earth, with the promise of rewards after death (Jamieson and Sewall, 1950).

The Persians absorbed much of the culture of their conquered lands, including the medicine and surgery of Egypt. They had great confidence in Egyptian medicine, as demonstrated by the emperor Darius, who renovated an old school to be used for the training of priest-physicians. This is thought to be the first case of a medical center's being established as a royal, or governmental, foundation.

Three types of physicians evolved from the medical center: those who healed by the knife, those who used plants, and those who healed by exorcism and incantations (Nutting and Dock, 1937). No mention is made of nurses, although descriptions of various surgical and medical procedures are given, some of which could well have belonged to the province of nursing. In retrospect, little attention has been given to the medical history of the Persian Empire. It may be that Persia contributed little to medicine in comparison to other countries.

THE FERTILE CRESCENT

A series of civilizations developed in the Fertile Crescent, an area that stretched from the Isthmus of Suez, up through Palestine and Syria, east through the region of Damascus, and down the Euphrates River valley. This land has also been called the Cradle of Civilization. In this region, thousands of years ago, the first cities in the world were built and the first attempt at developing a system of writing occurred. Three great rivers—the Tigris, the Euphrates, and the Jordan—were situated in the area. The combination of well-watered soil and a warm climate encouraged habitation. Successive peoples came and conquered their predecessors in the fertile valleys. Most of them spoke the Semitic languages.

Agriculture flourished in this area, and wealth and economic changes led to the building of memorable cities. Progress was similar to that of Egypt, with one significant difference: structures were built with clay or bricks instead of stone. Therefore natural phenomena and time caused these ancient cities to crumble into dust. Fortunately, records were kept on hardened clay tablets, and from these tablets information about religion, business, and medical practice has been deciphered. These cuneiform (wedge-shaped) writings frequently referred to practices performed by royal physicians that today would be carried out by nurses.

Babylonia. As Egyptian civilization was developing in the Nile valley, a comparable advance was occurring in the region between the Tigris and Euphrates valleys, now known as Iraq. This area was originally known as Mesopotamia, a Greek word meaning *between the rivers.* City-states that developed in southern Mesopotamia were dominated by temples where priests represented the patron deities of the city. Each ancient city was a community center with schools, li-

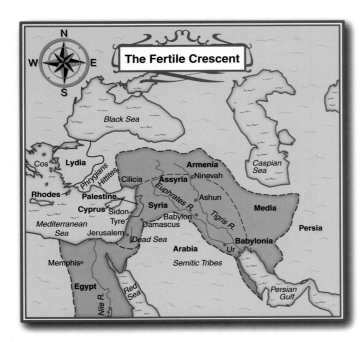

The Fertile Crescent of the Pre-Christian Era, **map**, Mosby.

braries, granaries, and workshops. Each was governed by a divine ruler and a priest-king who was the actual ruler. The most prominent of these city states was Sumer, regarded as the finest and earliest civilization of humankind. The Sumerians made significant contributions to human civilization in the development of morals, learning, and the arts. They were eventually conquered by the Babylonians, a Semitic people. The conquered lands ultimately became known as the Babylonian Empire, which was established by about 2100 BC.

The religion of the Babylonians comprised magical and superstitious principles and a strong astral influence. These people believed in polytheism, a plurality of gods, the majority of whom were nature gods. "The three greatest were the gods of the sky, the earth, and the sea. Next in rank were the moon god; the sun god; the god of thunder, lightning, wind, rain, and storm; of the planet Venus; Marduk or Merodak (light), who is also called Bel, the quickener of the dead, who fought and vanquished the dragon or 'Chaos' (darkness); Nebo, the god of arts, science, and letters, and others" (Nutting and Dock, 1937, p. 57). Local deities were also numerous. Disease was believed to be evoked by the wrath of the gods and by evil spirits; this resulted in the creation of hierarchies of good and evil spirits. Survival was dependent on securing aid from the good spirits. Ceremonies incorporating the use of fire, water, and incantations became important in this process, and various occult practices were cultivated.

The Babylonians were learned mathematicians and astronomers. They originated the division of time into months, days, and minutes; used a system of weights and measures; and followed the signs of the zodiac. Their study of sun, moon, and planets became the basis for scientific astronomy. Astrological interpretation became closely connected with physiological phenomena; the position of the stars and the motions of the planets and the moon were believed to affect humans directly. "As their lore accumulated, they began to 'cast horoscopes' in terms of an individual's birth, for

the position of the planets at this time was supposed to cast a spell over a man thereafter" (Shryock, 1959, p. 28). Eventually medicine became interwoven with astrology, and the result was the practice of a magic medicine carried out by astrologer-priests. These individuals practiced medicine by using a combination of magic, religion, and science. Sources of epidemics were ascribed to inauspicious astral influences. Human ailments were diagnosed through examination of the livers of dead animals. The art of divination (foretelling events or discovering hidden knowledge through the interpretation of omens or with the aid of supernatural powers) was practiced by means of a variety of methods, including palmistry, crystal gazing, and communication with the dead.

A very primitive stage in Babylonian medicine was recorded in which the sick were brought out into the marketplace. Passers-by were required to stop and render advice based on their own personal experiences. It is difficult to determine how long this empirical stage lasted and whether it occurred before or after there were physicians. What becomes clear, however, is that lay physicians were also prominent in Babylonia. The practice of medicine by these physicians was divided into two basic areas, surgery and internal medicine. Surgery was considered to be the more advanced field. "Their surgeons understood nasal tamponing for bleeding, cataract couching, the use of facial applications in cases of erysipelas, and blood-letting. Bodies of sacrificed animals supplied the only opportunity for anatomical research" (Jamieson and Sewall, 1950, p. 26). Circumcision is known to have been performed by Abraham, a native of Babylonia.

Internal medicine remained primarily in the realm of magic and was concerned with magical formulas to banish demons, the gods of evil spirits. Illness was thought to be caused by sin and the displeasure of the gods, so methods of treatment consisted of ridding the human body of these demons by means of incantations and other remedies. Vile-tasting plant and mineral concoctions, powders, enemas, and human and animal excreta were used. But the clinical observations of the physicians were fairly accurate

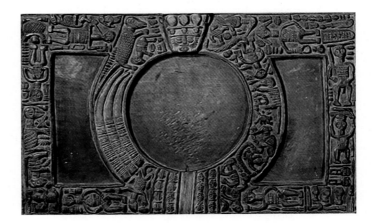

The art of divination (foretelling events or discovering hidden knowledge by the interpretation of omens or by the aid of supernatural powers) was practiced through a variety of methods. Palmistry, crystal gazing, and communication with the dead were frequently used.

Ifa Divination Tray, 16th-17th century, wood engraving, 13½" × 21⅞". Copyright Ulmer Museum—Weickmann Collection, Ulm.

portrayals of symptoms. Numerous diseases were described, including fevers, plague, abscesses, heart and skin diseases, tuberculosis, tumors, jaundice, and venereal disease.

The lay physicians and surgeons of Babylonia had to be careful about their practice. The legal codes of this country were more advanced than those of any other ancient culture and held individuals and groups responsible for their actions. Particularly significant was the Code of Hammurabi, inscribed about 1900 BC on a single great shaft of black stone and placed in one of the temples of Babylon. This code was developed by Hammurabi, sixth king of Babylonia, who was considered the greatest king and statesman during his reign of approximately sixty years. Hammurabi collected older laws and customs and systematically arranged them into a comprehensive code of law. Justice and consideration for the poor and defenseless classes were evident in this document, which was intended to be humanitarian. The code dealt with both civil and criminal law and contained regulations for various circumstances, for example, business contracts, thefts, rents, loans, property rights, dowries, adoption of children, employment policies, sanitation, and public health. In addition, the Code of Hammurabi contained provisions for the veterinarian, a clear indication that the two specialties (physician and veterinarian) were distinct. More important, it addressed medical and surgical practice, with control of the surgeon being the most severe aspect. Fees due practitioners, severe penalties for failures of treatments, and compensations to patients injured during treatment were outlined. In essence, the physician's conduct was regulated by the government, and penalties could result in cruel physical punishment: "If a physician has treated a free-born man for a severe wound with a lancet of bronze and has caused the man to die, or has opened a tumour of the man with a lancet of bronze and has destroyed his eyes, his hands one shall cut off" (Code of Hammurabi).

This eye-for-an-eye, tooth-for-a-tooth philosophy presumably deterred unnecessary surgeries and fostered precautionary measures among the practitioners.

A table of fees for operations was also set and varied from 2 shekels for surgery on a slave to 10 shekels for operating on a freeman:

If a doctor has treated a freeman with a metal knife for a severe wound, and has cured the freeman or has opened a freeman's tumour with a metal knife, and cured a freeman's eye, then he shall receive ten shekels of silver.
If the son of a plebeian, he shall receive five shekels of silver.
If a man's slave, the owner of the slave shall give two shekels of silver to the doctor.
[For the veterinarian] If a doctor of oxen or asses has treated either ox or ass for a severe wound, and cured it, the owner of the ox or ass shall give to the doctor one sixth of a shekel of silver as his fee.

— CODE OF HAMMURABI

The Code of Hammurabi was the greatest legal masterpiece of ancient civilization. It advanced the common good of Babylonia, and for nearly 3 centuries the country experienced increasing prosperity.

The history of Babylonia reveals little mention of nursing as a separate occupation. The writings, however, frequently

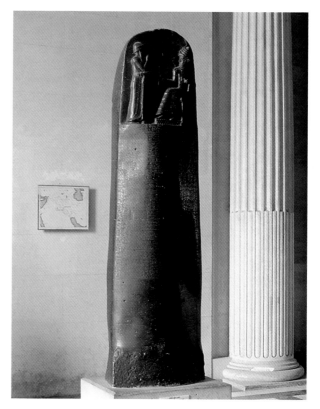

The Code of Hammurabi, which dealt with both civil and criminal law, was the greatest legal masterpiece of ancient civilization.

Code of Hammurabi, 18th century, sculpture. Image from Ancient Art and Architecture Collection Ltd.

refer to practices that are currently performed by nurses. The Babylonian nurse was probably a domestic servant or a slave, either male or female. Accounts of wet nurses, midwives, and children's nurses, who often had great affection for their charges, have been rendered. In addition, in some pictorial scenes the role of the nurse in assisting the patient has been portrayed.

Assyria. The Assyrians, who succeeded the Babylonians, were a hardened, warlike Semitic race who held the balance of power in the Near East from approximately 745 to 635 BC. Their little kingdom of Assur arose in the middle of the Fertile Crescent. Its location afforded protection of its boundaries, with mountain ranges on three sides and a river on the fourth. Nineveh, the capital city, eventually became the center of art and commerce in the Near East. Its walls, which stretched about two and a half miles along the Tigris River, provided the setting for the ruling king.

The Assyrian laws were severe. Mutilation was inflicted as a punishment for many offenses, and the death penalty was used frequently. Absorbed in war, the Assyrians made the "god of the battlefield" their supreme god. Their intensity in military tactics resulted in the production of stronger weapons (the Assyrians were the first to use weapons made of bronze) and new techniques of warfare. However, Assyrian power was short-lived; it suddenly lost vitality, and Nineveh fell to a coalition of powers in about 612 BC.

Assyria preserved the theory of demonology, which held that a sick person's body was possessed by evil spirits. Even further, the Assyrians fostered the belief that illness was a punishment for sin and could be cured only by repentance, magic, or a combination of magic and religion. The aspects of sin and repentance, however, may have been another way of stating that those who broke physiological laws would become ill and could be cured only by resuming the practice of hygienic rules (Nutting and Dock, 1937). The entire theory thus would have been predicated on the natural laws of health. Whatever is accepted as the basis for their belief, the fact remains that the Assyrians practiced only magic and empirical medicine, which was consistent with their superstitious nature. They believed in the influence of lunar changes, and charms and amulets were used extensively. Numbers were regarded as lucky and unlucky; for example, the number seven was so sacred that the seventh day was reserved for rest. Many regulations existed about the gathering of medicinal herbs: some should be gathered by night, some at dawn, and others at a certain time of the moon. Ceremonies were adopted whereby one could be purified by fire and water. Sacrifices involving the offering of human life were sometimes also required.

Medical texts were handed down by the Assyrians on clay tablets with cuneiform script. The greatest number came from Nineveh and were supposedly from the library of King Asurbanipal (668-628 BC). These texts exhibit a mixture of rational therapeutic remedies with purely magical devices:

> If a man's head is full of scabies and itch thou shalt bray sulphur, mix it in cedar oil, anoint him.
> . . . a thread thou shalt spin, double it twice, tie 7 knots. As thou tiest (them) thou shalt recite the charm, bind on his temples and he shall recover.
> If a man has a burning headache affecting his eyes, which are bloodshot, take one third of a measure of *sikhli* crushed and powdered, and knead with cassia juice; wrap it around his head, attach it (with a bandage) and do not remove it for 3 days.
>
> — *SEYMER, 1932, P. 6*

Unfortunately, nothing about nursing is revealed in the history of Assyria, nor is there any evidence that buildings were used as hospitals. In regard to women in Assyria, it can possibly be assumed that they were not accorded very high status.

Palestine. As tribes of the Semitic race were moving into Babylonia and Assyria, other tribes were moving into the region of Palestine at the western side of the Fertile Crescent. The geographical position of the latter tribes, between Egypt on one side and Assyria and Mesopotamia on the other, significantly affected the development of their own culture. These people were given the name Hebrews by the natives, whom they eventually dominated. The literal translation of the word *Hebrews* is "the people from beyond" (Reinach, 1930). The Hebrews were well established in their towns by the time Hammurabi was king of Babylonia (c. 1955 BC). Agriculture became their chief endeavor, although the mountainous character of this portion of the Fertile Crescent provided less than desirable conditions. The terrain comprised narrow, gorgelike valleys; the soil was lacking in minerals; and rainfall was inadequate, resulting in an insufficient water supply. The industrious Hebrew people, however, overcame these obstacles. They built towns, raised sheep, collected water in cisterns, and patiently cultivated olives and grapes. The country flourished, and the city of Jerusalem became the center of religious and political activities.

The Jews (Hebrews or Israelites) were the first to develop the art of writing historical narratives, and their early histories are preserved in the Old Testament. Thus they traced their descent from Abraham, who was born in Ur, Chaldea, and migrated to Palestine with his family. Abraham was the 1st of the patriarchs, his son Isaac was the 2nd, and his grandson Jacob was the 3rd. In the 18th century BC famine drove the Jews into Egypt, where they lived for a time in prosperity. Ultimately, they were taken into captivity, where they remained as slaves for more than 400 years. It was not until the 15th century BC that the Jews left Egypt under the leadership of Moses. Their reentry into Palestine took place after 40 years of wandering. At that time the people were divided into 12 tribes (based on the 12 patriarchs). Jacob had 12 sons and a daughter. However, his favorite son, Joseph, had no tribe; instead, Joseph's two sons Manasseh and Ephraim received his birthright. Because the tribe of Levi had a priestly role and did not bear arms, it was neither counted in the general census of the Israelites in the wilderness nor allotted tribal territory in the land of Canaan. State and church were under the same head, a theocratic government. The chiefs of the tribes and the elders possessed the power of civil authority. A tribal assembly approved or rejected decisions.

The Hebrews embraced a theocentric philosophy, a belief in a personal God. This philosophy held that humans have free will and an immortal soul created by God, and that a human being is a body-mind-spirit unity. Hebrew religious belief was theocratic and monotheistic. The Hebrew people

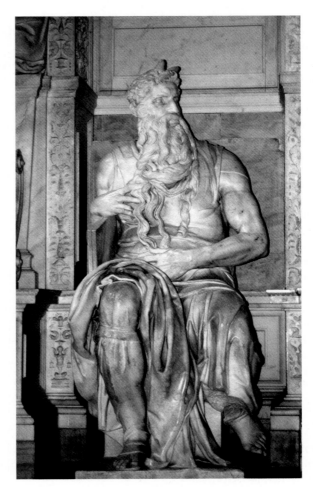

Michelangelo, *Statue of Moses*, 1513, sculpture, Rome. Image from Ancient Art and Architecture Collection Ltd.

abhorred the innumerable deities of other nations. They denounced superstitious and magical practices to the extent that death was the penalty for performing them. Yet they held the extreme view that disease was a punishment for one's own sins. Their strength was derived from belief in the one true God. This monotheistic view had been formed in Egypt earlier but had exerted only temporary influence there. All power over life and death was in the hands of Jehovah. God became the source of health, and its preservation was to be found in "keeping pure before the Lord." A way of living emerged that did not necessitate specific medical practices.

Religion and medicine were combined, and responsibility for the public health centered on the priest-physicians drawn from the priestly tribe of Levites. These men were held in high esteem: "Honor the physician for the need thou hast of him: for the most High created him. For all healing is from God: and he shall receive gifts of the king. The skill of the physician shall lift up his head: and in the sight of men he shall be praised (Ecclesiastes 36:1-4).

It is possible that much of the knowledge of the Hebrew people was borrowed from the Egyptians. Moses, the adopted son of the pharaoh's daughter, had led the enslaved people out of Egypt. Undoubtedly, he was well acquainted with Egyptian wisdom and received a sophisticated education, most likely at the University of Heliopolis (now Cairo). Although Moses' learning took place in a pagan atmosphere, he was taught the religious beliefs and traditions of his Hebrew heritage by his mother, who had been selected as his nursemaid. Mosaic Law was given to the Hebrew nation by Moses upon God's command. It contained civil specifications similar to those of the Code of Hammurabi. Yet the Mosaic Law exhibited consideration for the poor and the weak. As a result, justice became one of the most important characteristics of Hebrew social thought.

The laws ascribed to Moses, although expressed in religious terms, had definite hygienic significance. Regulations were provided for the general public health. Every detail of personal, family, and national hygiene was specified and directed toward the maintenance of health and the prolongation of life. A method for prevention of disease included personal hygiene, cleanliness, rest, sleep, and hours for work. Definite provisions were established for women during menstruation, pregnancy, and childbirth. Other provisions dealt with the inspection and selection of food, the disposal of excreta, the notification of authorities in cases of communicable disease, along with quarantine and disinfection. It is interesting to note that the health regulations were planned to improve the endurance of the race, which was in keeping with the thought that the Israelites were the chosen people (Deuteronomy 14:2).

The priest-physicians also functioned as health inspectors. Contagious diseases had to be reported and isolation was compulsory. The orders for treatment and isolation came from the priest, who also initiated the disinfection of the body, clothing, and environment. Permission had to be secured from the priest to reenter the camp after being quarantined. The acceptance of these practices demonstrates the ancient Jewish belief in infection by contact (contagion), the idea that epidemic diseases were spread from one individual to another. It is remarkable that the Jews not only pioneered the concept of contagion but also the notification and isolation measures necessary to combat and

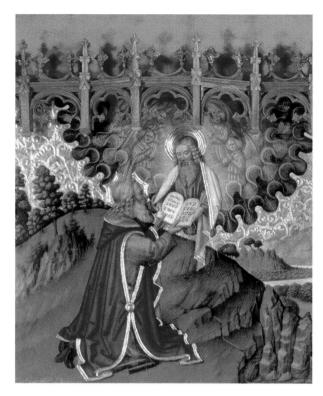

Moses Receives the Tablets of Law at Mount Sinai, 15th century, painting, Tortosa, Spain. Image from Ancient Art and Architecture Collection Ltd.

prevent it. This early approach to the management of public health, however, had little influence on other ancient races. It was eventually revived during the Middle Ages.

Dietary laws were a significant part of the Mosaic Law. Four cardinal rules were to be observed about animal food. First, blood was forbidden as food. Meats were to be drained of their blood before cooking (animals were scientifically bled). Second, animals torn by wild beasts or accidentally killed were not to be used as food. Third, animals that died naturally were not to be used as food. Fourth, the pig was forbidden as unclean. Cloven-hoofed animals that chew their cud and are not scavengers, birds that are not birds of prey, and fish that have fins and scales were permitted in the diet. According to Lyons, there may have been explanations for food prohibitions other than those with a medical basis. He renders this account:

> One recent suggestion is that the taboo against pigs was originally related to their competition with humans for water and grain (scarce commodities in a barren land), in contrast to cattle and sheep which consume relatively little water and graze on forage inedible to man. Since transmissible parasitic diseases and infestations such as tapeworm are also found in sheep and cows, singling out trichinosis in pigs would not be wholly logical. However, to discourage the raising of swine so as to conserve water and grain resources for human consumption, a strict religious taboo may have been necessary—considering man's nearly universal agreement on the delectableness of pork. Medical observations may indeed have been at the core of hygienic codes, but the Biblical listing of seemingly unrelated creatures prohibited as food is difficult to associate with purposes entirely hygienic.

— *Lyons, 1978, p. 71*

Knowledge of ancient Jewish medicine is derived almost entirely from the Old Testament of the Bible and the later Talmud, the authoritative compilation of Jewish tradition. The two Talmuds, the Jerusalem and the Babylonian, were written between approximately the 2nd and 6th centuries AD. In addition to exhibiting remarkable medical observations, they incorporate the attitudes, influences, and methods of the various peoples with whom the Jews lived. References to nurses in the Talmud and the Old Testament suggest wet nurses or children's nurses rather than nurses who were caretakers of the sick. The Jewish midwife was important, but more attention was given to the hygiene of pregnancy than to the actual assistance of the mother at the time of delivery. A woman was usually delivered while sitting on a stool designed in a circular fashion; the midwife sat on a lower stool before her. If complications arose and all known methods failed to improve the situation, religion dictated that she be cared for and comforted until she died. Deborah was the first nurse to be recorded in history, as described in the 24th chapter of Genesis. She is included in the story of Rebekah, who sets out by camel train with her nurse (Deborah) to meet her future husband, Isaac. Deborah was a child's nurse and a companion but at times may have been called upon to perform other nursing duties.

Ancient Jews believed that all people should have access to medical care, regardless of their social status. With an emphasis on human brotherhood and social justice, the duties of hospitality to strangers and relief for widows, orphans, the aged, and the poor were constantly urged as being righteous. Visiting the sick was a prominent feature of everyday life and was a designated duty. Houses for strangers, called xenodochia, were instituted and later expanded to include the care of the sick. These xenodochia were supported financially through a system of tithing. Whether these institutions had nurses is unknown. They did, however, become predecessors of the modern inn and the modern hospital. Overall, the Hebrews recorded achievements in the practice of hygiene and sanitation and in the systematic and organized prevention of disease.

THE FAR EAST

As the great civilizations of ancient times were developing in the Near East, others were developing on a vast continent that eventually became known as Asia. This region included current-day India, China, and Japan, an area usually designated by modern historians as the Far East or Orient. Little evidence of human progress in primitive times is available from this area. It is believed, however, that the stages of development were similar to those experienced by other cultures.

INDIA

India lay in the southern part of the Far Eastern continent. This triangular region was almost completely isolated from the rest of the world by two chains of mountains (the Himalayas) along its northern border and by waters (the Arabian Sea, Bay of Bengal, and Indian Ocean) on its other three borders. It is thought that an advanced civilization existed in the Indus River valley by approximately 3000 BC. Migration from central Asia occurred through the mountain passes on the north by Aryan peoples of Indo-European stock. This group found in India a warm climate, extremely rich vegetation, and a race darker-skinned than themselves. The difference in skin color may have been the basis for the formation of a caste system that developed gradually and had far-reaching consequences for health and well-being. The immigration continued over a long period, and the descendants, Indo-Aryans, were a vigorous people whose wealth consisted of cattle and whose amusements included hunting, gambling, and chariot racing. Eventually the native peoples of this area were conquered by the Aryans. An advanced culture developed, and it had direct access to Persia on the west and indirect contact with China on the east.

Excavated remains indicate that during the first civilization in India (2500-1500 BC) there were large cities and a highly developed culture. Within the carefully planned cities were baths, shops, multiroom buildings, and temples built with burned brick. An exceptional feature of this pre-Aryan culture was its system of public sanitation. Drainage systems, wells, bathrooms, public baths, and collection chutes for trash were in evidence. Practical arts included the cultivation of soil, domestication of animals, and smelting of metals. The script used in the writings left by this civilization has yet to be totally deciphered.

The Vedic Age, beginning after 1500 BC, produced the classical Indian civilization and Brahmanism (also known as Hinduism). Agriculture became the principal occupation at this time, although crafts were also practiced. Organized labor appeared in the form of guilds. The Jumna and Ganges rivers became sacred to the Hindus. India became a home of architectural beauty populated by a people who were well versed in war and politics and were inventors of the decimal system and discoverers in the fields of geome-

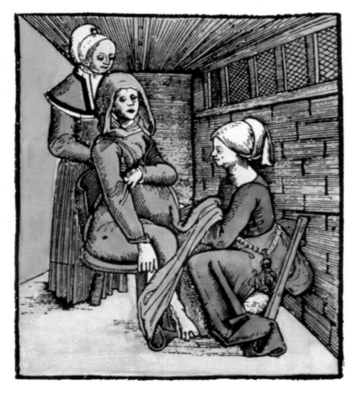

In ancient art, only two types of scenes illustrate women caring for the health of others: childbirth and the bathing of infants. During childbirth, the midwife functioned while sitting or kneeling in front of the woman. Rueff's *Trostbuechle* was a sixteenth-century book of instruction for midwives.

Obstetrical Chair (Birthing Stool), 1513, page from a book, from *Roslin's Garden of Roses for Pregnant Women*, The Granger Collection, NY.

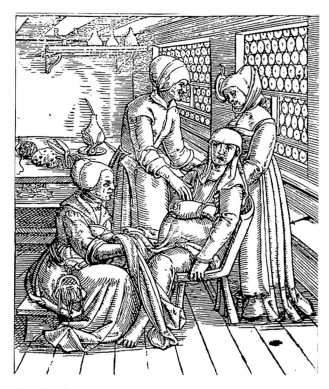

Jacobus Rueff, *Midwife*, 1554, etching/engraving. Image courtesy of National Library of Medicine, Bethesda, MD.

try and trigonometry. A priesthood was established, and the population was divided into tribes ruled by elected chiefs. In time, the state replaced the tribes, and kings replaced the chiefs.

India was known as the Land of the Temples. Its temples were masterpieces of artistry and were vitally important to the Hindu people. The idols, however, were usually hideous. Worship was directed to one or more of the prominent deities. Uppermost was the Trimurti, or divine triad of gods: Brahma, the power and spirit of the universe; Vishnu, the preserver of the world; and Shiva, the destroyer and conqueror of death. The other principal deities included Lakshmi, goddess of life, beauty, and good fortune; Soma, personification of the hallucinatory plant used in Aryan rituals; Indra, god of war and weather; Agni, god of sacrifice and fire; Varuna, god of justice and cosmic order; and Dhanvantari, patron god of medicine. The twin Ashvins were also medical gods, patrons of eyesight, who acted as physicians to the gods themselves.

Two philosophical systems strongly influenced the lives of the people of India: Brahmanism and Buddhism. Both were closely connected with deep religious beliefs, and both were pantheistic and nihilistic. Pantheism is the belief that reality is a single being of which everything else is a part. (The deities were parts of the eternal whole because Brahman permeated everything in the universe.) Nihilism is the belief that conditions in the social organization are so poor as to make destruction desirable. It holds that existence is senseless and progress involves destruction for its own sake.

Brahmanism, the religion of the Aryan conquerors, provided religious development during 30 centuries. It revolved about Brahma, the eternal spirit, who permeated everything in the universe. The ideal of perfection rested in absolute unity with Brahma. This was attained by sacrifice, penance, and contemplation. Transmigration of the living soul, the

doctrine of reincarnation, was affirmed. A person might be reborn into a lower or higher rank of human being, or even into the form of lower animals, after death. Ancestor worship was encouraged, and reverence for animals, especially cows and monkeys, was advocated. Consequently, consumption of products from these animals was forbidden. Inherent in Brahmanism was stratification of the society into four distinct castes: Brahmins (priests and their descendants); Kshatrityas (warriors); Vaishyas (merchants, farmers, and artisans); and Shudras (menial workers).

The religious and moral codes within Brahmanism were written in the Vedas (Vedic, the parent language of Sanskrit, was used), which served as the sacred books, or scripture, and were the historical documents of India. These doctrines, presented in the form of hymns, prayers, and teachings, were administered by the priestly class. The priests retained a very high position and were responsible for the interpretation, enforcement, and preservation of the dogma.

The Vedas, usually dated to about 1600 BC, consisted of four books. The Rig-Veda, the Yajur-Veda, and the Sama-Veda were almost entirely religious. In the Rig-Veda, disease was regarded as the result of divine wrath. The Atharva-Veda contained innumerable incantations and charms for the practice of magic; disease, injury, sanity, health, and fertility were mentioned. They were reinforced in the Sushruta-Samhita (Introduction, p. xiv): "In India, as in all other countries, curative spells and healing mantras (charms) preceded medicine; and the first man of medicine in India was a priest, a Bhisag Atharvan (i.e., magic doctor), who held a superior position to a surgeon in society."

Supplemental Vedas (Upavedas) were also developed. Of these the Ayur-Veda, or Science of Life, was supposed to have been derived from Brahma himself. It contained eight parts that dealt with subjects such as medicine, surgery, and children's diseases and stressed hygiene and prevention of illness. From these writings various authors made Samhitas, or compendiums, for which they claimed divine origin. Two of these contributors were regarded as the most influential: Sushruta and Charaka. The dates of origin of these documents vary widely—from the 4th century BC to the 5th century AD.

Sushruta represented the surgical aspect of Indian medicine; Charaka symbolized the medical aspect. Charaka was believed to have wisdom inherited from a serpent-god with a thousand heads who was the caretaker of all the sciences, especially medicine (Stewart and Austin, 1962). Both authors reveal a highly developed medicine and surgery, which no doubt evolved slowly after the writing of the Vedas and was incidentally influenced by contacts with the cultures of the Near East.

Indian surgery was the most highly skilled surgery of any ancient culture. Operations such as tonsillectomies, which were unknown to the later Greeks and Romans, were performed in India. Furthermore, Hindu surgeons performed amputations, excised tumors, repaired hernias and harelips, removed bladder stones, couched cataracts (displaced the opacifying lens down and away from the line of vision), reconstructed noses, and delivered babies by cesarean section. In addition to the procedures related to surgery, approximately 125 different surgical instruments were described. Hindu physicians drugged their patients with hyoscyamus, henbane, and *Cannabis indica* and used hypnosis in an attempt to provide anesthesia. Great care was taken in the washing and bandaging of wounds (fifteen principal varieties of bandage were available). The ideal doctor was identified in the following way:

> He should be cleanly in his habits and well shaved, and should not allow his nails to grow. He should wear white garments, put on a pair of shoes, carry a stick and an umbrella in his hands, and walk about with a mild and benignant look as a friend of all created beings. . . . A physician should abjure the company of women, nor should he speak in private to them or joke with them.
>
> — *Bhishagratna, 1907, p. 74*

Many illnesses, such as tuberculosis, typhoid fever, leprosy, hepatitis, neurological disorders, and cholera, were described. The epithet *mellitus* (honeylike) was applied to diabetes, and its symptoms were identified as languor, thirst, and foul breath. Variolation was practiced. About fifteen scarifications were made with a needle on the upper arm of a person to be immunized; the area was then covered with cotton dipped in pock material. Transmitters of specific diseases, such as mosquitoes in connection with malaria, were described. *It was believed that the prevention of disease was more important than the cure.* Indian medicine also displayed ideas about pathology, the most notable being that disease might be caused by impurities in the body fluids, or humors. This humoral pathology was later emphasized by Greek physicians and ultimately became a basic concept of European medicine.

An interesting portrayal of a team concept of medical care was presented in one Indian document:

> The Physician, the Drugs, the Nurse, and the Patient constitute an aggregate of four. Of what virtues each of these should be possessed, so as to become causes for the cure of the disease, should be known.
> *Physician.* Thorough mastery of the scriptures, large experience, cleverness, and purity (of body and mind) are the principal qualities of the physician.
> *Drugs.* Abundance of virtue, adaptability to the disease under treatment, the capacity of being used in diverse ways, and undeterioration are attributes of drugs.
> *Nurse.* Knowledge of the manner in which drugs should be prepared or compounded for administration, cleverness, devotedness to the patient waited upon, and purity (both of mind and body) are the four qualifications of the attending nurse.
> *Patient.* Memory, obedience to direction, fearlessness, and communicativeness (with respect to all that is experienced internally and done by him during the intervals between visits) are the qualities of the patient.
> As in the task of cooking, a vessel, fuel, and fire are the means in the hands of the cook; as field, army, and weapons are means in the victor's hands for achieving victory in battles; even the patient, the nurse, and drugs are the objects that are regarded as the physician's means in the matter of achieving a cure.
> Like clay, stick, wheel, threads, in the absence of the potter, failing to produce anything by their combination, the three others, viz., drugs, nurse, and patient, cannot work out a cure in the absence of the physician.
>
> — *Kaviratna, n.d., pp. 102-103*

This document is quite remarkable in that it stresses high standards for all members of the team, including the patient. That the patient is defined as a team member is even more surprising, considering this period of history. The document also specifies the patient, nurse, and drugs as the physician's means of achieving a cure. These three, however, cannot manage a cure without the physician. It is also important to note that the nurse is responsible for all aspects of drug usage, in essence acting as a pharmacist as well as a nurse. It is interesting that the virtues (characteristics or standards) required of the nurse include knowledge as well as skill, a factor that is still debated in contemporary society.

As time passed, the people of India became dissatisfied with the religion of the Vedas. There had long been those who had chosen the life of a recluse to attain a more intimate relationship with the spiritual. Among them was Siddhartha Gautama (560-480 BC?), from the caste of princes, who left home, wife, and child at the age of twenty-nine to find salvation. After wandering and speculation, he announced himself as Buddha, the Enlightened, and offered a new religious philosophy that came to be known as Buddhism. The major premise of Buddhism was based on the idea that perfection consisted of attaining nothingness, which was to be accomplished by severe penances.

"The long period of India's Golden Age was a period in which the religion of Buddha prevailed. Mercy, compassion, and justice were the tenets governing humane treatment of animals as well as man." Buddhism was, however, more of a moral discipline than an organized religion, and it encouraged the development of social institutions. India's greatest convert to Buddhism was King Asoka (269-237 BC), but he was unsuccessful in instituting its acceptance on a permanent basis. During Asoka's reign the greatest advances in charitable and sanitary work were made. Among many generous works, he established hospitals, which are considered to be the first in world history. The exact number of hospitals he developed is not known. Evidently there was difficulty with the Sanskrit word for *hospital* because it could also be interpreted as *pharmacy* or *dis-*

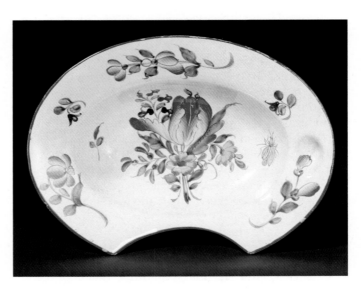

18th Century German school, *Bleeding Bowl,* 1760, porcelain bowl, Strasbourg, Germany. Photo courtesy of the Bridgeman Art Library.

pensary. However, there is no question that hospitals of some type were built during this period. These hospitals were constructed periodically by government order, serviced by government-paid physicians, and supplied by government stores. Consequently, state medicine had become a reality in India.

The early physicians came from the priestly or Brahmin caste. Later, physicians were drawn from the upper castes, and eventually all practitioners came to be known as Vaidya. High moral standards were expected of those who chose the care of the sick as a life's work. Permission to practice was obtained from the king, a procedure similar to the current licensing system. Appearance, dress, speech, and manners had to be above reproach. Rules for ritual and daily life were dictated by the Laws of Manu, which were compiled between 200 BC and AD 200. These laws have been compared to the Mosaic Law because they include ordinances for the regulation of family and personal hygiene and dietary practices. According to the Laws of Manu, physicians could be penalized for improper treatment of patients.

The history of India reveals a more complete description of nursing principles and practice than that of any other ancient civilization. Throughout the historical documents of India, frequent references are made to nurses. In most instances these nurses were men; however, in rare cases they were old women. Three main qualities of character—high standards, skill, and trustworthiness—were also required of these attendants. The specific requirements are described in the following passages:

> After this should be secured a body of attendants of good behaviour, distinguished for purity or cleanliness of habits, attached to the person for whose service they are engaged, possessed of cleverness and skill, endued with kindness, skilled in every kind of service that a patient may require, endued with general cleverness, competent to cook food and curries, clever in bathing or washing a patient, well conversant in rubbing or pressing the limbs, or raising the patient or assisting him in walking or moving about, well skilled in making or cleaning beds, competent to pound drugs, or ready, patient, and skillful in waiting upon one that is ailing, and never unwilling to do any act that they may be commanded (by the physician or patient) to do.
>
> — *CHARAKA-SAMHITA, VOL. 1, PP. 168-169*

> *Nurse.* That person alone is fit to nurse or to attend the bedside of a patient who is cool-headed and pleasant in his demeanour, does not speak ill of anybody, is strong and attentive to the requirements of the sick, and strictly and indefatigably follows the instructions of the physician.
>
> *SUSHRUTA-SAMHITA, VOL. 1, PP. 305-307*

It is interesting to note that in the above passage, the word *his* is used to refer to the nurse, consistent with the fact that the majority of nurses in India were men. Many of the nurse's requirements are still part of modern nursing although "strictly and indefatigably following the instructions of the physician" no longer fits with more contemporary concepts, such as the accountability, advocacy, and liability inherent in the current practice of nursing.

It was apparently the existence of hospitals that created the need for this special group. Although it is certain that nurses were employed in the hospitals of India, it is unclear whether they were viewed as glorified servants or as professional personnel. Women were midwives and in some cases, experts in drug lore. They held a high position in India, and their activities centered about the management of the home. It is assumed that women functioned as nurses when members of their families became ill.

CHINA

Ancient China was cut off from the Mediterranean world by the great range of the Himalaya Mountains. It lay far to the northeast of India and remains somewhat a mystery because accurate records are not available before the Shang dynasty (c. 1776-1122 BC). The inhabitants of China are believed to have come from central Asia in about 3000 BC, settling along the banks of the Yellow River. The land in this region was fertile. Grain became the staple crop, fruit trees were prevalent, and vegetation was so luxurious that the title The Flowery Kingdom was conferred upon China.

Information about this early civilization is primarily legendary, yet it emerged in possession of social, religious, and political institutions. China's history became authentic with the appearance of the second Chou dynasty (1122-249 BC), a rule that lasted almost 900 years. Civilization spread south from the Yellow River to the Yangtze River during this time. The people belonged to the Mongoloid race and had great respect for social order. A creative people, they carved in wood and ivory, produced works of art in bronze and lacquer, and used irrigation systems for their fields. Poetry and history were written, although the Chinese writing was slow, complicated, and difficult. It contained symbols that represented objects (pictograms), ideas (ideograms), and sounds (phonograms). Sacred books were also written, and they were comparable to the papyri of Egypt and the Vedas of India.

The Chinese form of government was patriarchal rule. The family was the fundamental unit of the society, so the government was concerned with the social group rather than the individual. Local government comprised a group of elders who were representatives of the various families making up a particular village. The elders, who met in the local temple to manage the village affairs, were the liaison between the people and the monarch. Shang, the first known dynasty, was followed by the Chou dynasties, which had a feudal form of government. These were succeeded by the Ch'in in the 3rd century BC, when various feudal states were united into one empire.

Four social classes were recognized in China: scholars, farmers, artisans, and traders. In reality, however, two classes functioned; these were the officials (mandarins) and the nonofficials. The officials were selected on the basis of talent rather than by class, because civil service, an ancient institution in China, opened examinations to all who could qualify.

Three religious systems influenced China: Taoism and Confucianism, which were indigenous, and Buddhism, which was imported from India. "Taoism was characterized by freedom from desire within one's self and an absence of self-determined actions for particular ends in things exterior to one's self" (Frank, 1953, p. 26). It was a religion concerned with obtaining long life and good fortune, often through magical means. The value of charms was emphasized as a method to combat the demons of disease. These charms were written on paper that was burned, and the ashes were then administered in a liquid such as tea. The study of alchemy arose from the practice of searching for the elixir of life and the transmutation of base metals into gold. Taoism ultimately yielded to Confucianism and Buddhism.

Confucius entered the lives of the Chinese about 500 BC. He had studied the sacred books as a child and later emerged as one of the greatest reformers and teachers the world has ever known. Confucius was a political reformer rather than a religious originator. His political reforms were based on moral principles, and he sought to relieve oppression by returning to ancient customs as the basis of government. Confucius stressed family cohesion, the value of knowledge, right conduct (etiquette), and ancestor worship, which prevented the dissection of bodies. (No worship was accorded to female ancestors.) Confucius' philosophy was the negative version of the Golden Rule: What you do not wish done to yourself do not do unto others. On the whole, Confucianism did not promote progress because it failed to stimulate ambition for better things. Yet some progress was achieved in China. By 200 BC Buddhism had become the religion of the land, having been brought from India into the Far East.

The religious practices of China were polytheistic, animistic, and idolatrous. Images of painted wood were adored, and sacrifices were offered to these images because the people believed them to be inhabited by souls. The evil spirits responsible for disease and disaster were frightened off by loud noises. Sacrifice to the gods was an official state function. Only distinguished social groups were permitted to participate in the ceremonies; the people could participate only in ceremonies for worship of their own ancestors.

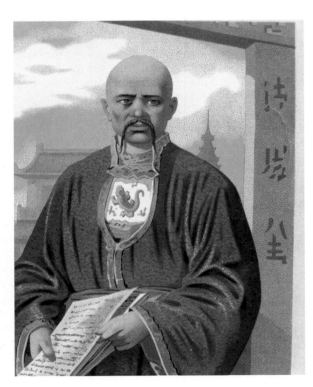

Confucius, 19th century, engraving. Image from Ancient Art and Architecture Collection Ltd.

Chinese medicine was focused on prevention. Health was considered to be a state of harmony or equilibrium within the individual and the universe. This state was accomplished through the interplay of nature's basic duality: the yang (male principle), which was positive, warm, dry, light, and full of life; and the yin (female principle), which was negative, passive, dark, cold, moist, weak, and lifeless. An improper balance of these energies resulted in discomfort and disease. Illness could also be caused by evil spirits and animistic forces.

The works of three legendary emperors provided the basic foundation for Chinese medicine. Fu Hsi (c. 2900 BC) created the *pa kua,* a symbol with yang and yin lines combined in eight separate trigrams. They could represent all yin-yang conditions. Shen Nung (Hung Ti), the Red Emperor, wrote the *Pen Tsao (Herbal),* which was the result of his investigations into medicinal herbs. The effects of 365 personally tested drugs were reported. Shen Nung is also thought to have drawn the first charts of acupuncture. Huang Ti (Yu Hsiung), the Yellow Emperor, was credited with writing the great medical compendium *Nei Ching (Canon of Medicine).* According to this work, four steps in examination were necessary to determine a diagnosis: look, listen, ask, and feel (observation, auscultation, interrogation, and palpation). These four steps are still used in health care, although they are now supplemented by the newest technological advances. In essence, this canon of medicine recorded all phases of health and illness, including prevention and treatment.

Medical knowledge in early China included techniques of dissection, studies of the circulatory system, massage, the therapeutic use of baths, and the significance of pulse rates. Diagnoses were often made on the basis of a complicated pulse theory in which the pulse of the patient was studied over a period of several hours. Some two hundred types of pulse beat were listed.

> The physician felt the right wrist and then the left. He compared the beats with his own, noting precise time as well as day and season since each hour affected the nature of the pulsations. Each pulse had three distinct divisions, each associated with a specific organ, and each division had a separate quality, of which there were dozens of varieties. Moreover, each division or zone of the pulse had a superficial and deep projection. Thus literally hundreds of possible characteristics were obtainable. In one treatise, *Muo-Ching,* ten volumes were necessary to cover all the intricacies of the pulse.
>
> — LYONS, 1978, P. 127

Five methods of treatment were identified in the *Nei Ching:* cure the spirit, nourish the body, give medications, treat the whole body, and use acupuncture and moxibustion. Acupuncture consisted of inserting needles an inch or so into areas along the twelve meridians that traverse the body and using a twisting motion. Moxibustion used the same meridians. However, this treatment also involved a powdered plant substance (cones of mugwort) that was fashioned into a mound on the patient's skin and burned slowly. This method of counterirritation caused blisters to form on the area.

Smallpox was a widely known disease in China. A more

primitive form of variolation than that used in India was performed by the Chinese. Crusts of diseased pustules were ground into a powder and blown into the nostrils through a bamboo tube. Surgery was limited to the castration of males seeking advancement at court (eunuchs) and to the treatment of wounds. The limited development of surgery may have been a result of the belief that mutilation of the body would remain in evidence in life after death. Chinese medicine spread into Korea, Japan, and Tibet, where superstition mixed with these practices.

Little mention is made of hospitals in ancient China, although Halls of Healing are described. These were adjuncts to the temples where the sick prayed for recovery. Berdoe

(1893) correlates the absence of hospitals with the duty of the Chinese people to care for their families at home. Even more striking is the lack of reference to nursing in the literature of the ancient Chinese. If there were nurses, they were probably not women because the woman's position, as defined by Confucius, was inferior. A woman's work was confined to the keeping of the home and the building of families. Her value was greatest when she produced sons. It is also possible that the belief that disease could be caused by evil spirits' taking up residence in a patient's body had a distinct impact on care of the sick. The fear that these spirits could enter anyone who touched a sick person would have made nursing almost nonexistent.

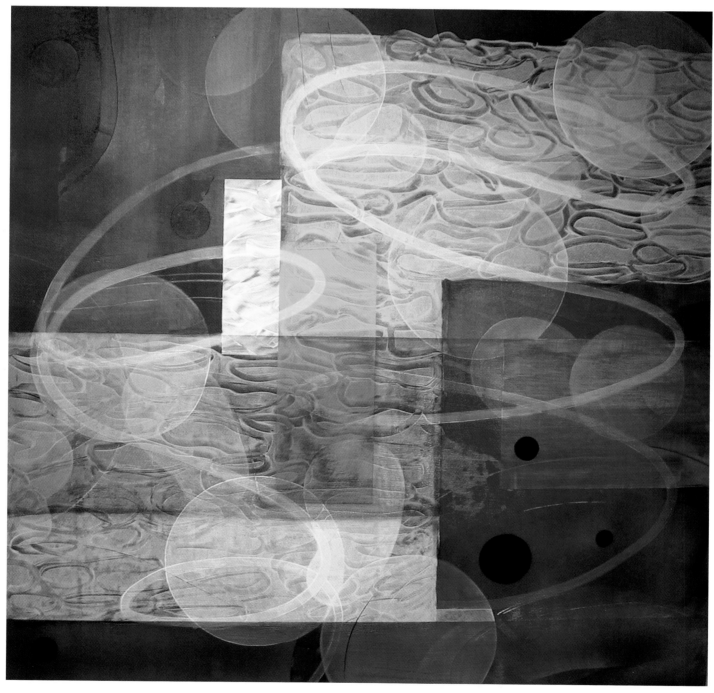

Carol Mode, *Harmonies*, 2006, acrylic/wood panel, 40" × 40", private collection, Davidson, TN.

THE MEDITERRANEAN WORLD

GREECE

Ancient Greece was a peninsula that jutted out into the Mediterranean Sea from the southeastern part of Europe. Surrounded by gulfs and ocean, its indented coastline provided good harbors, which led to the establishment of trade. The interior of the country was mountainous; the climate was warm and sunny. This topography led to a particular political organization in which small groups of people settled in the plains and valleys between the mountains. Cities were built within areas of two hundred to three hundred square miles. A location with a commanding view was chosen in each city for use during attacks by enemies. Temples and other buildings were also erected on these sites. Eventually, governmental functions were assumed by the cities, which became the ruling authorities in areas approximating a radius of ten miles. Each area was designated an independent city-state and had a king, a council, and an assembly.

Civilization entered Greece through the island of Crete by way of Egypt and Phoenicia and was not unlike that of the peoples of the Near East. Its growth was nourished partly by the inhabitants of Crete, the other Aegean islands, and the mainland and also by communication with the ancient civilizations of Egypt and Mesopotamia. The Greek people, or Hellenes, as the Greeks called themselves, who migrated into the area were of Indo-European stock. They assimilated the preexisting civilization. The Greeks were unlike other ancient peoples because they were keen observers, not experimenters; they were philosophers, not scientists. Their sense of beauty encompassed proportion and spatial relationships, resulting in architecture and temples of the high-est artistic caliber. The scattered nation was unified by language, literature, and religious worship. The Panhellenic, or Olympic Games, held every four years starting in 776 BC, brought the people together to compete for prizes. In addition, every family aimed to produce participants with healthy bodies.

Recorded Greek history begins with the Homeric Age, or Age of Heroes. The writings of Homer, *The Iliad* and *The Odyssey,* became the sacred books of Greece. Through mythology the origins of the peoples were traced, and health, illness, and medical practice were discussed. "In the Homeric poems, one gets a glimpse of commonsense remedies and of simple wound surgery, of charms against sickness, and of appeals to this god or that to protect a warrior against injury" (Shryock, 1959, p. 41).

The Greeks had the ancient gods of the earth and the underworld as well as special healing agents such as snakes and moles. Apollo, the sun god, was the god of health and medicine. Asklepios (in Rome, called Aesculapius), son of Apollo and a human mother, was the chief healer in Greek mythology. His fame may have been created on the basis of a mortal of fame and skill, for it is traced to about 13 centuries before Christ. This mortal was supposedly a Greek physician who was raised to the rank of a god. Two of his sons accompanied the Greek army to the Trojan War. Machaon was a surgeon with "skilled hands to draw out darts and heal sores"; Podalirius was an internist who was "given cunning to find out things impossible and cure that which healed not." Asklepios was represented holding the wand of Mercury, a wayfarer's staff entwined with the sacred serpents of wisdom. The medical caduceus is derived from this portrayal.

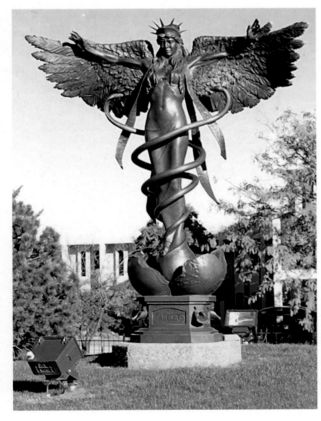

James Muir, *Caduceus,* 1997, sculpture, 12' × 9', J. N. Muir Sculpture Studios, Sedona, AZ. Copyright 1997 by James Muir.

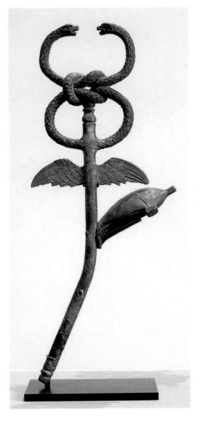

Caduceus Rod, 2nd century, bronze sculpture, 26¹/₈" × 12¾" × 5¾", Minneapolis Institute of Arts, The William Hood Dunwoody Fund.

The women also shared the work of health conservation in the myth of Asklepios. Epigone, the wife, was revered as the soothing one. The six daughters included Hygeia, the goddess of health; Panacea, the restorer of health, who personified miraculous all-healing herbs; Aegle, the light of the sun; Meditrina, the preserver of health (supposedly the ancient forerunner of the public health nurse); and Iaso, who personified the recovery from illness. "The whole family of Asklepios has significance for the medical and nursing arts, for if its members were only symbolic, they must have been meant to depict those arts as they existed at that time, and if they were actual persons they combined in their careers all the main lines of specialism that we consider modern (Stewart and Austin, 1962, p. 28).

The myth of Asklepios became highly complex. Temples were built to him on sites of great natural beauty that had pure spring water (often this water had already been noted for its medicinal properties) and refreshing breezes. The buildings, masterpieces of architecture, were exquisitely decorated. The temples that became famous for cures would emerge as great social and intellectual centers. Theaters, gymnasiums, a stadium, places for worship, a hospital, living quarters for patients, baths, lodgings for visitors and attendants, housing for priests and physicians, and libraries were built nearby and were surrounded by gardens and parks. These health resorts were frequented not only by people who were ill but also by those who enjoyed the beauty and contentment of the surroundings and the brilliance of the cultural life and entertainment. The most famous of these centers was Epidauros, situated a few miles from Athens. It accommodated about five hundred patients and was serviced by a chief administrator and various grades of attendants, including priestesses.

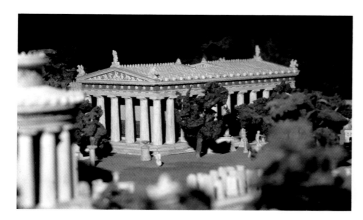

Epidauros Temple (Temple of Aesculapius Healing Centre), R Sheridan/Ancient Art & Architecture Collection Ltd.

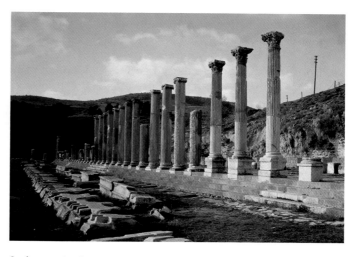

Scala, *Temple of Aesculapius*, photograph, Pergamon, Turkey. Image from Ancient Art and Architecture Collection Ltd.

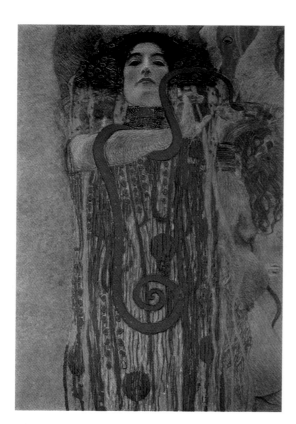

Gustav Klimt (1862-1918), *Hygieia* (detail from *Medicine*), painting, 430 x 300 cm. Copyright Scholl Immendorf, Austria/The Bridgeman Art Library Nationality/copyright status: Austrian/out of copyright.

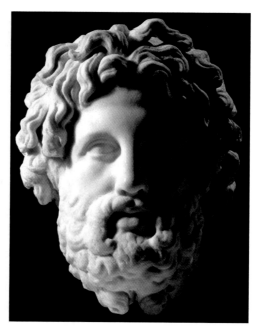

Colossal Marble Head of Asklepios, c325-300 BC, sculpture, 61.00 cm. Copyright the Trustees of the British Museum. All rights reserved.

Upon arrival, patients offered sacrifices of animals to Asklepios and underwent a cleansing or purifying process consisting of a series of baths and a period of abstinence from certain foods and wines. After several days in the outer courts, the patient was admitted to the inner court to participate in religious ceremonies that included elaborate rites and rituals. Finally, the patient was admitted to the *abaton* to sleep in full sight of a great statue of the god. This incubation, or temple sleep, would reveal through a dream or hypnotic state the treatment to be administered. Votive tablets were left behind that attested to innumerable cures. Yet maternity patients and the incurably ill were not admitted to the temples for medical assistance.

Two other institutions offered care to the sick: the *xenodochium* and the *iatrion*. The xenodochium was similar in function to the Hebrew xenodochium and first provided care for travelers, then for people who were sick or injured. In the later centuries of Greek history, it was placed under municipal management and may have been the forerunner of the modern city or county hospital. The iatrion was a facility where ambulatory care was received. It corresponds most closely with the dispensary or outpatient clinics of present-day hospitals.

The cult of Asklepios, which evolved from Greek mythology, provided religious healing and offered a blend of natural and supernatural remedies. Eventually, the priests of Asklepios branched into two specialized areas, one strictly medical and the other purely occult. From the medical branch, a group of lay physicians developed.

> While the shrines of Aesculapius continued to offer religious healing, lay physicians accumulated factual knowledge about common illnesses and how to handle them. These men moved from one town to another as skilled artisans and learned much from the bedside. They practiced both general medicine and surgery, and the experience of a number of them was finally incorporated in a collection of writings ascribed to Hippocrates. Although there probably was a physician of that name, he did not write all these works; as his name became legendary, it was applied to the whole collection. This became the first general text on medicine and was long viewed as a sort of Bible by the medical profession.
>
> — SHRYOCK, 1959, PP. 46-47

As Greek civilization progressed, many changes took place. The healing arts were particularly affected during the Golden Age of Greece, between the 6th and 4th centuries before Christ. This was the birth of the age of reason, which culminated in the classical philosophy of Socrates, Plato, Aristotle, and others. These days of the philosopher-scientists were devoted to attempts to attribute natural rather than supernatural explanations to phenomena. Truth was sought through clear thinking and close observation of physical and social phenomena. This study of nature was eventually called natural philosophy, the first clear expression of what is now known as science. The results of these scientific and philosophical investigations provided the fundamentals of good living. It was Aristotle (384-322 BC), however, who had a profound influence on medicine. He was credited with laying the foundation of biology and comparative anatomy. His contributions in the field of both plant and animal biology greatly aided the development of medical

thought. In addition, Aristotle dealt with ethical matters in a scientific manner.

Despite the fact that rational medicine had been developing before his time and magical medicine persisted long after his time, Hippocrates of Cos (460-370 BC?) was given credit for the establishment of rational, or scientific, medicine. He belonged to the order of Asklepiades and was believed to have been a direct descendant of Asklepios himself. Hippocrates is considered to have been one of the greatest physicians who ever lived, and he became known as the Father of Medicine. He taught that disease was not the work of spirits, demons, or deities but the result of the breaking of natural laws. The true art of the physician, therefore, was to assist nature to bring about a cure. The writings attributed to Hippocrates relate to nearly all aspects of medicine—pathology, anatomy, physiology, diagnosis, prognosis, mental illness, gynecology, obstetrics, surgery, therapy, bedside observations, hygiene, and professional ethics. Epilepsy, tuberculosis, malarial fever, ulcers, and other diseases were described. Perhaps the most interesting and significant portions of these writings were the case histories, which were preserved in the *Epidemics*. They included a compilation of the details of the patient who was ill, the patient's environment, and the complete examination. Even today, these case histories could serve as models for succinct clinical records because they are comprehensive, concise, and direct.

The practice of hygiene was more than a medical specialty. It was a way of life that was depicted in part by Hippocrates' discussion of diet, the avoidance of sexual excesses, and the importance of exercise. His emphasis on the role of environment in the spread of disease, as presented

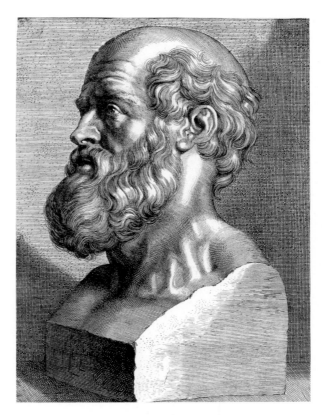

Although the "Hippocratic Oath" is one of the greatest early documents dealing with medical ethics, most scholars believe that it is not really a part of the Hippocratic teachings.

Paulus Pontius, *Hippocrates*, early 17th centruty, etching/engraving, 304 × 220 mm, National Library of Medicine, Bethesda, MD.

in *Airs, Waters and Places,* provided a basic epidemiological text in which the concepts of endemic diseases (those always present) and epidemic diseases (those that broke out at certain periods and involved large numbers of people) were illuminated (Rosen, 1958). Therapy was related to the elements of fire, air, earth, and water. In different combinations these exhibited the four basic qualities of heat, cold, dryness, and moisture. Everything, including the body, was composed of one or more of these elements. This led to the classic theory of disease, the four humors (blood, phlegm, yellow bile, and black bile). When these humors were in balance, the result was a healthy body; excess or deficiency of one or more caused illness.

The Hippocratic method basically rested on the following principles: observe all; study the patient rather than the disease; evaluate honestly; assist nature. These principles were to be combined with a professional spirit, or ethical conduct. The true physician had to be devoted to his profession and his patients and was to abstain from all that would dishonor the one and injure the other.

The literature of the Greeks contains many references to nurses. However, they were primarily children's nurses, wet nurses, and midwives. (Midwives provided most of the obstetrical care; physicians assisted with difficult or abnormal childbirth.) In historical accounts, discrepancies exist about who performed the other nursing functions because the activities of a Greek woman were confined to the home unless she was a priestess, a slave, or a harlot. Greek women could not be admitted to the "mysteries" of any art. Thus, if the Greeks had nurses, they would probably have been men. Even Hippocrates, the master of medical art, left no direct reference to nurses.

> A most remarkable feature of the ancient medical writings is the scant attention paid to that very important factor in modern treatment—the nurse. Professional nurses were, apparently, unknown (Note: midwives were common enough), and the general impression that the reader forms is that the physician did not consider the work of the attendant to be of great value. In some cases, doubtless, the household slaves acted as nurses. . . . But the burden of nursing fell chiefly upon the wife. . . . It is clear then that in ordinary cases it was the duty of the wife to nurse the whole household, with the help no doubt of her daughters and maid servants.
>
> — JONES, 1909, PP. 123-126

Yet in the Hippocratic writings, what we now call nursing is taught in minute detail, and the assistant or attendant is indicated as the coworker of the physician. Specific directions about poultices; cold sponging; fluid diets; warm baths; light and regular nourishment for heart cases; large amounts of fluid for kidney cases; the use of mouthwashes; and clean, smooth bed linen are given. It is clear from these writings that nursing care existed in ancient Greece. However, what nursing care was actually like is left to the imagination.

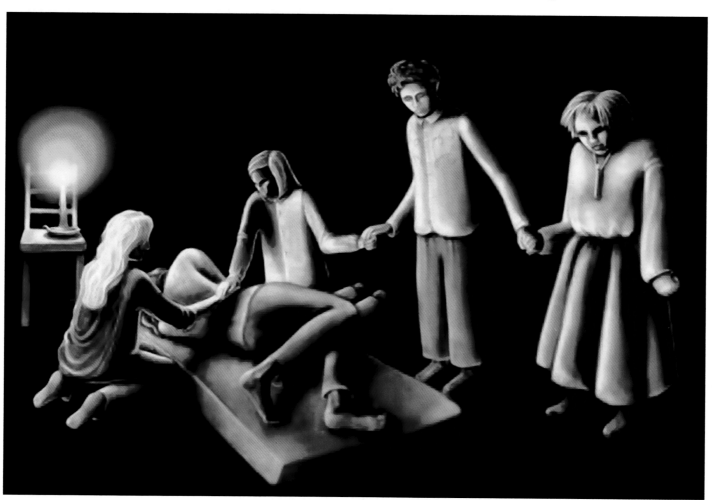

Stephanie Crooty Noverraz, *Healing,* 2005, digital image.

ROME

While civilization was progressing in the East, and Greece was emerging in the realms of art and thinking, a new power began to form in the West. This occurred in the peninsula we now know as Italy, where an agricultural people known as Latins resided. Italy was separated from Greece by water and was divided into two sections by a chain of mountains. The level plains on the western side were initially chosen by the Latins for the location of their homes. This area was occupied in ancient times by various peoples, the oldest of whom were the Etruscans, who had migrated from Asia Minor. The Etruscans achieved a higher degree of culture than other tribes in this area. They were later conquered and absorbed by the Romans.

The Gauls, or Celts, of western Europe originally occupied the northern part of Italy. The Greeks began to settle in southern Italy in about the 8th century BC in an area that became known as Magna Graecia (Greater Greece). Eventually the Romans, who were excellent warriors, conquered and absorbed them all. This Latin tribe had occupied the central and northern portions of Italy. In time, they succeeded

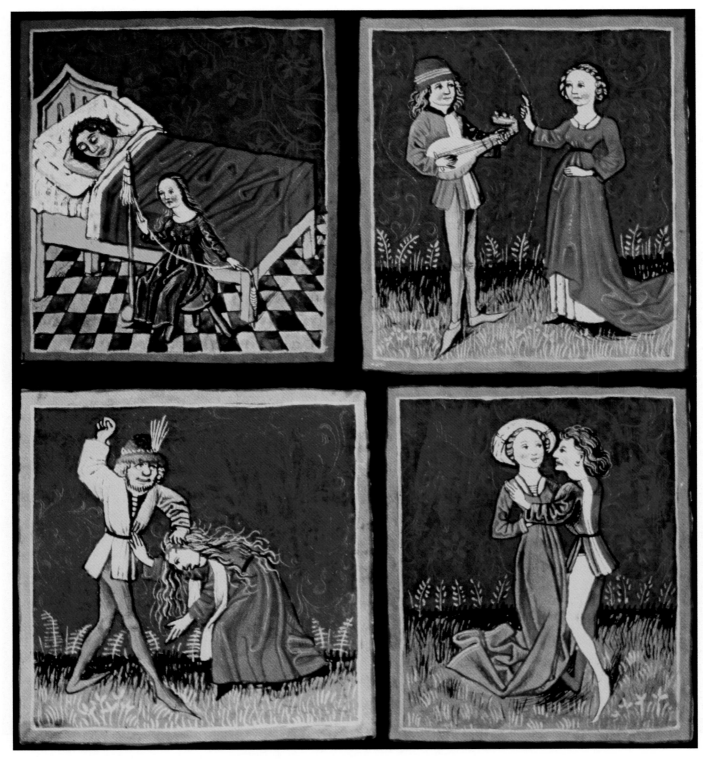

The Four Humors, 15th century, The Granger Collection, NY.

in bringing unity to the country under their rule. As a result, the village of Rome passed from a simple farming community to a thriving commercial center.

Legend places the birth of Rome at 753 BC. Located at the mouth of the Tiber River, Rome progressed through the stages of a kingdom, a republic, an empire, and a city. The event of its founding is intertwined with a variety of mythological interpretations. One account is told by Virgil in his great epic poem *The Aeneid,* which describes the wanderings of Aeneas and his companions in the period between the fall of Troy and the founding of Rome. It is also said that the site of Rome on seven hills "appears to have been the choice of twin brothers, Romulus and Remus, themselves indebted for life to the nourishment and care given them by a kindly wolf who found them on a mountain top, abandoned by a goddess mother" (Jamieson and Sewall, 1950, p. 74).

The Romans did not develop a religion, a medical system, or an art of their own. All were borrowed from their conquests, from other peoples and nations. From Greece, which was under Roman control by 146 BC, tangible things such as money, textiles, and sailing ships were acquired. Eventually Greek ideas were also absorbed, as were art and religion. The Greek alphabet was adapted to the Latin tongue.

Early Romans possessed gods whose functions were highly practical. Jupiter guarded the welfare of the city, Juno was the women's patroness, Mars was the god of war, and Janus was the god of openings and beginnings. Prosperity occurred if one pleased the gods; failure resulted if the wrath of the gods was incurred. During this early period, no distinctive gods of healing were identified. However, in a later period, gods were borrowed from the Greeks and polytheism prevailed. These gods included Hygeia and Asklepios. It is also said that there was a god or goddess for almost every known physiological function or disease process; for example, Scabies, Angeronia, Fluonia, Uterina, and Febris. Febris became particularly significant in Rome for the power of reducing the fevers associated with malaria. Yet the ancient Romans were free from the superstition that the sick and insane were possessed by demons.

The Roman population was divided into two classes: the patricians (the wealthy or privileged group), who were given civil and legal privileges and whose right to citizenship was hereditary; and the plebeians (the poor or lower class), who were denied the right of citizenship. Work was given over to home slaves who were brought from conquered countries. Homes became luxurious, dress elaborate, and social functions extravagant. The demarcation line between the rich and the poor broadened. Internal decay emerged and continued. The Roman Empire lasted about 5 centuries, from 31 BC to AD 476. The first 2 centuries were spent in peace and prosperity; the 3rd century was marked by frequent disorder within the empire; the last 2 centuries were characterized by internal rebellion and external attack. The decline and fall of Rome was unavoidable. The church founded by Jesus Christ was the one institution that remained unshaken during this time.

Before the conquest of Greece, Roman medicine combined folk, magical, and religious practices. After 200 BC the Greek physicians, who had been made slaves, did the medical work, and their practices filtered throughout Rome. The most skillful of these physicians were given Roman citizenship during the rule of Julius Caesar. Legend, however, indi-

cates that Greek medicine was introduced to Rome in a year when pestilence was devastating the city (293 BC). Sibylline books were consulted, and the oracle replied that Asklepios be brought from Greece to Rome. A galley was sent and returned with a staff of physicians and attendants. As it came up the Tiber, a sacred serpent sprang out on the little island in the river and established itself there. This was a divinely chosen spot, so a temple to Asklepios (Aesculapius) was erected there.

Several medical practitioners achieved fame during the rise of the Roman Empire: Dioscorides Pedanius, Aretaeus, Asclepiades, and Galen. Dioscorides Pedanius was a Greek physician and a surgeon in the army under Nero. His *De Materia Medica* contained descriptions of more than six hundred preparations of medicinal herbs. He observed these herbs as he accompanied the armies.

Aretaeus refocused the study of medicine on the methods of clinical observation used by Hippocrates. His writings rendered vivid descriptions of such diseases as pneumonia, empyema, epilepsy, tetanus, diphtheria, and a type of diabetes.

Asclepiades of Bithynia was a Greek physician from Asia Minor who assisted in the establishment of Greek medicine in Rome. He repudiated the teachings of Hippocrates, for he believed that the physician, not nature, cured disease. Asclepiades proposed an atomistic theory in which disease resulted from a disturbance of the movement of atoms in the body. Treatment consisted of diet, baths, exercise, massage, soothing medications, music, and singing. Tracheostomies were commonly performed for respiratory distress. Asclepiades' theory paved the way for the development of the system of methodism, which was founded about 50 BC.

Galen (AD 130-201), a Greek physician from Asia Minor, was probably the most renowned and influential medical writer of all time. He became a physician to the gladiators and athletes in Rome and was also connected with the army. Consequently, he developed great skill in surgery; this is reflected in his writings, which are based on physiological functions. Galen's knowledge was acquired through per-

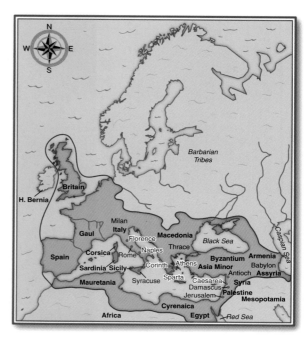

Roman Empire, map, Mosby.

sonal observations and experiences. His system for using drugs lasted through the medieval period in history. Galen is considered to be the great experimental physiologist of ancient times. His volumes of writings contributed greatly to medical knowledge and represent a preservation and amalgamation of Aristotle's teachings and the Hippocratic tradition, with additions by Galen himself (Taylor, 1922).

Two other individuals recorded much of the available information concerning medical practice in Alexandria and Rome: Cornelius Celsus and Caius Pliny. Known as encyclopedists, they lived during the 1st century AD. Celsus wrote the first organized medical history, translated works from Greek into Latin, and described the characteristics of inflammation as "redness and swelling with heat and pain" (rubor et tumor cum calore et dolore). These are still considered to be the four cardinal symptoms of inflammation. According to most scholars, Celsus was not a physician, yet he provided detailed accounts of surgical procedures and the ligation of blood vessels. The *De Medicina* of Celsus included such topics as pharmacology, dietetics, psychiatry, surgery, the preservation of health, and the history of medicine. Celsus also recognized the importance of basic research and fostered anatomical knowledge through animal dissections.

Pliny wrote extensively in the areas of history, biology, chemistry, physics, philosophy, magic, folklore, plants, food, and medicine. Some of this information is regarded as superstitious or inaccurate. Pliny's *Historia Naturalis* contained every piece of information he could gather from the past or the present (Lyons, 1978).

The genius of the Romans found its expression not in medical achievement but in works of public hygiene. It is quite possible that public health had its beginning in Rome. Of greatest importance were the colossal engineering feats accomplished by the Romans: the creation of drains, aqueducts, good roads, a system of central heating, proper cemeteries, and the draining of marshes. Massage and baths reached perfection among the Romans. "Rubbing and washing, warm and cold baths, both for cleanliness and for therapeutic uses, steam, oil, hot sand, steambox baths, and sitz baths were all in use, and there was a class of professional masseurs, the *iatralepta*" (Nutting and Dock, 1937, p. 88). Public and private bath houses were developed and assumed the character of clubs or social centers. Roman cities were cleaner than those of any other ancient civilization. Yet Rome had many epidemics, probably because of a number of factors related to conquests and modernization. For example, tenements were introduced in Rome to solve the rapid growth of the city.

The Romans had advanced military medicine and provided excellent care for their soldiers. First aid was rendered on the battlefield, and a field ambulance service was devised. Originally, wounded soldiers were carried to private homes. Later, they were cared for in tents or separate buildings and nursed by women and old men of upstanding character. Eventually, many military hospitals *(valetudinaria)* were erected, some of which could accommodate two hundred sick or wounded soldiers. A class of orderlies, the *nosocomi,* acted as nurses. Valetudinaria were also established for sick slaves of rich homes or estates, because slaves were considered to be a most valuable commodity. It is probable that slaves functioned as nurses in these institutions.

Roman women were independent and became involved in many activities outside the home. The care of the sick was no doubt undertaken by the mistress and by the male and female slaves of the household. Children's nurses and midwives were still the chief nursing roles for women.

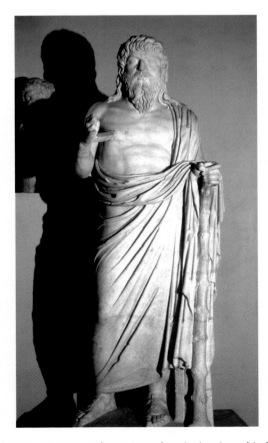

Galen Physician, 129-199 AD, sculpture. Image from Ancient Art and Architecture Collection Ltd.

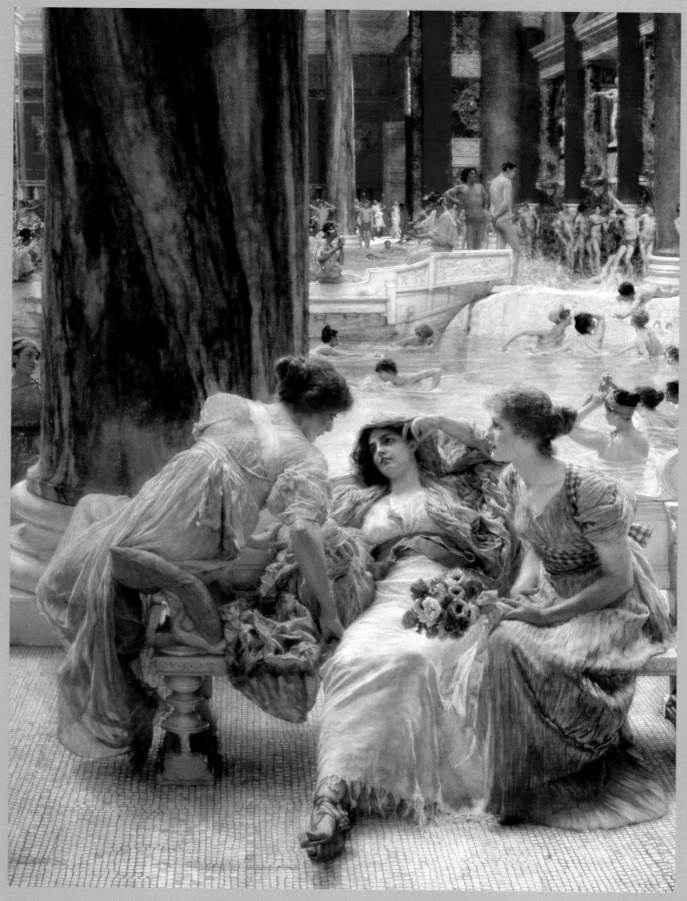

The Caracalla baths had a temple at each end; one was dedicated to Apollo, the other to Aesculapius. Aesthetics was an important aspect of this bath. Outside gardens featured grottoes and nymphs watered by fountains and springs. Shaded porticos displayed masterpieces of sculpture. There were tree-lined promenades for walking. The hypocaust, a room with a cavity beneath the floor where hot air circulated, provided an efficient form of central heating. Mixed bathing eventually became acceptable, and the baths provided social gathering places where friends could meet and talk, business could be conducted, and entertainment could be enjoyed.

Sir Lawrence Alma-Tadema (1836-1912), *Baths of Caracalla*, 1899, oil on canvas, 152.5 × 95 cm. Copyright private collection/The Bridgeman Art Library Nationality/copyright status: English/out of copyright.

THE FAR WEST

THE AMERICAS

The New World, as the Americas were titled by historians, was really an old world in which highly developed cultures had thrived. It may even be that some cultures in the Near East, the Far East, and the Mediterranean had begun and ended before it became known that a rich land lay across the endless sea. It may be that civilization was reached earlier in the Americas than in Egypt. Although the exact date for the habitation of this area is not agreed upon, "it may be assumed with some certainty that highly evolved cultures flourished on the soil of the New World from 2000 to 1000 BC" (Hermann, 1954, p. 188). Some individuals believe it began ten thousand or even twenty to thirty thousand years ago.

It is thought that the earliest inhabitants of the American continents came from Central Asia. Access was gained by crossing the Bering Strait into the territory currently known as Alaska. The people (Indians) followed the pattern of other primitive tribes by migrating toward food, water, and acceptable climates. They tended to move toward the east and south, and traces of their occupancy have been found as far east as the Atlantic coast. Mexico, Central America, and Peru eventually became the primary sites of their settlements. Hunting and agriculture became the way of life. In addition, the creativity of these tribes resulted in the development of various processes, such as basket weaving, the tanning of leather with oak bark, and the manufacture of cleaning powder from wood ashes and of glue from fish. The numerous American Indian nations in North and South America eventually decreased the consequence of tragic events.

Several tribes attained a high degree of civilization: the Mayas, the Incas, the Aztecs, and the Toltecs. Religion, magic, medicine, nursing, and pharmacology were frequently combined in these tribes; these activities were carried out by one individual who was set apart from the rest of the tribe. The medicine men (or shamans and, later, priests) attempted to cure the ills of both mind and body. As in other ancient cultures, it was believed that disease was caused by the displeasure of the gods. The sun god in particular was recognized and worshipped by many of these groups.

Health was simply a matter of balance among the person, nature, and the supernatural. Although the systems of healing might have varied from tribe to tribe, rituals or ceremonies, prayers, chants, herbal therapy, plans for prevention of disease, and the use of protective devices such as charms and fetishes were integral parts of the process. In some tribes human sacrifice was a significant part of the religious ceremonies; in others the transference of disease to animals was a magical ritual. Various other practices emerged that were significant to Indian health care and therapy.

Sweat baths or sweat huts were used to purify the body and maintain health. Various methods were used to achieve this goal. Water might be poured or sprinkled over hot stones, aromatic substances were used, and the body was sometimes beaten with bunches of twigs to stimulate circulation and hasten the sweating process (Dolan, Fitzpatrick, and Hermann, 1983).

Sand painting was another form of therapy. Intricate designs were created by the medicine man for a specific individual and a certain occasion. These designs took form through a process in which the medicine man allowed varieties of colored sand and crushed minerals to trickle from between his thumb and forefinger onto a pattern drawn on the ground. The natural color of the sand provided the background. These paintings were done on the floors of hogans or specially built medicine huts and were believed to promote healing. As in other ancient civilizations, many types of treatments were used. They included massage, tooth extractions, bloodletting, trepanning, bandaging, suturing, and amputation. In addition, herbal therapy was used extensively.

Significant contributions to modern-day medicine and medical practice were made by American Indians. Little mention, however, is given to nursing as a separate entity. Yet the position of Indian women was unusually good. It is said that they held complete authority over the home, took part in women's councils, and declared war once it had been agreed upon. One may assume that their role included the nursing of children, assistance with childbirth, and some type of involvement with the care of the sick and the elderly.

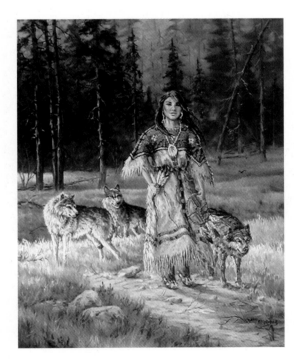

Mary Selfridge, *Medicine Woman of the Wolf Clan*, painting. Private collection of Randy Belmont, Finksburg, MD.

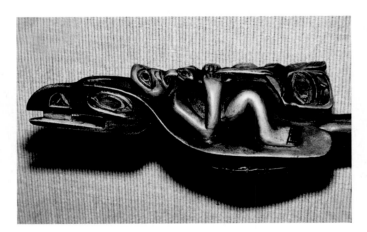

American Indian Shaman's Rattle. Image from Ancient Art and Architecture Collection Ltd.

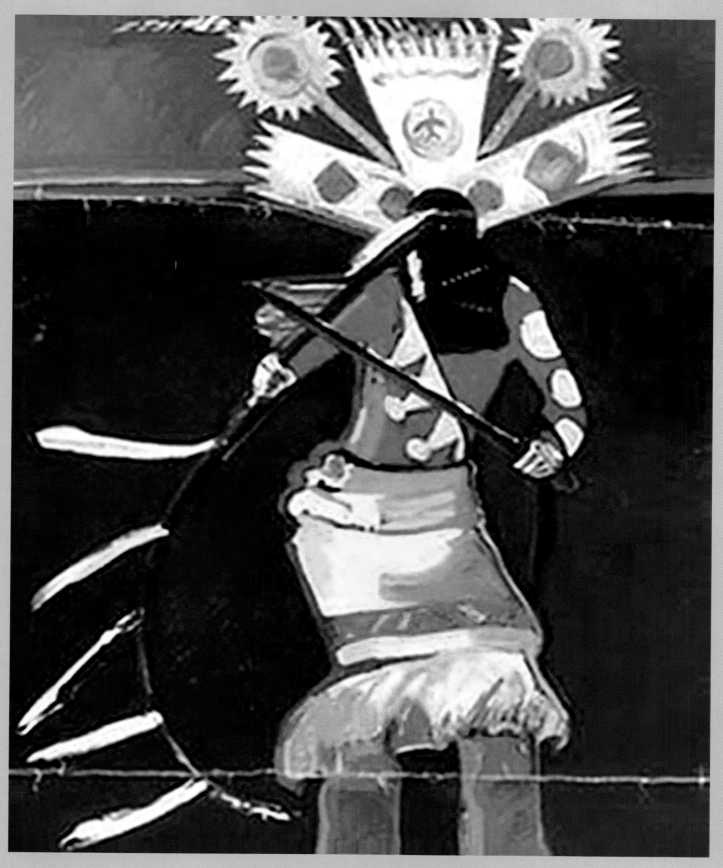

John Nieto, *Apache Mountain Spirit Dancer*, painting, 60" × 48".

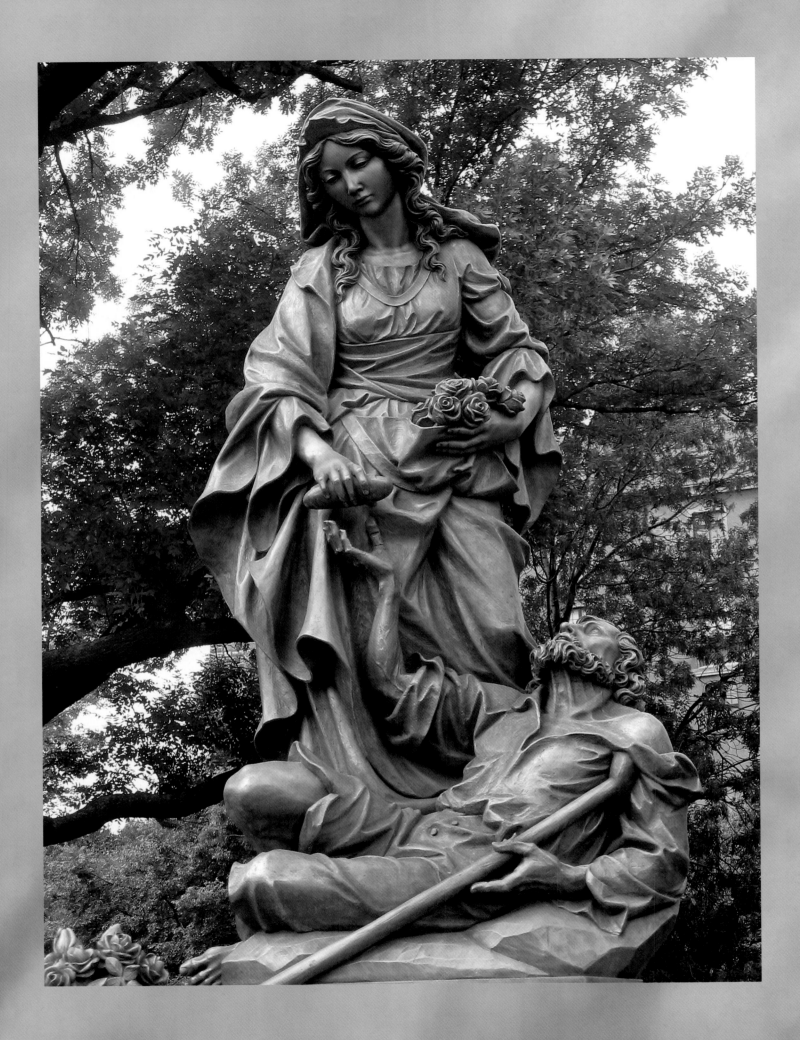

UNIT Two

Nursing in a Christian World

The care of the sick was only one of many forms of charity undertaken by the Church, but it was always given a place of honor because of the emphasis put on it by the founder of the Christian faith. In the first and second centuries, the visiting of the sick was a part of the duty of all Christians but especially the deacons and deaconesses, who took the poor and homeless members of the group into their own homes and cared for them there. No technical preparation was considered necessary for such service. All that was asked was devotion to the faith, brotherly love, and obedience to the Christian law of hospitality and service. Later, much of this charitable work was centered in hospitals or guest houses requiring full-time staffs. Such institutional workers were chosen, as a rule, from among the widows and virgins and other members of the Church most free from domestic ties. With the rapid growth of the monastic movement, after the sixth century, large numbers of voluntary celibates—men and women—joined religious orders, and the care of the sick, helpless, and infirm became in many cases their permanent vocation.

— ISABEL MAITLAND STEWART

St. Elizabeth Durinska, along with many healing saints, is portrayed in 15th- and 16th-century art. However, in contrast to other saints, she is shown performing some of the Seven Works of Mercy—visiting or nursing the sick, giving bread to the hungry, and giving her jewels to the poor. She was born in Bratislava during the time Slovakia was part of the Hungarian Kingdom. There she established an Elizabethan convent in 1738. Since January 1996, the Oncological Hospital of St. Elizabeth located in Bratislava provides a vital service.

St. Elizabeth Durinska (of Hungary), sculpture, Slovak Chamber of Nurses and Midwives, Bratislava, Slovak Republic. April 1, 2008 photo courtesy of JUDr. Martina Sekacova.

	1 AD	125	300	500	700
Nursing	**1-500** Rise of religious and social movements leads to systematic development of nursing **1-500** Patients in large numbers cared for by deaconesses, widows, Roman matrons, and other followers of Christ's precepts **60** Phebe (Phoebe) credited as first visiting nurse and deaconess		**300** Parabolani Brotherhood founded **347-404** St. Paula establishes monasteries and a hospital in Bethlehem **390** Fabiola establishes first free Christian hospital in Rome **410** St. Marcella, considered first nurse educator, dies	**End of 6th century** St. Dymphna organizes plan for mentally ill and retarded in Belgium **500-600** Monks and nuns serve as nurses **500-600** Nursing and charitable works develop in monasteries under famous abbesses **500-1000** Feudal chivalry brings nursing careers to highborn ladies outside of monasteries	**700** Monastic nursing orders flourish
Medicine and Health Care	**1-100** Houses of deacons and deaconesses become hospitals called Diakonoia **100-200** Military medicine in Rome well organized	**130-201** Galen, regarded as most renowned and influential medical writer	**370** Most famous Xenodocheion, the Basilias, founded by St. Basil in Caesarea	**542** Hôtel Dieu of Lyons established **651** Hôtel Dieu of Paris established	**717** Santo Spirito Hospital in Rome established **850-932** Rhazes, one of the greatest Arab physicians **857** Ergotism epidemics in western Europe **900** Founding of medical school at Salerno **936** York Hospital founded by Athelstane **962** Founding of the Hospice of St. Bernard, Switzerland
Science and Technology	**14** Pont du Gard Aqueduct built in France	**132** First seismograph invented by Chang Heng	**400-800** Gold and bronze coins minted in Axum, Ethiopia	**600** Book printing in China **700** Water wheels used for mill drive **750** Pharmacology and medicine become two separate sciences	**850** Salerno University founded **861** New nilometer built to measure height of annual Nile flood **868** Earliest complete woodblock-printed book, *Diamond Sutra,* in China
The Visual Arts	**100-200** Buddha depicted in human form **100-200** Three-dimensional sculptures in China	**150** Pyramid of the Sun constructed in Teotihuacan, Mexico **212-217** Baths of Caracalla built in Rome	**300** Christian symbols seen on sculpture and tableware	**500-600** Coptic art develops **550** Crucifix developed as an ornament **600** Porcelain produced in China **650** Weaving developed in Byzantine Empire	**814** Building of Doge's Palace is begun **900** Ethiopian Christian churches decorated with frescoes **900-1000** Great era of Byzantine Art
Daily Life	**1-33** Life of Christ **1-100** Chariot races popular in Roman festivals **64** Persecution of Christians begins	**161-181** Marcus Aurelius encourages the establishment of charitable funds to support and feed the poor **164** Great plague in the Roman Empire **200** Cotton grown in southwest North America **226-642** Silk weaving industry important in Persia	**325** Council of Nicea held **350** Stirrup invented in China	**500** Beginning of the Dark Ages **500** Incense introduced into Christian church services **500** Church bells used in France **500-1000** Feudalism and monasticism develop **542** Plague reduces Europe's population by half **550** Chess invented in India **570-632** Mohammed, founder of Islam	**700** Easter eggs come into use **750** Beds become popular in France and Germany **800-900** Monasteries become centers of alms giving **870** Calibrated candles used to measure time in England **993** First canonization of saints

1000	1100	1200	1400	1500
1000-1500 Midwives, not physicians, deliver infants **1000-1500** Rich period of nursing saints and mystics **1095** Antonines founded and devoted to sufferers of "St. Anthony's Fire" **1096-1272** Military nursing orders (Knights Hospitallers) carry chief burden of nursing	**c. 1100** The Benguines movement begins **1170-1221** St. Dominic establishes Order of Preachers and other orders involved with nursing **1182-1226** St. Francis of Assisi establishes three religious orders involved with nursing **1194-1253** St. Clare of Assisi, abbess of Poor Clares	**1207-1231** St. Elizabeth of Hungary, patron saint of nursing **1244** Misericordia functions primarily as volunteer ambulance society **1347-1381** St. Catherine of Siena, hospital and visiting nurse **1348** Alexian Brothers form to care for bubonic plague victims	**1400** Great extension of nursing by secular orders occurs	
c. 1098-1179 St. Hildegarde, considered leading medical authority	**1100** Barber-Surgeons form guilds **1101** St. Giles' Hospital built for the care of lepers **1123** St. Bartholomew's Hospital founded in London	**1200** Alcohol used for medical purposes **1213** St. Thomas' Hospital founded in London **1247** Bethlehem Hospital founded in England **1300** Urine examination used in medicine as means of diagnosis **1350** Fallopio discovers "fallopian tubes"	**1400** Rise of municipal hospitals **1451** Ospedale Santa Maria degli Innocenti built as asylum for abandoned children in Italy	**1500** Civil authorities take over all hospitals in Protestant countries **1510-1590** Ambroise Paré, French surgeon **1514-1564** Andreas Vesalius, founder of modern anatomy **1557** Influenza epidemic spreads over all of Europe
1000 Vikings sail to Nova Scotia **1041-1048** Earliest movable type for printing invented in China **1044** Exact formula for gunpowder published **1090** Chinese develop first water-driven mechanical clock	**1100s** Magnetic compass invented in China **1180** Windmill with vertical sails invented in Europe	**1233** Coal mined in Newcastle, England **1337** Attempt made at scientific weather forecasting	**1452** Metal plates used for printing **1480** Leonardo da Vinci develops the parachute **1492** First terrestrial globe constructed	
1000 Artistic revival in Italy with frescoes and mosaics **1000-1100** Illustrated books in Iran **1050** English monks excel in embroidery **1078** Tower of London built	**1100** Appearance of Gothic architecture **1174** Leaning Tower of Pisa built		**1440-1513** Bihizad, most famous artist for illuminated manuscripts **1450** Florence becomes center of Renaissance **1452-1519** Leonardo da Vinci, Italian artist and universal genius **1471-1528** Albrecht Dürer, German artist **1475-1564** Michelangelo Buonarroti, Italian sculptor **1477-1576** Titian, Italian artist **1483-1520** Raphael, Italian painter	
1066 First record of comet later called Halley's **1094** First record of gondolas in Venice **1096** First Crusade occurs	**1151** First fire and plague insurance (in Iceland) **1180** Glass windows appear in England	**1200** Engagement rings become fashionable **1215** Magna Carta signed **1230** Leprosy introduced into Europe by Crusaders **1290** Spectacles come into use **1348** Worst occurrence of Black Death devastates Europe	**1464** Royal mail service begins in France **1492** Columbus lands in America **1495** Syphilis epidemic spreads throughout Europe	**1500** Black lead pencils used **1509** African slave trade begins **1517** Coffee drinking begins in Europe **1532** Sugar cane cultivated in Brazil **1547** Moscow destroyed by fire **1596** Water closets installed in England

The beginning of the Christian era revealed a Roman Empire that extended over most of Europe, part of Britain, and areas of Asia Minor and Northern Africa. In essence, Rome was an eminent power that exerted control over nearly all the peoples of the known world. This empire continued for approximately 5 centuries after it replaced the republic (about 31 BC to AD 476). During this time the Roman Empire became distinguished for its political, legal, and administrative organization as well as for advances in sanitation and hygiene. Its pagan religion was, in general, tolerant and free from ignorant superstitions. The fact remains, however, that it was superior as a conquering military empire. Conquered freemen were permitted freedom of thought and action except in two areas: politics and economics. Slavery, which ultimately undermined the empire, became the basis for the political economy of Rome.

THE DAWN OF CHRISTIANITY

The first 2 centuries of the Roman Empire, known as the *pax Romana,* were marked by relative peace and prosperity. This interval included the period between the accession of Augustus, the 1st emperor, to the death of Marcus Aurelius in AD 180. Order was achieved through power, which served to conceal the basic and emerging weaknesses in the Roman social order. A minority of people became rich and powerful and enjoyed control of the lands. Theirs was a life of luxury, extravagance, and idleness. The masses were either poverty stricken or indentured slaves. A middle class was nonexistent, and the division between rich and poor was evident. The value of life was lessened by slavery. Exhaustion, misery, and corruption added to the gradual erosion of the empire.

After the death of Marcus Aurelius, disorder prevailed within the empire. Economic crises occurred frequently and taxation became oppressive. The government was often overthrown and its power declined. "Religion had come to represent formal duties imposed upon worshippers who had other religions" (Jamieson and Sewall, 1950, pp. 88-89). Rebellions threatened the city of Rome itself. Invasions occurred and took their toll on an already declining society. The 4th and 5th centuries gave way to increased plagues and pestilences, which may well have been the final ingredient necessary for the collapse of Roman power.

It was during this period of social change and confusion that Christianity spread throughout the European world. Christianity was based on the teachings of Jesus Christ, who was born in Judea when Rome was at the height of its power under Augustus Caesar. With the culmination of Christ's public life, his crucifixion, resurrection, and ascension, his teachings were spread throughout the empire by his apostles. The concept of a loving God of all humankind was the basis of the teachings of Jesus as preached in the 1st century of this era, and it became one of the principal tenets of Christianity.

Ultimately, Christianity prevailed over the other religions and philosophies of the empire. It embraced the customs, rituals, ideals, and ideas that were closest to the hearts of the people. Consequently, what began as a simple religion with minimal ceremony, ritual, or doctrine expanded into a complex religion with many sacraments and a complicated, rigid hierarchical structure. Initially forbidden by law, Christianity became the state religion into which people were born. In AD 313, 1 year after his own conversion to the faith, the Emperor Constantine proclaimed freedom for the Church. By AD 400 it was probably as dangerous not to be a Christian as it had been to be one in AD 100. Thus, as the Roman Empire declined, Christianity was bringing Christ into the personal and community life of the people.

THE CHRISTIAN MOTIVE AND NURSING

The emergence of a Christian world began the continuous recording of nursing history. Pre-Christian records of nursing are fragmentary and scattered; however, records of nursing are continuous from the days of the early Christian workers to the present day. Christ's teachings of love and brotherhood transformed not only society at large but also the development of nursing. Organized nursing was a direct response to these teachings and epitomized the concept of pure altruism initiated by the early Christians. The term *altruism* was derived from the Latin *alter,* meaning other; hence, altruism means thought for and interest in others. Altruism at this time was not a new idea but an old idea with a new motive.

Pure altruism was disinterested service to humanity and devotion to others without the hope of any sort of reward (material or spiritual) and was performed solely for the love of God and the desire to be like him. From this development of the concept of altruism evolved the care of the sick and disabled as a corporal act of mercy. The Corporal Works of Mercy encompassed basic human needs as well as scientific and humanistic objectives for caring. In addition, they recognized the needs of a variety of groups within the society and reflected the desire for human compassion:

- To feed the hungry
- To give water to the thirsty
- To clothe the naked
- To visit the imprisoned
- To shelter the homeless
- To care for the sick
- To bury the dead.

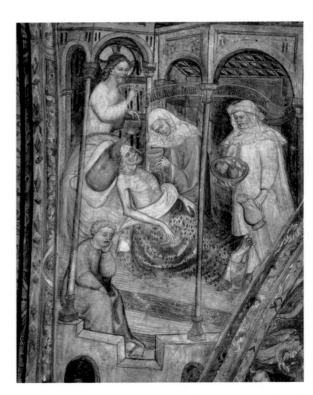

Caring for the Sick, Following Christ's Teaching, 15th-16th century, painting. Image from The Picture Desk Image Library.

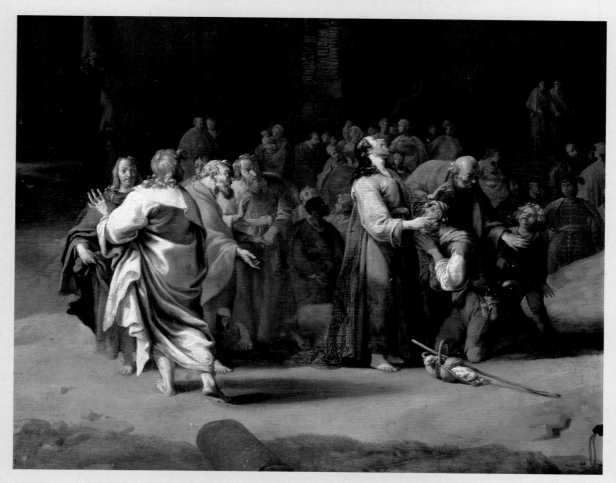

Bartholomeus Breenbergh, *Jesus Healing a Deaf-Mute*, 1600, painting, Musee du Louvre Paris. Image from The Picture Desk Image Library.

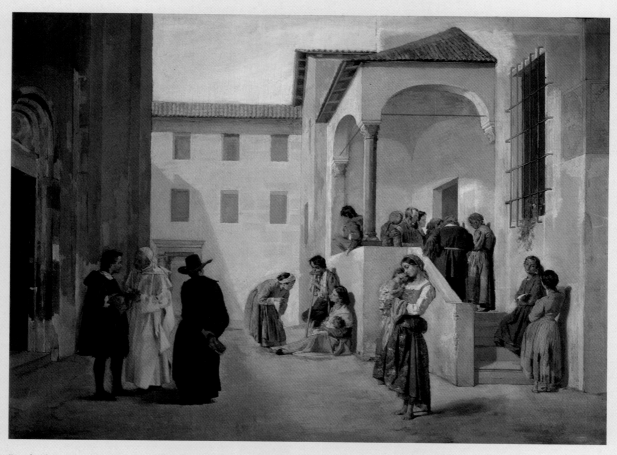

Ezechiele Acerbe, *Distribution of Medicine to the Poor*, 1873, painting, Civiche Racc d'Arte Moderna Pavia. Image from the Picture Desk Image Library.

A spiritual meaning became deeply attached to the care of the sick and the suffering. This flowering of Christian idealism was to have a deep and significant impact on the practice of nursing forever.

The original inspiration of Christians to care for the sick stemmed directly from the teachings of Christ himself. The motive for nursing thus became the marvelous activity of love and mercy embraced by men and women who responded to the teachings of Christ. Many instances are cited of Christ's healing the sick and raising the dead by direct intervention and without the use of any medicine or treatment. Faith healing, therefore, became a part of the Christian belief. In addition, conditions that would promote natural healing were added, and eventually they supplied the impetus for the establishment of centers for nursing care. Caring for the sick became an activity that was considered especially pleasing to God and through which an individual might inherit eternal life. Inherent in such a philosophy was a life of charity in a world of selfishness and hatred: "A new commandment I give you, that you love one another: That as I have loved you, you also love one another. By this will all men know that you are my disciples, if you have love for one another" (John 13:34-35). As explained in the epistles of St. Paul, "There is neither Jew nor Greek; there is neither slave nor freeman; there is neither male nor female. For you are all one in Christ Jesus" (Galatians 3:28).

Charity was love in action. It was taught most significantly in the parable of the Good Samaritan. This parable was a plea for sympathy, generosity, kindliness, brotherly love, and the dignity of all human life. It taught character development and purification of the soul as the aims of the givers of care.

A certain man was going down from Jerusalem to Jericho; and he fell among robbers, who both stripped him and beat him, and departed, leaving him half dead. And by chance a certain priest was going down that way: and when he saw him, he passed by on the other side. And in like manner a Levite also, when he came to the place, and saw him, passed by on the other side. But a certain Samaritan, as he journeyed, came where he was: and when he saw him, he was moved to compassion, and came to him, and bound up his wounds, pouring on them oil and wine, and he set him on his own beast, and brought him to an inn, and took care of him. And on the morrow he took out two shillings, and gave them to the host, and said, "Take care of him; and whatsoever thou spendest more, I, when I come back again, will repay thee."

— *LUKE 10:30-36*

The practical test of the new faith was "not to be ministered unto, but to minister." This golden rule later appeared on the seats of benches in hospitals. The care of the sick was lifted to a higher plane; what had once been an occupation primarily of slaves, or a necessary service of any household, became a sacred vocation. Service to others was an avowed duty of all Christian men and women.

The entry of women into nursing after AD 300 was affected by at least three factors: "First, the improvement in the social position of Roman women; second, the Christian teaching of the equality of men and women before God—and therefore in God's work; and, third, the Christian appeal to carry on His work in behalf of all who were in distress" (Shryock, 1959, p. 77). The position of women was indeed an extremely important factor. Yet discrepancies exist in writings that refer to this matter. Some writers indicate that the status of women was strikingly elevated by Christianity (Dolan, Fitzpatrick, and Hermann, 1983). Others (Dock and Stewart, 1925; Nutting and Dock, 1937) caution that one cannot assume this to be true, stating that the position of women, socially and legally, was not always low under the old religions. All agree, however, that the essential element was that Christianity vastly enlarged women's opportunities for useful social service by opening the door to honorable, active careers, particularly for unmarried women. In addition, Christ's teachings tended to place men and women on an equal plane, which led to the assumption of leadership positions by women engaged in charitable and social endeavors. Finally, the freedom to engage in humanitarian efforts led many men to the field of nursing. Caring activities were shared by men and women and at times included a carryover of the magic, empirical remedies, and home treatments of the earlier periods of history.

From a chronological point of view, there was a vast difference between nursing during the Christian era and nursing during the ages that preceded it. A superior type of care was given by those who understood the best medical and surgical techniques of the times. The rich and the powerful who converted to Christianity and engaged in charitable works were socially, culturally, and intellectually endowed.

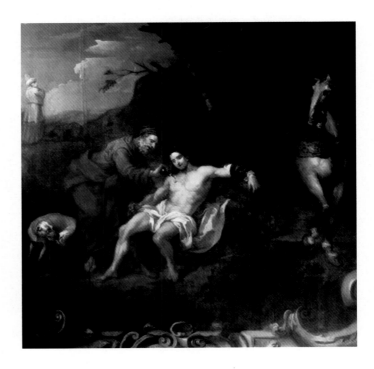

The parable of the Good Samaritan taught that charity was love in action. Service to others, providing care to strangers, was to become a duty of all Christian men and women. The parable is particularly significant to nursing in that nurses literally "care for strangers." With this new faith emerged the golden rule, "Not to be ministered unto, but to minister."

William Hogarth, *The Good Samaritan*, 1737, painting, St. Bartholomew's Hospital, London, UK.

Some were recognized scholars. The educationally prepared included members of the clergy who, for several centuries, had been the only group exposed to any type of formal training. Furthermore, a true integration of services was in evidence because medical and nursing care was seldom separated from other forms of charity for the poor (Sellew and Nuesse, 1946).

Many benefits were derived from the Christian effort. Chief among them was a distinctly humanitarian approach to the care of the sick and the poor and the development of organized nursing services. The positive aspects of nursing's heritage from the Christian teachings are evident and have been specifically identified. Yet this religious thought also handicapped progress in nursing well into the second half of the 20th century. As nursing became closely identified with religion and religious orders, strict discipline became a way of life. In a sense, religion forced nurses to make a strong commitment but a commitment at the expense of money, family, and personal freedom. Those engaged in the nursing work were eventually trained in docility, passivity, humility, and total disregard for self. Unquestioning obedience to the decisions of others higher in rank, usually the priest or physician, was promulgated. An individual nurse's accountability, the personal responsibility for decision making in regard to patient care, was thus bypassed and remained totally alien in nursing for many years to come.

It is not difficult to see the parallels to the training schools for nurses of the late nineteenth and early twentieth centuries. Indeed, one need only read some of the very early writings of our own American nursing educators who advocated a zealous dedication to the work, a selfless denial of personal comfort, and an unquestioning loyalty to the physician (Robb, 1901). Nursing as an occupation was likened to a religious vocation by many and was often referred to as a special "calling," which required selfless service to man and God. The essential characteristic of the "good" nurse was that of obedience, and the rigor with which this quality was developed is common knowledge among those nurses who graduated from nursing schools prior to the last decade. . . . The "good" student was the student who did as she was told, and she soon learned that the classmate who questioned too much often fell into a general category termed "personality unsuitable to nursing," a category that usually led to dismissal from the school. The greatest proponents of the concept of unquestioning obedience were physicians, but faculty members aided and abetted this attitude since they too had been indoctrinated with these ideas.

— *CHRISTY, 1976, P. 3*

THE EARLY CHRISTIAN ERA: AD 1-500

The Christian era is one of the most significant to understanding nursing's historical development. The first 5 centuries of this era witnessed the rise of a religious and social movement that enabled the systematic development of organized nursing. This marvelous activity of love and mercy was embraced by many men and women who responded to the teachings of Christ. More important, the right of the single woman to acquire a position of usefulness and responsibility was established, thereby opening the door to respected careers, particularly in the area of social service. Indeed, the foundations of the nurses' calling and of all modern works of charity were laid down and perpetuated.

From the earliest point in its history, the Christian Church assumed the care of the sick, the poor, and the helpless. This activity was in keeping with Christ's refusal to accept human suffering. Other religions had viewed suffering as deserved, as something to be left alone; Christ specialized in relieving it. Thus spiritual meaning became attached to the care given to humanity and to the suffering endured by it. The care of the sick and distressed became an avowed duty of all Christian men and women.

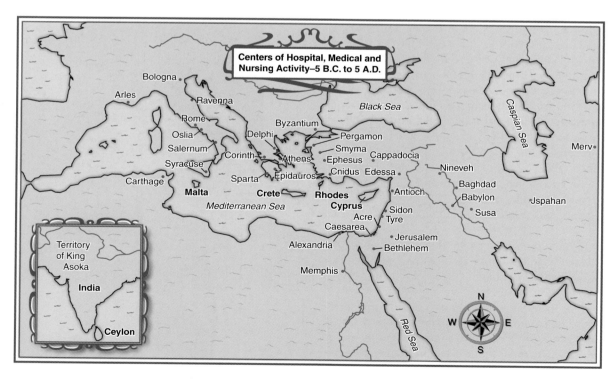

Centers of Hospital, Medical and Nursing Activity—5 BC to 5 AD, map, Mosby.

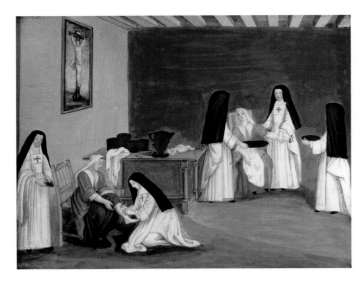

Madeleine De Boulogne, *Nuns Caring for the Sick*, 1700, painting, Musee de l'abbaye de Port-Royal-des-Champs Magny-les-Hameaux. Image from The Picture Desk Image Library.

The women of this early church shared activities with men in all works of the community. Chief among these was the care of the ill and infirm. Information about the various groups of women that developed, however, is confusing and contradictory; at times it is difficult to distinguish between what is actually known and what is surmised (Dock and Stewart, 1925; Frank, 1953; Nutting and Dock, 1937; Sellew and Nuesse, 1946; Seymer, 1932; Shryock, 1959). What is definitely known is that women in these groups concentrated on social work and nursing, which paved the way for the present role of the public health or community health nurse. These nursing groups (orders) flourished and became expressions of philanthropic desires for some and a kind of security for others. They were to be hospitable, pious, and committed to the relief of the afflicted. According to Tuker and Malleson (1900), the earliest orders of women workers were the Deaconesses and Widows. Later, the Virgin, Presbyteress, Canoness, and Nun appeared. Only deaconesses, widows, and nuns were involved with nursing (Nutting and Dock, 1937). It is apparent that the titles of these groups in themselves presented some difficulty because the primitive deaconess could be married, a widow, or a virgin. "The terms 'Widow,' 'Deaconess,' and sometimes also 'Virgin' are used with bewildering inexactitude by all the ancient authors, and pages of learned controversy have been written as to whether the Deaconess was the same as the Widow, or above her, or subordinate to her" (Seymer, 1932, pp. 23-24). What is important here is that organized nursing became a reality within society and a major turning point occurred in nursing's history.

DEACONESSES

It is difficult to trace the origin of the deaconesses because the Greek word *diakonos* could refer either to a special group, Christians who served their "brothers in Christ," or to those who served their masters. The verb *diakonein,* to serve, was used to refer to serving tables and to distributing alms. The nun, according to some writers, was also used by Christ to imply a minister. Consequently, confusion exists about what the term actually meant, but it would appear that the word was used in its generic sense of one who ministers to the needs of another.

Phoebe (Phoebe, c. AD 60), a friend of St. Paul, is the only woman called a deaconess in the New Testament: "I commend unto you our sister Phoebe, a deaconess of the church at Cenchrae, that you may receive her in the Lord as befits the saints, and help her in whatever she may require from you, for she has been a helper of many and of myself as well" (Romans 16:1-2). Phoebe was thus credited with being the first deaconess and the first district or visiting nurse. The latter term referred to the thought that she nursed the poor in their homes, which eventually became a major part of the work of deaconesses. Documents are sometimes contradictory with reference to the status of these individuals. According to the Bible, Phoebe was entrusted with the letters of St. Paul and was considered to be a woman of importance and dignity. Mention is made of her education, wealth, and position and of the fact that her travels to Rome were associated with her work.

Very early, the Church, in accordance with Christ's teachings, created officers to carry out acts of service for the members of the Church community. Bishops and other officers were empowered by the allocation of church funds for charitable purposes. Ministration to the sick was a vital component of the personal service that was emphasized. Men and women who became involved rapidly developed into ecclesiastical orders in a very definite hierarchy. The deaconesses were made popular during this time by the type of woman who joined—the rich, the able, and the well born, who commonly were the sisters of bishops or the wives or daughters of emperors. Nursing as such was not their chief occupation; nursing was a way to assist in the salvation of their souls.

The deaconesses were usually ordained to service, worked on an equal basis with the deacons, and were required to be unmarried or widows. They were usually mature women who could make judgments based on life experiences. The primary function of deaconesses was to attend the female catechumens at their baptism by immersion and

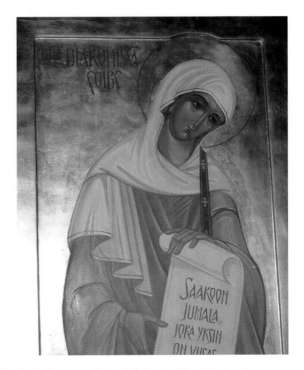

St. Phoebe the Deaconess, Finland. Orthodox Church in America, www.oca.org.

to anoint them with oil. Their visiting and charitable duties appear to have been a secondary function in which they carried the Church into the home by visiting the poor and caring for the sick. Deaconesses provided food, money, clothing, medicines, and physical and spiritual care to those in need.

Ecclesiastical histories have provided knowledge of the nursing carried out by these early workers of the church. Letters have included the names of many deaconesses. St. John Chrysostom gave the names of five: Olympias, Sabiniana, Pentadia, Amprucla, and Procla. Olympias (or St. Olympias, as she is frequently called), the most famous, was a daughter of a count of the Roman Empire who inherited a fortune from her parents. She became the wife of the prefect of Constantinople, a widow at the age of eighteen, and an ordained deaconess at twenty. Eventually, Olympias became the head of a community of deaconesses who resided in a convent, strengthening their religious lives as well as tending the needs of the community.

The deaconess orders held a position of importance for many years. However, as adult baptisms became uncommon and deaconesses were no longer needed to assist women catechumens, gradually this group faded and had all but disappeared by the 11th century. The growing importance of the monastic movement may have also contributed to this occurrence. Yet these orders never entirely died out. Periods of revival occurred throughout history in connection with religious movements, particularly in the 19th century, when the order became active in the Lutheran and other Protestant churches.

WIDOWS AND VIRGINS

The characteristics and duties of the widows and virgins, who were early Church officers and perhaps more important than the deaconess, were frequently identified. At certain periods they wore distinctive dress, lived either in their own homes or in monasteries, and took the vow of chastity. They were closely related to deaconesses in duties, and they shared in the work of relief and in nursing. In addition, they were not always clearly distinguished from deaconesses because those appointed to the diaconate were often chosen from the groups of widows and virgins.

The widows were the second classification of women recognized as having special functions among the poor in the early Church. They were not necessarily women whose husbands had died; the title of *widow* was also used as a designation of respect for age. If the woman had been a widow, however, she had to vow never to marry again. Qualifications were explicitly defined by St. Paul in his first epistle to Timothy (5:6): the woman must be pious, devoted in hospitality to strangers and saints, and anxious to relieve the afflicted; the age requirement was 60 years. Younger widows, in the opinion of St. Paul, were too anxious to marry and were inclined to be idle, to indulge in gossip, and to talk too much! Considerable numbers of women joined, despite the restrictions, and engaged in work with the sick and the poor, eventually taking an important part in the development of hospitals. In the 3rd century, the widows' work was greatly curtailed as the result of jealous disapproval on the part of men (Nutting and Dock, 1937; Stewart and Austin, 1962). The vow of chastity, which originally had been spoken in private, became a public function and led to the absorption of the widows into the community life of the *monastriae,* or nuns.

There are discrepancies in the literature regarding the duties and responsibilities of the virgins. In some instances they are credited with responsibility for religious exercises and church duties rather than with charitable work. In others they are ascribed with the visiting or nursing of the sick or the pursuit of missionary labors. It is clear that the virgins were highly respected and ranked with the clergy. This rank, originally shared by both men and women, was comparable to that of the consecrated nun, the lineal descendant of the virgin. The virgin was ". . . distinguished by a white veil, but in Rome the earliest distinguishing mark of her dress was a gold fillet, the symbol of virginity. At a much later date a ring and bracelet were added" (Tuker and Malleson, 1900, vol. 3, p. 34). In this way virginity began to be interpreted as essential to purity of life. The virgins were also eventually absorbed into community life as nuns (*non nuptae,* not married).

ROMAN MATRONS

Deaconesses were rarely mentioned in the Western or Roman Church. Yet illustrious women of Rome devoted themselves to the care of the sick and other charitable works. The noble Roman matrons were active during the 4th and 5th centuries after converting to Christianity. Roman women of the upper classes had, by that time, attained considerable social and legal freedom. They had proven themselves to be successful managers of their wealthy husbands' estates and had participated in public affairs. The names and histories of these matrons, some fifteen in number, have been preserved in the writings of St. Jerome. Their independent positions and great wealth were used to establish community life and to initiate the groundwork for charity and nursing work. The ascetic lives of these women were held in high regard. Three of these matrons, Marcella, Fabiola, and Paula, were particularly significant to continued progress in nursing.

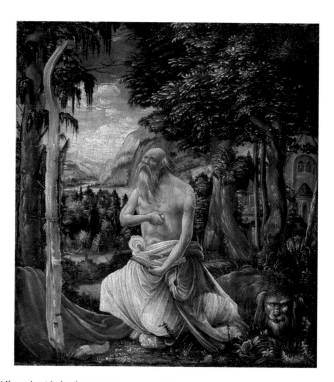

Albrecht Altdorfer, *The Penitence of St. Jerome,* 1507, painting, 23.5 × 20.5 cm, Staatliche Museen zu Berlin. Bildarchiv Preussischer Kulturbesitz/Art Resource, NY.

The most famous woman, who was considered leader of the Roman matrons, was Marcella. She converted her palace, located in a most exclusive part of Rome on the Aventine, into a monastery (the prototype of the later convent), which led to her being called Mother of Nuns and Founder of Convents in the West. She encouraged other intelligent and spiritually inclined Roman matrons to join her. One of the chief interests of this religious community of women was the care of the sick poor. Marcella was considered to be extremely intelligent and possessed of great virtue and purity. She devoted herself to the study of the Scriptures, and the clergy often consulted with her about scriptural passages. Marcella instructed her followers in the care of the sick, while also devoting her time to charitable works, prayer, and study. She was attacked during the raid on Rome by the Visigoths under Alaric in 410 and died soon after. She is referred to as St. Marcella by some authors (Dolan, Fitzpatrick, and Hermann, 1983; Sellew and Nuesse, 1946); others identify her simply as Marcella (Jamieson and Sewall, 1950; Nutting and Dock, 1937).

One of the most charming, and perhaps the most worldly, of the Roman matrons was Fabiola. A member of the patrician Fabian family, she married, divorced, and remarried, again unhappily. After the death of her second husband and her conversion to Christianity, Fabiola acknowledged her "evil ways" and joined the ranks of penitents. She renounced her earthly pleasures and bestowed her immense fortune on the sick and the poor. The first free Christian hospital in Rome was founded by Fabiola in her own palace in 390. It was described by St. Jerome as a *nosocomium,* a place for the sick, as distinguished from objects of charity who were simply poor. Fabiola sought out the poor and the sick in the streets of Rome and cared for them herself. It is said that she was particularly skilled in the dressing of wounds and sores that were ugly and repugnant. She has been viewed almost as the patron saint of early nursing, and her idealized portrait is well known. Fabiola not only nursed but also shared

in the poverty of her patients. Some reports also indicate that she helped to establish a great hospice for pilgrims and strangers at Ostia, a seaport of Rome. Some writers have made the supposition that this hospice was a home for convalescent patients (Haeser, 1857). The entire life and works of Fabiola were related in a famous eulogy by St. Jerome upon her death in 399:

> There she gathered together all the sick from the highways and streets, and herself nursed the unhappy, emaciated victims of hunger and disease. Can I describe here the varied scourges which afflict human beings?—the mutilated, blinded countenances, the partially destroyed limbs, the livid hands, swollen bodies, and wasted extremities? . . . How often have I seen her carrying in her arms these piteous, dirty, and revolting victims of a frightful malady! How often have I seen her wash wounds whose fetid odour prevented every one else from even looking at them! She fed the sick with her own hands, and revived the dying with small and frequent portions of nourishment. I know that many wealthy persons cannot overcome the repugnance caused by such works of charity; . . . I do not judge them, . . . but, if I had a hundred tongues and a clarion voice I could not enumerate the number of patients for whom Fabiola provided solace and care. The poor who were well envied those who were sick.
>
> — ST. JEROME, LETTER TO OCEANUS (LXXVII)

Paula traced her descent to some of the oldest, noblest families, and her husband, Toxotius, was of the Julian family, who claimed descent from Aeneas. Her family was immensely wealthy and owned, among other things, the entire town of Actin. Paula was the wife of a pagan and the mother of five children, four daughters and one son. Her worldly life ended with the death of her husband, when she began to devote herself to strict asceticism. Paula and her daughter Eustochium adopted Christianity, shared in charitable work, and studied with Marcella. Paula was particularly respected for her intellectual ability, which enabled her to develop a relationship with the recognized scholars of the day. This example of colleagueship between the sexes was described by Lord as an important advent of Christianity: "If to her [Paula] we do not date the first great change in the social relations of man with woman, yet she is the most memorable example that I can find of that exalted sentiment which Christianity called out in the [relationship] of the sexes, and which has done more for the elevation of society than any other sentiment except that of religion itself" (Lord, 1885, p. 63).

Paula was one of the most learned women of this period of history. She studied Hebrew and Greek and assisted St. Jerome with his Latin translations of the Scriptures, known as the Vulgate. In 385, Paula and Eustochium sailed for Palestine. Eventually they settled in Bethlehem, where they attracted a following of devout women and founded a monastery. In addition, Paula built hospices for pilgrims and hospitals for the sick along the road to Bethlehem. The design and construction of the buildings were the plainest, which demonstrated the philosophy that it was better to spend money on the poor than on fine buildings. For approximately twenty years, Paula managed the institutions and personally nursed the weary travelers and the sick. St. Jerome's account of her life emphasized her caring and compassion: "She was marvellous, debonair, and pietous to

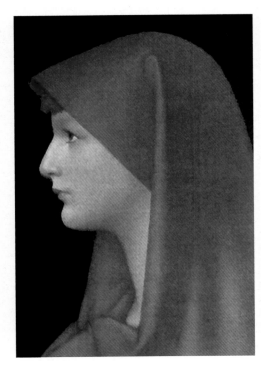

JJ Henner, *Fabiola,* 19th century, oil on velvet, author's collection.

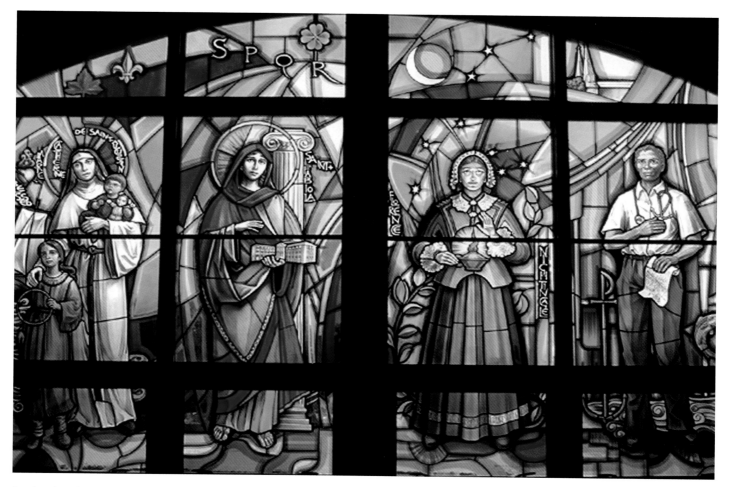

Panel 1: Blessed Marie-Catherine of St. Augustine, a French nursing sister of St. Augustine who dedicated her life to the sick in Quebec.
Panel 2: Saint Fabiola, a Roman matron of nobility who devoted herself to the needs of the church and the care of the poor and suffering.
Panel 3: Florence Nightingale, the creator of modern nursing, a pioneer in nursing education, a reformer of hospital sanitation methods, and a leader in the development of applied statistics.
Panel 4: Villanova University student.

Vetrate Artistiche Toscane, Driscoll Hall Stained Glass Window, 2008, window, 13' 3" × 9' 3", Villanova University, Villanova. PA.

them that were sick, and comforted them, and served them right humbly; and give them largely to eat such as they asked; but to herself she was hard in her sickness and scarce. . . . She was often by them that were sick, and she laid the pillows aright and in point; and she rubbed their feet, and boiled water to wash them; and it seemed to her that the less she did to the sick in service, so much the less service did she to God." It is thought that Paula was the first to train nurses in a systematic way, to teach nursing as a distinct art rather than as a generalized service to the poor. The following description of nurses at work is thought to explain the origin of the tradition of hard manual labor as an expression of good nursing: "They trim lamps, light fires, sweep floors, clean vegetables, put heads of cabbage in the pot to boil, lay table cloths and set tables, hand cups, help to wash dishes, and run to and fro to wait on others" (St. Jerome, letter to Pammachius).

In the late 4th century in Rome, the place in good works was taken by this notable group of women, all friends of St. Jerome. All were Christian converts and lived not too many years after Constantine gave freedom to the Church. They were a striking contrast to the decadent, selfish, and apathetic Roman society. Probably no group of women has surpassed them in intellectual powers and commanding characters. Many individuals benefited from their services, including St. Sebastian. Sebastian was company commander in the Praetorian Guards during the reign of Emperor Diocletian (AD 284-305). His public declaration of his faith in Christianity and his affiliation with the Christian Church resulted in his being fastened to a stake and shot by arrows. Later that night, St. Irene, the widow of his martyred friend St. Castulus, found him still alive. She and her associates provided the nursing care that has been documented and portrayed through the years by many artists. Consequently, St. Sebastian became a popular subject of medieval art. The idea that contagious or infectious diseases were shot into the body by invisible arrows fostered the practice of praying to St. Sebastian for prevention or cure.

MEN IN NURSING

Men have always occupied an important position in the care of the sick. They have been nurses and care givers in all cultures and throughout the history of humankind, a fact well documented by history and traditions. What is of particular interest is that nursing was considered as much a male profession as a female one prior to the late 19th century. A glimpse into the past reveals that "in the early Christian period, and for centuries thereafter, men of the priestly class, or belonging to military or religious orders, have been responsible for at least one half of the nursing service through mediaeval times up to a very recent period" (Nutting & Dock, 1907, p. 101). Military and other male nursing orders

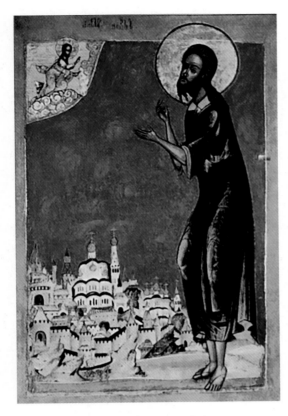

St. Alexius, 17th century, painting.

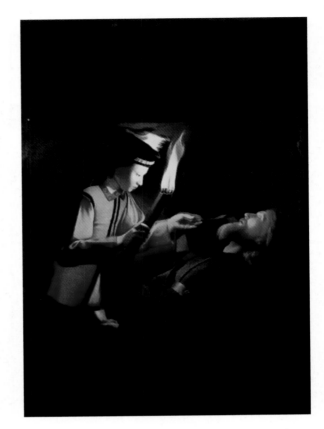

Etienne de La Tour, *The Discovery of the Body of St. Alexis*, 1640s, oil on canvas, 143.5 × 117 cm, The National Gallery of Ireland. Copyright The National Gallery of Ireland.

have left their mark on nursing and at times carried the chief burden of nursing. Along with the Knights Hospitallers, the Benedictines, the Order of the Santo Spirito, the Antonines, the brotherhood of Misericordia, the Alexian Brothers, numerous other orders of men distinguished themselves as caring and competent nurses. Individual men also contributed markedly to the progress of nursing during various periods in history, as is demonstrated by St. Francis of Assisi and St. Dominic, who founded orders to take nursing out among the people (Donahue, 2004). Additional information related to male nursing orders and individuals is discussed in the section on the Late Middle Ages.

An early organization of men in eastern Rome was the Parabolani brotherhood. The name referred literally to those who risked their lives by coming into contact with the sick. The duties of these members of a minor religious order included searching for the needy sick and taking them into hospitals. The members also acted as bodyguards of the bishop and became a burying detail as well. They were forbidden in public places and theaters, perhaps as a way of reducing contagion. It is believed that this group originated during the 3rd century, when the black plague depleted the population of the entire Mediterranean area. When this dreaded disease was at its peak in Alexandria, the Parabolani reportedly organized a hospital and traveled throughout the city nursing the sick. These several hundred men and their nursing work were vividly described in *Hypatia,* a novel written by Charles Kingsley (n.d.).

PHYSICIANS AND MEDICINE

In the early centuries of Christianity, approximately 16 Christian physicians reached the level of distinction. The majority

of them came from Syria, and the group included Aetius of Amida, Paul of Aegineta, and Alexander of Tralles (Frank, 1953). Two of the most prominent ones, St. Cosmas and St. Damian, were twin brothers who were born in Arabia and educated in Syria. They were the youngest of five brothers from a Christian family of some distinction. They became known as the moneyless ones because they did not charge for professional services as they traveled to provide services for those in need. It was their hope that this practice would gain converts to Christianity. Although they specialized in both medicine and pharmacology in Asia Minor, St. Cosmas and St. Damian were chosen as the patrons of the medical profession. They suffered martyrdom in 278 during the reign of Diocletian and soon achieved a following as the result of numerous miraculous cures during their lives and after their deaths. Their legendary undertakings included the idea of limb transplantation.

Facing page, In the foreground, Saints Cosmas and Damian prepare to transplant the leg of an Islamic Moor onto a recent amputee. These twin traveling physicians, who offered their services without charge to those in need, became known as the "moneyless ones." During the reign of Diocletian and the Christian persecution, they were tortured and beheaded. They received sainthood and were chosen as the patron saints of the medical profession. In the background of this painting appear a cripple, a patient in a sickbed, a physician examining a urine flask, and another surgeon treating a wounded man.

Ambrosius Francken, *Sts. Cosmos & Damian—Transplantation of Leg,* late 16th century, painting, 237 × 89 cm, Koninklijk Museum.

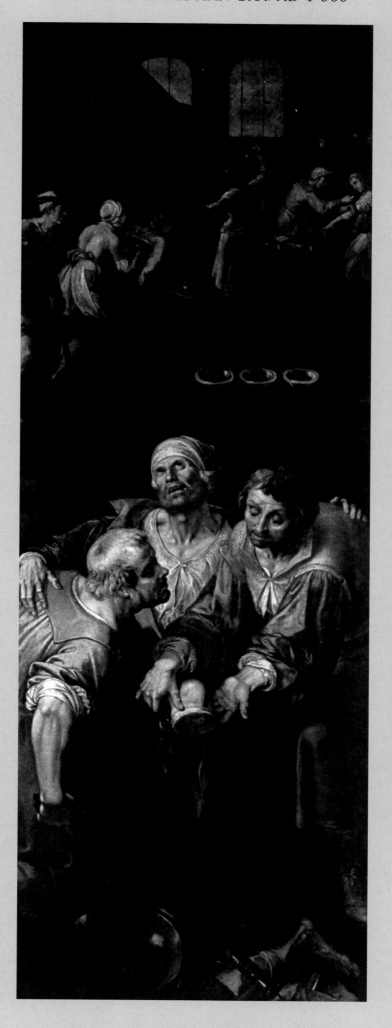

Perhaps the best known of the physicians of this era was St. Luke, the Evangelist. St. Paul called him "the beloved physician." It has been suggested by several writers that Luke had some type of medical preparation, that he may have studied at the famous school at Tarsus. His writings demonstrate an interest in medical subjects. He traveled extensively and at one point may have been a ship's physician. His several talents included literary and artistic ability.

St. Pantaleon, like Luke, Cosmas, and Damian, practiced free medicine among the sick poor. This, as well as the fact that he was a Christian, created hostility among his pagan friends. Eventually, he was put to death and regarded as a healing saint. Later, Pantaleon was associated with the image of the comic in Venetian commedia dell'arte, and his name provided the term *pantaloon* for men's trousers (Petrucelli, 1978).

Aetius (502-575), who studied in Alexandria, wrote of treatments for varicose veins, hypertrophied tonsils, hydrophobia, goiter, and aneurysm of the brachial artery (ligation is described). His extensive collection of surgical writings, the *Tetrabiblion,* was first published in 1534 and included some accounts of conditions considered to be the most exact of the time period. Paul (625-690) discussed dietary regimens, pathology, pharmacology, surgery, and medicine; his writings include discussions of cancer, particularly of the uterus and breast. Little is actually known about him, although he, too, studied in Alexandria and was greatly admired for his surgical skills. His *Seven Books,* published in 1528, was a complete, concise synopsis of the medical and surgical literature of the day.

Alexander (525-605) wrote of internal medicine and pathology. His excellent powers of observation led to accurate deductions about diseases, such as ascites, the origin of epilepsy in the brain, and the detection of an enlarged spleen by palpation. Alexander made a study of diseases of the nervous system and described melancholia as a state of being that could terminate in mania, which he classed as an advanced state of dementia. He traveled extensively and achieved great fame as a skilled physician and an independent scientist. His comprehensive writings on medicine, the *Practica,* also contained magical cures that involved the use of amulets and incantations.

During the period of the Roman Empire and the early centuries of Christianity, medicine experienced a gradual loss of the scientific knowledge that had been attained by the Greeks. This decline was consistent with the deterioration of Roman civilization after the 2nd century. Another contributing factor was the invasion of barbarians into the empire after 400, which helped to bring about the disintegration of Roman culture. Medicine and all of the sciences were affected; medical knowledge practically disappeared. Of all the Roman institutions, the Church alone survived intact. In addition, the idea that work with the hands was degrading then began to be applied to medicine.

HOSPITALS

The development and construction of early Christian hospitals was not left entirely to the charity of individual women. As the Church became freely established, the bishops also assumed responsibility for the expansion of charitable facilities as well as the responsibility for the care of the sick. Consequently, one reads of houses for the sick, for strangers, for the poor, and for the aged that existed in the 4th century. The original rooms in homes for hospitality and the care of the sick were called *diakonia.* The title was indicative of the close association of the nursing care of the sick poor in private homes with the activities of the diaconate. The term *diakonos* later became synonymous with the term *hospital* or *nursing director.*

An expectation of Christianity was that all who needed help would be received. As the congregations grew, it became necessary to expand the social services of the Church. As a result, the original diakonia became too small, and new rooms, wings, and buildings were added. "Usually it seemed more economical to gather all classes of unfortunates into one institution known as a *xenodocheion,* which was the ancestor of the modern hospital as well as of most other types of charitable institutions" (Shryock, 1959, p. 79). Inns for strangers (hospitality centers); hospitals for the sick, the insane, and lepers; homes for the aged; almshouses; asylums for foundlings, orphans, the maimed, and the deformed; dwellings for nurses and physicians; and offices were included in these institutions. As early as the First Council of Nicaea (325), it was decided that each bishop should establish a xenodocheion. These institutions were administered by deaconesses and visited by widows of the Church. They were financed by Church alms and direct gifts from wealthy Christians. Eventually names for the various special divisions that were found in these charitable institutions arose: *xenodochia,* inns for strangers or travelers; *nonsocomia,* wards or rooms for the sick; *brephotrophia,* foundling asylums; *orphanotrophia,* orphan asylums; *gerontokomia,* homes for the aged; *cherotrophia,* homes for widows; and *ptochotrophia,* almshouses for the poor. According to Nutting and Dock (1937, p. 119), the evolution of the earliest forms of Christian care of the sick proceeded with the "diakonia, or rooms in private houses; xenodochia, amplifications of the diakonia; and finally, hospitals; while the forms of the earliest nursing organizations, beginning in the congregation, passed through the diaconate, the widows' sisterhoods, the parabolani, to monks and nuns."

Controversy exists regarding the exact date of the earliest xenodocheion. It is said, for instance, that one was built in Constantinople in the reign of Constantine but also that those built during the time of Julian the Apostate were the earliest. What is certain is that the most famous of them is the one founded by St. Basil the Great in Caesarea (370), often referred to as the Basilias. St. Basil's institution was almost a second city and was as self-sufficient and self-supporting as it was possible to be. All individuals who were able to work were given employment in blacksmith shops, in the foundry, in the laundry or the dairy, in shoe and clothing shops, or in the kitchen. Out of gratitude the public officials of the city of Caesarea remitted taxes on the property. This gesture became an important aspect in the development of the precedent of allowing properties used for religious or charitable purposes to be exempt from taxation.

The Basilias was an outstanding example of Christian charity that embraced total hospital care—prevention, treatment, and social services. In the hospital were resident physicians, resident nurses, and carriers of the sick (Walsh, 1929). There was an orphanage; a place of hospitality for strangers; an asylum for infants and children; a building for the aged, lepers, and those with contagious diseases; a trade school for the physically impaired; and a hospital that cared

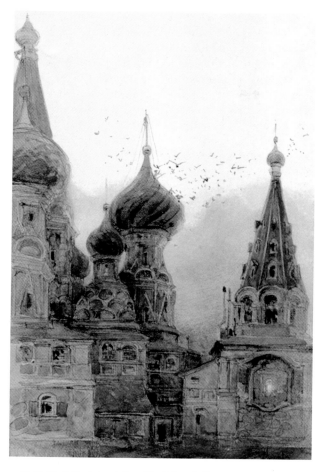

St. Basil's Cathedral, painting, The Palma Collection. Getty Images.

THE EARLY MIDDLE AGES (DARK AGES): AD 500-1000

The term *Middle Ages* is used by historians to denote the time between the middle of the 5th century (the fall of Rome occurred in 476) and the middle of the 15th century (the fall of Constantinople occurred in 1453). The thousand-year period that followed the collapse of the Roman Empire is also referred to as the medieval period of history, the division between ancient and modern times. Although this is a useful term because it is fairly well understood, it must be remembered that no period in history has hard-and-fast boundaries. In addition, this period can be subdivided into the early and later Middle Ages. The early centuries are collectively known as the Dark Ages, a title that clearly demonstrates the prevalent social destruction of the times, the deteriorating world.

During the Dark Ages the domination of society by the Church was practically unchallenged. As the Roman Empire was slowly disintegrating, the Church had been developing into a well-integrated and highly organized institution. Its organization followed a pattern similar to that of the Roman government. Each ecclesiastical province paralleled a civil province. Dioceses were formed under bishops, and they corresponded to a Roman governmental unit. Over all was the bishop of Rome, the Pope, who corresponded to the emperor. Finally, when the emperor removed himself to Constantinople in 330, the Pope was left the most powerful figure in the West. The bishops emerged as the natural leaders of the people, and the empire was perpetuated through the Church. All of these events contributed to the evolution of the image of the nurse as a saint. The activities of nursing itself became honored because many royal, noble, and distinguished people engaged in it and regarded it as the work of God. Nursing became a penitential activity that was used as a means of purgation and purification. It was a work calling for unceasing toil without expectation of earthly reward.

Three large classes of people dominated society in the early Middle Ages. The majority were serfs, who were farmers living under primitive conditions. Above them were the aristocratic and warlike lords. Finally, there was the clergy, both secular and monastic, who were bound by celibacy so they could give undivided devotion to the religious life. Women had again fallen into a subordinate position, but positions in religious orders were open to them as well as to men. It was possible to acquire dignity as a nun. "There were even joint monasteries of men and women, living in separate houses but ruled over by a woman superior. Certain of the orders, both for men and for women, came to devote themselves to nursing; and it was this trend that brought women into such service for the first time on a large scale. By the modern period, indeed, nursing began to be viewed as primarily a woman's field" (Shryock, 1959, p. 89).

The early Middle Ages revealed a crumbling world. Chaos reigned supreme because of the impact of the onslaughts of barbarian tribes and extreme moral decay. The middle class disappeared because of exorbitant taxes, widespread epidemics, natural disasters, and wars. Money and cities disappeared along with trade, commerce, and industry. The population declined, crime waves occurred, poverty was abysmal, and torture and imprisonment became prominent as civilization seemed to slip back into semibarbarianism. In

for the sick, the crippled, and the poor. In addition, Basil's hospital had a special department for the insane.

The early Christians combined the sacred custom of hospitality with loving service. This resulted in an effective system for the care of the sick and the destitute. Little, however, is known of the specific nursing services that were provided in these hospitals. (Correspondingly, knowledge of medical services is also limited. This perhaps explains why a revival in faith healing occurred.) It is reasonable to assume that deaconesses may have served as nurses. It is also possible that servants did the ordinary labor under the direction of Church authorities. Certainly, no indication is given of any type of formal training for the women or men who did participate in the nursing work. Eventually, nursing orders were formed in the Church to serve in the hospitals. The practice of clustering buildings was adopted by monasteries and continued until the 12th century, when it became customary to separate hospitals from other branches of relief service and build them separately. This intimate connection between the Church and the care of the sick during this period in history is an important factor in understanding of the organization and functions of the hospital. "At the outset it will be well to make clear what the hospital was, and what it was not. It was an ecclesiastical, not a medical, institution. It was for care rather than cure; for the relief of the body, when possible, but pre-eminently for the refreshment of the soul. . . . Faith and love were more predominant features in hospital life than were skill and science" (Seymer, 1932, p. 36).

essence, the Greco-Roman culture stumbled to a halt. Medieval life became increasingly dangerous and necessitated the formation of protective groups by the populace. The people had lost their sense of security and gathered together in search of safety. This phenomenon was characterized by three great movements that arose during this early period of the Middle Ages: feudalism, monasticism, and Islamism. These movements developed simultaneously and were thought to be possible solutions to the chaos of the times.

FEUDALISM

Feudalism was a new system of land tenure that had complex social arrangements in which self-sustaining groups prepared themselves to resist attacks by bands of fighting men sworn to uphold the might of their leaders. It involved cooperative farming units that were isolated from each other and governed by individuals known as knights, counts, earls, barons, or lords. Feudalism was a type of patriarchal rule that provided men with homes for their families, food, and bodily protection. In return for these services, the tenants worked the land as farmers and became soldiers in the case of war. These serfs could not be sold as slaves. Political, economic, and social life were based on the holding of land. The typical edifice was the rural manor or estate owned by the lord. It was usually set high in an inaccessible location, and massive turreted walls enclosed the manor, which was also encircled by a moat.

Feudalism did, however, have drawbacks that eventually led to many abuses within the society. This was particularly true for most women who were forced to marry young, often without their consent. Their chief value to society was their breeding power and the ability to manage a home. The lord's wife, the lady of the manor, was faced with a difficult life. She was responsible for the supervision of the entire establishment, for bearing and caring for children, for riding and hunting, for whatever needed to be done. She was frequently called upon to nurse family guests or villagers. The lady was in charge of the care of the sick of the manor and was a combination of doctor and nurse. She applied first aid, faced surgical emergencies, and had an extensive knowledge of home remedies for all types of illnesses. Empirical medicine was almost entirely in the hands of such women. The number of doctors was small, and only a few of them were located in the manors.

> The lady was thus obliged not only to be housewife in her own capacity, but also amateur soldier and man of the house in her husband's absence and amateur physician when no skilled doctor could be had. She was supposed to be manager of the household and know how to choose, to air and mend and keep moths out of clothes and furs, to know the best recipes for catching flies and other "familiar beasts to man," and for keeping bedrooms free of mosquitoes and barns of rats. There is even an injunction to his [the lord's wife] "If one of your servants fall ill, do you yourself lay aside all other cares, very lovingly and charitably care for him or her."
>
> — WALSH, 1929, P. 35

MONASTICISM

The idea of finding the ineffable love of God by renouncing the world found a practical outlet in monasticism. The dangers of medieval life led many men and women who were spiritually minded to the monasteries to escape worldly chaos. Others probably entered the monasteries to obtain security and protection. From the efforts of St. Basil in the 4th century, the monastic movement spread to the West and assumed prominence in the social structure of the early Middle Ages. Through the 5th century the movement spread slowly because the majority of monasteries were weak, poor, and disorganized. By the 6th century, however, monasticism provided great practical and spiritual value to concerned individuals and to society at large.

The basic concept of monasticism was withdrawal from society for the sanctification of one's soul. Asceticism was also a marked feature of this religious life, particularly in the earlier periods. All degrees of self-mortification, self-denial, and strict discipline were observed. The monks and nuns were governed by rules—the constitutions, bylaws, and directives by which they were to live. Four rules were recognized by the Church for the government of monastic orders: those of Basil, Augustine, Benedict, and Francis. Monasteries were not established to care for orphans, to educate children, or even to nurse the sick. These were secondary works that arose serendipitously and were done well by the monks and nuns who performed them; they were not an essential part of their calling.

The credit for the organization of many of these institutions is given to St. Benedict of Nursia (480-543), who founded the order of Benedictines in the 6th century. St. Benedict became a hermit who practiced the most excessive and excruciating asceticism, which led to his ultimate fame. His followers were formed into twelve communities of 12 monks. St. Benedict established the most influential monastery in western Christendom at Monte Cassino. This monastery became a Nazi stronghold during World War II and was bombed by the Allied forces.

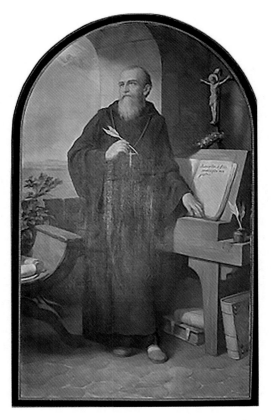

Hermann Nigg, *St. Benedict of Nursia Writing the Benedictine Rule,* 1926, painting, church of Heiligenkreuz Abbey near Baden bei Wien, Lower Austria.

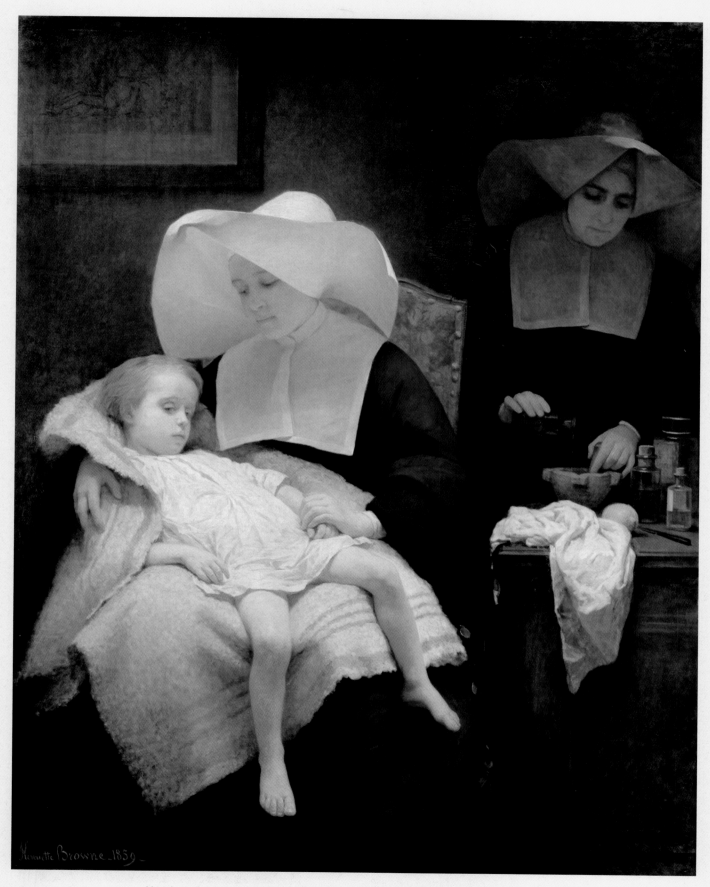

Henriette Browne (1829-1901), *The Sisters of Mercy*, 1859, painting, 39.94 × 30.99 cm, Bridgeman.

In about the year 529, St. Benedict composed his rule, the Benedictine Rule, which had a strong influence on Western civilization:

> Before all things and above all things care must be taken of the sick so that they may be served in the very deed as Christ Himself; for He has said: "I was sick and ye visited me" and "As long as ye did it to one of these my least brethren, ye did it to me." But let the sick themselves consider that they are served for the honor of God, and not grieve their brethren who serve them by their importunity. Yet must they be patiently borne with, because from such as these is gained more abundant reward. Therefore the Abbot shall take the greatest care that they suffer no neglect.
>
> — ST. BENEDICT

The success of the Benedictine Rule lay in its moderation, an adaptation of monastic tradition to Western conditions. It helped to bring stability and organization out of chaos, to bring calm out of panic. The rule provided for reasonable and moderate conditions, which included adequate sleep, rest, diet, and clothing and a balance of study, prayer, and manual labor, both indoors and out. Members, after a year's probation, vowed never to return to the world, to render complete and unquestioning obedience to their leader, and to deny themselves totally through humility and service. It was, therefore, possible for persons of ordinary spiritual gifts to follow the rule. Communities were able to retain monks, to be physically, spiritually, and socially healthy and, most important, to be effective.

The Benedictine monasteries became centers of influence, learning, and culture. The monks revived agriculture through labor in the fields, orchards, and vineyards. They improved the plow and invented the windmill, the waterwheel, and the horse collar. They not only labored for souls but tilled the soil and made barren lands bountiful. The excess food produced was used to feed the poor. The monks increased the available knowledge in many ways. They were scholars, librarians, and teachers and opened schools so that all, not only their own members, could read and write. They laboriously copied, clarified, and illustrated precious manuscripts, thereby being the official chroniclers of the history of their times. They used their knowledge of medicine and herbs to care for the sick. The monasteries offered hospitality and shelter to the homeless and refuge to the persecuted.

Nursing the sick eventually became a chief function and duty of the community's life. This command was stated in the rule "Before all things and above all things care must be taken of the sick." Every monastery provided an *infirmarium* for its members and a *hospitalarius* just inside or outside the gates for the needy of the community. These were at first hospices rather than hospitals. They were refuges for the poor and were devoted more to shelter and comfort than to cure. More affluent monasteries later sought to divide the sick from the poor and to offer more than food and shelter to those who needed help. As time elapsed, it was not only the sick poor who requested assistance. Monks were called from their monasteries to the courts of kings and nobles and to the homes of the wealthy. From the original refuges, city hospitals grew and became the responsibility of a monastic order. In most instances, the nursing in these institutions was done by a monastic sisterhood.

Information about the nursing personnel in these earliest monastic hospitals is scanty. It is possible that deaconesses were still active as nurses. In some cases religious societies were instituted to meet the needs of specific situations. It was also the custom for the monks and nuns of related orders to serve the hospitals. Monastic orders for women had developed concurrently with those for men and followed the same pattern. Monks did nursing in the men's wards and nuns in the women's wards, an arrangement that became common toward the middle of the 13th century. In some cases the nuns were in charge of an entire hospital and the monks of the same order acted as priests. It is doubtful, however, that all the nursing work was done by the nuns and priests because they had many lay attendants and perhaps volunteers.

Little is known about the actual care given the sick during the Dark Ages. Secular medicine had become almost completely extinguished, and there was little impetus toward advancement in the science and art of nursing or of medicine. In fact, little distinction was made between medicine and nursing. The monks and the nuns practiced medicine as well as nursing and for long periods seemed to have been the only practitioners. Medical historians report that the medical practice was almost entirely confined to the members of these monastic orders. Considerable folk and drug lore, mysticism, religious faith and, at times, superstition crept into the care of the sick. Bloodletting, diet, and baths were common treatments of the day, along with the application of cups and leeches and the use of blisters, cautery, scarification, and enemas. "The main advancement in nursing during this period probably came through the internal organization and operation of monastic institutions and the discipline and training of large groups of sisters and brothers in their cooperative undertakings" (Stewart and Austin, 1962, p. 50). The nursing in those times was done partly by monks and nuns and partly by servants. It is difficult, however, to determine the division of

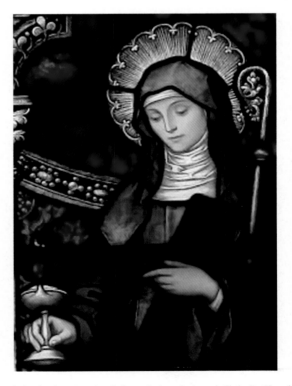

St. Brigid of Ireland, 1903, stained glass window, St. Joseph Catholic Church, Macon, GA.

labor between the two and whether either received much formal training or training of any kind.

Monastic Nurses

Monastic houses for women grew in number in the 6th and 7th centuries. Many of the women who entered these houses were wealthy and had great influence in the community. The two primary reasons given for women's entry into these orders were the prevailing need for protection and the opportunity to follow the occupational career of one's choice. The women in these monasteries were sheltered by a rule, granted by the Church, that afforded the freedom and safety to pursue intellectual studies or practical interests. Many famous women of the early Middle Ages were connected to the monastic life. They included Hrotswitha, who knew the Latin classics and wrote dramas; Lisba, Walburga, and Berthgythe, who went from Ireland and England to evangelize Germany; and Hildegarde, whose medical knowledge and political insight were remarkable. Other women carried on hospital nursing and medical work.

Large twin communities, or double monasteries, of men and women were also a feature of early monastic life. They were under the direct control of an abbess, who held a position of great importance. The two related houses, one of monks, the other of nuns, were usually kept rigidly apart. The opposite system, the rule of women's orders by an abbot, met with failure; the groups did not flourish or survive (Tuker and Malleson, 1900). A sense of joint ownership united the members of these religious settlements and resulted in the emergence of centers of culture and of art. Famous abbesses who ruled the twin communities were Radegunde at Poitiers; Hilda at Whitby in England, who had some of the great bishops as her scholars and taught Caedmon, the first English poet; and Hersende at Frontevrault, who ruled a vast establishment of 3000 members. Each abbess administered the property of the monastery and maintained discipline. The monks and the nuns swore obedience to her.

The most famous double establishment was founded and ruled by St. Radegunde (519-587) at Poitiers in 559. Radegunde, the daughter of a Thuringian king and a descendant of Theodoric, experienced numerous tragedies in her young life. Her father was murdered by her uncle; she was captured and forced to marry Clotaire, the Frankish king of Neustria, becoming one of his six wives; and she fled to Noyan after her husband murdered her brother. Eventually Radegunde made her way to Poitiers, where she took refuge in the Christian Church. She founded the Holy Cross Monastery, a religious settlement of about 200 nuns.

Scripture reading, the study of ancient literature, the transcription of manuscripts, and the performance of dramas (the mystery plays of the Middle Ages) were important activities in this community. The care of the sick, however, was the chief function. Radegunde nursed the patients herself in the hospital she established. She was particularly sensitive to the lepers, who were social outcasts, and was seen giving a kiss to their diseased bodies. There is no indication that physicians were connected with this hospital. Nursing care seems to have been the key to the restoration of health. Baths were built at the instigation of Radegunde. This was particularly significant because Christian monasticism had destroyed the cult of the Roman bath. Stimulation of the skin was condemned as provocative of sexual desire in this age of asceticism. In a sense, Radegunde carried on the forgotten tradition of the baths of Caracalla (Robinson, 1946).

The monastic ideal of humility led to the use of plain, coarse materials for clothing. This ideal was perpetuated by the poverty of many of the earliest convents. Yet abbesses and nuns of royal birth wore beautiful clothing, as depicted in the following description: "A vest of fine linen of a violet colour is worn, above it a scarlet tunic with a hood, sleeves striped with silk and trimmed with red fur; the locks on the forehead and temples are curled with a crisping iron, the dark head-veil is given up for white and coloured headdresses which, with bows of ribbon sewn on, reach down to the ground; the nails, like those of a falcon or sparrow-hawk, are pared to resemble talons" (Putnam, 1921, p. 85).

Criticism of this costume as incongruous with monasticism paved the way for a clothing reform that ended in uniformity. A distinctive dress for religious women became a custom. The veil as part of convent dress symbolized humility, obedience, and service. Regulations were developed that governed the use of the veils. They came to be a part of the prescribed habit and were always white during the probationary period of the novice. Various forms of the veil were worn by women to distinguish social position. The cap of the modern nurse was a modification of the religious veil and has been associated with humility and the rendering of service to humankind.

St. Brigid (452-523) introduced female monasteries into Ireland as early as the 5th century. She was the daughter of an Ulster prince and a disciple of St. Patrick. Brigid became a famous abbess in Ireland at Kildare and was respected as a scholar, educator, and counselor and an expert in the healing arts. References are made to the miracles of Brigid, who was also known for her healing of lepers and her care of the sick. She was labeled "the patroness of healing." The monastery at Kildare became a center for culture, the arts, learning, and spirituality.

St. Scholastica, the twin sister of St. Benedict, founded a Benedictine community for women. This order was established near Monte Cassino, and Scholastica became its abbess.

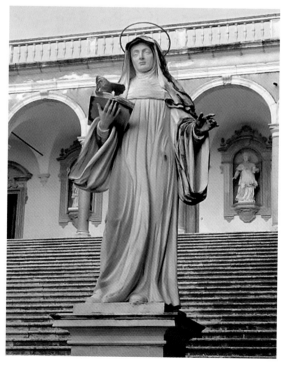

Santa Scolastica Montecassino, 2006, sculpture.

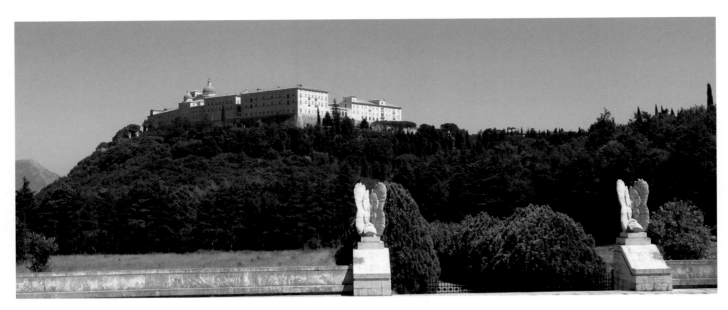

Monte Cassino Abbey and the Polish Way Cemetery in Italy.

ISLAMISM

During the early centuries of the Christian era and into the early Middle Ages, Arab kingdoms extended from Spain through northern Africa and into western Asia. The Arab influence was felt as far away as India and China. The conquests of the Arab people exposed them to a variety of native cultures, and they developed a certain tolerance for different beliefs and ways of living. They learned from the achievements of the Egyptians and the Greeks. They built universities where experimental research and scientific studies in astronomy, mathematics, and chemistry were conducted.

Muhammad (570-632) was born at Mecca, the religious and commercial center of Arabia. His tribe was one of the most influential and guarded the sacred Kaaba, the idolatrous shrine to which heathen Arabs made an annual religious pilgrimage. He was considered to be the first and only prophet of a new world religion: "There is no God but Allah, and Muhammad is his prophet." At Muhammad's command, primitive gods and native animism were abandoned. Submission was the core of the religion and the basic ideal that led to the name of Islam (surrender to the will of Allah). The followers of the monotheistic religion were called Muslims. The teachings of Muhammad were written down and incorporated in the Koran. Both the civil and the religious lives of Muslims were directed by the tenets of this new religion. Muhammadanism has been called "a religion of the sword" because the followers of Islam were inspired by the creed to spread their conquests throughout the Mediterranean and to threaten the gates of Europe.

Medicine was an interest of the Arabs, and they strongly encouraged its study. They translated many Hellenic works into Arabic, particularly those related to medicine, including the works of Hippocrates and Galen. The Arabs studied hygiene and developed an extensive *materia medica*. Their belief in the uncleanliness of the dead forbade dissection, so knowledge of anatomy and physiology was hampered. Surgery, however, was practiced, and the Muslims are credited with the use of catgut for sutures. Physicians were held in high esteem and were required to pass qualifying examinations.

The Arabs built large, well-constructed hospitals and introduced new methods of caring for the sick. The hospital at Cairo had chief physicians who held clinics for medical students. Some of the unusual features of this hospital included classified wards, male and female nurses, streams of running water in some of the wards, and fever wards cooled by fountains.

> The great Al-Mansur hospital of Cairo was a huge triangular structure with fountains playing in the four courtyards, separate wards for important diseases, wards for women and convalescents, lecture rooms, an extensive library, outpatient clinics, diet kitchens, an orphan asylum and a chapel. It employed male and female nurses, had an income of about $100,000, and disbursed a suitable sum to each convalescent on his departure, so that he might not have to go to work at once. The patients were nourished upon a rich and attractive diet, and the sleepless were provided with soft music or, as in the Arabian Nights, with accomplished tellers of tales.
> — GARRISON, 1913, pp. 92-93

Alexandria and Damascus also had well-equipped hospitals under the control of expert physicians. The one at Damascus gave free treatment and drugs for more than 3 centuries. The hospital at Baghdad employed 60 salaried physicians on its staff, probably the earliest instance of a paid staff. A system of care of the patient incorporated spiritual and mental aspects as well as attention to the body. Yet the care of a woman during childbirth and in the case of gynecological disease remained in the hands of untaught midwives.

Among the many outstanding physicians, three in particular are remembered: Razes, Avicenna, and Maimonides. Rhazes (Razi-abu-Bakr Muhammad ibn-Zakariya al-Razi, 850-932) was one of the greatest of the Arab physicians. He was especially known for his writings on measles and smallpox and contributed material to an encyclopedia of medicine. Rhazes was respected for his clinical descriptions of illness, his observations, and his pragmatic approach to treatment.

Avicenna (abu-Ali al-Husayn ibn-adallah ibn-Sina, 980-1037) was considered to be both a philosopher and a scientist. He received his medical education in Baghdad and eventually was made the physician-in-chief of its largest hospital. Although he may have practiced medicine, his principal contribution in the field was his writings. The *Canon of Medicine,* in use for centuries after his death, was considered one of the most important textbooks in the field of medical education. Until the middle of the 17th century, medical curricula of the Christian universities were based on his writings.

Maimonides (Rabbi Moses ben Maimon, 1135-1204) was the most famous Jewish physician in Arab medicine. He was born in Muslim-controlled Cordova, Spain, but fled with other Jews to Fez in, Morocco, when nonbelievers began to be harassed. Later he went to Palestine and then to Cairo, where he entered medicine for financial reasons. He finally became court physician to the sultan Saladin. Maimonides aimed at practical therapeutics and gave advice on such things as hygiene, poisons, diet, and first aid. However, he was basically a philosopher who attempted to reconcile scientific reasoning and religious faith. He is remembered specifically for codifying the Talmud. Although credited by some with composing the Morning Prayer of the Physician, Maimonides probably was not the author (Lyons, 1978). This section of the prayer is often quoted:

> O God, let my mind be ever clear and enlightened. By the bedside of the patient let no alien thought deflect it. Let everything that experience and scholarship have taught it be present in it and hinder it not in its tranquil work. For great and noble are those scientific judgments that serve the purpose of preserving the health and lives of Thy creatures. Keep far from me the delusion that I can accomplish all things. Give me the strength, the will, and the opportunity to amplify my knowledge more and more. Today I can disclose things in my knowledge which yesterday I would not yet have dreamt of, for the Art is great, but the human mind presses on untiringly.
>
> In the patient let me ever see only the man. Thou, All-Bountiful One, hast chosen me to watch over the life and death of Thy creatures. I prepare myself now for my calling. Stand Thou by me in this great task, so that it may prosper. For without Thine aid man prospers not even in the smallest things.
>
> — *Morning Prayer of the Physician*

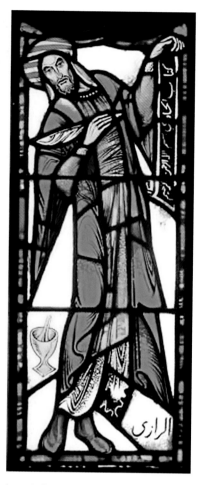

Al-Razi, stained glass window, Princeton Chapel, Princeton University, Princeton, NJ.

School of Salerno

The earliest universities were established at Salerno, Bologna, Paris, and Oxford. The circumstances of the founding of each remain obscure. Their growth, however, was gradual. Salerno, near Naples in Italy, began as a medical center and served a vital role in the transition from monastic to lay medicine. The date of its founding and its origins are unclear. Some speculate that the Benedictines had a monastery and a hospital there in about 820. Legend states that the school was started by four physicians: one Jew, Elinus; one Greek, Pontius; one Latin, Magister Salernus; and one Arab, Adala. Until the 12th century it prevailed as the leading medical institution in Western Europe under secular authority.

Salerno became an important center of medical learning and assisted in the revival of medicine in Europe. It was open to female students, and women physicians were on the faculty. Trotula and Abella were the two most famous women of this school. Trotula was supposedly the author of an obstetrical and gynecological treatise titled *Trotulae Curandarum Aegritudinum Muliebrum (Trotula on the Cure of Diseases of Women).* She was also the head of the department of diseases of women. Throughout the early Middle Ages, however, midwifery was the province of women, and other medical concerns were generally forbidden to them. Women physicians usually specialized in diseases of women and children, even though they were licensed for general practice.

The standard requirements of the school of Salerno included three years of premedicine at the college level in the study of logic, philosophy, and literature; five years of medicine and surgery; and one year's practice with a reputable physician. A law was enacted in about 1140 to prohibit anyone from practicing medicine without a license. *Regimen Sanitatis Salernitanum* or *Flos Medicinae* was the most famous work of the Salernitan school. This Latin poem, consisting of rational dietetic and hygienic precepts, underwent many versions, more than three hundred editions, and numerous translations. It appeared in the form of verse so that it could be easily memorized:

> If thou to health and vigor wouldst attain,
> Shun weighty cares—all anger deem profane,
> From heavy suppers and much wine abstain,
> Nor trivial count it, after pompous fare,
> To rise from the table and to take the air.
> Shun idle, noonday slumber, nor delay,
> The urgent calls of nature obey.
>
> — *Portion of a verse*

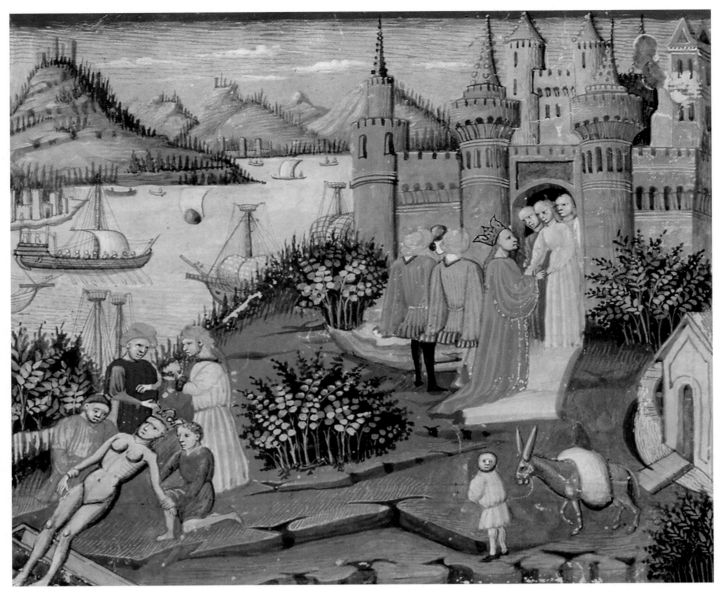

Salerno won the title of the "Town of Hippocrates." People from all over the world flocked to the "Schola Salerni," both the sick (in the hope of recovering) and the students (to learn the art of medicine). In the school, besides the teaching of medicine (women were also involved), there were courses in philosophy, theology, and law.

Avicenna, *School of Salerno,* from the book *Canon Maior Sec. XIV-XV,* 1025, Biblioteca Universitaria di Bologna, Bologna, Italy.

MEDIEVAL HOSPITALS

Three famous medieval hospitals, the Hotel Dieu of Lyons, the Hotel Dieu of Paris, and the Santo Spirito Hospital of Rome, were built outside monastic walls and are still in existence. The most complete records dealing with the nursing arrangements are available for the Hotels Dieu of Lyons and of Paris. The name Hotel Dieu, meaning God's house, was generally used to indicate the principal hospital in a French town or city (Nutting and Dock, 1937). The original hospitals were established as xenodochia, or almshouses, and attended to the needy and infirm as well as to the sick.

The Hotel Dieu of Lyons was founded in 542 at the request of Sacerdos, the archbishop of Lyons. It was originated on the almshouse plan and was managed by lay groups. Including other charitable works besides nursing, it was designed to shelter pilgrims, orphans, the poor, the infirm, and the sick. Its earliest nurses were laywomen who were recruited from penitents (fallen women) and widows. Eventually, men who were originally called servants and later,

brothers, assisted with the nursing work. This particular hospital provided a striking contrast to other institutions of the time in that it was free of clerical control.

The Hotel Dieu of Paris dates from 650 or 651. It was founded by Bishop Landry (Landericus), whose statue stands in its courtyard. This house of God was built with an open door to all who suffered. Also patterned after the almshouse, it was governed by a lay administration. The Hotel Dieu began as a small hospital and grew to immense proportions. The original group of laywomen who cared for the sick were organized into a religious body by Pope Innocent IV. They became known as the Augustinian Sisters because they adopted the Rule of St. Augustine. Brothers, too, belonged to this strict order. The sisters were responsible to the clergy and for all practical purposes were about the same as cloistered nuns. They are considered to be the oldest purely nursing order of sisters in existence. The importance of the Hotel Dieu of Paris is noted in the following description.

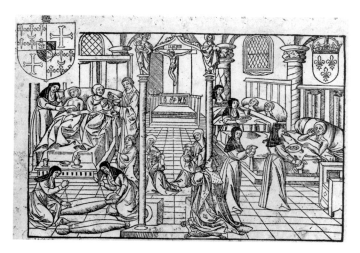

Paul Lacroix, *A Ward in the Hotel-Dieu, Paris*, 19th century engraving, Biblio-teque des Arts Decoratifs, Paris, France.

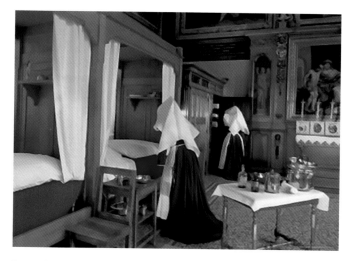

Gene Chandler, *Hotel Dieu, Beaune,* 2008, photograph, Hotel Dieu, Beaune, France.

No other ancient hospital has bequeathed to posterity a nursing history so extensive or one that has thrown so much light on internal hospital management. For the publication of these interesting records we have mainly to thank the un-remitting and bitter contest which for centuries was carried on by the clerical and civil powers over the administration of the important and extensive institution. In this, as in ev-ery similar contest, the nursing service was the chief storm centre, and to gain control of the nursing staff the main point of vantage sought. The story of this struggle points anew to the elemental importance of the nursing factor in the composition of hospitals, and many useful lessons may be taken therefrom.

— *NUTTING AND DOCK, 1937, P. 294.*

Both the brothers and the sisters were assigned specific activities that fell into the categories of exterior work, hospi-tal administration, care of the sick, and religious services. Some nursing was done by the brothers in the general wards, but in the women's wards only sisters performed the nursing care. The Augustinians went through three stages of training. Their nursing role included the admission and dis-charge of patients, responsibility for the kitchens and the laundry (all the washing was done on the banks of the nearby Seine), and the burying of the dead. In addition, re-ligious rites were an essential part of the hospital routine, with services conducted for both patients and staff.

The Santo Spirito Hospital in Rome, established in 717 by order of the Pope, was probably the largest of the medieval hospitals. It was built for the primary purpose of care for the sick. By 1500 it possessed a main hall that contained nearly 1000 beds. Several distinct wards were included for men, women, and convalescents. As the revival of a lay medical profession in the later medieval period brought physicians into the hospitals, Santo Spirito encouraged this connec-tion. It is said that more than 100 physicians and surgeons were eventually in attendance at this hospital. The institu-tion became a well-known prototype for the development of other medieval hospitals.

THE LATE MIDDLE AGES: AD 1000-1500

The roots of a movement toward the creation of religious orders of men and women with the primary motivation of nursing the sick began to occur in the late Middle Ages. It was accompanied by a marked tendency toward the secular-ization and commercialization of nursing. Numerous inter-acting forces were activated in this period. As a result of these forces, society would never be the same again. By this time many barbarian tribes had settled in various areas of Europe, had staked claims to lands, and in many cases had been Christianized and civilized. It was a period of history that was characterized by mobility of the population and, eventually, by the detachment of individuals from protective units. It was a time in which surprising progress was made, not only in the arts and writing (greatly aided by the inven-tion of printing) but also in architecture and the healing arts. In some ways it was marked by a spirit of optimism and en-thusiasm that would be shattered nearly 5 centuries later by war, plagues, famine, and instability.

Trade promoted the development of inland cities and a middle class of merchants, bankers, shop owners, and shop-keepers; craftsmen arose and became as wealthy and pow-erful as the land barons. New inventions in crafts and trades occurred in relation to these changes. Learning was revived, and university education became a privilege of the middle class. This middle class grew as social forces freed the serfs from their manor duties and set them adrift in the cities to seek paid employment. The protection that the castle or monastery walls had previously offered was replaced by the building of town walls. The gates in the walls were secured at sundown; the bridge was raised in the cities surrounded by moats. In many instances the walled cities were over-populated. There were limited, if any, facilities for sanitation and for the provision of pure water and food. Slums became hotbeds of disease, crime, violence, and death.

A new spirit challenged the domination of the Catholic Church, which remained the chief influence on the people. This spirit was characterized by an emerging interest in the things of this earth and the life of the present rather than the focus on life after death, with its emphasis on the soul. The Church had grown rich and powerful, and this caused criticism of the priesthood and monastic orders as well as of the Church itself. Wealth, laxity, and greed failed to exem-plify the teachings of Christ. Unrest occurred as the middle class grew more independent, knowledgeable, and sophisti-cated. Various reform movements, which included new pat-terns of religious thought and action, tended to divert the unrest, at least for a time. Eventually, a new interpretation of the doctrine of the Church was demanded. Individuals such as Peter Abelard (1079-1142) broke from the rigid Augustinian doctrine of predestination. In the Augustinian doctrine, the life of the body was held to be of little importance except as an opportunity for the soul to find unity with God. This unity could be achieved by suppressing physical desires and appetites, having faith in Christ, and obeying the commands of Christ. Life in this world was a journey between life and death. Each person would struggle with the forces of good and evil and would be rewarded in the next world on the basis of his or her success. Reason and logical analysis as the means to truth began to be advocated as an alternative. The writings of St. Thomas Aquinas (1225-1274) became a part of this new ideology and the basis of Catholic doctrine for many centuries thereafter. Aquinas, also known as "the angelic doctor," expressed his interpretation of the whole doctrine of Catholicism in *Summa Theologica*.

A resurgence in religious fervor demonstrated itself in reforms of the monasteries and priesthood, crusades against the heretics of the Near East, and an increase in the number of pilgrimages to the Holy Land. Nursing was affected by these events because crowded living conditions and the resulting increase in the spread of disease created the need for the establishment of new and different types of orders to care for the sick. The redistribution of the population and urban growth brought nursing out of the institutions and back into the home. The individuals who were drawn to nursing continued to be of high intellectual and social backgrounds. Great numbers of men became nurses, and the military ideal of discipline and order entered nursing. This era was rich in nursing saints, several of whom were widely acclaimed and highly honored. There is no doubt that momentous forces such as the Crusades and societal developments related to the care of the sick influenced health practices generally and nursing in particular during this period.

GUILDS

The earliest guilds, initially mentioned in the 8th century, were specifically religious and social in orientation. This was an attempt to balance the spiritual and temporal needs of the members. The guilds were commonly named for a saint whose patronage the members sought. Activities included the building of chapels, the founding of schools, and the presentation of mystery plays. Eventually, hospitals were maintained and social insurance (distress assistance for sickness, poverty, and death) was provided through dues paid by the members. Other types of guilds also developed. They included peace guilds for the maintenance of justice in the town and merchant guilds for the purpose of carrying on trade. Frequently, the law of the guild became the law of the town, as exemplified in London in the 10th century.

The first associations of workers arose in the form of guilds and were extremely important in the late Middle Ages. They were usually known as craft guilds, which divided workers into three levels of vocational training: the apprentice, who remained under the direction of a master craftsman for three to ten years; the journeyman or craftsman, who hired his services to another; and the master craftsman, who was required to make an original contribution to the craft, pass an examination, and be economically stable in order to achieve this status. The craft guilds were the vocational training schools of the era. Under the apprenticeship method, learners worked with experts, were motivated to become masters, and recognized the value of their crafts. These guilds were also the labor organizations of the day and as such protected and improved the status of the members. Wage scales and prices were fixed, hygienic working conditions were demanded, reasonable hours of labor were established, and high quality of the work of the craftsmen was demanded.

Men in the same crafts and professions thus banded together to promote high standards. Ultimately, physicians' guilds were established, and they fostered the separation of surgeons from medical practitioners. This was necessary because of the inclination to draw individuals together according to the similarity of their tools and materials rather than the consideration of their purposes. For example, surgeons' guilds admitted barbers who were able to perform such services as routine bleeding; physicians were joined with apothecaries and artists because of their common use of powders.

In general, the guild system provided an element of stability in the larger social order. It was a viable method of regulating economic life and providing for the discharge of personal responsibility to the community as a whole. It was a system whereby the consumer and the worker could be protected, and a quality product could be ensured. In addition, the medieval apprenticeship system survived and affected the development of some types of workers throughout various periods in history. The apprenticeship form of nursing prevalent in the United States until the 1940s was probably influenced by the pattern of the craft guilds. This type of system did not foster a bona fide educational process; rather, it encouraged a strong aspect of service, which impeded the progression of nursing for many decades.

THE CRUSADES

The Crusades have been identified as "the supreme folly of the Middle Ages" in one source (Nutting and Dock, 1937). This statement, however, is in direct opposition to the idea that throughout history people have regarded certain places, events, and objects as sacred and have journeyed long distances to revere them. From the 4th century, people had made pilgrimages to shrines and to the Holy Land. By the 11th century, both the numbers and the sizes of these pilgrimages had greatly increased, until some were made up of thousands of individuals. There are records of 6 pilgrimages in the 8th century, 12 in the 9th century, 16 in the 10th century, and 117 in the 11th century.

Pilgrimages to Palestine started soon after the Crucifixion. Initially, these journeys were made by the inhabitants of the Holy Land itself but they eventually included inhabitants of distant lands. By the late 11th century, however, a series of military and political changes had taken place in the Middle East, and the Seljuk Turks, who had embraced Islam, captured Jerusalem. Mosques were erected in the Holy City of Jerusalem, and Christians who had been making pilgrimages there were persecuted. Therefore, a united effort to stop the actions of the Turks was launched in the form of military expeditions known as Crusades. Hundreds of thousands of men answered the call of Pope Urban II to initiate this movement. Each Crusader was identified as a soldier of Christ by a red cross on his head or breast. The first expedition of these crossbearers began in 1096.

Numerous Crusades occurred between 1096 and 1291. (The dates vary somewhat according to the reference used.) They are generally divided into four major expeditions and four minor ones. The major expeditions included the First Crusade (1096-1099), led by knights of France and the Normans; the Second Crusade (1147-1149), under the direction of the kings of France and Germany; the Third Crusade (1189-1192), led by the kings of France, England, and Germany; and the Fourth Crusade (1202-1204), led by French nobles and the doge of Venice. The minor Crusades took place from 1216 to 1220, 1228 to 1229, 1248 to 1254, and 1270 to 1272. Jerusalem was captured during the First Crusade but was lost once again to the Turks in 1187. It was never regained by the Western world until the First World War.

The Crusades were extensive expeditions to conquer the Holy Land, which had been in the hands of the Muhammadans for several centuries. Among the participants were members of the clergy, adventurers, pious individuals, and others who sought an opportunity to satisfy a variety of motives. The Crusades, indeed, represented many things to many people: aristocratic and military ideals in social life, political ambition, economic gain, the desire for adventure, and the extension of Christianity by means of war, a holy war.

These enterprises extended over a long period and increased the need for hospitals along the Crusader and pilgrim routes and in Syria and Palestine. An acute demand arose for hospitals and for providers of health care because of the effects of the war, which became more and more deadly as disease was carried wherever armies were sent:

> That the Crusades were turned back by epidemics much more effectively than they were by the armed power of the Saracens can hardly be questioned. The history of the Crusades reads like the chronicle of a series of diseases, with scurvy as potent as infections. In 1098, a Christian army of 300,000 men besieged Antioch. Disease and famine killed so many and in such a short time that the dead could not be buried. The cavalry were rendered useless within a few months by the death of 5000 of their 7000 horses. Nevertheless, the city was captured, after a nine months' siege. On the march to Jerusalem, the hosts were accompanied by an enemy more potent than the heathen. When Jerusalem was taken, in 1099, only 60,000 of the original 300,000 were left, and these, by 1101, had melted to 20,000.
>
> — *Zinsser, 1934, p. 155*

The response to these identified needs resulted in the development of military nursing orders, knighthood, additional hospitals, mendicant orders, and the rise of several great nursing saints. In addition, with the advent of the military order a harsher element entered nursing. Emphasis was now placed on rank, deference to superior officers, and the vow of unquestioning obedience. All of these would profoundly affect the progress of nursing and nursing education for many years.

MILITARY NURSING ORDERS

The military nursing orders were an outcome of the Crusades to the Holy Land. They were a special type of nursing order that appeared in the military brotherhoods. These orders combined the attributes of religion and chivalry, as well as militarism and charity, in their dedicated services. The

chronicles and histories of this period contain little information about how the knights cared for the sick and the wounded because the primary emphasis in these documents was on the military aspects of the pilgrimages. However, they do indicate that great hospitals were built and equipped and that knights nursed patients (Austin, 1957). So great was the influence of these orders on nursing that Nutting and Dock devoted an entire chapter of the *History of Nursing* to the origin and development of them. There is no doubt that the religious zeal that called forth groups of knights to care for the wounded and the sick was important to the organization and structure of European hospitals and to the pattern of nursing service that was established and standardized by them. The majority of what was written about these orders is good; the members were benevolent, brave, and charitable. Yet the accumulation of vast riches and large land holdings proved to be the eventual downfall of the orders. Soon after the Holy Wars ended, devotion to the calling of nursing diminished, works of mercy dwindled, and warfare against unbelievers became the sole focus. "The pride of riches and power, with the gradual abandonment of the humbler humanitarian duties for a spiritual dominance, had made the once peerless order of serving brothers a menace to the secular power" (Nutting and Dock, 1937, p. 206).

Great orders were formed, all called by the name hospitallers. The membership in these orders consisted of three classes—knights, priests, and serving brothers. The knights were men of patrician birth who bore arms, protected pilgrims, and fought in the Crusades. When they were not engaged in battle, they helped to nurse the sick. The priests attended to the religious duties in churches, camps, and hospitals. The serving brothers (*serjeus,* or half-knights) were responsible primarily for weary travelers and the care of the sick. Three of these nursing orders stand out as being the most famous and the most important in history: the Knights Hospitallers of St. John of Jerusalem; the Teutonic Knights (der Deutsche Order); and the Knights of St. Lazarus. Both the Hospitallers and the Teutonic Knights formed women's orders that were subordinated to the men's communities, as was often the case. Frequent references are also made to the Knights Templars, or Red Cross Knights, although this group was always purely military.

Knights Hospitallers of St. John of Jerusalem. Rich merchants of Amalfi, Italy, established two hospitals (one for each gender) in Jerusalem in about 1050. They were placed under the protection of St. John the Almoner (neither the Evangelist nor the Baptist, but a Cypriot) and St. Mary Magdalene. These hospitals originally tended any individual who was sick, including the pilgrims and the insane, but they became crowded with wounded and dying Crusaders during the siege of Antioch and the battle for Jerusalem. Many Crusaders of noble birth laid aside their arms to help with the work of tending the sick in the Hospital of St. John. Thus was born the order of the Knights Hospitallers of St. John of Jerusalem.

Until 1099, when Godfrey was made King of Palestine, the order was secular and was directed by Peter Gerard, who was considered to be a pious and saintly man. Gerard developed a code of rules; major decisions were voted upon in adherence to a democratic constitution. A female branch of the order, the Hospitaller Dames of the Order of St. John of Jerusalem, served the Hospital of St. Mary Magdalene. The women met at first on terms of equality with the knights;

both nursed, ate, and worshiped together. Eventually, the men and women formed a religious fraternity and dedicated themselves as servants of the poor and of Christ to function under the rule of St. Augustine. Later, segregation occurred, and the sisters were subordinated to the brothers. Solemn vows of poverty, chastity, and obedience were taken, and a black robe that had a white linen Maltese cross embroidered on the left breast was donned. (In subsequent years, the Knights of St. John were differentiated from other hospitallers by wearing a white cross on a red background.) The order became extremely wealthy through gifts of grateful benefactors, which enabled the building of additional hospitals, hostels, and hospices. Rules were drawn up for hospital management, and they were followed by the best city hospitals, or Maisons Dieu, of Europe for many centuries.

The career of this order was one of distinction in nursing until the expulsion of the Christians from Palestine. Nursing was gradually neglected when the Sisters of St. John disappeared temporarily and the men's order fled to Cyprus and then to the island of Rhodes, where they remained for approximately two hundred years. With the conquest of Rhodes by the Turks, the care of the sick became a secondary objective. In 1522 the Knights were forced out of Rhodes and were without a headquarters until Emperor Charles V granted them the isles of Malta, Goza, and Tripolis in 1530. Finally the Knights were turned out of Malta by Napoleon in 1798. The name of the order changed as its geographical locations shifted. The members were successively known as the Knights of St. John of Jerusalem, the Knights of Rhodes, and the Knights of Malta. The significance of this organization in nursing history is great:

The most important and the largest of the many hospitals of the order was established in 1575 at the seaport town of Valetta in Malta. In its early days this hospital was a model for all of Europe, but by the time of John Howard's visit in 1786 it had fallen into a deteriorated state. The hospital, which remains a magnificent monument of architecture,

initially accommodated somewhat fewer than a thousand patients. A well-defined organizational structure provided for department heads, nursing, almsgiving, distribution of food to the poor, mending of clothing, and foundling care. Acute cases and cases of hemorrhage, lithotomy, and insanity were isolated. Visitors to the hospital frequently remarked about its cleanliness and expressed their surprise that the knights actually cared for the patients. Chaplains attended to spiritual needs; paid physicians assisted the knights in anatomy and the care of disease. "A peculiar interest attaches itself to this institution because of the remarkable splendour of its equipment and service. They were unrivaled in their day, and indeed, with all the improvements in hospital service which modern progress has brought, we would find it hard to better some of these old regulations of 1533. In reading them over one is struck with the careful arrangements made for the division of labour, and the proper conduct of the work" (Nutting and Dock, 1937, p. 196).

The Knights of St. John were finally suppressed but later continued their activities in a modified form. Branches were developed in several countries, including England and the United States. Continuing a semimilitary tradition, the Hospitallers functioned as units in Europe, supplying ambulance and other medical services during times of war. "But their original functions have been largely taken over and expanded during the last century by the International Red Cross" (Shryock, 1959, p. 109). The order lives on in the St. John's guilds and ambulance corps and in societies that provide first aid to the injured. The hospital buildings established by the Knights of St. John can still be seen on Rhodes and Malta.

The Maltese cross, once worn by the Knights of St. John, survived the period of the Crusades and became a part of the insignia of many groups caring for the sick. It was on the banner of the United States Cadet Nurse Corps and was

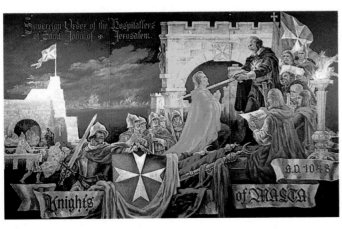

The first duty of knights, or men-at-arms, was to fight; those who were expected to serve in the hospital wards when not engaged in battle wore a white cross on their habits. Frequent references are also made to the Red Cross Knights (Knights Templars), although this group was always purely military.

Knights of Malta, painting. Photo courtesy of Knights Hospitallers of the Sovereign Order of St. John of Jerusalem, Knights of Malta, the Ecumenical Order.

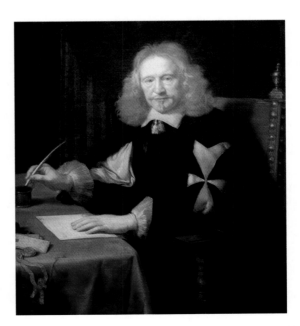

The Knights of St. John of Jerusalem became known as the Knights of Malta when Emperor Charles V granted them the Isles of Malta, Gozo, and Tripolis in 1530. The Knights of Malta are famous as the only military order that cared for insane patients.

Pierre Mignard, *Knight of Malta,* 17th century, painting, National Museum La Valletta Malta. The Art Archive/National Museum La Valletta Malta/Gianni Dagli Orti.

worn on the shoulders of nurses' uniforms. The eight points of the cross signify the beatitudes that knights were expected to exemplify in the works of charity in their daily lives: to express spiritual joy; to live without malice; to weep over their sins; to humble themselves to those who injured them; to love justice; to be merciful; to be sincere and pure of heart; and to suffer persecution.

The Teutonic Knights. The German order of Knights Hospitallers, formed in 1191, was called the Deutsche Orden, or Teutonic Knights. During the Third Crusade German pilgrims set up a temporary hospital beside the walls of Acre, engaged religious knights for defense, and originated this group. The Teutonics followed the hospital rules of the Knights of St. John and the military structure of the Templars. The first members were from noble families. They took the usual vows of poverty, chastity, and obedience but added a fourth vow that required them to care for the sick and defend the faith. They, too, were divided into three classes—warriors, nurses, and spiritual brothers. The Teutonic Knights had from the very beginning both nursing and military duties. They were distinguished by a black habit over which was worn a white cloak with a black cross embroidered in gold on the shoulder.

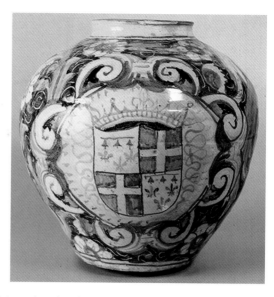

Coat of Arms of Knights of Malta, late 16th century, ceramic vase, National Museum La Valletta Malta. From the Picture Desk Image Library.

Dan Escott, *The Defeat of the Order at Wahstadt by Mongols in 1241,* September 11, 1971, gouache on paper, private collection. Copyright Look and Learn/The Bridgeman Art Library.

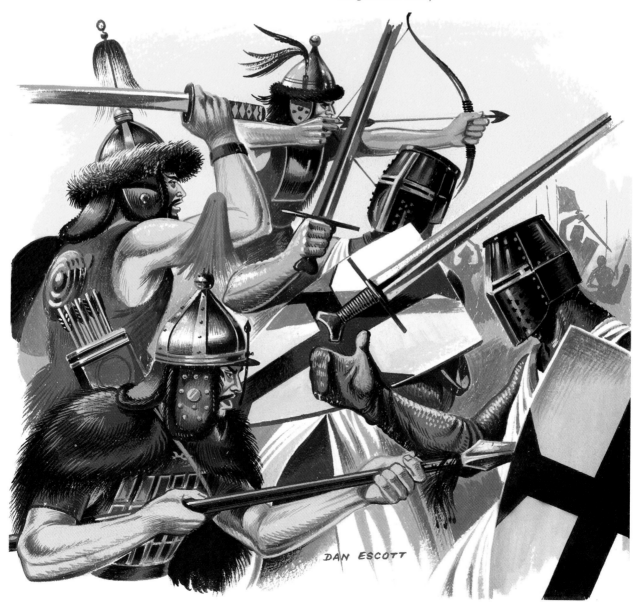

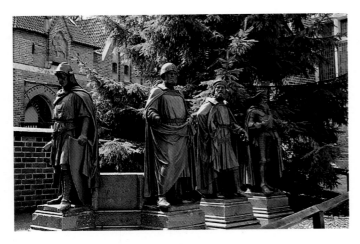

Rudolf Siemering, *Teutonic Knights*, 1877, sculpture, UNESCO World Heritage Site, Malbork Poland, Polska. Photo courtesy of Janusz Leszczynski, August 17, 2006.

A women's order was founded in Germany specifically to perform hospital work. The women were not, however, admitted to full membership and were called consorores (lay sisters). They took vows but lived outside the monastic precincts. Their nursing duties were perhaps regarded as menial, because the Rule of 1280 says that women are to be admitted "because services to cattle and to sick persons in hospital are better performed by the female sex."

The Teutonic Knights became powerful in Germany, and many hospitals were given over into their hands. From various princes they received rich possessions in a number of countries, particularly in Sicily. According to reference material, their history is similar to that of the Knights of St. John, but their nursing services were not as effective. By the 14th century, they had fulfilled their destiny.

The Knights of St. Lazarus. According to some historians, the Knights of St. Lazarus were the oldest of all the orders of hospitallers. It is speculated that this order originated from the hospital built by St. Basil at Cesarea, which kept a separate house for lepers. Attempts have also been made to trace it back to the days of Christ's raising of Lazarus, the brother of Mary and Martha. Whatever the origins of this order, the fact remains that leprosy, which had always been a problem in society, became its special cause. Lepers had been excluded from society and confined to institutions called *lazarettos* in honor of the leper spoken of in the parable of the rich man. Those who were not confined to institutions were obliged to wear a distinctive dress and carry a wooden clapper to warn of their approach; they were isolated and considered to be incurable. At that time the term *leprosy* was also applied to syphilis and many chronic skin diseases.

The members of the Knights of St. Lazarus were not only knights who had participated in the wars of the Crusades but were also those who had been stricken by leprosy, which was endemic in the Near East. Initially, the order was a purely nursing order, but by the 13th century it had added armed combatants to its membership. This action created two categories of knights—the warriors and the hospitallers, who were headed by a grand master of a noble family who was himself a leper. This rule was in effect until 1253, when permission was given by Pope Innocent IV to elect a non-leper to this office. With the addition of the warring aspect, care of the lepers became secondary and the order became purely military. Decay and deterioration set in until Pope In-

nocent VIII suppressed it in the 15th century. The order had ceased to exist by 1830.

Details about the work of the order are obscure. There is little information regarding what real service was rendered to the sick poor or to the lepers. After the Crusades, however, the incidence of leprosy began to decrease and the need for the special work of the order diminished. As with the other hospitallers, the Knights of St. Lazarus received lavish gifts and rich possessions. According to Nutting and Dock (1937), there were also sisters in the order, but few sources mention the existence of a female branch.

The first Knights of St. Lazarus varied both their habits and their crosses in different countries. The color of the original cross is unknown, but its form was distinguished by four arms of equal length, somewhat flared at the ends. The French cross was an eight-armed golden and green or purple-red cross with tiny golden lilies in the corners. The Italian cross was white and green. The emblem of the order of St. Lazarus was adopted by the German Nurses' Association.

THE RISE OF MENDICANT ORDERS

Social groupings for nursing and neighborhood work occurred with the rapid spread of sickness and disease and the fear associated with the plagues. Religious fervor escalated and led to the development of types of care different from that required when monasteries were the focal points of the communities. Emphasis began to be placed upon the great reward that could be achieved through total withdrawal from the world. Religious missionary bodies arose and pledged themselves to literal poverty. These groups exemplified the democratic and secular tendencies that developed along with the military orders. However, the extension of Christianity in this case transpired through peaceful means. Many devout individuals took part in this movement.

Success in this endeavor meant taking religion and nursing out among the people. The mendicant orders were founded to accomplish this goal. The members lived as part of the world, owned no property, gave their possessions to the poor, and followed the teachings of Christ. They depended on begging for sustenance, a practice that earned them the name of mendicants. The personification of this approach was St. Francis of Assisi (1182-1226), who instituted three religious orders. The first order, Friars Minor (Little Brothers), was for friars; the second, called Poor Clares, was for nuns; the third order, Tertiaries, was for laymen and laywomen who wished to continue to lead secular lives. (St. Dominic also founded three orders and patterned them after these.) The members lived outside the monastery walls and were guided by an order or rule. Care of the sick as well as the poor, the needy, and the outcast became a primary duty. The Franciscans, the Dominicans, the Carmelites, and the Oblates of St. Benedict became the most famous of these third orders.

St. Francis of Assisi. St. Francis became one of the best-known and best-loved saints in history. Born to a life of wealth and ease as the son of a cloth merchant in Assisi, he spent his youth as an exuberant, carefree cavalier. Francis' style of living changed after he suffered a serious illness in his early twenties. Even before the illness, however, he looked with aversion upon the miseries that were prevalent in the society and was particularly affected by the plight of

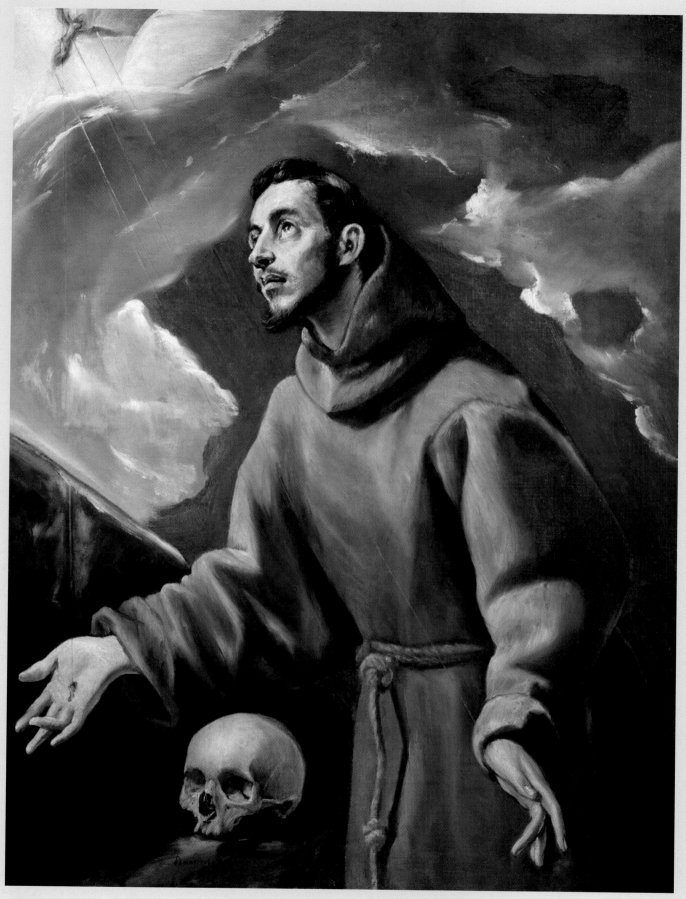

With St. Francis came the emergence of the nun from her cloister and her close association with nursing in hospitals. St. Francis stressed the need for care for the homeless and the poor sick of the towns as a matter of Christian duty. Nursing care of the sick expanded beyond the hospital walls.

El Greco, *St. Francis Receiving the Stigmata*, 1590-1595, painting, Bridgeman Library.

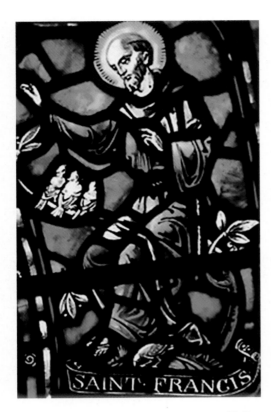

Ralph Ohmer (D'Ascenzo Studios, Philadelphia, PA), *World Christian Fellowship Window—St. Francis*, 1959, stained glass, entire window is 8' x 20'; St. Francis located in upper right arch. Used with permission of The Upper Room Chapel and Museum, Nashville, TN.

the lepers. A variety of circumstances, particularly his giving of great amounts of alms to the poor, led to Francis's being disinherited by his father. Rejected by his family, Francis set out alone, barefooted, and clothed in a rough brown tunic tied at the waist with a heavy white rope, to travel the countryside. Appalled by the sufferings of the poor and the sick, he devoted his life to their ministrations. Most important, he provided a necessary example of considering human beings as individuals:

> What distinguishes this very genuine democrat from any mere demagogue is that he never either deceived or was deceived by the illusion of mass-suggestion. . . . To him a man was always a man and did not disappear in a dense crowd any more than in a desert. He honored all men; that is, he not only loved but respected them all. What gave him his extraordinary personal power was this; that from the Pope to the beggar, from the sultan of Syria in his pavillion to the ragged robbers crawling out of the wood, there was never a man who looked into those brown burning eyes without being certain that Francis Bernardone was really interested in *him;* in his own inner life from the cradle to the grave; that he himself was being valued and taken seriously, and not merely added to the spoils of some social policy or the names in some clerical document.
>
> — *Chesterton, 1924, pp. 141-142*

St. Francis became known for his great compassion and capacity for love. He became the champion of lepers and urged his followers to go to leper hospitals. He frequently visited the leper houses, where the lepers were always waiting for him, knowing that he brought not only alms but also love. Initially, St. Francis became the jest of the town because the people could not understand his close association

with the lepers. Adults and children flung mud at him and shouted, "Pazzo! Pazzo!" According to Robinson (1946), the pale, gaunt appearance and cadaverous face with the burning eyes probably did make him look like a madman. Francis's work for these sufferers eventually influenced and inspired others to improve their conditions.

Slowly, disciples began to gather around and follow Francis of Assisi. When they numbered twelve, they went to Rome to seek permission of Pope Innocent III to preach and follow an ascetic life. With papal sanction, the Franciscans, or the Order of Friars Minor (Brothers Minor), grew rapidly. The habit of the Franciscans was the same rough tunic with rope girdle that St. Francis himself had worn. The shade of the garment might be brownish or grayish, and the wearers were called Gray Friars. Poverty and humility were emphasized in the Franciscan order; begging was done for the members themselves and for the poor.

St. Francis ultimately became a victim of a barbaric medical practice. His vision began to fail and it was believed that he would become blind. His eyes were cauterized with a red-hot iron, a treatment conducted without the benefit of any type of medicine or herbs that would allay or prevent discomfort. He died in 1226, aware that his order was departing from his original concept of complete poverty and simplicity. Leadership passed into other hands and a new rule was established. The structure of the order became more elaborate and properties were acquired. Some of the brothers had established themselves in universities even before the death of St. Francis, despite his great opposition to scholarship. Both Francis and Clare were canonized, and the bodies of these two saints repose in their native Assisi.

St. Dominic. While the Franciscans were achieving success, St. Dominic (1170-1221) established the Order of Preachers, the Dominicans. A member of the noble family of Guzman in the village of Castile, Dominic had given up his plan of becoming a monk in a monastery so he could have closer contact with the rich and the poor who needed spiritual assistance. He set forth to restore to the Church those who had fallen away and to convert others. Both men and women gathered about him, and this led to the development of the Dominicans. The followers were sent abroad as traveling preachers in an effort to make Christianity the one religion. The order practiced both individual and corporate poverty. The Dominican robe was made of white wool and topped by a black cape with a hood. The hood could be pulled over the head for warmth. This cape led to the title of Black Friars.

Eminent scholars arose from the Franciscans and the Dominicans. Many of them taught at great universities such as Padua, Cologne, Vienna, Prague, and Paris. Among them were the Dominican Albertus Magnus; the Franciscan Roger Bacon, who stressed the value of observation, experimentation, and inductive reasoning, which assisted in the development of experimental science; and the Dominican St. Thomas Aquinas, who studied under the Benedictines at Monte Cassino and completed the *Summa Theologica,* his greatest work.

St. Clare of Assisi. The life of St. Clare of Assisi (1194-1253) was closely interwoven with that of St. Francis. Clare, a beautiful daughter of the knightly family of Sciffi, at the age of sixteen heard St. Francis preach in the churches of Assisi. She became convinced that his way of life, extreme poverty, was what the Lord wished for her. She believed that the adoption of this type of life would provide her with contentment, peace, and joy. Clare remained in the household of her father until the age of eighteen, then ran away to the chapel of the Franciscans where she exchanged her expensive dress and jewels for a rough woolen robe. Francis cut off her long hair and received her vows of poverty, chastity, and obedience. Clare lived in a Benedictine convent for a brief period until a special convent was established for her. Other women who wished to share this simple life joined her. Thus began the second order of St. Francis, more commonly referred to as the order of Poor Clares (Clarisses), with Clare as its abbess. A short time later Clare was followed by her younger sister Agnes.

It is said that the Poor Clares cared principally for lepers, whom they housed in small mud-and-wattle huts around their convent in San Damiano. Accounts vary, however, about the actual services they provided. One author (Austin, 1957) suggests: "It would probably be a mistake to ascribe to the Poor Ladies any widespread activity in the care of the sick. Their chief preoccupation seems to have been with the contemplative life" (p. 67). Austin adds that "the Rule of 1253 indicates that the Poor Clares cared for their own members, but whether their care extended to the surrounding community is uncertain" (p. 69). Other authors (Jamieson and Sewall, 1950; Nutting and Dock, 1937; Robinson, 1946; Shryock, 1959) discuss the nursing activities of this order of Franciscan nuns.

Clare outlived St. Francis by more than twenty-five years. After her death, the order experienced many changes. It has been known at various times and in various countries by a variety of names: Order of Poor Ladies, Clarisses, Minoresses, and Poor Clares. It eventually became a strictly cloistered order whose members functioned under the most austere conditions. Professed sisters living under rule did not go outside the walls, nor were they in contact with the outside world until after the Protestant Revolt. Since its original founding, the Poor Clares, as well as numerous other sisterhoods that have adopted Franciscan rule, have founded many hospitals and other institutions for the sick.

Tertiaries: Third Orders of St. Francis and St. Dominic. The Tertiaries, or Third Orders, were founded for the laity of both sexes who wished to continue their ordinary lives in the world. They were to practice charity and devotion to God in a manner similar to that of the religious orders. Several communities of tertiaries lived almost the same lives as the religious members without being cloistered. These orders attracted thousands of people of all classes and were a powerful force for a number of years. Some were later formed into communities (convents arose in a number of

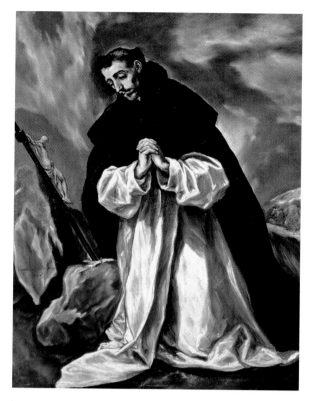

El Greco, *St. Dominic in Prayer*, 1585-1590, painting, Bridgeman Library.

countries) that often undertook nursing as their main work. The idea became so popular that many tertiary orders emerged, and this prompted Gregory at the Council of Lyons (1272) to reduce them to four: the Dominicans, Franciscans, Carmelites, and Augustinians.

The Third Order epitomized the ideals of St. Francis. It represented a revival of the early Christian spirit. Religion was carried into everyday life, and unselfish and useful service was rendered to humanity. Many famous nursing saints were enrolled in this order of St. Francis: Elizabeth of Hungary (1207-1231); Louis of France (1214-1270); Elizabeth of Portugal (1271-1336); Isabelle of France; Anne of Bohemia; and Bridget of Sweden (Tuker and Malleson, 1900).

St. Elizabeth of Hungary was probably the most renowned among the women tertiaries of St. Francis. Her virtues have been set forth in prose, poetry, art, and music. Elizabeth, the daughter of the Hungarian king Andreas II, was married at the age of 14 to Ludwig of Thuringia, and she became the mother of 4 children. With her husband's support she built hospitals in Thuringia and humbly ministered to the sick with her own hands. Daily she distributed alms to the poor, fed the hungry, nursed the lepers, and bathed newborns and comforted their mothers with special tenderness. Hers was a life of extreme piety, asceticism, and austerity. Elizabeth was the heroine of beautiful tales, which were accepted as either fact or fiction. The story of the miraculous roses is perhaps the most well known. It is said that one winter day while Elizabeth was carrying a basket of food to the poor, she met Ludwig. (In some accounts it is her father-in-law whom she met.) Irritated by complaints against Elizabeth by his family, Ludwig demanded to see what she was carrying. When she opened her cloak, Ludwig saw an armful of blooming white and red roses.

Upon Ludwig's death during the Crusades, Elizabeth was driven from her husband's castle, the Wartburg, by her in-

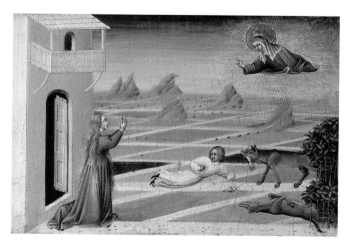

Giovanni di Paolo, *St. Clare of Assisi Saving a Child from a Wolf*, 1455, tempera, 20.6 × 29.2 cm, Museum of Fine Arts, Houston, TX.

laws. She became a member of the Third Order of St. Francis and built the Franciscan hospital at Marburg, where she spent the remaining years of her short life nursing the sick. Elizabeth was considered to be an excellent organizer, administrator, and nurse. Her conception of social service carried a modern ring because her service to the needy "was tempered with discretion; and instead of encouraging idleness in such as were able to work, she employed them in a way suitable to their strength and capacity" (Butler, 1934, vol. 10, p. 43). Always frail, Elizabeth died at the age of 24. Considered the patron saint of nursing, she is honored on November 19. Elizabeth is regarded by some as the forerunner of the visiting and public health nurses of the 20th century. The Gray Nuns of the 13th century, who were also Tertiaries of St. Francis, were often called Sisters of St. Elizabeth because they had chosen her as their patron saint.

St. Louis IX was another saint whose work with lepers was well known. His special care of their needs was recognized and respected by his subjects, who mourned his death in 1270 during the Eighth Crusade. France flourished under Louis' rule and experienced peace and prosperity. Louis personally tended to the sick and devoted his life to promoting humane treatment for all individuals. He was interested in education, particularly for health care workers, and attempted to assist in its provision. He built Sainte-Chapelle in Paris and founded the Sorbonne College of the University of Paris. Louis belonged to the Franciscan Tertiaries.

The Third Order of St. Dominic was originally formed to recover Church property. The Tertiaries, however, performed other services as well and assisted the poor and the ill as regular functions of their religious duties. They were patterned after the Third Order of St. Francis. There are at least hints that some competition existed between the two groups. Robinson presents an interesting account of this rivalry:

> Dominic was the imitator, Francis always the originator; and the story of Dominic lacked the emotional fire of the Francis legend. Moreover, the Franciscans had the inestimable advantage that only upon the body of their founder had been miraculously inflicted the Five Wounds which Christ received at his crucifixion: after the death of Francis, Clara saw the wounds in his feet, but could not extract the nails which had been driven through them. In the contemporary rivalry between the Franciscans and the Dominicans, Catherine came to the rescue of the latter: Christ put a ring on her finger as proof that she was to be his heavenly spouse; and, as she knelt in a church in Pisa, she received the crowning glory of the wounds of the Lord. . . . The Franciscans coldly denied, while the Dominicans fervently accepted, the stigmatization of St. Catherine.
>
> — ROBINSON, 1946, PP. 46-47

The first members of the Third Order of St. Dominic were known as the Mantellate. They wore the Dominican habit—a white tunic bound by a leather belt, a white veil, and a black cloak (mantella). Margaret of Metola (1287-1320) was the first young woman to join the Mantellate. She was the daughter of wealthy parents who abandoned her because she was blind and deformed. Margaret gave her life to the needs of others. She had a special affinity for prisoners and visited them daily, giving them food, clothing, medicines, and bedding. Other remarkable personalities joined the Dominican Tertiaries.

During the famine of 1226, Elizabeth organized food distribution and devoted her life and strength to helping the sick and poor. She had hospitals built where she cared for lepers and comforted prisoners. When her husband of six years died, she moved to Marburg and spent the rest of her young life nursing the sick. She died at twenty-four years of age.

Bartolome Esteban Murillo, *St. Elizabeth*, 1670-1674, painting, Hospital de la Caridad.

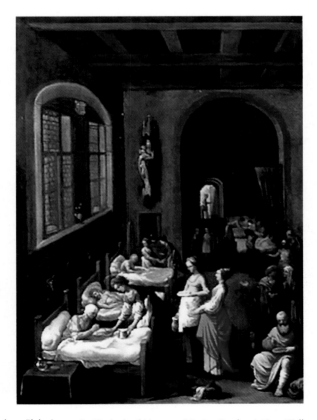

Adam Elsheimer, *St. Elizabeth of Hungary Bringing Food*, painting, Wellcome Library.

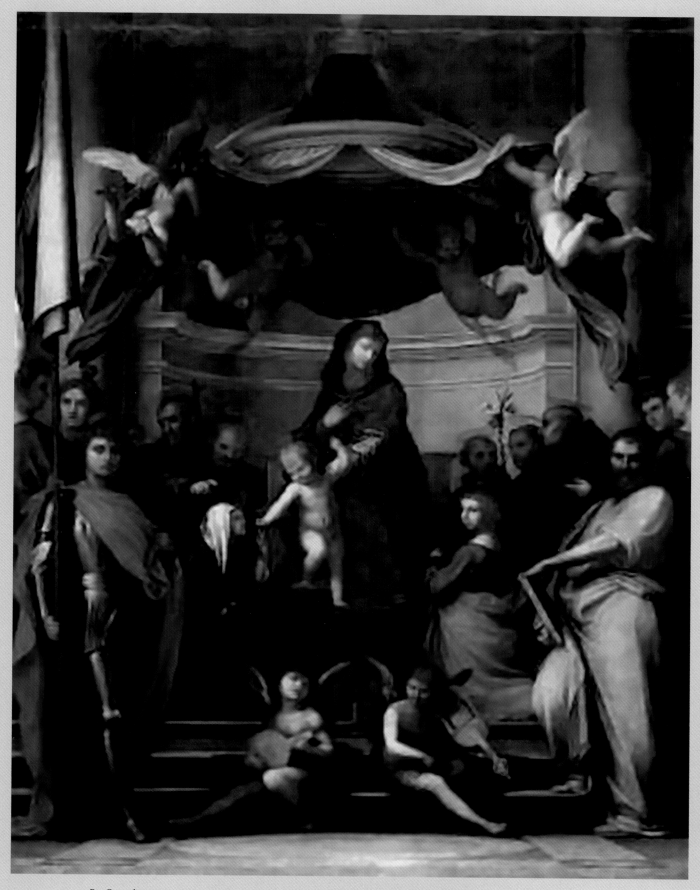

Fra Bartolommeo, *The Mystic Marriage of St. Catherine of Siena, with Eight Saints*, 1511, painting, 257 × 218 cm, The Louvre.

St. Catherine of Siena (1347-1380), a favorite subject of painters, is often portrayed in the act of expelling demons or in an ecstatic state, holding a lily, thorn, or book. She is also frequently pictured with a lighted lamp, which she carried on her nightly visits to La Scala hospital. (Her lamp was as famous as the Nightingale lamp of later years.) Catherine Benincasca was the daughter of a wealthy merchant and the last of twenty-five children. Her twin died at birth. At the age of seven, Catherine devoted herself to Christ. She became a member of the Third Order of St. Dominic when she was eighteen. The literature identifies Catherine as a hospital and visiting nurse, social welfare worker, reformer of society and of the Church, peacemaker, stateswoman, and great mystic.

When the Black Death (bubonic plague) swept over Siena, Catherine personally cared for the victims. For more than a year she rarely went home but spent her nights and days in the La Scala wards tending to the afflicted. Although there was little that could be done for the victims of the plague, she exhibited her willingness to comfort them. She organized groups of young men as stretcher bearers to transport the stricken from all over the city to wards of the hospital, which she supervised. Catherine's prominence, however, lies in her influence in the political affairs of the day. She never hesitated to speak out to the highest and mightiest in the land and had some part in persuading the Pope to end the Babylonian Captivity and to return to Rome from Avignon. Catherine attempted to start another Crusade to rescue Jerusalem from the Muslims. She was also instrumental in healing breaches between members of prominent families in Genoa.

SECULAR NURSING ORDERS

At the same time that the military knights and the first, second, and third orders were developing, groups of workers banded together in semireligious orders. These orders were not bound by vows to monastic life and have been referred to as secular nursing orders. They made many contributions to nursing and served the sick, the poor, foundlings, and orphans in their own communities. At times they also did hospital nursing. The development of these orders marks a significant step in the secularization of nursing. Their success was in part a result of their freedom in the community.

Another order of men in this period was the Antonines (Hospital Brothers of St. Anthony), founded in about 1095 and issued a rule in 1218. Houses were established in France, Spain, and Italy. The members devoted themselves to sufferers of "St. Anthony's Fire," which was probably the condition of ergotism. This disease is caused by a fungus that grows on rye, which was a staple grain of the Middle Ages. Hospitals were developed for the victims of this disease, who were lovingly cared for by the brothers. The hallucinatory manifestations of ergotism have been vividly described in the literature. An interesting account of an outbreak of ergotism in 1951 in Pont Saint-Esprit, France, is described by Fuller (1968) in his book *The Day of St. Anthony's Fire.* Eventually this order cared for victims of other diseases as well, and they were also in charge of the papal household until their suppression in the 18th century.

The origin of the Beguine movement is uncertain, and the derivation of its name is obscure. It is usually credited to a priest of Liège, Lambert le Begue, who encouraged the settlement of Mulières Sanctae around his church—among them the daughters of barons, knights, and nobles—in what has come to be regarded as the first beguinage. The Mu-

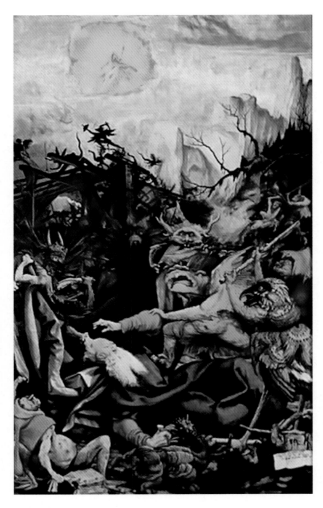

Matthias Grunewald, *The Temptation of St. Anthony,* 1515, painting, 265 × 141 cm, Musee d'Unterlinden, Colmar.

lières Sanctae were individual women who identified themselves with a monastery by donating a part of their substance (if they were rich) or voluntary service (if they were poor). They took no vows and lived in their own homes. Eventually these women gathered together into a communal life. They took vows of chastity and obedience for the time they were in residence but did not give up rights to property or possessions. They were free to marry and leave at any time. The Beguines of Flanders were one of the most prominent secular nursing orders. Later, many of these communities became Tertiaries of St. Francis or St. Dominic.

The organization was extremely simple. Two to four women lived together in small houses built in an enclosed precinct and grouped around a church or hospital. Such beguinages were picturesque in their simplicity. Those at Bruges (c. 1184) and Ghent (c. 1234) in Belgium are well known. Each community was self-contained and fixed its own rules, which were approved by the bishop of the diocese. Because there was great diversity among the Beguines, it is difficult to render an adequate description of their work. Their original objective seems to have been religious; they strived for the perfection and reform of the Church and the saving of souls. Members ranged from the rich to the poor, the noble to the humble. Their work and their dress varied according to location.

The Beguines supported themselves by teaching, spinning cloth and making other handicrafts, and caring for the sick in hospitals. They started a visiting nursing service in the neighborhood homes, and fees were charged if the

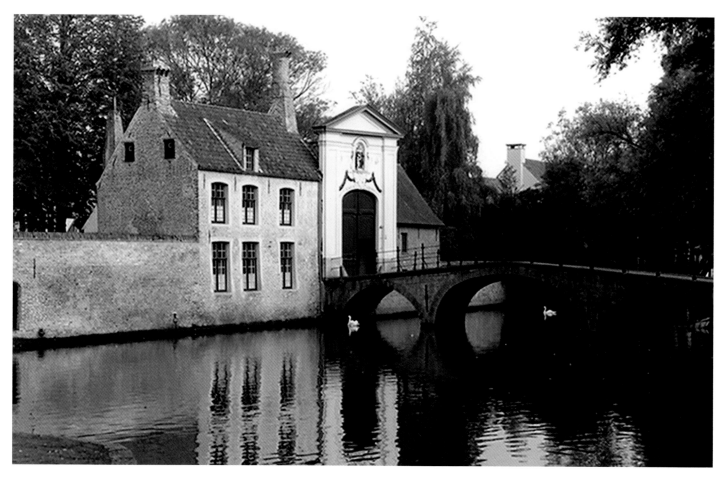

The Flemish beguinages can be compared with monasteries for women. However, in the beguinages the sisters (or beguines) never made vows for life. They were free to leave the beguinage again if they wanted to do so. The Beguinage of Bruges is certainly one of the most beautiful examples of its kind in Belgium.

Daniel Suy, *The Beguinage of Bruges—Unesco World Heritage*, photograph. Copyright Daniel Suy-Dotodansaert.com.

families were able to pay. Hospital work became one of their chief interests and led to the erection of their own hospitals, where they nursed. One of the most famous is the Hôtel Dieu in Beaune, France, which was founded in 1443. These hospitals were also staffed by the Sisters of Matilda, an order established specifically for this purpose by the Beguines. During wars, famines, and epidemics, members of the order converted their cottages into hospitals; they also served as nurses on battlefields.

The Beguines were always popular with the people, but they met with resistance and suffered a certain amount of persecution from ecclesiastical authorities. Clerics could not tolerate their independence and the striking innovations they made in community life. The Beguines were accused of heresy and in 1215 were forbidden by the Pope to found any additional groups. Despite several periods of persecution, they flourished and expanded. By the end of the 13th century there were few communities without a beguinage, and the order had spread to neighboring countries. It is estimated that there were 200,000 Beguines by that time. Gradually a decrease in numbers and size of these organizations occurred for various reasons. The Beguines retain a corporate existence in Belgium today.

Other groups of women appeared somewhat later. The Sisterhood of the Common Life gathered about Gerhard Groot, who was an idealist and a leader in new thinking. These sisters, like the Beguines, took no binding vows, but they held no private property. They lived together in a conventional manner and were preeminently visiting nurses in the cities along the Rhine. Their habit was a simple gray dress, and they were self-supporting. The order of men, the Brothers of the Common Life, was also founded by Groot. The brothers devoted themselves to the sick poor and taught children who were bedridden. They became known as the schoolmasters of the time. Thomas à Kempis lived and studied with this community.

Another interesting confraternity was the brotherhood of Misericordia, which was started about 1244 in Florence. Founded primarily as a volunteer ambulance society, it was composed of a group of religious laymen. The members functioned in many Italian cities and became known as the Masked Brotherhood. This name arose from the members' belief that their contributions would gain spiritual reward only if they prevented themselves from being recognized by others.

The order of the Alexian Brothers was formed in 1348 to assist with the care of the victims of the bubonic plague in the Netherlands. This group of laymen also undertook the burial of the dead. St. Alexius, a 5th-century Roman who nursed the sick in a hospital at Edessa, was chosen as their patron saint. This occurred in 1469, when the group organized under Augustinian rule. The sick continue to be cared for by this order. Several large general hospitals for men and boys, a rest home, and a home for elderly men are supported and serviced by its members. The Alexian Brothers also staff Memorial Hospital and Clinic at Boys Town, Nebraska. At one time, the Alexian Brothers' Hospital School of Nursing in Chicago was the largest male nursing school in the United States.

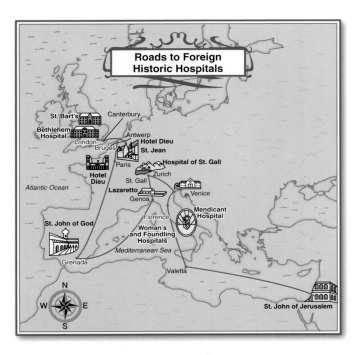

Roads to Foreign Hospitals, map, Mosby.

THE GROWTH OF HOSPITALS

During the late Middle Ages, Pope Innocent III encouraged the development of hospitals in European cities. Church executives and influential citizens who visited with him were invited to study the model Santo Spirito Hospital and were encouraged to organize similar institutions in their own communities. This idea of city hospitals was met with support and approval, and in some cases hospitals passed amicably from ecclesiastical to secular control. The number of hospitals rapidly escalated, but the size of the institutions varied greatly. Several factors contributed to the demand for more hospitals: existing hospitals had been organized as orphanages, hospices for travelers and the sick, and almshouses; communicable disease was uncontrolled; and urban life had been hastily developed and crowded living conditions were contributing to the spread of disease.

In general, the hospitals were erected to care for the sick poor. The wards were large, and privacy was commonly provided by the use of cubicles. The structures were usually beautiful, having been constructed at a time when every public building was to be a work of art. The larger ones were similar in architectural form to the churches of the period. "Indeed, the appearance of a main hall or ward would have suggested an ecclesiastical interior to a modern observer. Straw pallets were replaced by wooden beds, and curtains or partitions supplied some privacy. Linen and woolen supplies became more ample, and a large place would have its own farms to provide food and its own wind or water mills to prepare 'corn' (wheat) for the patients. Although the buildings were still cold and dark by modern standards, they were a great improvement over the bare and humble dwellings of the 'dark ages' " (Shryock, 1959, pp. 109-110).

Management and hygienic practices varied from hospital to hospital; they were sometimes good and sometimes bad. The hospitals, which were usually well endowed, were built on carefully chosen sites. Medieval hospitals were a place to keep, not cure, the patients. The aspect of cure evolved slowly and did not become widespread until the late 19th century. Nursing care, which was largely custodial, was provided 24 hours a day, primarily by monks and nuns, although servants were used part of the time. It is difficult, however, to determine where the division of labor actually occurred. As centuries passed, there were not always enough nurses. Other changes began to occur: the sickbed began to hold more than one patient; patients were sometimes not only dirty but ill fed; and the practice of using individuals of low character to augment inadequate nursing staffs became more common. At least a hint of a decline in nursing was present, a decline that would ultimately occur and persist for a long, dreadful time.

A custom of this period was to display paintings in the hospitals as diversional therapy for patients. St. John's Hospital in Bruges, Belgium, offers an example of this practice. Established in 1118 by Augustinian monks and nuns as a hospice for travelers, its older buildings are preserved as a museum. Six paintings by the Flemish master Hans Memling hang in this hospital.

The first English hospital was doubtless that at York, built by Athelstane in about 936. It was also a poorhouse and had a ward for lepers. St. Giles' Hospital was built by Queen Matilda in 1101 for the care of forty lepers. The queen was also instrumental in the building of the Hospital of St. Katherine in London in 1148. Women of noble birth did the nursing in these hospitals, and they did district nursing in the homes of the poor. The charters of these hospitals incorporated both types of nursing service.

St. Bartholomew's Hospital probably has the longest continuous record of service of any hospital in the British Empire. It was founded in 1123 by Rahere, who rose to fame as a jester to Henry I and then joined the Augustinian monks. Rahere became a convert after a pilgrimage to Rome, where he became critically ill. He promised to build a church and hospital in honor of St. Bartholomew if he recovered and reached England safely. During the Reformation the hospital was seized by Henry VIII. The pleas of the lord mayor and citizens of London resulted in a new charter that allowed it to become a hospital once again. Originally a poorhouse and orphanage, St. Bartholomew's was exclusively a hospital by the 13th century.

St. Thomas's Hospital was founded in 1213 by Richard, Prior of Bermondsey. This institution was made famous in the 19th century, when the first school of nursing was established there by Florence Nightingale. Because of its strategic location in a densely populated area of London, on the main route to Rome and other cities, St. Thomas's became a hospital for the sick, a refuge for the poor, and a hospice for travelers and pilgrims. Lepers were not admitted but were sent to the nearby Lock Hospital. (St. Thomas's Hospital paid their bills.) There was a "foule" ward for contagious diseases and men's and women's wards; children were also admitted. In addition, there was a lying-in ward for unmarried women, which had been donated by the famous Richard Whittington.

Bethlehem Hospital was the first English institution for the mentally ill. It was founded in 1247 by Simon FitzMary, sheriff of London, as a priory. Originally a hospice of St. Mary of Bethlehem, it was designated a hospital in about 1330. During the 14th century it was mentioned as a lunatic asylum that rapidly became infamous for the brutal treatment of its inmates. It has been said that once patients responded to treatment they were sent out into the streets to beg for a living. They wore metal armbands to identify

St. Thomas Hospital was described as ancient in 1215. It was a mixed order of Augustinian monks and nuns, dedicated to Thomas Becket, that provided shelter and treatment for the poor, sick, and homeless. The hospital was located in Southwark, just south of London Bridge. In the fifteenth century, Richard Whitington endowed a laying-in ward for unmarried mothers. In 1859, Florence Nightingale became involved with St Thomas Hospital, setting up her famous nursing school on the site.

Samuel Wale, *St. Thomas Hospital*, 1748, oil on canvas, Copyright Coram in the care of the Foundling Museum, London/The Bridgeman Art Library.

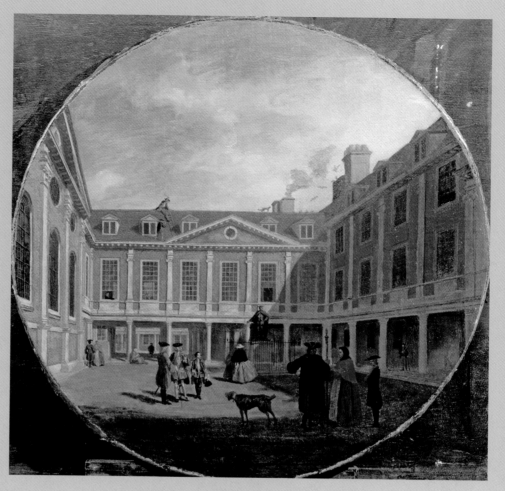

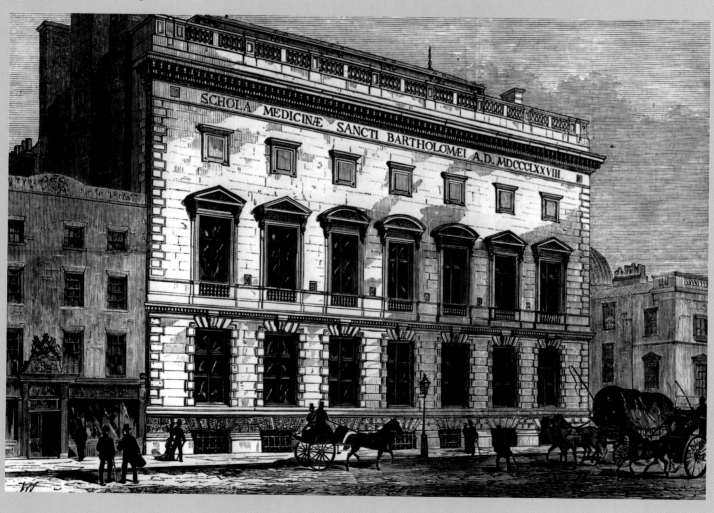

Bart's Hospital, 1879. Getty Images.

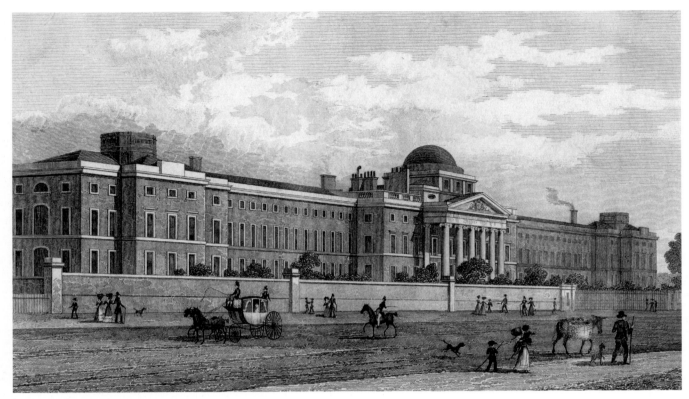

Drawn by Tho. H. Shepherd   Engraved by J. Tingle.

NEW BETHLEM HOSPITAL, ST. GEORGE'S FIELDS.

The Hospital of St. Mary of Bethlehem, St. George's Fields, London, was first founded as a hospital in 1247. The term "bedlam" originates from this mental asylum.

Hulton Archive, *Bethlehem Hospital*, January 1, 1800, photograph, London. Getty Images.

themselves as mental patients and were called Tom o'Bedlams. Violent patients were chained in cells, and they became one of the tourist attractions of London in the 18th century. Admission fees provided a source of revenue for the hospital. The name of the hospital was gradually contracted into Bedlam. This word is used today to describe a place where fools chatter.

Ospedale Santa Maria degli Innocenti was built in Florence in 1451 as a foundling asylum for abandoned children. Such children either died or became the property of the person who had found them. Many times the children were picked up and sold for money, and they were constantly at the mercy of the slave traders. This hospital was built with funds donated by a guild of silk merchants. The structure, designed by Brunelleschi, embodied beautiful architecture and was adorned with the famous medallions of Andrea della Robbia (1435-1525), a nephew of Luca della Robbia. Luca had created a kind of glaze combined with clay that became known as Robbia ware, and he produced artworks of enameled terra-cotta for which the della Robbias became famous. Andrea designed figures of infants that fit into the arches of the long arcade in the hospital building. A type of foster-parent plan was initiated by the institution, in which the parents promised to treat the orphans as their own children. Either the hospital or the foster parents taught the children a trade.

MEDICINE IN THE LATE MIDDLE AGES

As hospitals were built in the cities of Europe, the universities and their medical schools were also developing. The revival of a lay medical profession brought physicians into the hospitals during the later medieval period. The most reputable physicians were those who had attended universities and had received the degree of doctor of medicine. The beginning of a connection between physicians and hospitals occurred as physicians were called into the institutions to see or follow patients. The physician might even be paid a retainer fee if summoned on a regular basis.

Medicine saw its darkest days in the early medieval period. During the later medieval period, the foundation of scientific medicine was being laid by the more common use of dissection of human bodies. This facilitated the study of human anatomy and disease processes in human tissues. Prior to this time, the teaching of anatomy was based almost entirely on the work of Galen, whose observations had been derived from animal dissections. Yet there also continued to be an enormous amount of faulty knowledge and superstition during this time. Undoubtedly, the majority of it had been passed down from the ancient world and from tribal ancestors.

The use of astrology and alchemy were accepted practices; physicians consulted the horoscopes of their patients as well as medical books to determine treatments. Humoral

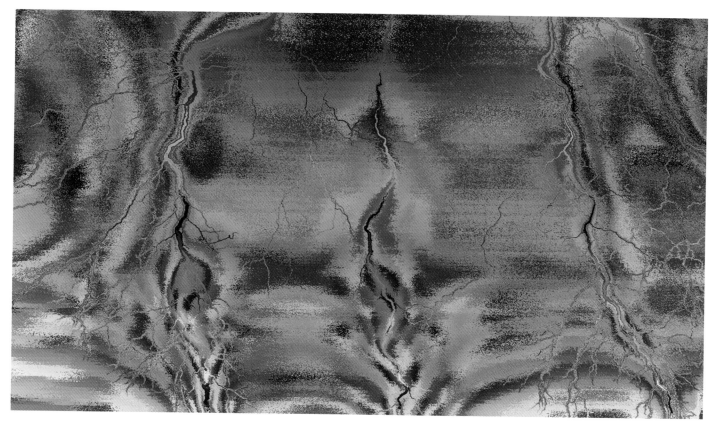

Hildegard of Bingen was the great Christian mystic of the Middle Ages. She was a Benedictine prioress, a nurse and physician, a composer and lyricist, an author and playwright, a scientist, a linguist, a philosopher, and a psychologist. This art piece was dedicated in honor of Hildegard's divine presence and powers of divine transformation. Hildegard has undergone a remarkable rise in popularity in the last 40 years because many readers have found in her visions, or read into them, themes that seem to speak to many contemporary issues.

Fred Casselman, *Fires of Saint Hildegard*, January 1998, digital image.

therapy was still trusted. The astrological signs were used to determine when to administer medicine and when to bleed because the humors were thought to be controlled by the planets. Various other techniques were developed and put into practice by physicians in this period, including the use of extraordinary medicines such as the horn of the unicorn, a narcotic inhalation for anesthesia, the use of spices as drugs and leeches for blood-letting, and the examination of urine.

St. Hildegarde (1098?-1179), the "Sybil of the Rhine," was a leading medical authority during this time. She was born at Bockelheim of noble, wealthy, and religious parents. At the age of eight, she was sent to be educated at the Benedictine cloister at Disibodenberg. Hildegarde entered this monastery and eventually became its abbess at the age of 30. She established another Benedictine cloister near Bingen on the Rhine.

During her life of 81 years, Hildegarde accomplished many things. Considered to be one of the greatest women of the 12th century, she was a mystic, poet, prophetess, musician and composer, artist, and physician. She ascribed her extraordinary intellectual powers to a kind of revelation granted to her frequently while she was in a trancelike state. In fact, her writings are among the earliest important mystic works of the Middle Ages. Hildegarde foretold such things as the downfall of the German Empire, the approach of the Reformation, and the disasters of the papacy (Nutting and Dock, 1937). She consistently communicated with kings and princes. Pilgrims frequently sought her advice and counsel; invalids came to her to be cured.

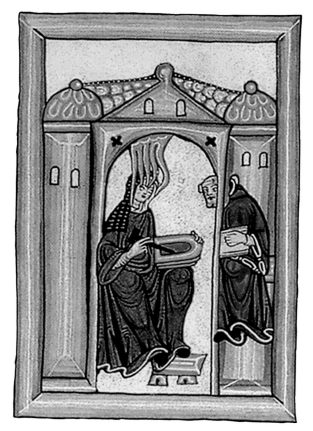

Hildegard von Bingen, the Seeress, 1165, from the book *Scivias*.

77

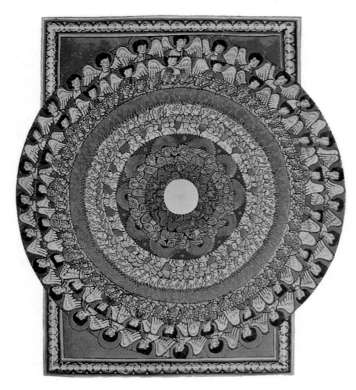

This is the sixth vision of Hildegard: the nine choirs of angels, each with their specific characteristics shown in the form of a celestial chorus encircling the light. Hildegard's work is dominated by circular forms.

St. Hildegard of Bingen, *Nine Choirs of Angels,* 12th century. Photo taken by Erich Lessing/Art Resource, New York.

Hildegarde's knowledge embraced medical science, nursing, music, herb gardening, natural science, and spiritual and religious philosophy. She was a prolific writer on many subjects, including theology and physiology. Her greatest achievement, however, was her knowledge of medicine. Hildegarde was more conspicuous as a physician than as a nurse, although she combined the arts of both in her work. (No account of nursing work as such or mention of the care of the sick, however, is found in her biographies.) Whether she actually practiced medicine or nursing is unknown, yet her vast knowledge is certain (Eckenstein, 1896). Hildegarde wrote 2 medical books between 1151 and 1159, when she was nearly 60 years old. One of these, *Liber Simplicis Medicinae,* which contained 9 books, was edited in the 16th century under the title *Physica St. Hildegardis.* The other, *Liber Compositae Medicinae,* contained five books that dealt with the causes, symptoms, and cures of disease. Normal and abnormal psychology were also discussed. Hildegarde referred to anxieties, obsessions, idiocy, phobias, and mental illness, and stated, "When headache, vapours, and giddiness attack a patient simultaneously they make him foolish and upset his reason. This makes many people think that he is possessed by an evil spirit, but that is not true" (Butler, vol. 9, 1934, p. 234). Another important work by Hildegarde was *Liber Operum Simplicis Hominis,* which was concerned with anatomical and physiological subjects. The range of subjects contained in these works is amazing. Hildegarde foretold autoinfection, recognized the brain as the regulator of all the vital processes, understood the influence of the nervous system, and discussed the vibration and pulsation of blood in the veins. Her mental distinction gave her a natural supremacy over her contemporaries.

Obstetrics. The care of the pregnant woman and the infant has always been a sensitive index of social progress. Contrary to popular opinion, childbearing has become more difficult as civilization has advanced. This has been particularly true among city populations. The simple outdoor life of primitive women and wives of serfs on feudal manors was substituted in the city by monotonous work that taxed one part of the body. In addition, city life was unhygienic in many ways. In countries where rickets prevailed, a woman's pelvis was often deformed, and cesarean operations were thus necessary to save the mother and child. Often the mother died because medieval surgery was crude. Returning Crusaders spread syphilis, which became an important cause of infant, and sometimes maternal, fatality. Intermarriage occurred and often resulted in the union of a man and woman of different body structures. Thus a woman might give birth to a child too large for the size of her pelvis.

During the Middle Ages the midwife, not the physician, delivered infants. Only in difficult cases was a barber-surgeon asked to help with the delivery. The unborn child was sometimes killed and the body removed with crude instruments introduced through the vagina. Reputable physicians attended pregnant women only in rare instances, usually if the woman was of noble birth or was the king's mistress. In fact, the services of a physician in this area were not valued, and strong prohibitions existed against their use. A Doctor Wertt of Hamburg was burned at the stake in 1522 for attending a delivery dressed as a woman.

Numerous paintings depict the practice of obstetrics by midwives. The delivery is portrayed in a variety of ways, and various themes are depicted: the guarding of the lying-in chamber from medical interference; the presence of the midwife and the child's nurse; the various positions used for delivery, such as sitting or squatting; and the types of appliances used—the obstetrical chair, the V-shaped stool, and beds.

Shortly after 1500 several events occurred that affected obstetrical care. The first book on obstetrics, *The Garden of Roses for Pregnant Women,* was written by Eucharius Roslin in 1513 at the request of the Duchess of Brunswick. In it, the best-known practices of obstetrical care were reinforced; full of superstitions, this book sanctioned the crudest practices of midwives (Haggard, 1929). The "podalic version" was introduced in France by Ambroise Paré. In this technique, used when a child was not in the proper position for a normal delivery, the surgeon inserted his hand into the uterus and the child was grasped by the feet and turned. A school of midwifery was opened at the Hotel Dieu in Paris in the 16th century. The Chamberlen brothers invented the obstetrical forceps in 1588. This instrument was kept a secret and passed on to the son of one of the brothers.

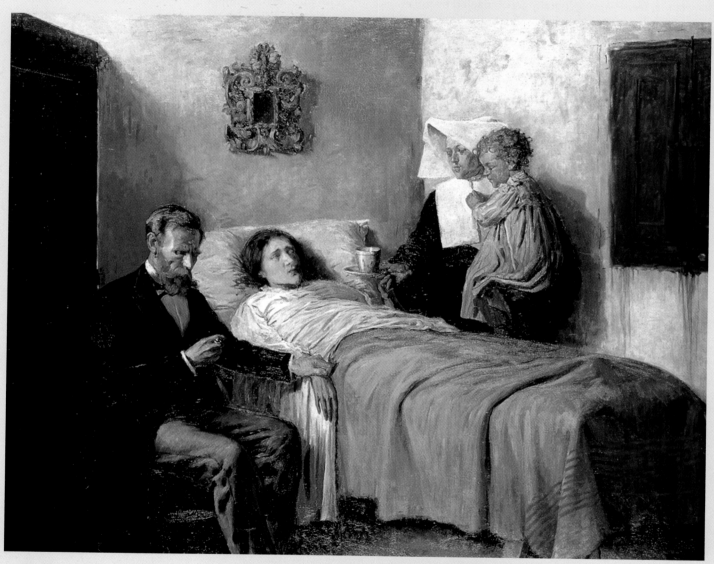

In this work, a contrast is presented: the detachment of the attending physician with the warmth of a nursing nun as they aid a sick woman. Numerous discussions about this work were held between Picasso and his father. To represent the sick woman, they chose a poor woman who had been begging with her child in her arms. The nun is probably a young boy in disguise, but the habit was possibly lent by Sister Josefa González of the order of St. Vincent. Picasso's father posed as the physician. The title originally chosen for this painting was "The Visit to the Sick Woman." Painted when Picasso was 15, it shows a doctor taking the pulse of a bedridden woman. A nun with a child in her arm stands on the other side of the bed, offering a cup to the sick woman.

Pablo Picasso, *Science and Charity*, 1897, painting, 197 × 249 cm. Copyright 2009 estate of Pablo Picasso/Artists Rights Society (ARS), New York.

EPIDEMICS AND PLAGUES

In the 14th century a catastrophic disease, the Black Death, swept over the European continent and England four times. The worst occurrence was in 1348. The Black Death is generally believed to have been a plague of the bubonic type, which results from the bite of an infected parasite. Primarily a disease of rodents, particularly rats, it is transmitted to humans by parasites such as fleas that have fed on the diseased rodents. Direct contact with an infected person can also transmit the disease. Rats on vessels that were being used to transport supplies spread the disease over the greater part of Europe. The name Black Death derived from the dark hemorrhagic spots that appeared under the skin of its victims. These were generally accompanied by inflammation of the lungs, unquenchable thirst, burning sensations, and inflammation in a variety of body parts. The outbreak of bubonic plague in the 14th century is considered one of the most devastating crises that ever occurred in human history. The sudden and unusual character of the disease brought terror to the people.

The Black Death, which caused the unprecedented mortality of one-fourth of the population of the earth (over sixty millions of human beings), appeared in Europe about 1348, after devastating Asia and Africa. . . . Sweeping everything before it, this terrible plague brought panic and confusion in its train and broke down all restrictions of morality, decency and humanity. Parents, children and lifelong friends forsook one another, everyone striving to save only himself and to come off with a whole skin. Some took to vessels in the open sea only to find that the pestilence was hot upon them; some prayed and fasted in sanctuaries, others gave themselves up to unbridled indulgence, or . . . fled the country to idle away their time in some safe retreat; others lapsed into sullen indifference and despair. The dead were hurled pell-mell into huge pits, hastily dug for the purpose, and putrefying bodies lay about everywhere in the houses and streets.

— *GARRISON, 1913, PP. 127-128*

The sweating sickness began in England and spread over the continent about the same time. This virulent disease is thought to have been influenza. Large numbers of people died within a day or a few hours after the first symptoms appeared. The onset was accompanied by chills, fever, headaches, stupor, cardiac pain, vomiting, fatigue, and profuse sweating. Some of the care that was rendered probably hastened patients' deaths. It was believed that the patient must sweat continuously for twenty-four hours. Therefore windows and doors were closed, stoves were lighted, and furs were piled on the ill person. Attendants stayed with the patients, attempting to keep them awake so that they might retain their senses. Various techniques were used to accomplish this, such as whipping the body with branches or dropping vinegar into the eyes. It has been remarked that the patient was "stewed to death" (Jamieson and Sewall, 1950).

Tremendous changes took place in the last centuries of the Middle Ages. The feudal system deteriorated. Cities and a middle class society developed. Luxury and misery, learning and ignorance existed side by side. The changing needs of society prompted the beginning of great social changes, revolutions, and reforms that would greatly impact the healing arts and the history of nursing.

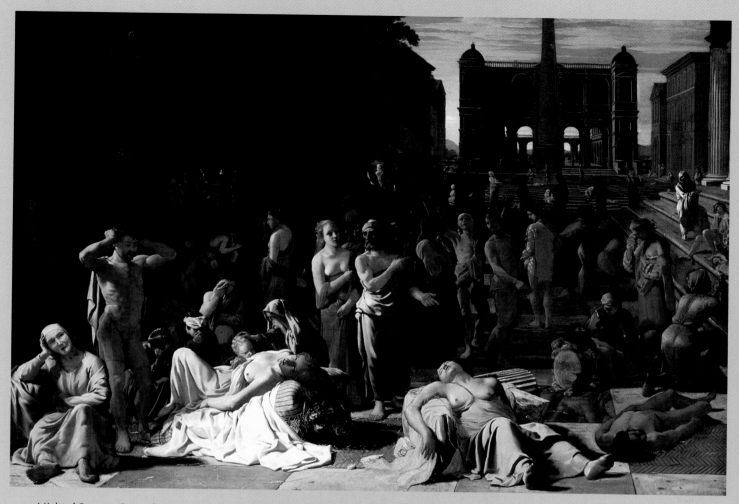

Michael Sweerts Brussels (1618-1664), *Plague in an Ancient City*, 1652-1654, painting, 118.75 × 170.82 cm, Los Angeles County Museum of Art, AC1997.10.1.

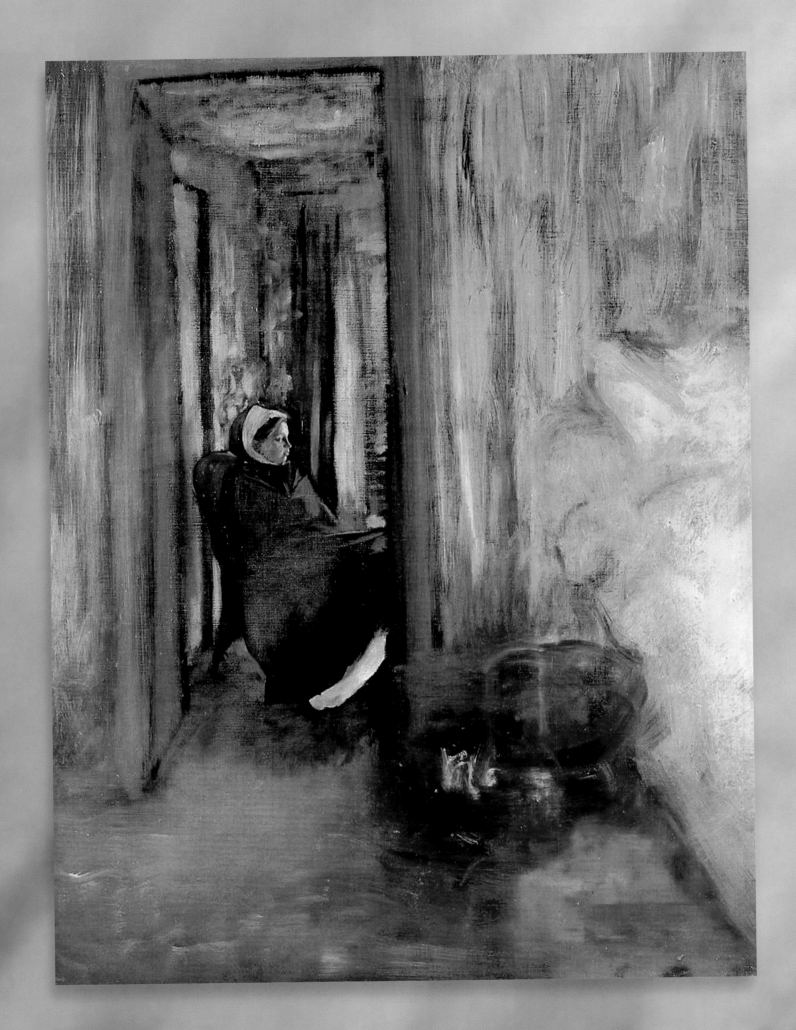

Nursing in Transition

The Dark Period and the Dawn of Modern Times

The transition from medieval times becomes quite evident toward the close of the fifteenth century. Among the momentous forces that again changed the existing social order were movements whose seeds had been planted in preceding centuries and that came to fruition in this era. Those forces were the Renaissance, the Protestant Revolt or Reformation, nationalism, the discovery of a new world, oceanic commercial enterprise, and diffusion of knowledge through the printed word. All of these forces influenced the healing arts in one way or another.

– SISTER CHARLES MARIE FRANK

Edgar Degas, *Garde Malade (Nurse)*, 1872-1873, painting, private collection.
Photo courtesy of the Athenaeum.

	1400	1500	1600	1700
Nursing		**1538** Jean Ciudad (John of God) founded Brothers of St. John of God in Spain **1550-1614** St. Camillus De Lellis founds Nursing Order of Ministers of the Sick **1550-1850** "Dark Period of Nursing" **1576-1660** St. Vincent de Paul founds Dames de Charité	**1633** Sisters of Charity founded **1634** St. Louise de Marillac becomes first Sister of Charity of St. Vincent de Paul	
Medicine and Health Care		**1514-1564** Andreas Vesalius, founder of modern anatomy	**1619** William Harvey describes circulation of blood **1632-1723** Anton van Leeuwenhoek discovers protozoa, bacteria, and human spermatozoa **1641** Arsenic prescribed for medicinal purposes in the United States **1668-1751** Thomas Coram labors to establish the Hospital for Foundlings in London	**1775** F.A. Mesmer uses hypnosis for health purposes **1798** Edward Jenner discovers a vaccine against smallpox
Science and Technology	**1473-1543** Nicholas Copernicus' discoveries precipitate Intellectual Revolution	**1561-1630** Henry Briggs promotes use of logarithms **1564-1642** Galileo	**1600** Dutch opticians invent the telescope **1642-1727** Isaac Newton discovers laws of gravity	**1742** Celsius invents centigrade thermometer **1752** Benjamin Franklin invents lightning conductor **1793** Eli Whitney invents cotton gin
The Visual Arts	**1400** Renaissance begins in Italy **1450** Renaissance spreads throughout Europe **1452-1519** Leonardo da Vinci, Italian artist who drew illustrations of human body **1475-1564** Michelangelo Buonarroti, Italian sculptor **1483-1520** Raphael, Italian painter	**1577-1640** Peter Paul Rubens, Flemish painter **1580-1666** Frans Hals, Dutch painter **1599-1641** Antony Van Dyck, Dutch painter	**1603** Carlo Maderna builds facade at St. Peter's in Rome **1606-1669** Rembradt van Rijn, Dutch painter **1656** Academy of Painting established in Rome **1697-1764** William Hogarth, British painter and engraver	
Daily Life	**1454** Guttenberg Bible printed	**1500** Suppression of monasteries occurs **1517** Reformation begins **1517** Martin Luther pins his 95 theses to castle church door at Wittenburg **1545** Council of Trent meets in Trentino, Italy	**1600** Wigs and dress trains become fashionable **1618-1648** Thirty Year's War **1665** Great plague in London	**1700** Factory system of production gains popularity **1738** First cuckoo clocks developed in Black Forest district of Germany **1750** Industrial Revolution begins in England **1789-1795** French Revolution **1797-1815** Napoleonic wars

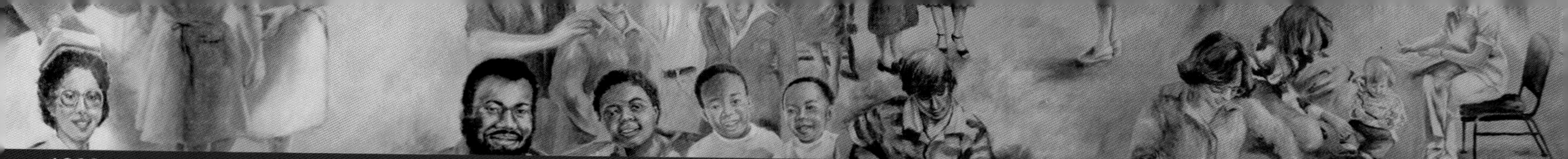

1809 Mother Elizabeth Seton establishes Sisters of Charity in America

1815 Mother Mary Aikenhead establishes order of Sister of Charity in Ireland

1820-1910 Florence Nightingale, pioneer and founder of modern nursing

1836 Deaconess Institute, Kaiserswerth, established

1840 Elizabeth Fry establishes Society of Protestant Sisters of Charity as visiting nurses

1844 Dickens' *Martin Chuzzlewit* depicts nursing conditions through characters of Sairey Gamp and Betsy Prig

1854-1856 Death rate of British Army reduced from 42% to 2% with nursing care

1857 Longfellow immortalizes Nightingale in poem *Lady with a Lamp*

1859 *Notes on Nursing* published

1860 Nightingale training school for nurses opens at St. Thomas Hospital, London

1861 Dorothea Dix appointed Superintendent of Female Nurses of Union Army

1881 Clara Barton and associates establish the American Red Cross

1881 Institute of Midwives established in London

1886 *The Nightingale,* first nursing journal, published

1893 Nightingale Pledge recited for the first time in Detroit, MI

1893 American Society of Superintendents of Training Schools for Nurses is created

---

1802-1887 Dorothea Dix focuses on care of criminals and the mentally ill

1805 Sartürner isolates morphine

1818 René Laënnec develops the stethoscope

1822-1895 Louis Pasteur lays foundation for science of bacteriology

1843-1910 Robert Koch discovers causes of cholera and tuberculosis

1849 Elizabeth Blackwell first woman to qualify as a doctor in U.S.

1861 U.S. Sanitary Commission created

1899 Aspirin introduced into medicine by Heinrich Dresser

1865 Gregor Mendel enunciates Law of Heredity

1806 Claude Clodion begins Arc de Triomphe, Paris

1846 First painted Christmas card designed by John C. Horseley

---

1800-1825 Latin American Revolution

1817 Elizabeth Fry establishes association to improve Newgate Prison conditions

1846 Irish potato famine

1848-1849 Extensive immigration to America from Europe

1854-1856 Crimean War

1864 Treaty of Geneva signed by twelve governments, establishing International Red Cross

1865 First carpet sweeper comes into use

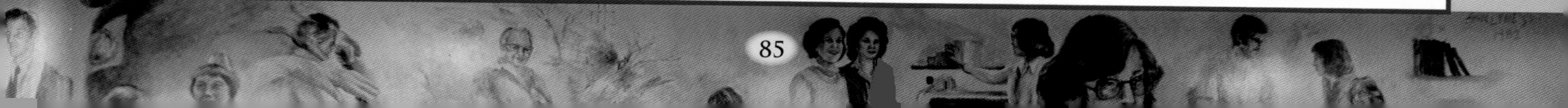

The centuries that immediately followed the Crusades were marked by great social changes. These changes began as early as 1250, tended to accelerate in about 1450, and by 1750 had become dominant as the modern characteristics of Western Europe. Between the fall of Constantinople (1453) and the Battle of Waterloo (1815), a variety of revolutions served to expand people's ideas about the universe and the meaning of human life. Yet these forces also threatened to destroy the social recovery that had been accomplished so far. The economic, industrial, intellectual, political, and religious revolutions inevitably had far-reaching effects on every aspect of life, including the treatment of the sick and the sick poor, the management of hospitals, and the status of nursing. These movements demonstrated the currents of popular feeling that increased tensions in most of Europe: the dominant Church, with its large temporal power, had become oppressive; the intellectuals were criticizing the doctrines of extreme ecclesiasticism; the laboring classes were bitter toward serfdom and oppression; and the religious were yearning for a return to a simpler faith with greater observance of ceremonials. The time was ripe for change.

RENAISSANCE AND REFORMATION

Two great movements, the Renaissance and the Reformation, occurred during the 16th century. Each was a result of the spirit of revolutionary change and the human quest for beauty and new knowledge. Probably the same social forces that produced the intellectual movement known as the Renaissance brought a split within the Church that eventually divided Christianity into warring sects. Together, these movements ushered in the "modern era," in which society was aware of the new world of Columbus, the old world of the Near and Far East, the new laws of Newton, and the old learning of the Greco-Roman ages. The scientific method of inquiry was initiated, and secularism became the modern spirit. All established institutions were affected during this transition period, which produced new institutions and also modified the old ones. Those having to do with the care of the sick were, perhaps, affected the most. Reforms promoted by the changing needs of the society began to occur, although in some instances they were slow in coming.

THE RENAISSANCE

The chaos of the Middle Ages subsided with the unparalleled phenomenon known as the Renaissance. Its exact time frame varies slightly depending on particular source materials, but the dates span a period from 1400 to 1700. Changes, although fairly rapid, came about at different times in different countries. The Renaissance is generally viewed, however, as the primary period of transition from medieval to modern times. This period in history was called a *rinascita,* or rebirth, by Giorgio Vasari (1511-1574), a Florentine artist and architect who believed that the major motivation for its evolution was a return to the cultures of ancient Rome and Greece. It was a period characterized by shifts in standards that were evident in literary and intellectual circles. Of primary importance was the decline in the power of the Church in temporal matters, which was accompanied by a rise in intense secular interest in worldly affairs. The dominant

spirit of the Renaissance was an interest in the things of the earth without reference to God. This notion was captured quite well by Devane (1948): "In the sixteenth century men rejected the Church but held on to their belief in Christ. In the seventeenth century the intellectuals rejected the divinity of Christ but retained their belief in the Deity. . . . In the eighteenth century, the Age of Enlightenment, the 'philosophers' openly rejected God Himself and substituted Reason. In the nineteenth century, religious indifferentism, materialism, general unbelief, and atheism spread among the masses" (p. 55). With this lost sense of relationship to God, the movement became characterized by both gullibility and skepticism, which led to a renewal of pagan superstitious practices and witchcraft. Yet outstanding Christian humanists emerged during this time, and renowned saints lived exemplary lives.

The Renaissance, indeed, has been viewed as both a blessing and a curse. It brought about a tremendous renewal of interest in learning in the areas of classical literature, humanism, and expressions of beauty. It was therefore also known as the period of humanism or the revival of learning. This renewal of interest in the arts and the sciences had a positive influence on the medical advancement during the Renaissance period. The learning, however, engendered materialistic, secularistic, and individualistic tendencies in the people. The society divided into two classes, the intelligentsia, who lived luxurious lives, and the working classes, who were oppressed because of their lack of knowledge and worldly possessions. Intellectual superiority and moral laxity emerged and drastically affected the political and religious character of the European people.

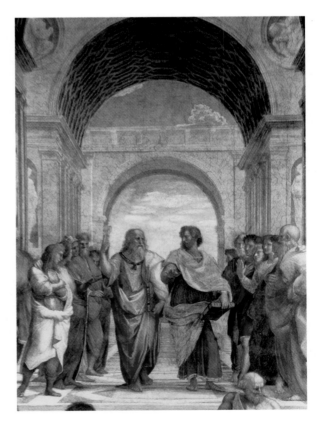

Leonardo da Vinci and Aristotle (in the center).

Raphael, *School of Athens*, Italy. Image from Ancient Art and Architecture Collection Ltd.

The Renaissance began in Italy in about 1400 and permeated Western Europe during the ensuing century. The new state of mind reflected itself in literature, painting, sculpture, and architecture. In addition, increasing wealth made it possible for art to penetrate the middle class. Painting, which had been limited to religious subjects and idealized themes from the Christian tradition, expanded to include the depiction of contemporary life. It was a realistic type of painting that sought to represent natural objects as they actually appeared. Artists even began to devote themselves to scientific studies. In Italian Renaissance painting, however, religious subjects still predominated. Renaissance painting, noted for its human quality, was "realistic" and attempted to reproduce natural objects as they actually appeared. During this era, prominent and innovative artists portrayed real people with increasing skill in perspective and color. Students from the school of Florentine art who left indelible marks in this field included Leonardo da Vinci (1452-1519); Michelangelo (1475-1564), who painted frescoes in the Sistine Chapel; and Raphael (1483-1520). Titian (1477-1576) led a second group of students from the Venetian school. The Florentine school was noted for form and grace of line; the Venetian school, for its mastery of color.

Leonardo da Vinci was perhaps the most versatile of the artists of the Renaissance. His masterpiece, *The Last Supper,* was painted on a wall of the refectory in a monastery in Milan. Although not a physician, he belonged to a guild comprising artists, apothecaries, physicians, and surgeons. Da Vinci was the first artist to consider anatomy for reasons other than its practicality.

> Leonardo himself made anatomical preparations from which he produced drawings, of which more than 750 are extant, representing the skeletal, muscular, nervous, and vascular systems. The illustrations were often supplemented with annotations of a physiological nature. Leonardo's scientific accuracy was greater than that of Vesalius, and his artistic beauty remains unchallenged. His correct assessment of the curvature of the spine went otherwise undiscovered for more than a hundred years. He depicted the true position of the *fetus in utero* and first noted certain anatomical structures. The sketches were seen by only a few contemporaries and were not published until the end of the last century.
>
> —*PETRUCELLI, 1978, P. 410*

Da Vinci painted marvelous variations in the expressions on the faces of his subjects. Reactions of fear, frustration, pain, joy, and happiness appeared natural and lifelike. His anatomical drawings and sketches were advanced for his time, perhaps because of the one hundred human dissections he performed.

The northern schools of painting, notably the Dutch and the Flemish, gave rise to artists such as Peter Paul Rubens (1577-1640), Anthony Van Dyck (1599-1641), and Rembrandt van Rijn (1606-1669). The Dutch and Flemish masters tended to abandon religious themes and devote themselves to merchants, princes, or scenes from everyday life. In addition, the Dutch masters were interested in human dissection and left excellent examples of it, as in Rembrandt's classic *Lesson in Anatomy.* Dissection was practiced in their medical schools.

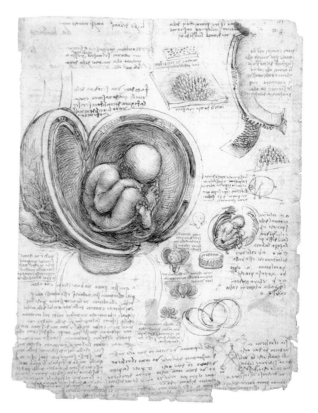

Da Vinci was the first to draw the single-chambered uterus at a time when it was generally believed that it was made up of several compartments, which was thought to explain the mystery of twin births. He was also the first to correctly describe the fetus in utero tethered by an umbilical cord. His ideas, however, that the cord was equal in length to the body at each stage of the child's development and that the child did not breathe since it was in water proved to be wrong. The majority of da Vinci's anatomical drawings were produced between 1506 and 1513.

Leonardo da Vinci, *The Foetus in the Womb*, 1510-1512, pencil and ink, 12.04" × 8.56" (30.1 × 21.4 cm), Windsor Castle, UK. The Royal Collection. Copyright 2008 Her Majesty Queen Elizabeth II.

THE REFORMATION

The Reformation (Protestant Revolt), which began in 1517, started as a reform and ended as a revolt. It was a religious movement that resulted in the division of Christianity. The Reformation was precipitated by two major factors: (1) the widespread abuses that had become a part of Church life and practice, such as the selling of indulgences and pardons, the veneration of relics, and the ignorance and depravity of the clergy; and (2) doctrinal difficulties. Essentially, a showdown occurred between the philosophy of St. Augustine, which dominated the early Church, and that of St. Thomas Aquinas, which gained preeminence in the 13th century. The more liberal doctrine of Aquinas permitted humans free will to choose between good and evil and to achieve grace through both good works and faith. Reform had been advocated for many centuries by influential individuals within and outside of the Church. Erasmus scoffed at the ridiculous abuses, and Thomas More prayed for internal

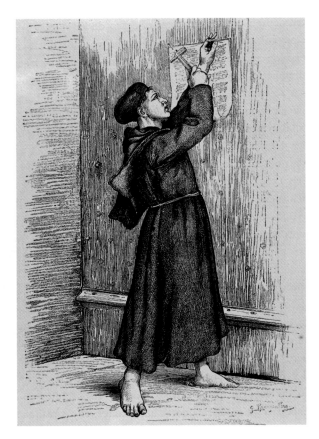

Martin Luther Posting the Principals of Lutheranism, Germany. Image from Ancient Art and Architecture Collection Ltd.

revision. The Church, however, did not take action and thereby paved the way for drastic intervention. By the time Martin Luther (1483-1546) pinned his Ninety-Five Theses to the castle church door at Wittenburg in 1517, many people were ready to oppose the established regime.

The rebellion against the Pope and the patriarchal rule of the Church was led by Martin Luther. Formerly a German mendicant monk, he became the leader of a group of dissatisfied people who broke away from the Catholic Church. These separatists were called Protestants ("those who protested"), a group that was to comprise many religious denominations. The followers of Luther were called Lutherans, and the Lutheran Church of today still adheres to his doctrine. The Lutherans rapidly declared both the independence of their congregations from the Pope and the right of each state to choose between the new Church and the old. Where there had been only one Europe, there were henceforth two. The Western world was divided into Catholics, who adhered to the teachings of Christ as dictated by the Church, and Protestants, who adhered to the teachings of Christ but rejected the authority of this Church. "The ground gained by Protestantism in that period brought to a climax influences that had been previously at work weakening the monastic system, and the changes resulting from the decline of monasticism had a distinct influence on nursing work and hospital organization" (Dock and Stewart, 1920, pp. 87-88).

Within a few years, northern Germany, Norway, Sweden, and Denmark were Lutheran. In addition, the success of Lutheranism encouraged other revolts against Catholic authority. During the next century, many sects arose, such as Anabaptists, Mennonites, Quakers, Calvinists, Presbyteri-

ans, Puritans, and Anglicans. Each interpreted the doctrine in a slightly different way; each was certain of the absolute truth necessary for salvation. Although this division weakened Protestantism, it enhanced society by insisting upon each individual's right to think for himself or herself. Some of these groups ultimately established churches that were as intolerant of opposition as was Catholicism.

Correction of abuses within the Church finally came with the Council of Trent, a general council of church authorities called at Trentino in northern Italy, in 1545. To identify means of removing causes of criticism and clarify the Church's position, this council continued its sessions for 18 years, until 1563. Serious abuses were altered, a popular and simple prayer book was adopted, and an even more rigorous discipline pervaded nursing orders and other groups. However, efforts to reconcile Catholicism and Protestantism failed, and Europe drifted into a tragic struggle between the two groups. The result was an era of hatred, civil conflict, the development of multiple factions that fostered individuality, and an international conflict known as the Thirty Years' War (1618-1648). People had also begun to depart for the New World, where they might ensure for themselves true freedom in religion.

The Reformation had no direct effect on hospitals in Catholic countries, and some hospitals did, indeed, survive in Protestant countries. Yet the majority of hospitals operated by the Catholic religious orders were closed or controlled by the "reformers." Monks and nuns were driven out of the institutions, particularly in the Protestant countries, which caused a tremendous shortage of people to care for the sick and the poor. The plight of the unfortunates became unbearable as they were reduced to a state of disgraceful pauperism. (Under Catholicism, the poor had been esteemed.) Hospitals became places of horror because there was no qualified group to take the place of the nursing religious orders. The most serious consequences occurred in England, where Henry VIII suppressed all the religious orders and confiscated the property of some 600 charitable endowments. Women were recruited from all sources to fill the nursing ranks. Many of these women were assigned nursing duties in lieu of serving jail sentences. This Dark Period of Nursing, between 1550 and 1850, saw nursing conditions at their very worst.

The seeming ambivalence of Protestant countries toward their sick and poor was the result of two conflicting influences: the desire to make money, to be rich and powerful; and the desire to be the chosen of God by doing works that would provide a state of grace. Laws and customs discouraged the humane care of the downtrodden and the weak, yet tremendous efforts were made to raise money to open hospitals and provide the necessities of life. This dichotomy had the most serious effect on nursing which, for a time, was thrown into a state of utter disorganization because public authorities were not ready to take over the care of the sick poor (Dock and Stewart, 1920).

Ultimately, the Reformation had a profound effect on nursing. Nursing suffered a great setback as monastic institutions were closed and nursing orders were eliminated. Even in some Catholic countries kings seized monasteries to accumulate more wealth and possessions. The most extreme impact on nursing in both Protestant and Catholic countries, however, was the nearly entire removal of men from nursing. Thereafter, the majority of Catholic nursing

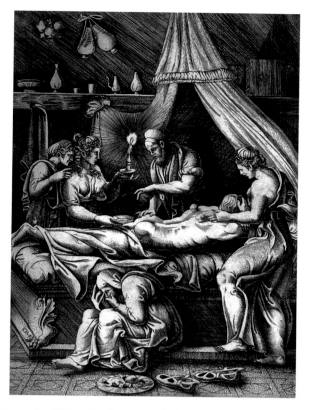

A large overhead fixture illuminates a surgical operation attended by more than 30 surgeons, anesthesiologists, physicians, and nurses, all of whom are presumably needed in the crowded operating room. There are also observers watching the surgeons at work. In the foreground, several cylinders of the anesthetic give the print its name.

Giorgio Ghisi, *The Allegory of Sickness*, Philadelphia Museum of Art.

orders were for women; nursing in Protestant countries became a woman's occupation.

THE AGE OF REVOLUTIONS

The intellectual, political, industrial, and economic revolutions were strong motivators for the change in human ideas and activities, as was the religious revolt. These movements—complex, varied, and interrelated—were influences that brought about the Renaissance. It was a time of flux, and these factors were crucial to the development of new necessities and new circumstances in the life that had evolved. The modern world was being born, but it would experience severe labor pains and harsh growing pains.

THE POLITICAL REVOLUTION

The political life that was characterized by feudal institutions in medieval times gave way to the establishment of national states during the Renaissance. These national states developed in the part of Europe that had previously been unified under the Holy Roman Empire. Unity was achieved through monarchs who gradually overthrew feudal lords. Authority was centralized in the monarchy; a system of private ownership and private enterprise took shape. Individuals and nations sought power through the accumulation of wealth and the grasping of opportunity.

Other changes occurred as nationalism progressed. The language and customs of the capital were spread through-

out the entire kingdom. The trend toward a national language had begun and fostered a growing pride in the land. Individuals in the literary field began to work in their own tongues instead of using Latin. This patriotism was also stirred by wars against other peoples, which were initiated by the ambition of kings. National competition developed and resulted in armed interventions. One great struggle followed another until the Seven Years' War (French and Indian War) in 1754, which earned first place for England. However, poverty and discontent followed the wars, and a series of revolutions erupted in an endeavor to create more democratic forms of government. The American Revolution (1775-1783), the French Revolution (1789-1795), and the Latin American Revolution (1800-1825) reflected a reaction against human inequality and placed an emphasis on individual rights. Finally, the Napoleonic Wars began in 1797 and ended in 1815 with the Battle of Waterloo. This particular conflict suppressed dictatorship for a time.

THE ECONOMIC REVOLUTION

The physical world was explored by England, France, Spain, Portugal, and Holland over the space of 3 centuries (1450-1750). New lands were discovered. North and South America, New Zealand, and the Oceanic islands were seized from less civilized peoples and colonized. India, China, and Africa were rediscovered and forced into trade with Europe. The world of humans had doubled in size, and humans' dreams of wealth expanded proportionately. Vast riches resulting from trade with the Old and New Worlds poured into Europe. Particularly significant was the bullion carried from the Americas by Spain, which put more gold and silver into circulation in Western Europe than ever before. It is estimated that the circulating gold and silver in 1500 was worth two million dollars; by 1600 its worth had increased to two billion. (Bullion could also have included precious stones.) A revolution in economic thought and practice was thus created. A capitalistic economic system, sometimes referred to as merchant capitalism, began to take form.

Mercantilism developed in response to economic activity for national ends. It began to emerge as early as the 14th century and was dominant during the 17th and early 18th centuries. This system held that a nation's wealth was determined by the amount of precious metals in its treasury. Government regulated industry, agriculture, and labor. Furthermore, government controls would ensure the maintenance of a stable economy and an increase in the stockpile, particularly through a favorable balance of trade. The state would create laws to force an excess of exports over imports and reap the profit in bullion. Businessmen became the dominant class in their community and were led by merchant princes. (Shakespeare's title character in *The Merchant of Venice* [1596] impressed men of England as the dynamic business leader.) Private enterprise, competition for markets, and expectations of gains were vital components of this system.

THE INDUSTRIAL REVOLUTION

The industrial revolution began in England in approximately 1750 and drastically upset traditional lifestyles. With the rise of the capitalist economic system, medieval craftsmen became dependent upon capitalists for wages. At first, craftsmen labored in their own homes, but by 1700 the factory system of production had gained popularity. This system required a centralized authority and elaborate financial expenditures.

A belief prevails that the industrial system was suddenly introduced during this time because of inventions in the textile industry. The real revolution, however, was under way before the occurrence of such inventions, which served to accelerate the process. Machinery did, however, standardize quality, and master craftsmen were forced to give up their crafts and lands and become laborers (factory hands) for rich individuals. All types of industries were affected, and efficiency became the key to success. In addition, as the era of invention unfolded, the number of manufacturing cities grew. Along with these cities came various social problems, including poverty, overcrowding, and disease.

THE INTELLECTUAL REVOLUTION

The intellectual, or scientific, revolution was precipitated by the discoveries of Copernicus (1473-1543), Galileo (1564-1642), and Newton (1642-1727). Their work demonstrated that the earth was not the center of the universe but revolved in accordance with universal laws over which humans had no control. Experimentation, measurement, and instruments to improve sight and hearing became important aids to observation and the development of the new science, experimental philosophy. The inductive method of thought was introduced as scholars began to observe facts and phenomena and determine solutions to the mysteries of life through a process of reasoning.

Numerous discoveries occurred in the physical sciences that seemed to revolutionize human thought. Nicholas Copernicus demonstrated that the earth turns on its axis and moves in an orbit around the sun. Johannes Kepler

(1571-1630) further developed this theory. Isaac Newton discovered the law of gravitation. Simon Stevin (1548-1620) developed the use of decimals. John Napier (1550-1617) and Henry Briggs (1561-1630) promoted the use of logarithms. René Descartes (1596-1650) invented analytical geometry. A number of other individuals were also instrumental in advancing the physical sciences. These 16th-century discoveries led to the invention of the telescope, microscope, thermometer, barometer, and pendulum clock.

The field of the biological sciences was also advancing and would become basic to the progress of medical science. The work of Andreas Vesalius (1514-1564), the founder of modern anatomy, was thought to be revolutionary. His findings were based on investigation rather than speculation. William Harvey (1578-1657) described the circulation of the blood, proof of which was published in 1628 in his *Exercitatio Anatomica de Motu Cordis et Sanguinis in Animalibus (On the Movement of the Heart and Blood in Animals)*. Robert Hooke (1635-1703) described the cellular structure of plants. Anton van Leeuwenhoek (1632-1723), using the recently invented microscope, discovered protozoa and bacteria and described human spermatozoa.

Advances in technology interfaced with progress in the sciences. This was particularly evident in the greatest of the Renaissance inventions, the printing press. Letters could be stamped on paper by movable type, and after the year 1500 manuscripts were rapidly superseded by printed volumes. The first complete book printed in this manner was the famous Gutenberg *Bible* (1454). Books became cheaper and more available to all educated persons. Scientists were thus able to read one another's books, exchange ideas promptly, build on published works, and communicate findings.

NEW DIRECTIONS IN MEDICINE

The birth of the scientific method of inquiry profoundly influenced the development of medicine in the Renaissance period. Medical scientists, like other scientists, benefited from the development of experimentation. Indeed, the majority of scientists were physicians. Yet the line between science and magic remained blurred. Quacks and charlatans continued to appear and to appeal to the poor and the ignorant, who depended on this type of "medicine man" and self-medication. This was necessary because physicians were the elite group during this period, and they took care only of the upper classes.

THE NEW ANATOMY

The first movement in the advance of medical science was the growth of anatomical knowledge and its application to surgery. The Flemish anatomist and surgeon Andreas Vesalius was undoubtedly the leader in this area. His work, which was based on human dissection, replaced crude medieval concepts and corrected more than two hundred mistakes in the works of Galen (Shryock, 1959). Vesalius's *De Humani Corporis Fabrica (The Fabric of the Human Body)* of 1543 illustrated in both words and pictures the dissected parts of the human body—the skeleton, muscles, vascular system, abdomen, and so forth. The findings of Vesalius were revolutionary but were not well received by his colleagues, who derided him and ignored his work. He eventually decided to leave academic life after suffering bitter disappointment and disillusionment. After Vesalius's death his

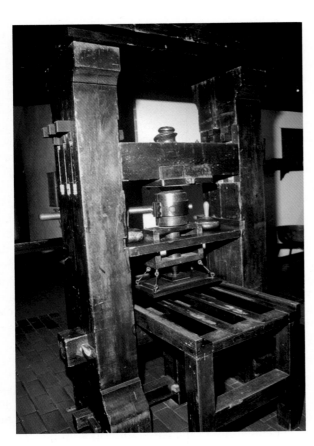

Gutenberg's Printing Press in Mainz, about 1450. Image courtesy of The Granger Collection, NY.

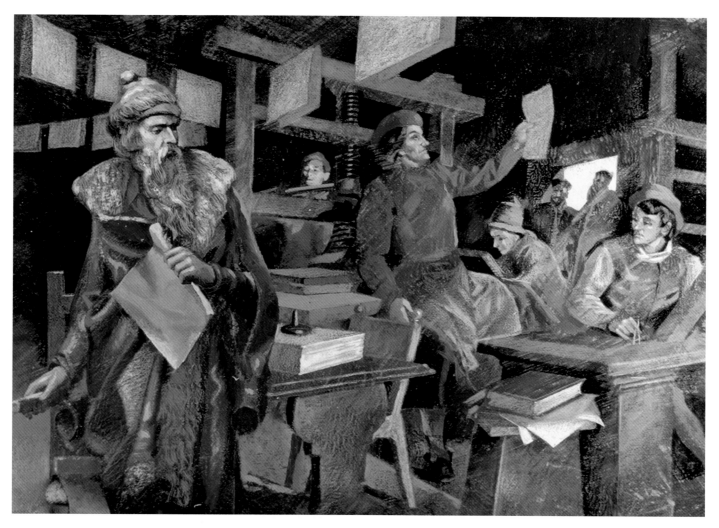

Gutenberg and his Press, Germany. Image courtesy of The Granger Collection, NY.

students continued his work. They included Gabriele Fallopio (1523-1562), the discoverer of the fallopian tubes.

Ambroise Paré (1510-1590), a Parisian surgeon, transformed the practice of surgery by applying anatomical knowledge with the scientific method. He began his career as a barber's apprentice, became an assistant at the Hôtel Dieu, and finally was a surgeon in the army. Based on his military experience, he reinstituted the use of ligatures for bleeding vessels caused by gunshot wounds. (His colleagues treated such wounds with boiling oil.) Paré brought together the surgeons of the universities and the barber-surgeons who were relied upon by the people. He believed that anatomy was a necessary prerequisite to a surgeon's skill. His practical genius included improvements in artificial limbs, trusses, hernia operations, and the glass eye. A man of many talents, he was also involved in dentistry; he restored missing teeth, reimplanted teeth, and invented a palatal obturator. His collected writings, *Oeuvres,* were first published in 1575. Paré always credited his success with patients to God, which was clearly evident in his motto: "Je le pansay. Dieu le guérit"; that is, "I treat him. God cures him."

Aureolus Theophrastus Bombastus von Hohenheim (1493-1541), better known as Paracelsus, was one of the most unusual individuals in medical history. Paracelsus viewed the body as a sort of glorified chemical retort and initiated

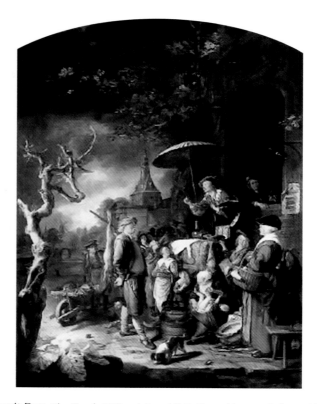

Gerrit Dou, *The Quack*, 1652, painting, 112 × 83 cm, Museum Boijmans Van Beuningen, Rotterdam.

the chemical approach to physiology. This often led others to view him as an ignorant, itinerant quack. He stressed that alchemists should stop attempting to make gold and start making medicines. Paracelsus particularly advocated the use of mercury, arsenic, lead, iron, sulfur, and antimony. He thus earned the title of Father of Pharmacology, even though he combined the use of chemicals with astrology. Paracelsus, an eccentric Swiss physician who had trained in Italy, consistently rebelled against authority. It is said that he publicly burned the books of Galen and other classical works. Paracelsus was one of the few surgeons of his time who renounced the accepted theory that pus was normal in the healing process. His was a daring approach to the field of medicine (Haggard, 1933). This transition from anatomy to physiology was clearly illustrated by work relative to the location of the heart and blood vessels. "Galen had declared that the vascular system centered in the liver and that blood ebbed and flowed through the body via a septum between one side of the heart and the other. But anatomists now found that no such septum existed, and this cast doubt on the whole theory" (Shryock, 1959, p. 140).

William Harvey (1578-1657) solved the problem by demonstrating in animals the actual circulation of the blood, with the heart acting as a central pump. These findings were published in his *Exercitatio Anatomica de Motu Cordis et Sanguinis in Animalibus (On the Movement of the Heart and Blood in Animals)*, one of the most important works in medicine and biology. He demonstrated that the heart was both a muscle and a pump, that blood flowed continuously in one direction along the arteries, and that the blood returned to the heart through veins, thereby completing a circle or cycle. Harvey was ridiculed and became known to some as "the circulator." To others, he was known as the Father of Modern Medicine because his most valuable contribution was the establishment of physiological experimentation.

The value of anatomical studies was demonstrated during the Renaissance. Wide-reaching effects of these studies oc-

curred in medicine, particularly in the areas of surgery and physiology. In addition, they logically led to the acceleration of the field of pathology.

THREE CENTURIES OF PROGRESS

The 17th century saw the beginnings of attempts to explain the mechanics of the human body. Jerome Fabricus (1537-1619) was the first embryologist. Athanasius Kircher (1602-

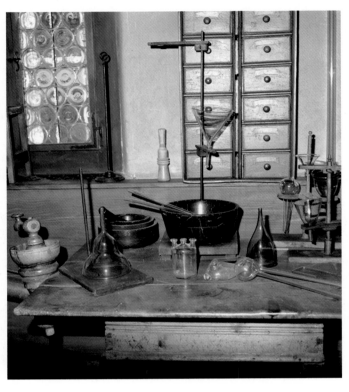

R. Sheridan, *Pharmacy Laboratory Used by Paracelsus, Basle,* items in the photo are from the 16th century, photograph, Switzerland. Image from Ancient Art and Architecture Collection Ltd.

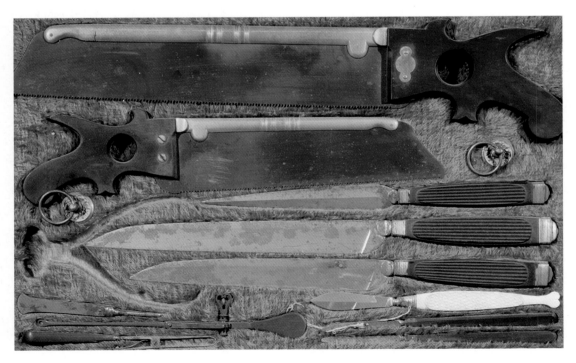

Set of Surgical Instruments for Studying Anatomy, 18th century, photograph, Museo Storico Nazionale dell'arte Sanitaria Rome.

1680), a Jesuit monk, used a microscope and connected microorganisms with contagion. Anton van Leeuwenhoek perfected the microscope and described bacteria and protozoa. The development of the clinical method was the contribution of Thomas Sydenham (1624-1689), who advocated the subjection of old theories to new scientific observation. His efforts to observe cases and to experiment with treatments led him to propose new methods of handling the sick. His thought was that specific diagnosis might lead to specific therapy. Sydenham provided detailed descriptions of prevalent diseases, such as dysentery and measles, and influenced the trend of medicine by emphasizing fresh air to replace the stuffiness of the sick room. Also during this period, the autopsy was found to be useful.

The real importance of these discoveries was the provision of frameworks for thought about normal and deviant functioning of the human body. These innovations served to illustrate a specific trend in medical thought, the readiness of enlightened persons to discard old ideas for new ones. Increasingly, medical and scientific names of renown began to emerge. In addition, this century witnessed the changing of alchemy into chemistry by Robert Boyle (1627-1691). His knowledge of the nature of a pure substance overturned the ancient, long-revered theory that the four elements are earth, air, fire, and water. With this change, the old humoral theory of health and illness was no longer relevant and a new theory was needed. One of the first new models was offered by René Descartes (1596-1650), whose *De Homine* was the original modern attempt at a physiology text. Descartes was perhaps the most influential intellectual of his generation.

It took the first 50 years of the 18th century for all of this new knowledge to be organized and digested. Advances continued to be made during this new century, but they were not as bold or as conspicuous as those of the previous one. They were, nevertheless, important in improving the standards of medical practice. Albrecht von Haller (1708-1777) systematized the new discoveries and made them available to practitioners. Giovanni Morgagni (1682-1741) correlated diseases of the organs with symptoms arising from impaired organic functioning. John Hunter (1728-1793) used his studies of comparative anatomy in new operative procedures and developed a simple, safe operation for aneurysms.

In the 18th century, smallpox was prevalent and took many lives. Edward Jenner (1749-1823), an Englishman, discovered a satisfactory method of vaccination against smallpox in 1798. This procedure, with certain modifications, is still used today. Despite its proven efficiency and effectiveness, however, vaccination has been avoided by some people.

Psychiatry developed as a separate branch of medicine in the latter part of the 18th century. The mentally ill had received cruel, inhumane treatment in the 16th and 17th centuries. Vicious practices were associated with the idea that the mentally ill were "possessed" of a demon or even the Devil himself. Hogarth, the English artist, vividly portrayed these conditions through such works as *The Rake in Bedlam*. Attempts were made to rectify conditions by certain physicians who protested that mental disease was a medical problem and that the mentally ill should be treated in a humane fashion. Vincenzo Chiarrigi (1759-1820) established sound treatment of the mentally ill in the hospital that he directed. A Quaker, William Tuke, introduced more understanding methods in a retreat (York Retreat, managed by the Society of Friends) that he had established.

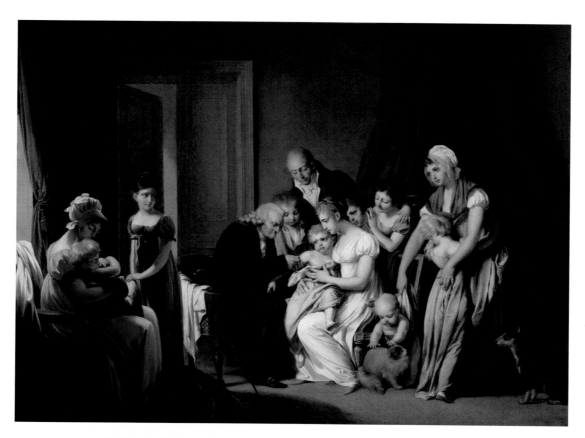

Louis-Leopold Boilly, *Vaccination*, 1807, painting, 60 × 49.7 cm, Bridgeman Art Gallery.

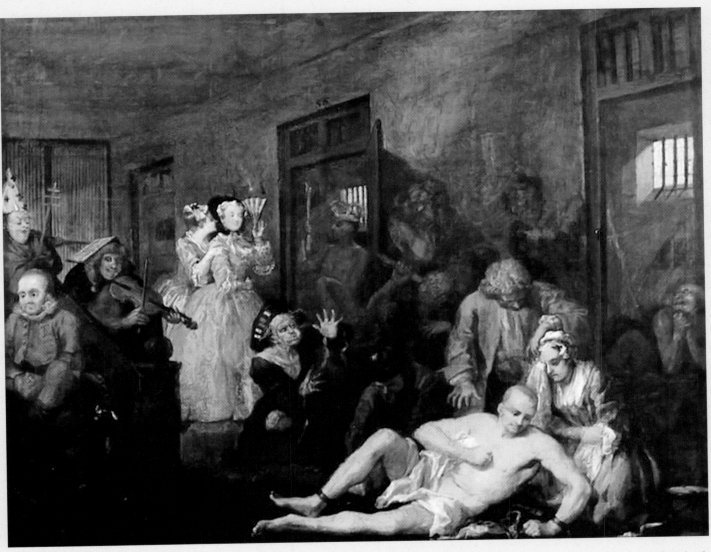

In the final painting of Hogarth's series *A Rake's Progress*, Tom ends his days in Bethlehem Hospital (Bedlam), London's celebrated mental asylum. Some of the details in the painting may appear disturbing to modern eyes but were commonplace in Hogarth's day (e.g., the fashionably dressed women who have come to the asylum as a social occasion to be entertained by the bizarre antics of the inmates).

William Hogarth, *The Madhouse*, 1733, oil on canvas.

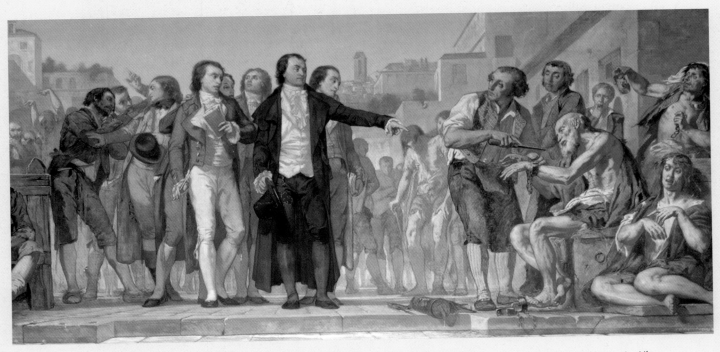

Charles Louis Muller, *Phillipe Pinel Has the Irons Removed from the Insane at Bicetre*, 19th century, mural, Giraudon. The Bridgeman Art Library.

Philippe Pinel (1745-1826), a physician and director of two hospitals in Paris, was probably the most famous leader in this area. He abandoned the use of restraining chains and advocated acceptance of the mentally ill as human beings in need of medical assistance, nursing care, and social services. His treatises on insanity were an effort to promote both scientific and humane treatment of the mentally ill.

During this same period, instruments were invented for the measurement and inspection of the body. A pulse watch was made by Sir John Floyer (1647-1734) in 1707. This watch ran for exactly one minute and then stopped, allowing the physician to obtain an accurate pulse count. Leopold Auenbrugger (1722-1809) initiated the use of percussion. Previously, this technique had been unique to innkeepers, who tapped wine kegs to determine the remaining volume. René Théophile Laënnec (1781-1826) devised the stethoscope after listening to heart sounds through a tube of rolled-up paper tied with a string. This was followed by a cylinder made of light wood, about twelve inches long, that could be taken apart by unscrewing it into two pieces. (Dr. Cammann of New York developed the binaural stethoscope.)

Advances in medicine continued into the 19th century. One of the greatest contributions was the result of the work of Louis Pasteur (1822-1895). His discoveries laid the foundation for the science of bacteriology. The principles relating to attenuation of viruses, preventive vaccination against disease-producing organisms, treatment of rabies, and the discovery of the process of pasteurization were all significant works that enhanced the practice of medicine and the prevention of disease. Robert Koch (1843-1910), one of Pasteur's contemporaries, discovered the causes of cholera and tuberculosis. Joseph Lister (1827-1912) became one of the greatest men in the history of surgery. He introduced the use of antiseptics in operating rooms as a preventive measure against infection. During Lister's time "hospitalism" was accepted as an unavoidable evil in surgery. This name was applied to the infectious epidemics that stalked the hospital wards and took many lives. Anyone who was fortunate enough to recover from surgery commonly regained only partial health. Such morbidity and mortality rates were not acceptable to Lister, who scientifically studied their causes and perfected his techniques. Other very important discoveries were facilitated by the work of Pasteur. In 1879, Neisser discovered the gonococcus; in 1880, Eberth described the typhoid bacillus; in 1882, Koch reported the discovery of the tubercle bacillus; in 1883, Klebs and Loeffier discovered the *Bacillus diphtheriae*, and Salvioli described the pneumonococcus that he found in thoracic exudates and tissues; in 1892, Welch and Nuttal first described Welch's bacillus (gas infection); and in 1897, Shiga discovered the dysentery bacillus. Other discoveries were equally important: Röentgen discovered x-rays in 1895; Marie and Pierre Curie isolated radium, and Widal introduced his agglutination test for diagnosing typhoid fever in 1896.

By the middle of the 19th century, other instruments of diagnosis had come into being. The stethoscope, the mercury thermometer, and x-rays had become important adjuncts to the practice of medicine. The introduction of ether and chloroform as general anesthetics greatly aided the practice of surgery. The science of bacteriology had become the basis of modern medicine and surgery. Indeed, medi-

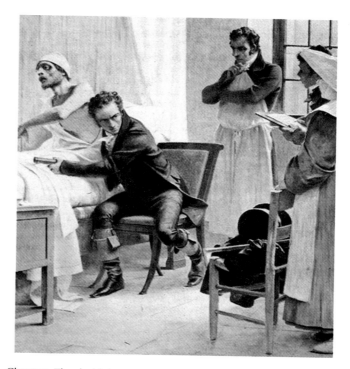

Chartran, Theobold, *Laennec Listening with his Ear Against the Chest of a Patient at the Necker Hospital*, painting. Photo courtesy of the National library of Medicine.

cine had made revolutionary progress. Many individuals, only a few of whom have been mentioned here, had made significant contributions. A rapid series of discoveries had occurred over the 3 centuries, and they would forever change the direction of medicine.

The development of the role of nurse-anesthetist as part of the increasing sophistication in surgery in the early 1900s was a major nursing contribution to this period in history. It was a response to the fact that it was no longer safe or satisfactory to have untrained medical students or attendants providing anesthesia. These early specialists were recruited from the available pool of trained nurses to meet very specific societal demands and needs. Opposition from particular specialty groups in medicine along with legal barriers to practice were among their greatest struggles. The same struggles continue to occur in current nursing specialization.

Obstetrics and Infant Welfare

The serious problem of infant and maternal death rates in the 18th century was tackled in Europe and the British Isles. Exact statistics are not available, so it is difficult to assess the change with any accuracy. The maternal death rate had many causes, including poor or no prenatal care, poor nutrition resulting from ignorance and poverty, infectious disease in early pregnancy, and the dreaded hospital infection—puerperal fever. In some instances it was also precipitated by delivery at the hands of ignorant, unwashed midwives.

In the 18th century, all but the wealthy used midwives for delivery in normal cases; surgeons were called in for difficult cases. The destruction of the child and removal of its body, however, were performed less frequently by the sur-

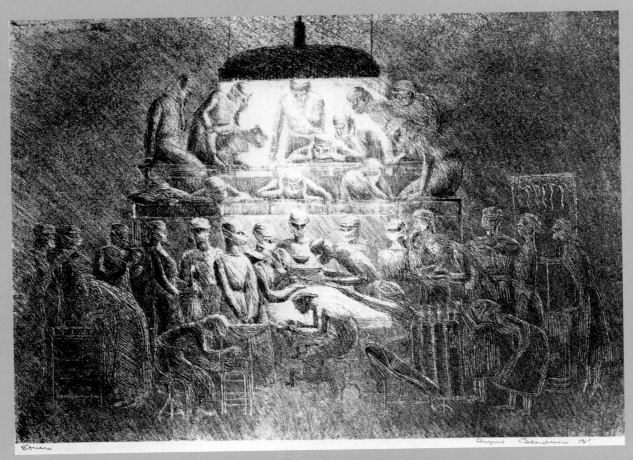

Alfred Bendiner, *Ether*, 1936, lithograph, Philadelphia Museum of Art.

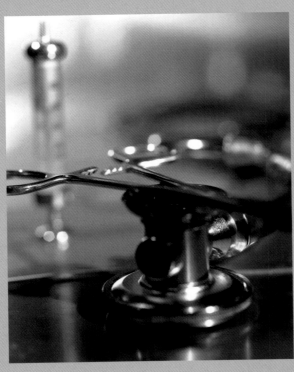

Nurses rely on a variety of common objects as well as their own knowledge to perform their work with excellence.

Nannette Bedway, *Implementation*, photograph, Nannette Bedway Studio, Cleveland, OH.

A
TREATISE
ON THE
ART of MIDWIFERY.
SETTING FORTH
VARIOUS ABUSES therein,

Especially as to the

PRACTICE with INSTRUMENTS:
THE WHOLE
Serving to put all Rational Inquirers in a fair
Way of very safely forming their own Judg-
ment upon the QUESTION;

Which it is best to employ,

In Cases of PREGNANCY and LYING-IN,
A
MAN-MIDWIFE;
OR, A
MIDWIFE.

By Mrs. ELIZABETH NIHELL,
PROFESSED MIDWIFE.

LONDON:
Printed for A. MORLEY, at Gay's-Head, near Beau-
fort Buildings, in the Strand.
MDCCLX.

Elizabeth Nihill, *A Treatise on the Art of Midwifery*, 1760, photo of front matter, London.

geons because of Paré's introduction of the podalic version and the invention of the obstetrical forceps by Peter Chamberlen. Yet surgeons tended to interfere with the deliveries, either with instruments or manually, so that their efforts to relieve mothers often brought death to both the mother and the infant. In the latter part of the 18th century, particularly in England, physicians assumed the care of pregnant women. They replaced surgeons in difficult cases and even attended some normal deliveries. The "consultant in midwifery," the predecessor of the obstetrician, became a specialist who was separate from both physicians and surgeons. Two other events occurred that assisted in the improved status of the mother: the addition of the study of obstetrics to the medical curriculum and the advent of lying-in hospitals. In the lying-in hospitals, however, improved maternal death rate was dependent on the conditions that existed. In some, where conditions were the worst, the rate fluctuated between 10% and 20% of the mothers who delivered.

As an answer to the problem of puerperal fever, William Hunter (1718-1783) proposed noninterference during delivery. During his time the number of cases of puerperal fever had increased to tragic proportions. The cause of the infection was unknown and the danger of contracting it was high, so Hunter's solution seemed plausible. However, some of his followers became so adamant about noninterference that some patients were allowed to die who might otherwise have been saved.

Ignaz Philipp Semmelweis (1818-1865) also became concerned about the problem of puerperal fever. Born in Budapest, he received his doctor's degree and the degree of master of midwifery from the University of Vienna. Semmelweis was granted a position as assistant director of the obstetrical clinic at the Lying-in Hospital in Vienna, where he was appalled by the high maternal mortality rate resulting from puerperal sepsis (childbed fever). He began to observe and analyze patient care and noticed a curious fact. He noted a difference between the maternal mortality rates in two clinics. The incidence of the fever and death was lower in the clinic where midwives practiced, but it was higher in the one where medical students practiced. Semmelweis determined that the spread of infection occurred because of the careless habits of the medical students, who went directly from the dissecting (autopsy) table to deliveries or to examinations of prenatal or postpartum patients. Therefore he demanded that the students wash their hands with soap and water, then wash them with chlorinated lime. As a result of this practice, there was a remarkable decrease in the death rate, from ten percent to a little over one percent. *The Cause, Concept, and Prophylaxis of Childbed Fever,* published in 1861, provided an account of this valuable research. The work of Semmelweis was ridiculed and was not accepted by his colleagues. The criticism he suffered apparently led to his eventual mental illness. In 1865 he died of blood poisoning, a condition that he had fought to eliminate.

Oliver Wendell Holmes (1809-1894), a graduate of Harvard, also fought to eliminate childbed fever. Holmes, who abandoned the study of law for medicine, in 1829 wrote the essay "The Contagiousness of Puerperal Fever," now considered a medical classic. This work was published five years before the research of Semmelweis became known and was bitterly attacked by the medical community. Like Semmelweis's theory, Holmes's idea regarding the cause of puerperal fever was correct. He republished the essay in 1855 with an introduction that criticized what he thought were unjust remarks. Gradually, the cause of the disease as identified by both Holmes and Semmelweis was accepted.

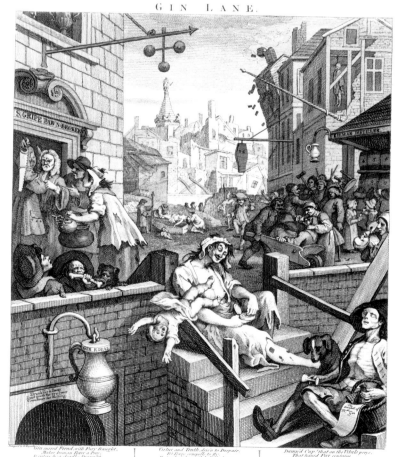

Hogarth's paintings vividly depict the frailties of human nature. His criticism focused on society's emphasis on a world in which people craved the "pleasures of life." Numerous activities are taking place in this illustration, which is a masterpiece of excess. One mother reaches for a pinch of snuff while another, at right, pours gin into her baby's mouth to pacify him; all around her are rowdy drinkers. The pawnbroker is extremely busy with those in need of money to buy liquor. In the background, a barber has hanged himself because no one in Gin Lane cares about personal grooming.

William Hogarth, *Gin Lane*, 18th century, engraving, England.

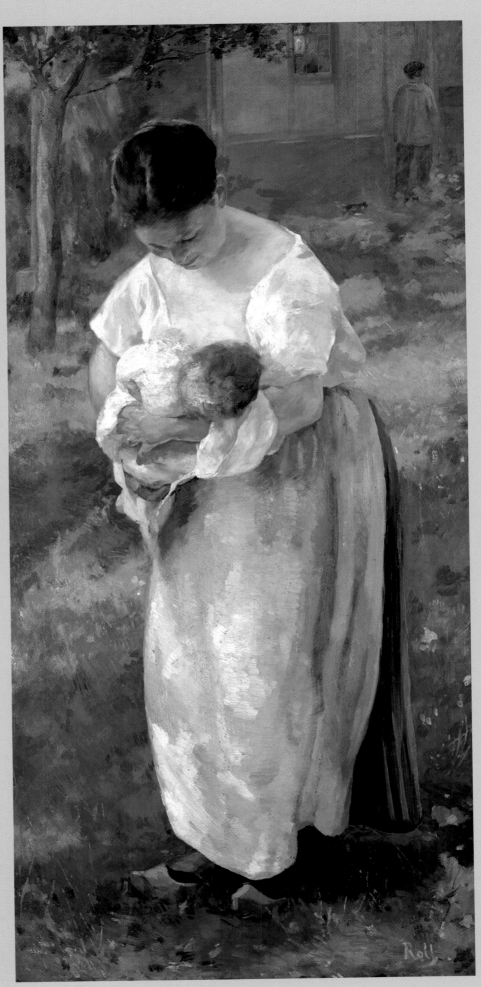

The rearing of children was often entrusted to a wet nurse, just as the children's births were often attended by a midwife. Since wet nurses and midwives were rarely adequately trained or supervised, at times their services were fatal for infants and, in the case of midwives, for the mothers as well. Nevertheless, midwifery and wet nursing were among the principal female occupations in the eighteenth century.

Alfred Roll (1846-1919), *The Wet Nurse*, oil on canvas. Copyright Musee des Beaux-Arts, Lille, France/ Lauros/Giraudon/The Bridgeman Art Library Nationality/ copyright status: French/out of copyright.

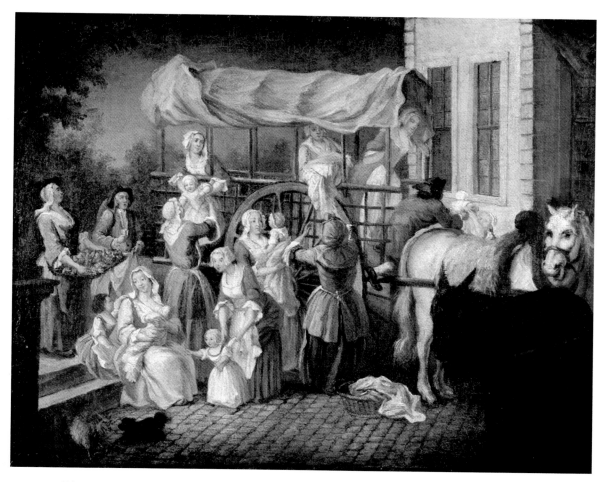

Etienne Jeaurat, *Arrival of the Wet Nurses*, painting, Musee Municipal, Laon, France. The Bridgeman Art Library.

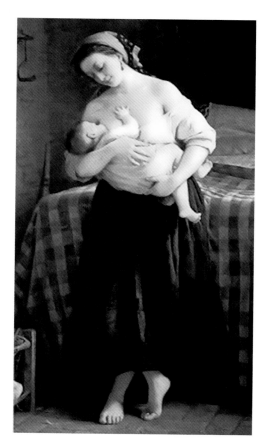

Mattia Pretti, *The Wet Nurse*, painting.

The plight of the child in this time was vividly depicted by the extremely talented British painter and engraver William Hogarth (1697-1764). Hogarth criticized the social problems of his day, which were present in a world craving the pleasures of life. His pictures were stories about the frailties of human nature, usually displayed in a scene of horrible devastation. In the *Works of Charles Lamb,* a section titled "On the Genius and Character of Hogarth" explains the extraordinary gift of this artist with the observation that most "pictures are looked at—his prints we read" (Lamb, vol. 1, 1818, p. 70).

The abandoned child had become a serious problem in the 18th century. There was public callousness and indifference to the practice of extensive infanticide. This attitude had to be changed before strides could be made in the reduction of infant mortality rates. Evidence was also available that demonstrated infant death resulting from neglect, cruelty, and illness. "The exact statistics are not available, but in the early part of the century, the infant mortality rate for children under five years of age was 50 percent. In London between 1730 and 1750, 75 per cent of all the babies christened were dead before the age of five. Of 10,272 infants admitted to the Dublin Foundling Hospital during 21 years (1775-1796) only 45 survived, a mortality rate of 99.6 percent. Many famous foundling hospitals of the period had similar records" (Dolan, Fitzpatrick, and Hermann, 1983, pp. 111-112).

The infant death rate was also caused by factors other than neglect and cruelty. They included *headmouldshot,* the overriding of the sutures of the cranium; *horseshoehead,* the separation of the sutures, usually associated with congenital cranial defects; and *overlying,* the practice in which nurses slept with infants. In addition, wet nurses were frequently hired, and they sometimes transferred disease to the child. Just as there were nurses who infected their sucklings, there were also infants who infected their nurses (Robinson, 1946). Bottle-feeding, too, was a potential contributor to infant death through the contraction of disease from contaminated milk and water. Some sources indicated the death rate of bottle-fed infants to be three times that of breast-fed infants. Another cause of infant death was the common occurrence of "dropping," the practice of abandoning infants on doorsteps of wealthy homes or simply leaving them to freeze or starve in the street. Infanticide continued into the 19th century.

As in most complex social movements, it is difficult to establish all the reasons for improvement in the infant death rate. However, this improvement was in no small part the result of the efforts of several individuals who wished to alleviate the high rate of infant mortality. Among them were Thomas Coram (1668-1751) of England, who labored to establish the Hospital for Foundlings in London (1738); Jonas Hanway (1712-1786), who was involved with the parish workhouse movement in England and persuaded Parliament to enact laws for the relief of infants of the poor; and George Armstrong (died 1781), one of the first English pediatricians, who was a staunch advocate of infant welfare and the prime leader in the dispensary movement that culminated in the establishment of the Dispensary for the Infant Poor on April 24, 1769. Perhaps the most significant development was a work titled "An Essay Upon Nursing and Management of Children," which appeared in London in 1750. It was written by William Cadogan (1711-1797), who became a physician at the Foundling Hospital after receiving master of arts, bachelor of medicine, and doctor of medicine degrees at Oxford. Cadogan was the first to write a simple, understandable book of instructions addressed to mothers about the care and feeding of infants and young children. Some might consider him the Doctor Spock of the era! A now-familiar passage dealt with Cadogan's plea for maternal feeding:

> There would be no fear of offending the husband's ears with the noise of the squalling brat. The child was it nurs'd in this way would be always quiet, in good humour, ever playing, laughing or sleeping. In my opinion a man of sense cannot have a prettier rattle (for rattles he must have of one kind or another) than such a young child. I am quite at a loss to account for the general practice of sending infants out of doors to be suckled or dry-nursed by another woman, who had not so much understanding, nor can have so much affection for it as the parents: and how it comes to pass that people of good sense and easy circumstances will not give themselves the pains to watch over the health and welfare of their children: but are so careless as to give them up to the common methods, without considering how near it is to an equal chance that they are destroyed by them. The ancient custom of exposing them to wild beasts or drowning them would certainly be a much quicker and more humane way of despatching them.
> — *QUOTED IN ROBINSON, 1946, P. 83*

Cadogan was an apostle of maternal breast-feeding; no other woman's milk was good enough for the child. He also stressed daily baths for infants and frequent changes of clothing. But of particular importance was his influence in removing all swaddling clothes from babies and emphasizing the use of loose clothing.

DISEASE AND EPIDEMICS

Epidemics continued to ravage Europe from the 16th through the 19th centuries. Devastating outbreaks of typhus and bubonic plague occurred and reduced the masses of the population to a pitiful state. These plagues were particularly ravaging because of the social decay that had resulted from urban industrialism. The epidemics of this early modern period forced physicians to accept a realistic view of medicine. Advances in medical knowledge and sanitation were frequently offset by the health hazards that existed in the large cities.

It is clear that health conditions were probably no better or worse than those that had existed in previous centuries. Yet urban living conditions facilitated the precipitation of diseases; sanitation was poor, sanitary facilities were lacking, sewage disposal was inadequate, cities were filthy, public health laws were lacking, water supplies were impure, and dirt and congestion inevitably brought pests such as rats, lice, and bedbugs, which carried infection. Congestion had increased, but its implications for health had been ignored. Epidemics of typhus were evidently spread to the European nations through foreign trade. Dark rooms served to increase the rate of tuberculosis. The value of fresh air was not understood, so doors and windows were closed when someone was ill. Windows in hospitals and homes were commonly blocked up or bricked over for economic reasons.

Approximately one third of the population of London died in the plagues that swept England in 1603 and 1625. Other diseases were equally destructive: typhus caused a large proportion of the deaths in the 18th century; smallpox was responsible for the death or disfigurement of one of every ten people in Europe. Conditions resulting from smallpox were even worse in new settlements, where immigrants

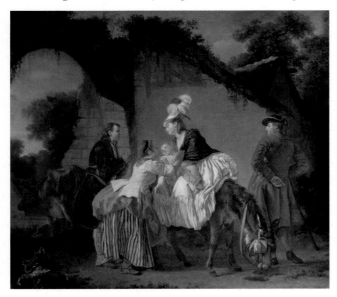

Etienne Aubry, *Farewell to the Wet Nurse,* 1776-1777, painting, 51.9 × 62.8 cm, The Clark Art. Copyright Sterling and Francine Clark Art Institute, Williamstown, MA.

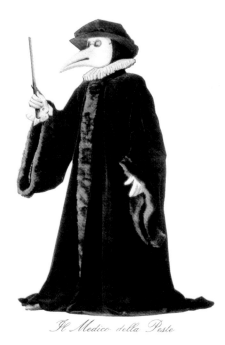

R. Sheridan, *Masked Plague Doctor from Venice*, 16th century, Italy. Image from Ancient Art and Architecture Collection Ltd.

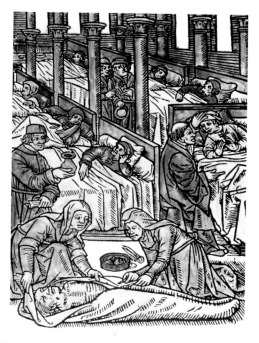

Plague victims.
Nuns and Monks Working in a Hospital, 16th century, wood engraving, France. Image from Ancient Art and Architecture Collection Ltd.

carried the infection to natives. At one point, Cotton Mather wrote that nine of ten, "nay 99 out of 100," of the American Indians perished of smallpox. Cholera epidemics occurred frequently, with the greatest severity in the slum areas. During the 19th century major outbreaks of this disease occurred in 1832, 1849, and 1866.

The home of the person who contracted plague was boarded up, and the well members of the family became prisoners of the house and the disease. The imprisonment usually lasted at least a month after all trace of the disease had disappeared. The plague physician wore an elaborate dress—a long red or black leather gown, leather gauntlets, a mask with glass-covered openings for the eyes, and a long beak filled with fumigants and antiseptics. He carried a container of sweet-smelling spices, a meager attempt to thwart the stench in the air. Fires were burned continuously in the streets to help purify the air. The dead were buried at night, usually with great precautions.

The spread of syphilis became so far-reaching that it could truly be called one of the great plagues. Although it had been differentiated from epidemic diseases by the close of the 15th century, it was thought to be spread in the same manner, through proximity to an infected person. At first the sexual nature of this disease was unknown, and no social stigma existed. Social attitudes changed very rapidly, however, as people became aware that syphilis was transferred through sexual relations. Secrecy was common among those who had contracted the disease, and it led to the forgoing of treatment and the spread of the disease through marriage. At that time, barber-surgeons treated syphilitic sores with salves that contained mercury; this treatment was extremely painful.

Urban life, trade, and industrialism contributed to the overwhelming health hazards that existed during these centuries. The situation was confounded by the lack of adequate means of social control. Reforms were desperately needed. Eventually, the organization of physicians, hospitals, and public health activities arose from the alterations incurred by the industrial revolution.

HOSPITALS AND REFORMERS

The Reformation brought about the widespread movement toward the suppression of monasteries that was led by Martin Luther and Henry VIII. The immediate result of monastic dissolution was that established hospitals and inns were taken away from the public, who had been dependent on them for many years. This was followed by a period of rapid deterioration in the care of the sick and the poor. A decline in the quality of public service, particularly for the sick, thus occurred and created a long period of stagnation and decay. As wars were waged about religious opinion, the sick and the poor were being neglected. The unselfish devotion of the religious orders was no longer available in countries where these orders had been oppressed. In this age of callousness and brutality, neither officials nor physicians took any particular interest in elevating nursing or in improving the conditions of hospitals.

HOSPITAL DECAY

After the Protestant Revolt, charitable activities were usually divided along religious lines or delegated to secular authorities. The religious struggles had no direct effect on hospitals in Catholic lands such as Spain and Italy. Many small institutions, however, were closed in countries in which the nursing orders were suppressed, and this led to the necessity of modifications in the large city establishments or the development of city hospitals. Severe utility replaced the beauty that previously had been associated with institutions for the sick. "The hospitals of cities were like prisons, with bare, undecorated walls and little dark rooms, small windows where no sun could enter, and dismal wards where fifty or one hundred patients were crowded together, deprived of all comforts and even of necessities. In the municipal and state institutions of this period the beautiful gardens, roomy halls, and springs of water of the old cloister hospital of the Middle Ages were not heard of, still less the comforts of their friendly interiors" (Nutting and Dock, 1937, p. 500).

The unsanitary conditions that prevailed in these hospitals led to outbreaks of epidemics. Diseases were seldom segregated. "It was not uncommon for the sick to be thrown into beds already occupied by several bedfellows—the dead or the delirious, side by side, perhaps, with those who still lived and retained their reason" (Jamieson and Sewall, 1950, pp. 268-269). Beds were so close together that cleaning was almost impossible. Consequently, all types of rubbish remained under them. Bed baths were not attempted; bleeding and purging were the usual treatments for all conditions. The following description of a late 18th century hospital was rendered by Max Nordau: "In one bed of moderate width lay 4, 5, or 6 sick persons beside each other, the feet of one to the head of another. . . . In the same bed lay individuals inflicted with infectious diseases beside others only slightly unwell; on the same couch, body against body, a woman groaned in the pains of labor, a nursing infant writhed in convulsions, a typhus patient burned in the delirium of fever, a consumptive coughed his hollow cough, and a victim of some diseases of the skin tore with furious nails" (Quoted in R. Dalton, 1900, pp. 17-27).

Mismanagement, inadequate staffing, and exploitation were common occurrences within these facilities. Men who were civil appointees assumed leadership and withheld authority from the women (matrons), who were placed in charge of the secular help doing the "nursing" of the day. Control of nursing was thereby lost by women. This was truly a period of the most complete and general masculine supremacy in the history of nursing. Women were without a voice in both hospital management and nursing organization. In addition, the typical nurses were usually the dregs of society, those individuals who were immoral, drunken, and illiterate. The actual squalor of the times is evident in a portion of the regulations (1789) of the Royal Hospital at Haslar, which were hung in the wards:

III. That no dirt, bones, or rags, be thrown out of any window, or down the bogs, but carried to the places appointed for that purpose; nor are any clothes of the patients, or others, to be hung out of any of the windows of the house.

IV. That no foul linen, whether sheets or shirts, be kept in the cabins, or wards, but sent immediately to the matron, in order to its being carried to the wash-house; and the nurses are to obey the orders of the matron in punctually shifting the bed and body linen of the patients, *viz*, their sheets once a fortnight, their shirts once in four days, their nightcaps, drawers, and stockings once a week, or oftener if found necessary.

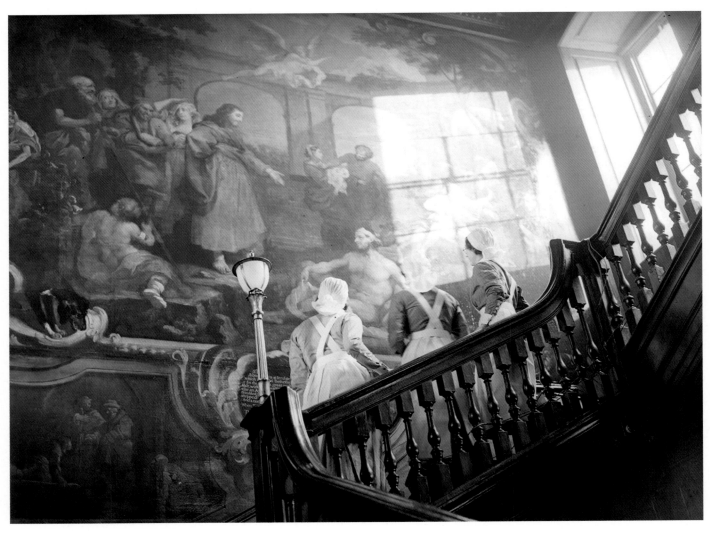

Nurses inspecting the wall paintings by Hogarth of "The Good Samaritan" and "The Pool of Bethesda" on the great staircase of St. Bartholomew's Hospital.

Fox Photos, *Hogarth Murals*, January 14, 1935, photograph, London. Getty Images.

V. That no nurse or other person do wash in the water closets. . . .

VIII. That no nurse do admit any patients, on any pretense whatsoever, into her cabin, nor suffer any person to remain in it at night, not even her husband or child.

IX. That any person concealing the escape of any patient from her ward, or that has not made due report, at the agent's office, of her having missed such patient, be discharged the hospital, upon proof thereof.

X. That all nurses who disobey the matron's orders, get drunk, neglect their patients, quarrel or fight with any other nurses, or quarrel with the men, or do not prudently or cautiously reveal, to the superior officers of the house, all irregularities committed by the patients in their wards (such as drinking, smoking tobacco in the wards, quarrelling, destroying the medicines, or stores, reigning complaints and neglecting their cure) be immediately discharged from the service of the house, and a note made against their names, on the books of the hospital, that they may never more be employed.

— HOWARD, 1791, PP. 180-182

In some hospitals, nurses were dismissed for abusing the patients. In other hospitals they were reprimanded or dismissed for abuses of various types, such as entertaining men at night in wards, scolding patients, or general patient neglect. Some attempts were thus made to develop qualifications for nurses or sisters who would function in the hospitals. Thomas Fuller (1654-1734), an English physician, developed the first set of qualifications, believing that the nurse should be:

1. Of middle age, fit and able to go through with the necessary Fatigue of her Undertaking.
2. Healthy, especially free from Vapours, and Cough.
3. A good Watcher, that can hold sitting up the whole Course of the Sickness.
4. Quick in Hearing, and always ready at the first Call.
5. Quiet and Still, so as to talk low, and but little, and tread softly.
6. Of good Sight, to observe the Pocks, their Colour, Manner and Growth, and all Alterations that may happen.
7. Handy to do every Thing the best way, without Blundering and Noise.
8. Nimble and Quick a going, coming, and doing every Thing.
9. Cleanly, to make all she dresseth acceptable.
10. Well-tempered, to humour, and please the Sick as much as she can.
11. Cheerful and Pleasant; to make the best of Every Thing, without being at any time Cross, Melancholy, or Timorous.
12. Constantly careful, and diligent by Night and by Day.
13. Sober and Temperate; not given to Gluttony, Drinking, or Smoking.
14. Observant to follow the Physician's Orders duly; and not be so conceited of her own Skill, as to give her own medicines privately.
15. To have no Children, or other to come much after her.

THE ENGLISH SCENE

The most serious consequences in health care occurred in England. It must be remembered, however, that an inward and religious revolution had taken place in England, especially in London, long before Henry VIII legalized its outward and visible form. Many people were ready for the break with Rome, the divorce between Henry and Catherine, and the suppression of the monasteries. This sovereign used the Protestant Revolt to free himself from papal authority with the excuse of the Church's refusal to sanction his divorce. An ulterior motive was based in the fact that monastic properties represented one fifth of his kingdom. Henry VIII suppressed all orders and confiscated the property of more than 600 charitable endowments. Many of them had been devoted to beggars, orphans, the elderly, and the poor, as well as to those who were acutely ill. Eventually, the civil government was forced to take over the general public relief, and this culminated in a "Poor Law" system, which was developed during the reign of Elizabeth I.

All the London hospitals were closed in two waves, the smaller ones in 1538 and the larger ones (income over 200 pounds per annum) in 1540. The fate of the larger English hospitals was particularly important because they essentially limited their work to the care of the sick. Decisions about their outcome ultimately affected the future of both medicine and nursing. The effect was immediate because "England alone among European countries possessed no hospital system" (Evans and Howard, 1930, p. 69). It was not long before the citizens begged that hospitals be given to the city to be financed and run by civil authorities. In 1547 the city of London petitioned Henry VIII's son, Edward VI, who reigned from 1547 to 1553, for permission to take over the largest hospitals—St. Bartholomew's, St. Thomas's, Bridewell, Bethlehem, and Christ's.

The city arranged to govern these hospitals through a court of governors, undertook to add to their endowments, maintained them through private subscription and rates (taxes), and assigned to each the specific responsibility for the solution of one social problem. St. Bartholomew's and St. Thomas's hospitals were to care for the sick poor; Bridewell, the unemployed; Bethlehem, the insane; and Christ's, the orphans. With the passage of time the individual functions changed. St. Bartholomew's and St. Thomas's hospitals progressed toward the cure aspect of the general hospital as opposed to the medieval custody function. Bridewell became a workhouse and a house of correction. Knowledge regarding treatment of the insane was lacking, and the conditions in Bethlehem Hospital were dreadful. Over time, the term *Bedlem*—a contraction of *Bethlehem*—came to indicate a state of confusion. Christ's Hospital became one of the leading schools of England. Such was the beginning of the civilian control of hospitals and the advent of lay nursing in England. Care of the sick in these institutions gradually deteriorated for about 300 years because England possessed no nursing class. Other Protestant countries followed trends similar to those in England, including reorganization of city hospitals.

RELIGIOUS NURSING ORDERS

The 16th century also saw renewed activity in nursing within the Church itself. Various religious orders devoted to this cause originated during this period. More than a hundred orders of females were founded specifically to do nursing. In fact, orders multiplied so rapidly, and some had so little permanence, that information about them is unavailable. Most prominent among them was an order of men, the Brothers of St. John of God, or the Brothers of Mercy. The name was derived from the inscription on their alms boxes:

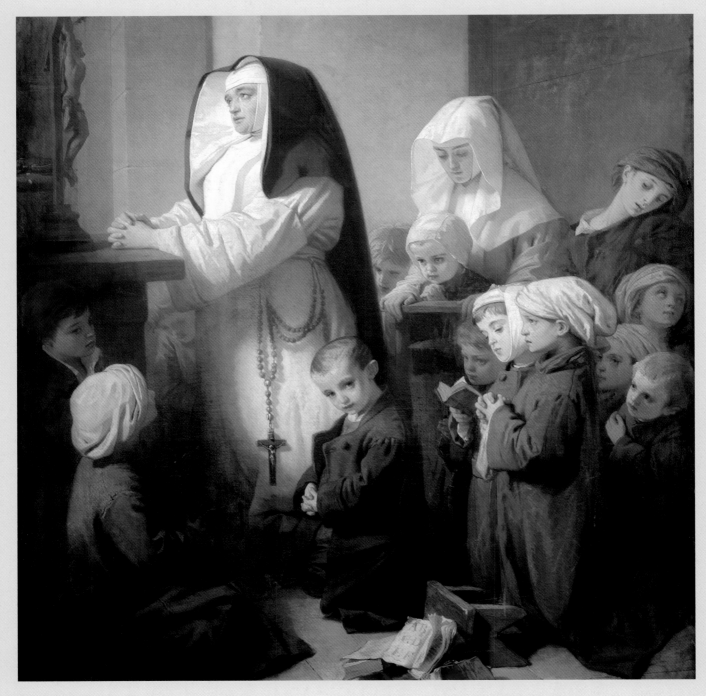

Isidore Pils, *The Prayer of the Children Suffering from Ringworm*, 1853, painting, Musee de l'Assistance Publique, Hospitaux de Paris, France. The Bridgeman Art Library.

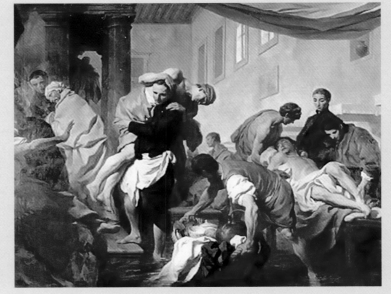

Saint Camillus de Lellis, founder of a religious order and universal patron of the sick, hospitals, and nurses.

Pierre Hubert Subleyras, *Saint Camillus de Lellis*, 1746, oil on canvas, 248 × 172 cm, Museo di Roma.

Brothers, do good *(Fate bene, fratelli)*. This order was founded in Spain in 1538 by a Portuguese man, Jean Ciudad (1495-1550), known as John of God (Juan di Dios).

After spending 18 years as a soldier, he vowed to devote his life to God if he recovered from a wound received in battle. In 1540, John opened a hospital in Granada and invited a group of friends to assist with the nursing care. At first these brothers were laymen, not monks, and they worked without a rule until 1570. They were mendicants who devoted themselves to nursing, hospital work, the distribution of medicines, the tender care of the mentally ill and abandoned children, and the visitation of the sick at home. Those in need were cared for in a very loving and special way. Homeless vagrants, the crippled, and even derelicts received devoted nursing service. It is said that St. John himself carried on his back the deformed who were unable to walk or crawl to the hospital. The Brothers of St. John eventually opened hospitals in Madrid, Cordova, Toledo, Naples, and Paris. This order spread over a large part of the civilized world within 50 years of its founding. Its members were probably the best-known nursing brothers *(baumherzigen Brüder)* in Catholic Germany by the 18th century. Paintings of Juan di Dios commonly show the wards of a hospital in the background.

Another notable nursing order of men, the Nursing Order of Ministers of the Sick, was founded by St. Camillus De Lellis (1550-1614). St. Camillus was totally committed to alleviating the sufferings of human beings, a service that was dependent on love. He achieved success in the care of the dying and eventually opened a hospital for alcoholics in Germany. His Nursing Order of Ministers of the Sick, an Italian order, did hospital work and in particular cared for those stricken with the plague in Rome in 1590. Conflicting information exists regarding the early life of St. Camillus. What is important, however, is that a series of illnesses that necessitated his hospitalization stirred him to devote himself to the care of the sick. The members of his order, popularly known as the Camillian Fathers and Brothers, took the three regular vows plus an additional one, a pledge to the work of nursing. They wore a red cross on their cassocks.

Perhaps the most interesting of these later organizations, and one that has maintained importance up to the present day, is the Sisters of Charity, founded by St. Vincent de Paul (1576-1660). With the creation of these Sisters of Charity, the beginning of modern nursing becomes apparent. This order developed at a time when destitution and disease resulting from continual wars were overcoming France. Political unrest was also pervasive. St. Vincent offered solutions to these problems that were both revolutionary and visionary. He was a quiet, unassuming French Catholic priest (Franciscan) whose experiences in his earlier life had prepared him to assist in alleviating the suffering of humanity. Of particular note were his capture by Barbary pirates and his sale as a slave to the Turks. St. Vincent described this experience in a personal letter:

This is how they set about disposing of us. After having stripped us naked, they bestowed on each of us a pair of breeches, a linen doublet and a cap, and marched us through the streets of Tunis, whither they had come in order to sell us. After having perambulated the town five or six times with chains round our necks, we were taken back to the boat for the dealers to come and see who could eat and

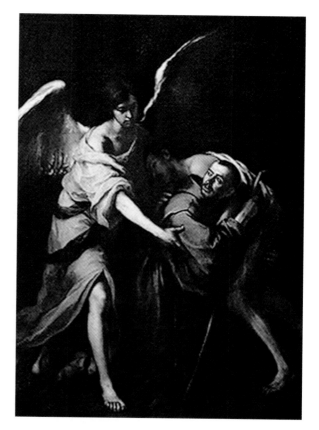

Bartolome Esteban Murillo, *St. John of God*, 1670-1674, oil on canvas.

who could not, by way of proving that our wounds were not mortal. When this was over they led us into the marketplace, where the dealers came and inspected us precisely as one does when one is buying a horse or an ox, opening our mouths to examine our teeth, feeling our sides, probing our wounds, making us walk, trot and run, carrying burdens the while, then setting us to wrestle in order to judge of our respective strength, and indulging in hundreds of other brutal proceedings.

— *QUOTED IN ROBINSON, 1946, P. 63*

Eventually, St. Vincent was able to return to Paris, where he was appalled at the conditions of the poor and the sick poor in such a large town. He began to assist the Brothers of St. John of God with the care of patients in the Charité Hospital in Paris. His interests soon reached out into provincial communities, and in 1617 he moved to the country parish of Châtillon-en-Bresse. Here St. Vincent was asked to appeal on behalf of a destitute family, and he became distressed by the indiscriminate relief that came forth. The family was inundated by well-meaning individuals. This event vividly demonstrated charity's waste because of the absence of control. It proved to be the motivating force for St. Vincent's institution of a society of ladies called the Confrérie de la Charité (Dames de Charité), whose members visited the sick in their homes to render both nursing care and spiritual consolation. This was the first society that dispensed organized aid in which service was offered to as many people as possible, with a minimum of duplication. The membership of eleven women took no vows and did not make any kind of promises. From this simple beginning, associations arose in numerous towns and villages. At first, all the branches were composed of women, but later a branch for men was

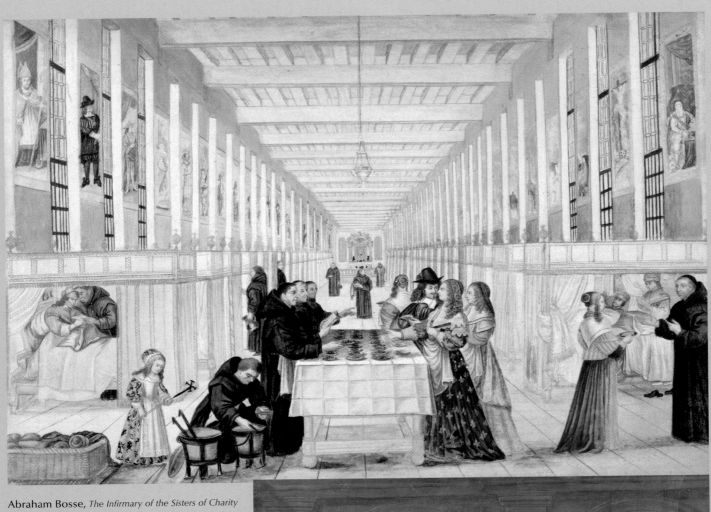

Abraham Bosse, *The Infirmary of the Sisters of Charity During a Visit of Anne of Austria*, 1601-1666, painting, Musee de la Ville de Paris, Musee Carnavalet, Paris, France. The Bridgeman Art Library.

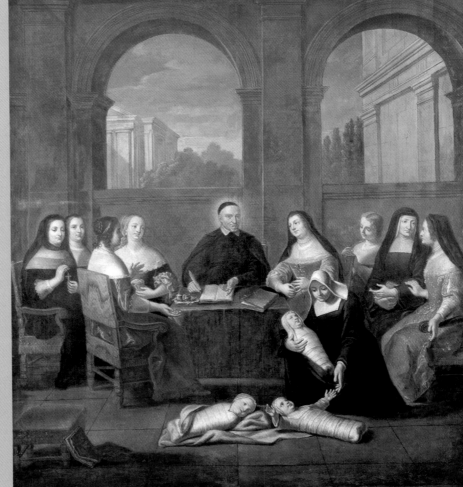

St. Vincent was instrumental in reforms for the poor and hospitals. Groups of men and women who formed under his counsel constituted the first societies for organized charity.

Jean Andre Frere, *St Vincent de Paul Being Shown Three Small Children*, 1729, painting, Musee' de l'Assistance Publique-Hopitaux de Paris, France.

founded at Folleville. With the extension of services into homes in the centuries that followed, St. Vincent became a regular feature in the work of certain communities. Sympathy for the poor was combined with a genius for organized reform, and that led to a system of social service, a method of helping people to help themselves.

Mlle Le Gras (1591-1660) became the first supervisor of these community nurses. Ste. Louise de Marillac, as she was later known, was a woman of noble birth and a widow when she became associated with the work of St. Vincent. In 1629 and 1631 she was sent on tours of the provincial associations to investigate their work and assist them with improvements in the care they offered. A secular nursing order called Les Filles de Charité, or the Sisters of Charity, was founded in 1633, and Ste. Louise became its superior. The Filles were initially under no written rule but merely followed a few regulations that had been drawn up by Mlle Le Gras. Young single girls were recruited; they were required to be intelligent, refined, and sincerely interested in the sick poor. An educational program was established to include experience in the hospital, in home visits, and in the care of the sick. Such was the modest and humble beginning of the now famous Sisters of Charity. (They perhaps should be called Daughters of Charity because St. Vincent always referred to them as filles.)

On March 25, 1634, approximately 1 year after this community was formed, Ste. Louise formally took a vow to devote herself to this life. She thus became the first Sister of Charity of St. Vincent de Paul. In the year 1642 the first four sisters took vows that were, and still are, only annual. This order was a tremendous innovation because it was active yet uncloistered. (The Church insisted that consecrated virgins be cloistered.) St. Vincent was adamant in this regard and expressed his ideal quite eloquently: "Their convent must be the houses of the sick; their cell the chamber of suffering; their chapel the parish church; their cloister the streets of the city or the wards of hospitals; in place of the rule which binds one to the one enclosure, there must be the general vow of obedience; the grating through which they speak to others must be the fear of God; the veil which shuts out the world must be holy modesty" (Nutting and Dock, 1937, p. 436).

The sisters' spiritual training was in the hands of St. Vincent, who provided a weekly lecture conference. These talks were written down by Ste. Louise, and about one hundred and sixty have been preserved. "They are a model of simplicity and clearness and remain the earliest as well as one of the best series of addresses on nursing ethics" (Seymer, 1932, p. 54). The organizational pattern of this order was composed of the following:

- A selected group, with set regulations restricting acceptance
- A common home with experienced supervision
- A system of instruction
- A probation of two months followed by a training period of five years
- Protection by the use of uniform dress of a type which would distinguish them from the people about them, and at the same time be secular
- Annual renewal of vows, or freedom to leave for marriage or change of occupation

— *Jamieson and Sewall, 1950, p. 323*

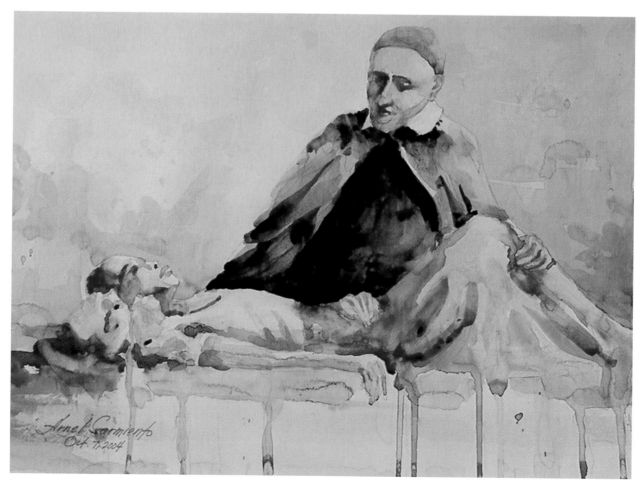

Arnel Sarmiento, *St. Vincent de Paul,* October 7, 2004, watercolor, 11" × 14", Santuario De San Vicente De Paul at St. Vincent Seminary Complex, Quezon City, Philippines.

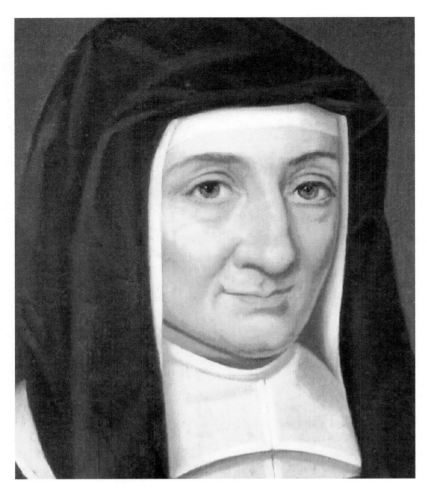

Gaspard Duchange, *Louise de Marillac,* 17th or 18th century, painting.

The dress of the Sisters of Charity did indeed become distinctive—a gray-blue gown and apron of rough woolen cloth, a stiff white collar, and a white, spreading headdress called a cornette. In 1809 the sisters were introduced into America by Mother Elizabeth Seton (1774-1821), the first American-born person to be canonized. A community was established at Emmitsburg, Maryland, after the rule of the Motherhouse in France had been obtained. It was not until 1815 that Mother Mary Aikenhead organized a community in Dublin.

The work of the society was ever expanding into new fields. One important role was the development of special skills in caring for abandoned children. With the encouragement of St. Vincent the women went into action to save these doomed children. They wandered the dark streets and gathered the babies who had been thrown away. Unwanted infants were frequently brought to the Hospice des Enfants Trouvés et Orphelins, established by Vincent's disciples, where the Sisters of Charity served as nurses. This organized relief for the foundlings of Paris led to the portrayal of St. Vincent with orphans in his arms, wrapped in his cloak. The sisters also took charge of hospitals, foundling asylums, and homes for the insane, and they engaged in general parish work. They taught in schools, gave heroic service during many wars, and offered care to lepers. The modern principles of visiting nursing and social service were sown during this time.

HUMANITARIAN EFFORTS

The existence of actual deterioration in hospitals during this time is beyond dispute. A period of stagnation had set in, and little or no progress in the art of nursing was made, particularly in Protestant countries. There is evidence of the squalor in the hospitals and the inferiority of the attendants within them. The era of reform, however, was on the horizon. A number of humane individuals were stirred by the painful social conditions of the 18th century and began to work for change. Of those reformers who lived before the 19th century, one of the best known was John Howard (1727-1789). An English philanthropist, Howard spent his life and fortune examining and reporting on the conditions of prisons, dungeons, pesthouses, hospitals, and asylums. His series of investigations were probably the most powerful factor in the improvement of public institutions in this era. Howard's writings depicted the story of the degradation of often forgotten human beings. Although prisons and lazarettos were his chief concerns, he left graphic notes about what he observed in hospitals. His reports on hospitals were the most authentic of the time and emphasized the necessity of fresh air and cleanliness. Howard's only praise was extended to the Sisters of Charity and the Beguines. His accounts varied, sometimes limited to a few sentences and other times consisting of long commentaries, as in the case of the Knights of St. John's Hospital at Malta:

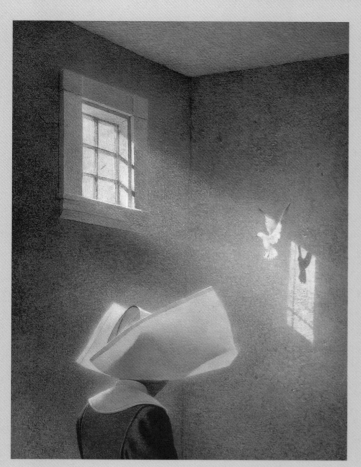

The Sisters of Charity were organized by St. Vincent de Paul and were perhaps the most widespread and best loved of all nursing orders. They took charge of hospitals, the poor, asylums, and parish work. They became widely known as visiting nurses because they also cared for the poor and the sick in their homes.

Robert Vickrey, *Trapped Bird*, 1970, painting. Copyright Robert Vickrey/Licensed by VAGA, New York. Used with permission from Visual Artists and Galleries Association.

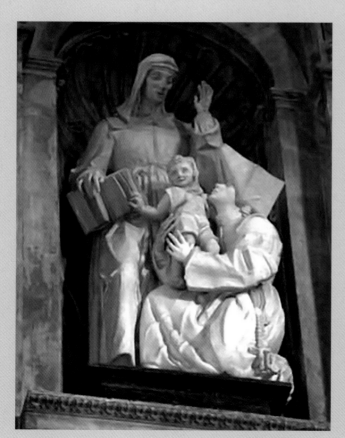

Antonio Berti, *Founder Statue of St. Louise de Marillac*, 1954, statue, St. Peter's Basilica. www.stpetersbasilica.org.

One ward is for patients dangerously sick or dying; another for patients of the middle rank of life; and the third for the lower and poorer sort of patients. In this last ward (which is the largest) there are four rows of beds; in the others, only two. They were all so dirty and offensive as to create the necessity of perfuming them; and yet I observed that the physician, in going his rounds, was obliged to keep his handkerchief to his face. . . .

From the kitchen (which is darker and more offensive than even the lower hall, to which it adjoins) the broth, rice soup and vermicelli are brought in dirty kettles first to the upper hall, and there poured into three silver bowls, out of which the patients are served. . . .

The number of patients in the hospital during the time I was in Malta (March 28th to April 19, 1786) was from five hundred and ten to five hundred and thirty-two. These were served by the most dirty, ragged, unfeeling and unhuman persons I ever saw. I once found eight or nine of them highly entertained with a delirious *dying* patient. The governor told me that they had only twenty-two servants, and that many of them were debtors or criminals, who had fled thither for refuge.

— *HOWARD, 1791, PP. 58-60*

The writings of John Howard were serious and had their effect. However, they penetrated society slowly, and for another generation or two, shameful conditions continued in both hospitals and nursing. Through Howard's efforts, vast prison reforms ultimately occurred and conditions were vastly improved.

Interest in reform grew steadily, and the movement brought about many changes that influenced health care and nursing. Humanitarian leaders emerged and dwelt on a sense of social responsibility for the welfare of others. One of these was the notable social reformer Elizabeth Gurney Fry (1780-1845), who was closely identified with practical reforms and the revival of nursing. Elizabeth Gurney was a deeply religious Quaker who married Joseph Fry and settled in London. She was beautiful, a gifted speaker, and the mother of eleven children. She, too, gave conspicuous service in prison reform based on principles similar to those of John Howard. She visited Newgate Prison in 1813 and was appalled by the conditions and treatment of the incarcerated prisoners. Murderers, sex offenders, thieves, and the mentally ill and retarded were all housed together in dark, damp, and poorly ventilated living quarters. Even children were inmates of this prison; they accompanied their parents if there were no relatives who could or would care for them. Such children were thus raised in an environment where there was a scant supply of food and little adequate clothing. Although the exterior of Newgate was beautiful, conditions within the walls were deplorable, as a description of the women's quarters illustrates:

> They occupied two long rooms, where they slept in three tiers, some on the floor and two tiers of hammocks over one another. . . . When I first entered, the foulness of the air was almost insupportable; and everything that is base and depraved was so strongly depicted on the faces of the women who stood crowded before me with looks of effrontery boldness and wantonness of expression that for a while my soul was greatly dismayed.
>
> — *WHITNEY, 1936, P. 193*

> The infirmary was not much better: On going up, I was astonished beyond description at the mass of woe and misery I beheld. I found many very sick, lying on the bare floor or on some old straw, having very scanty covering over them, though it was quite cold; and there were several children born in the prison among them, almost naked.
>
> — *WHITNEY, 1936, P. 184*

In *David Copperfield*, Charles Dickens vividly portrays Newgate using humorous, pointed descriptions of the existing evils. Few who read his story realized that it was one of personal experience. Dickens's father had been locked up in debtors' prison, where the entire family had resided until a fortunate legacy set them free. This novel brought the conditions of the English gaols to the attention of groups that might have ignored the reports of Elizabeth Fry.

In 1817, Fry established an association for improving the lot of women prisoners in Newgate Prison. She began a program of instruction for the children, arranged for sewing rooms for the women, found books for those who wanted to read, and was instrumental in developing a prison shop where materials produced in the prison could be sold outside. (Income from the sales would go to the workers.) In 1818, she visited other prisons in the British Isles and became known for her investigations of prison conditions and her attempts to arouse public opinion.

Fry, who became widely known as a philanthropist, eventually founded a society for visiting nursing that had its origin in her prison work. This group of ardent workers was called the Society of Protestant Sisters of Charity (1840). They were not, however, affiliated with any church and later were known as the Institute of Nursing Sisters. The members were prepared for private nursing only, to nurse the sick of all classes in their homes. These women received no classroom or theoretical instruction; for several hours a day for a few months' period, they visited Guy's Hospital in London, where they obtained a minimum of practical experi-

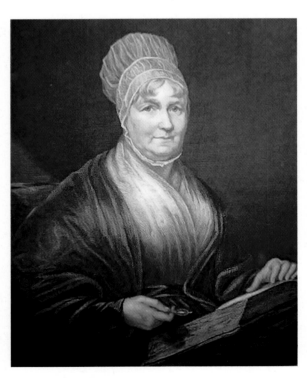

J.J. Hincliff, *Portrait of Elizabeth Fry*, 1850, engraving, book: (Chavannes, Herminie): Vie d'Élisabeth Fry : extraite des mémoires publiés par deux de ses filles et enrichie de matériaux inédits, Genève, V. Beroud et S. Guers, Paris, Librairie protestante, 1850.

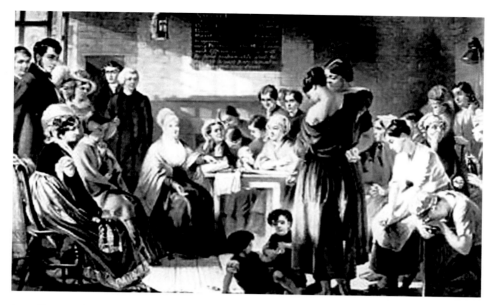

Jerry Barrett, *Elizabeth Fry Reading to Prisoners in Newgate Prison*, 1823, Religious Society of Friends, London, England.

ence. A similar organization was founded among the Quakers in Philadelphia at a later date.

Elizabeth Fry kept in close contact with other leaders of humane thought. Among them was Amalie Sieveking (1794-1859) of Hamburg, Germany, a well-known author who was prominent in the women's movement. Sieveking wished to develop a Protestant counterpart of the Sisters of Charity but was not successful. She therefore formed a group of volunteers, the Friends of the Poor, who visited the poor and the sick and gave nursing care in homes. Both men and women were originally included in this organization, and the women were called nurses rather than deaconesses. Amalie Sieveking was also interested in the establishment of better housing for low-income groups, the distribution of food, the finding of employment for the disabled, and other types of social services for the poor. She enlisted the aid of women who were interested in a larger sphere of women's work outside the home. From that time forward, social work and nursing became closely connected with feminist movements.

More than a century later, the efforts of Dorothea Lynde Dix (1802-1887) on behalf of the insane in the United States were comparable to the work of Howard and Fry. She focused on two distinct problems: the care of the criminal and the care of the mentally ill. Dorothea Dix found that many of the prisoners were actually mentally ill and that treatment for them was negligible. Her efforts, begun at the age of thirty-nine, eventually earned her the title of the John Howard of America. Her constructive work in surveying the needs of the mental patients and prisoners in Massachusetts led to the establishment of more than thirty psychiatric hospitals in the United States. One of these, Butler Hospital, was founded in Rhode Island with the backing of a wealthy and influential gentleman named Cyrus Butler.

The accomplishments of Dix were many, including the construction of the first state psychiatric hospital in Trenton, New Jersey; the elevation of standards of care for the mentally ill in the United States and Canada; and the systematic and careful recording of observations to be presented to the legislature to elicit support for humane treatment of the mentally ill. Dix had personally observed the incredible practices associated with these patients: some were confined in cages, closets, and cellars; other patients were

chained and naked; and some were beaten into submission with rods or other implements. Her crusades continued for approximately twenty years and resulted in a system of mental hospitals under government control. Legal commitment based on medical diagnosis as well as the abolition of restraints and the expertise of supervision provided the backbone of these institutions.

Dorothea Dix was the pioneer crusader for the mentally ill in the United States. Before her endeavors, few people realized that the mentally ill needed humane treatment or that they had been classified by law as being comparable to criminals. The mentally ill were commonly used as entertainment for the public, who paid a fee to witness their an-

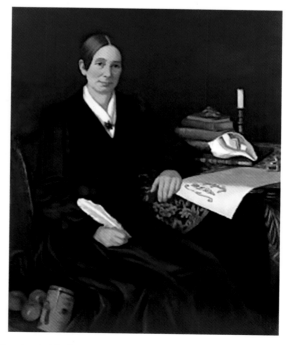

Dorothea Lynde Dix became well known for her crusades to reform insane asylums. She travelled thousands of miles to inspect existing mental institutions. Armed with evidence of shocking mistreatment, she appealed to state legislatures for improved treatment and improved facilities.

Susan Murray Stokes, *Dorothea Lynde Dix*, Worcester Women's History Project, Worcester, MA.

tics. In some locations they were kept in almshouses or jails. The most unfortunate aspect of this situation was that mental illness was thought to be incurable. Consequently, incentives for reform were lacking, and efforts toward change were not understood. So a persistent individual such as Dix was necessary to initiate a movement to correct an unpardonable situation.

SOCIAL REFORMS AND NURSING

The great revival of learning left the care of the sick untouched and unimproved. This was probably because of the prevailing thought that nursing was a religious rather than an intellectual occupation. Therefore, scientific improvement was not considered necessary. Yet the religious motive was lacking in the lay persons who were employed to care for the sick after the Reformation had occurred. Intelligent persons could not be persuaded to undertake nursing in the offensive municipal hospitals. Nursing slipped back into its ancient position of menial work, and the disagreeable features of nursing assumed prominence.

The latter half of the period between 1500 and 1860 saw nursing conditions at their worst. The Dark Period of Nursing had indeed arrived. In general, the lay attendants or nurses were illiterate, rough, and inconsiderate, oftentimes immoral or alcoholic. When a woman could no longer earn a living from gambling or vice, she might become a nurse. Nurses were drawn from among discharged patients and prisoners and from the lowest strata of society. They scrubbed, washed, cleaned, worked long hours (sometimes 24 to 48 hours at a stretch), and essentially led a life of drudgery. Roaches, other insects, and vermin plagued the nurses in the hospitals of this period. Pay for nurses was poor and was frequently supplemented in any way possible. The nurses expected and took bribes whenever they could

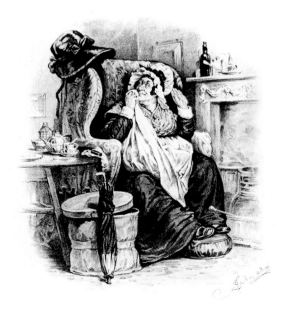

Sairey Gamp was the best-known literary image of a nurse until contemporary times. She clearly reflects Dickens' attitude toward nurses, those women who "care for the sick" by neglecting them, stealing from them, and at times physically abusing them. According to Dickens, Mrs. Gamp not only cared for the sick but also delivered babies and prepared bodies for burial. These functions were exclusively the function of women before the evolution of male obstetricians and funeral directors.

Frederick Barnard, *Mrs. Gamp*, circa 1894, etching/engraving, Corbis.

be obtained. This deplorable status of nurses and nursing continued throughout the period. Little organization was associated with nursing, and certainly no social standing was involved. No one would enter nursing who could possibly earn a living in some other way. As nurses, even the sisters of the religious orders came to a complete standstill professionally because of a persistent sequence of restrictions that started in the middle of the 16th century (Nutting and Dock, 1937).

The investigation of the social evils of the 18th century included an examination of nursing. Hogarth's cartoons and Charles Dickens' later descriptions of nurses were effective caricatures. In *Martin Chuzzlewit* (1844), Dickens depicted nursing conditions through the immortal characters of Sairey Gamp and Betsy Prig. Mrs. Gamp represents the hired attendant for the sick, the private-duty nurse; Mrs. Prig portrays the hospital nurse. Sairey Gamp was, in reality, not a fictitious character but an actual nurse Dickens' friend had hired for a member of his family. Both of these women cheated their employers, tricked their patients, and stole their rations and possessions. They demanded that the patients pay for extra little services, and they were deliberately cruel to the sick, who were at their mercy. In a later preface to the novel (November 1849), Dickens remarked: "Mrs. Sarah Gamp is a representation of the hired attendant on the poor in sickness. The Hospitals of London are, in many respects, noble institutions; in others, very defective. I think it not the least among the instances of their mismanagement, that Mrs. Betsy Prig is a fair specimen of Hospital Nurse; and that the Hospitals, with their means and funds, should have left it to private humanity and enterprise, in the year Eighteen Hundred and Forty-nine, to enter on an attempt to improve that class of persons" (Dickens, 1910, p. xxviii).

Mrs. Gamp's first appearance in the novel occurs when she is summoned by Mr. Pecksniff to prepare the body of Anthony Chuzzlewit for burial:

> She was a fat old woman, this Mrs. Gamp, with a husky voice, and a moist eye, which she had a remarkable power of turning up and showing the white of it. Having very little neck, it cost her some trouble to look over herself if one may say so, to those to whom she talked. She wore a very rusty black gown, rather the worse for snuff, and a shawl and bonnet to correspond. In these dilapidated articles of dress she had, on principle, arrayed herself, time out of mind, on such occasions as the present; for this at once expressed a decent amount of veneration for the deceased, and invited the next of kin to present her with a fresher suit of weeds: an appeal so frequently successful, that the very fetch and ghost of Mrs. Gamp, bonnet and all, might be seen hanging up, any hour in the day, in at least a dozen of the second-hand clothes shops about Holborn. The face of Mrs. Gamp—the nose in particular—was somewhat red and swollen, and it was difficult to enjoy her society without becoming conscious of a smell of spirits. Like most persons who have attained to great eminence in their profession, she took to hers very kindly; insomuch, that setting aside her natural predilections as a woman, she went to a lying-in or a laying-out with equal zest and relish.
>
> — *DICKENS, 1910, PP. 312-313*

Leigh Hunt, a contemporary of Dickens, also gave his version of the midwife specialist, which Sairey also professed to be. (Mrs. Gamp considered herself a monthly nurse or, as her signboard boldly stated, "midwife.")

> Her greatest pleasure in life is, when lady and baby are both gone to sleep, the fire bright, the kettle boiling, and her corns quiescent. She then first takes a pinch of snuff, by way of pungent anticipation of bliss, or as a sort of concentrated essence of satisfaction; then a glass of spirits—then puts the water in the teapot—takes another glass of spirits (the last having been a small one, and the coming tea affording a "counteraction")—then smoothes down her apron, adjusts herself in her arm-chair, pours out the first cup of tea, and sits for a minute or two staring at the fire, with the solid complacence of an owl—perhaps not without something of his snore, between sneeze and snuffbox.
>
> — HUNT, 1889

Help was needed for the prevailing nursing situation, and public interest in its improvement began to be demonstrated among various groups. Doctors, clergy, and philanthropic citizens advocated the establishment of nursing systems of a different character. Some favored a system under religious auspices, others a secular plan involving paid nurses. This public concern resulted in the beginning of significant changes that directed steady reform in nursing.

THE BIRTH OF MODERN NURSING

One of the most important factors in the regeneration of nursing was the Deaconess Institute at Kaiserswerth, Germany, established in 1836 by Pastor Theodor Fliedner (1800-1864). The deaconess orders, which had existed at the time of Christ, were revived by the Protestant churches during the 19th century. This movement was sparked by the recognition of the need for the services of women. In a number of instances, women were prompted by religious motives to perform social services, and the care of the sick became their chief duty. Kaiserswerth became the most significant organization of Protestant deaconesses for nursing service; it is credited with creating the first modern order of deaconesses.

This institute was started on a modest scale, but it made an indelible impression on the whole of nursing that was to follow. It indirectly influenced individuals such as Florence Nightingale, who stayed there for a brief time. Pastor Fliedner, who had been appointed to the parish of Kaiserswerth in 1822, began his social work by founding a German Prison Association (Rheinisch-Westfälischer Gefängnisverein) in 1826. The first of its kind in Germany, it was inspired by the work already achieved in prison reform in England and Holland. Fliedner had traveled abroad to raise money for his struggling parish and had observed these changes firsthand. He met Elizabeth Fry and was impressed with her work at Newgate Prison. He inspected hospitals, almshouses, and prisons in Holland, where he observed the work of deaconesses. He married Friederike Münster (1800-1842) in 1828, and their joint activities in prison reform led to the start of a small refuge for discharged prisoners in 1833. This asylum, as it was called, was the first of many units that formed the institute.

The Fliedners next turned their attention to the care of the sick and opened a small hospital with a training school for deaconesses. This hospital was started in a house, and the first deaconess, Gertrude Reichardt, the daughter of a physician, was admitted in 1836. By the end of the first year, six other women joined her for training. These deaconesses

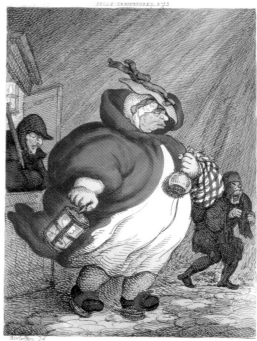

Thomas Rowlandson, *Midwife Going to a Labour*, 1811, etching with watercolor, 34.5 × 24.4 cm, The British Museum, London, England.

took no vows but simply promised to work for Christ. Although they received no salary, they were taken care of for life, an arrangement known as the motherhouse system. It was an offspring of the monastic system and offered security, because the deaconesses were provided with permanent homes and protection. They were sent out to district, hospital, and private-duty assignments or to distant mission fields. Their dress was a plain blue cotton gown with a white apron and a large turned-down collar. A white muslin cap with a frill around the face was tied under the chin with a large white bow. Outdoors, long black cloaks were worn and black bonnets covered their caps.

The institute expanded rapidly, and "by 1840 the work at the Kaiserswerth hospital had grown so much that two other adjoining houses were bought; by 1842 the total bed capacity was over two hundred, and the institute itself, now too small to house all the Deaconesses, had to be rebuilt" (Seymer, 1932, p. 63). The training of the deaconesses was designed to prepare them for both teaching and nursing. The program in nursing included a rotation in hospital clinical services (experience in wards for men, women, and children, as well as in wards for communicable diseases, convalescents, and sick deaconnesses); instruction in visiting nursing; theoretical and bedside instruction in the care of the sick; instruction in religious doctrine and ethics; and enough pharmacology to pass the state examinations for pharmacists. This program of study took three years. An interesting principle was enforced: the nurses were required to follow the physician's orders exactly, and the physician alone was responsible for the outcome.

> It is interesting to see how much of their system and detail our modern training schools have inherited from the Motherhouse—the probationary system, and the school for preparatory training; the letters from clergyman and physician as to character and health; the allowance of pocket-money; the grading of work, from easy to difficult; the chain

of responsibility; the grading of pupils from probationer to head nurse, with the superintendent at the head; the class-work and lectures; and every principle of discipline, etiquette, and ethics. The combination of a semi-military form of professional discipline with social equality, found in the Motherhouse, gave the pattern to the early American schools even more than did the English schools, whose system of class distinctions was never established in America.

— *NUTTING AND DOCK, VOL. 2, 1907, P. 40*

A framework of organization evolved at Kaiserswerth that incorporated many facets of service, which were divided into four areas: nursing, relief of the poor, care of children, and work among the unfortunate women who were prisoners and Magdalens. The institute became so well known that many individuals came to study its methods. Friederike Fliedner, the ambitious, energetic cofounder of Kaiserswerth, died in 1842. After her death, Pastor Fliedner married Caroline Bertheau (1811-1892), who had acted for three years as superintendent of the female surgical department of the Hamburg Hospital. Her nursing experience proved to be extremely valuable to the continuation of the work at the institute. The Kaiserswerth influence spread far beyond the German boundaries. In 1849, Fliedner escorted four deaconesses to Pittsburgh, Pennsylvania, where they were to assume responsibility for the Pittsburgh Infirmary (currently Passavant Hospital); other branches were founded in Jerusalem, Smyrna, Constantinople, Beirut, and Alexandria. Graduates of the program went to all corners of the globe to assist with the care of the sick and the needy. These beginnings set the stage for the founding of a new system of nursing by Florence Nightingale, whose reforms drastically changed the care of the sick throughout the world.

THE NIGHTINGALE REVOLUTION

It is doubtful that any woman's story has been repeated more often than that of Florence Nightingale. Yet existing accounts fall short in their efforts to document totally her place in the sphere of social progress. Unquestionably, she was a significant individual in nursing's history and has been identified as the pioneer and founder of modern nursing as well as a reformer of hospitals. Florence Nightingale pursued a mission of service to humanity throughout her lifetime. Her achievements are especially impressive when viewed against the background of the social restraints on women in Victorian England. Some still question which of her numerous contributions are the greatest. Certainly her efforts to reform the military health care system in Britain and her development of a solid nursing program built on sound professional standards are at the top of the list. Others of her endeavors are less well known, including her work in the area of statistical analysis. However, an article about Nightingale by Bernard Cohen identified her as "a pioneer in the use of social statistics and in their graphical representation" (Cohen, 1984, p. 128).

There is, indeed, controversy among biographers regarding the "true essence" of Florence Nightingale. For the most part, she is portrayed as a saint. Yet she has long been recognized by some of the principal authors to have had faults: Cook (1913) noted that she was hard on her friends and intolerant of other points of view; Strachey (1918) saw her as an eagle rather than a swan; Goldsmith (1937) depicted her with frankness; Woodham-Smith (1951) did not emphasize her faults but did not ignore them and considered her to be

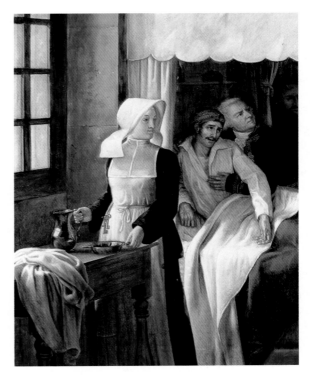

Alexandre Veron-Bellecourt, *Nurse*, 1800, painting, Musee du Chateau de Versailles. Image from The Picture Desk Library.

not only a saint but also a woman of the world. A contemporary author, however, F. B. Smith (1982), dismisses the earlier biographers as hagiographers who were blinded by the belief that those who do good deeds must be good themselves. It would seem that his purpose was specifically to malign Nightingale, to expose her as a fraud. Yet whatever is the truth regarding her personal side, it certainly does not detract from her many accomplishments. She was a "rarely versatile genius who starred in many roles and played them all with distinction" (Stewart, 1939, p. 208). In retrospect, there would probably be agreement that Florence Nightingale foretold the transition of nursing as it moved from a prescientific to a scientifically oriented era, as it now functions.

Florence Nightingale (1820-1910) was born in Florence, Italy, on May 12, 1820, to wealthy English parents who resided at Embley Park, Hampshire, in the summer and at Lea Hurst, Derbyshire, in the winter. The birth occurred during one of her parents' travels on the Continent, and they named the child for the city of her birth. Florence was raised in England with her elder sister Parthenope and received a thorough education. By the time she was seventeen she had mastered several ancient and modern languages, was well read in literature, philosophy, religion, history, political economy, and science, and had mastered higher mathematics. She was probably better educated than most men of her time. At a very early age she expressed a desire to enter nursing; her parents objected because of the hospital conditions of the day. Not surprisingly, they hoped that she would give up her unusual ambition, marry, continue in the social circles to which she was accustomed, and have children.

The details of Florence Nightingale's life at home, her education, her friends, and her travels are too extensive to relate in this book, but they have been amply dealt with in several biographies. This background is, however, important to an understanding of the driving force in her life—her struggle for independence and the freedom to pursue a

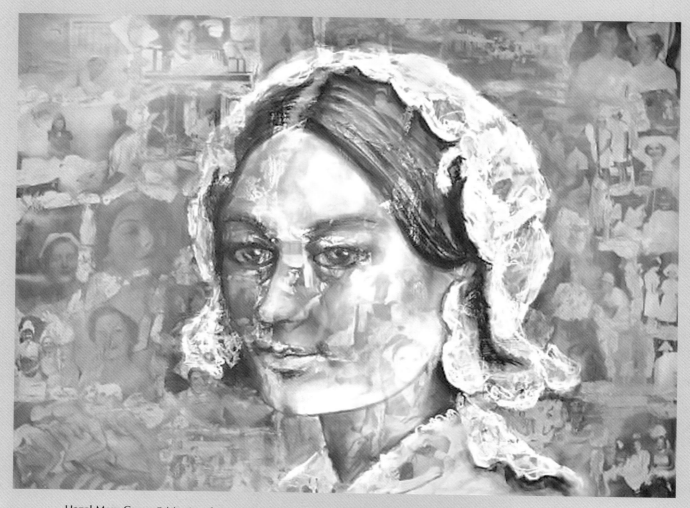

Hazel Mary Cope, *Celebration of Nursing in Queensland*, 2007, mixed on canvas, 92 × 122 cm. Photo courtesy of Hazel Mary Cope.

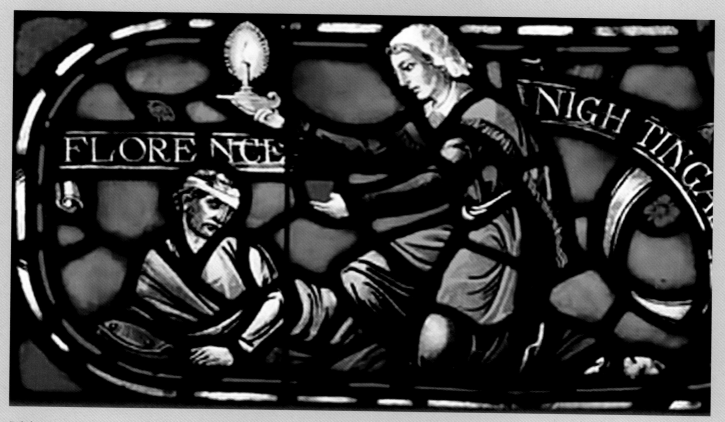

Ralph Ohmer (D'Ascenzo Studios, Philadelphia, PA), *World Christian Fellowship Window—Nightingale*, 1959, watercolor, entire window is 8′ × 20′. Used with permission of The Upper Room Chapel and Museum, Nashville, TN.

career in nursing. A series of events transpired during the sixteen years it took Nightingale to overcome family obstacles, some of which were particularly significant in her quest to become a nurse. She systematically studied various institutions she visited while engaging in Continental travel. Perhaps the crucial period of her career began with a visit to friends in Rome (1847), where she entered into a lifelong friendship with Mr. and Mrs. Sidney Herbert. Sir Sidney was to have the greatest influence on her life because it was through him that she later went to the Crimea and with him that she formed "the little war office." On this particular journey she also became familiar with the nursing of Roman Catholic sisterhoods. Her travels took her to Egypt, Greece, and eventually Germany, where she spent a fortnight at Kaiserswerth. Later in 1847 she enrolled in the program for nursing at Kaiserswerth and finished the three-month program. She spoke of this institute as her "spiritual home," although she would not admit that she had "trained" there. In her opinion the hospital work of the deaconesses was not on a level with the rest (Cook, 1913). In 1853, Nightingale studied in Paris under the Sisters of Charity at the Maison de la Providence. Returning to London, she assumed an administrative position as superintendent of the Establishment for Gentlewomen During Illness, a charity hospital for governesses that was run by titled ladies. She remained for a year and succeeded in creating a model institution by the standards of the day. However, she was disappointed that she was unable to initiate a formal training school for nurses. As she began to plan and prepare for the superintendent's position at King's College Hospital, British and French troops invaded the Crimea in support of Turkey's dispute with Russia. This event precipitated an unexpected opportunity for achievement.

The Hour and the Woman. In his biography of Florence Nightingale, Cook (1913) used the chapter heading "The Hour and the Woman" to express the period of Nightingale's life during the time of the Crimean War. No other phrase could better describe the union that occurred between the national need and the woman who was most fit to meet it. Soon after the outbreak of the Crimean War, England rang with the stories of the base at Scutari. With the British army was the first war correspondent, William Howard Russell of the *Times* (London), who quickly dispatched, in October 1854, vivid reports of the conditions of soldiers and the utter inadequacy of their care:

> It is with feelings of surprise and anger that the public will learn that no sufficient preparations have been made for the proper care of the wounded. Not only are there not sufficient surgeons . . . not only are there no dressers and nurses . . . there is not even linen to make bandages . . . it is found that the commonest appliances of a workhouse sick-ward are wanting, and that the men must die through the medical staff of the British army having forgotten that old rags are necessary for the dressing of wounds. . . . The manner in which the sick and wounded are treated is worthy only of the savages of Dahomey. . . . Here the French are greatly our superiors. Their medical arrangements are extremely good, their surgeons more numerous, and they have also the help of the Sisters of Charity, who have accompanied the expedition in incredible numbers. These devoted women are excellent nurses.
>
> — *WOODHAM-SMITH, 1951, P. 85*

An appalling picture of the army's inefficiency was thus presented to the public; it illustrated the high death rate from wounds, infections, cholera, and lack of adequate care. The country was seething with rage, and a letter in the *Times* demanded angrily, "Why have we no Sisters of Charity?"

Sir Sidney Herbert, by then the secretary of war, decided to defy precedent and for the first time in English history send a contingent of female nurses to military hospitals. He knew of one woman capable of bringing order out of the chaos and immediately wrote his remarkable letter (October 15, 1854) to Florence Nightingale, requesting her services. It contained a plea to supervise the military hospitals in Turkey:

> There is but one person in England that I know of who would be capable of organising and superintending such a scheme. . . .
>
> The selection of the rank and file of nurses will be very difficult: no one knows it better than yourself. The difficulty of finding women equal to a task, after all, full of horrors, and requiring, besides knowledge and goodwill, great energy and great courage, will be great. . . . My question simply is, Would you listen to the request to go and superintend the whole thing? You would of course have plenary authority over all the nurses, and I think I could secure you the fullest assistance and co-operation from the medical staff, and you would also have an unlimited power of drawing on the Government for whatever you thought requisite for the success of your mission. . . . but I must not conceal from you that I think upon your decision will depend the ultimate success or failure of the plan. Your own personal qualities, your knowledge and your power of administration, and among greater things your rank and position in Society give you advantages in such a work which no other person possesses.
>
> — *WOODHAM-SMITH, 1951, PP. 87-89*

Florence Nightingale was appointed Superintendent of the Female Nursing Establishment of the English General Hospitals in Turkey. She left for the base hospital at Scutari on October 21, 1854, accompanied by 38 nurses. (She realized that several were unfit, but time was of the essence.) They included 10 Roman Catholic sisters from Bermondsey, 8 Anglican sisters from the Sellonite order, 6 nurses from St. John's House, and 14 from various hospitals. The vast Barrack Hospital, which resembled a hollow square with a tower at each corner, was crowded with 4 miles of beds. It was designed to accommodate 1700 patients, but between 3000 and 4000 were packed into it. Candles stuck in empty beer bottles lit up endless scenes of human agony. An open sewer that attracted rats and vermin was immediately under the building. There was no water and no soap; there were no towels, few utensils of any sort, no knives or forks, and putrid food. It took 4 hours to serve a meal that for all practical purposes was not edible. Men lay practically naked or in ragged uniforms clotted with blood. When available, canvas sheets were used; these were so coarse that the wounded men begged to be left in their blankets. Essential surgical and medical supplies were lacking, and there was no dietary or laundry equipment of any kind. The death rate was 42.7 %.

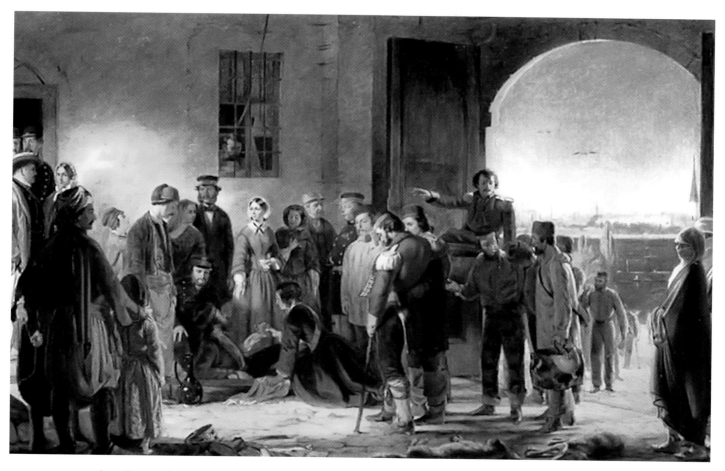

Jerry Barrett, *Florence Nightingale Receiving the Wounded from Scutari*, 1906, painting, 23½" × 35", National Portrait Gallery.

Nightingale demonstrated her skill as an administrator. She was, however, hampered by military authorities who resisted every change that she suggested. They resented that her authority was independent of the armed services, that she was a civilian, and that she was a woman. In addition, she had to reckon with the unreliability of many on her nursing staff. Yet none of her difficulties with doctors was as wearing as those with her nurses. In the midst of appalling horror, this type of situation occurred: "I came out, Ma'am, prepared to submit to everything, to be put on in every way. But there are some things, Ma'am, one can't submit to. There is the Caps, Ma'am, that suits one face and some that suits another. And if I'd known, Ma'am, about the caps, great as was my desire to come out to nurse at Scutari, I wouldn't have come, Ma'am" (Woodham-Smith, 1951, p. 119).

Overcoming these obstacles and obtaining the obvious necessities, Nightingale transformed a place of horror into a haven where patients could truly convalesce. She set up five diet kitchens, a laundry, coffee houses that provided music and recreation (canteens), reading rooms, and organized classes. In the evening, after the other nurses had retired, she made solitary rounds. She stopped to observe the condition of the sickest patients. These rounds were made with her famous lamp or lantern, which had a wind shield that prevented the candle within it (placed in a candlestick) from being extinguished. Henry Wadsworth Longfellow immortalized this Lady with a Lamp in his poem of 1857, "Santa Filomena":

Whene'er a noble deed is wrought,
Whene'er is spoken a noble thought,
Our hearts, in glad surprise,
To higher levels rise.

The tidal wave of deeper souls
Into our inmost being rolls,
And lifts us unawares
Out of all meaner cares.

Honour to those whose words or deeds
Thus help us in our daily needs,
And by their overflow
Raise us from what is low!

Thus thought I, as by night I read
Of the great army of the dead,
The trenches cold and damp,
The starved and frozen camp—

The wounded from the battle plain,
In dreary hospitals of pain—
The cheerless corridors,
The cold and stony floors.

Lo! in that house of misery,
A lady with a lamp I see
Pass through the glimmering gloom,
And flit from room to room.

And slow, as in a dream of bliss,
The speechless sufferer turns to kiss
Her shadow, as it falls
Upon the darkening walls.

As if a door in heaven should be,
Opened, and then closed suddenly,
The vision came and went—
The light shone and was spent.

On England's annals, through the long
Hereafter of her speech and song,
That light its rays shall cast
From portals of the past.

A lady with a lamp shall stand
In the great history of the land,
A noble type of good,
Heroic womanhood.

Nor even shall be wanting here
The palm, the lily, and the spear,
The symbols that of yore
Saint Filomena bore.

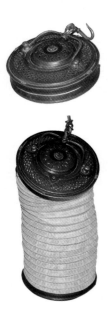

This rare Turkish candle lamp or "Kelly lamp" was donated to the AARN Museum and Archives by Dr. Winston Backus and Mrs. Backus of Sylvan Lake, Alberta. This lamp was carried by Mary Stanley, a nurse who, during the Crimean War, rather annoyed Florence Nightingale. The lamp was originally given by a patient (the granddaughter of Mary Stanley) to the late Mrs. Valmai Backus when she was a student at the London Hospital in London, England. Three lamps of this specific design are known in the world; an identical lamp to this one is located in the Florence Nightingale Museum Trust in London, and another is situated in a different museum in London and reported as "not being of the same quality." The lamp "has a circular shaped brass base linked by a linen concertina supported by wire to a circular shaped brass cover with a heat shield and hook. The cover contains some lattice design. The lamp is thus used as a lantern when extended or a candle holder when collapsed." Miss Nightingale used the folding candle lanterns, not the "Aladdin type" or "Greek lamp of knowledge" with which she is so often depicted.

Florence Nightingale Lamp, photo June 6, 1992, AARN Museum & Archives. College and Association of Registered Nurses of Alberta Museum and Archives P-650.

The greatest measure of Nightingale's success was the overall drop in the mortality rate—to 2.2 percent—that occurred within 6 months' time. When the conditions at the Barrack Hospital were reasonably satisfactory, Nightingale went across the Black Sea to the Crimea, where two British hospitals were located near the seaport of Balaclava. On horseback or in a carriage the army had given her, she covered the distances between them. She visited the front and the hospitals but contracted Crimean fever and nearly died. The English soldiers wept at the news of her illness, and all of England waited patiently for her recovery. The strain of the illness and the nursing care she had provided undermined her health to the point that she was never again able to work with her former vigor. For the rest of her life she remained a semi-invalid. Nightingale returned to England in July 1856, 4 months after the end of the war. By that time she had supervised 125 nurses. A testimonial was presented to her by the English public in the form of fifty thousand pounds. This sum was obtained by compulsory subscription from the soldiers of the Crimea and donations from the public. It was deposited into the Nightingale Fund, which later was used for a training school for nurses.

Two figures emerged from the Crimea as heroic, the soldier and the nurse. In each case a transformation in public estimation took place, and in each case the transformation was due to Miss Nightingale. Never again was the British soldier to be ranked as a drunken brute, the scum of the earth. He was now a symbol of courage, loyalty, and endurance, not a disgrace but a source of pride. . . . Never again would the picture of a nurse be a tipsy, promiscuous harridan. Miss Nightingale had stamped the profession of nurse with her own image . . . in the midst of the muddle and the filth, the agony and the defeats, she had brought about a revolution.
— WOODHAM-SMITH, 1951, P. 179

Before departing from the Crimean theater, Florence Nightingale made a pledge to the dead soldiers to fight for their cause. She insisted on a formal investigation of military health care, which led to the establishment of a Royal Commission on the Health of the Army in 1857. Nightingale published her own views in an 800-page book titled *Notes on Matters Affecting the Health, Efficiency and Hospital Administration of the British Army,* which included a section of statistics accompanied by diagrams. These polar-area charts (diagrams) depicted the statistics as represented in proportion to the area of a wedge in a circular diagram (Cohen, 1984).

Some individuals and articles referred to them as "coxcomb graphs" (Cook, 1914; Martineau, 1859), a title that was never used by Nightingale. She actually used the word *coxcomb* to refer to an 1858 book that included text, tables, and graphics. These statistics were Nightingale's most compelling argument for the improvement of medical care in military and civilian hospitals. After five years of hard fighting for reforms, her efforts were realized. Army hospitals and barracks were reconstructed on a sanitary basis, a sanitary code for the army was developed, a military medical college was established, recreational clubs were founded, and the army's procedures for gathering medical statistics were reorganized.

Florence Nightingale exercised a somewhat similar influence over British administration in India. Vast irrigation projects and economic reforms were enacted by the government on the strength of two of her reports, *Observations on the Sanitary State of the Army in India* (1863) and *Life or Death in India?* (1873). This revolution in the military hospitals was carried over into civilian hospitals. The work was aided by *Notes on Hospitals* (1859), an exhaustive study of hospital planning and administration. Nightingale also drew up a standard nomenclature of diseases and devised a Model Hospital Statistical Form that was approved at the International Congress of Statistics, held in London in the summer of 1860. As a recognized authority, she was frequently consulted about the plans for new hospitals in England, Australia, the United States, and Canada. Plans for the Johns Hopkins Hospital in Baltimore were taken to England for her critique.

The Forgotten Heroine. Mary Seacole is considered to be the forgotten nurse heroine of the Crimean War. Yet, she was a contemporary of Florence Nightingale and was celebrated for the care of soldiers during this conflict. At the outset of the Crimean War, she went to London and volunteered her services to the War Office, other military organizations, and Nightingale's nursing group. She was first ignored and then rejected on the basis that she was not needed, despite the shortage of suitable nurses available to go to the Crimea. Her autobiography, *The Wonderful Adventures of Mrs. Seacole in Many Lands,* first published in 1857 and reprinted in 1984, details her bitter disappointment. It was particularly difficult for Seacole to accept this situation because regiments from her home, Kingston, Jamaica, had been sent to join the fight. It is apparent that she was unable to understand the refusal and had searched for reasons to account for the decision: "Doubts and suspicions rose in my heart for the first and last time, thank Heaven. Was it possible that American prejudices against colour had some root here? Did these ladies shrink from accepting my aid because my blood flowed beneath a somewhat duskier skin than theirs?" (Alexander, 1984, p.124).

Mary Jane Grant Seacole was born in 1805 in Kingston, Jamaica, the daughter of a free black woman and a Scottish army officer. Her knowledge of diseases and treatments was acquired by observing her mother, a well-known herbalist, and military doctors caring for British soldiers and their families staying at her mother's boarding house. Prior to the Crimean War, Seacole had gained a reputation as a skilled nurse and doctress. Her expertise included preparing medi-

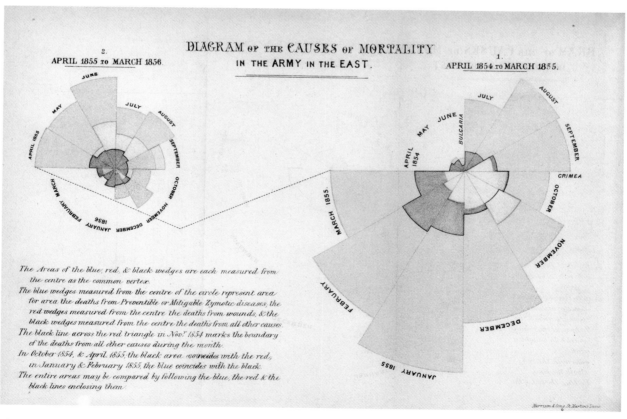

This causes of morality diagram was published in *Notes on Matters Affecting the Health, Efficiency, and Hospital Administration of the British Army.* The graph indicates the number of deaths that occurred from preventable diseases (in blue), those that were the results of wounds (in red), and those due to other causes (in black) during the Crimean War.

Florence Nightingale, *Diagram of the Causes of Mortality in the Army in the East,* 1858, page from a book, 20.8 × 47 cm, The Royal Collection. Copyright 2005 Her Majesty Queen Elizabeth II.

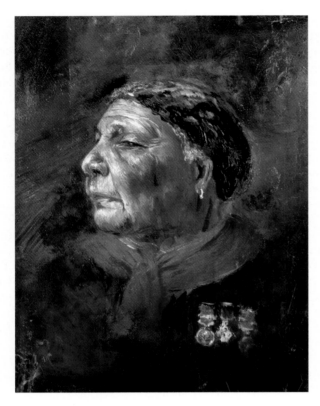

Albert Charles Challen, *Mary Jane Seacole (nee Grant)*, 1869, painting, 9.5″ × 6.25″, National Portrait Gallery London.

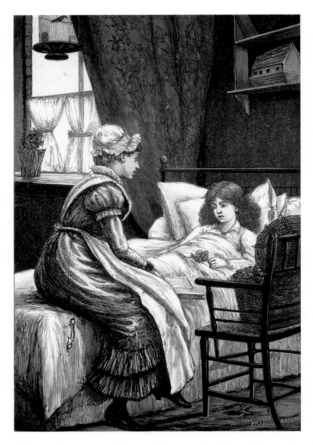

Francis James Barraud, *Sick Nursing*, 1880s, painting, 191 × 127 mm, Alexander Turnbull Library, New Zealand.

cines, applying herbal remedies, diagnosing illnesses, and performing minor surgical procedures. These skills were acquired as she cared for victims of cholera, dysentery, yellow fever and other conditions that occurred in countries where she traveled or in which she resided.

Mary Seacole was a remarkable woman who persevered under the harshest of circumstances. She went to the Crimea at her own expense, acquired a supply of food and medicine, and left for Turkey. She established a store and boarding house called The British Hotel at Spring Hill, which was located approximately two miles from Balaclava. It provided an eating establishment as well as a hospitable and comfortable accommodations for sick and convalescing officers. The money she received for these services financed her medical and nursing work. Seacole also tended the wounded on the battlefields wearing a colorful outfit of a "yellow dress and blue bonnet with red ribbons and her famous medical bag" (Alexander, 1984, p. 45). She soon became known as the Black Nightingale, a title of respect accorded by the soldiers who benefited from her care and praised her nursing skills.

Seacole spent the remaining years of her life traveling between Jamaica and London. She was eventually awarded the Crimea Medal by the government for services provided to the sick and injured (Carnegie, 1984). Her name and accomplishments faded from memory after her death in Paddington, London, on May 14, 1881. It was not until 1973 that attention turned to her once again. A special ceremony of reconsecration was held at Seacole's grave on November 20. Several other events occurred that provided a resurgence of interest in Mary Seacole: a touring exhibition "Roots in Britain"; a memorial service on May 14, 1981, marking the one hundredth anniversary of her death; and the *Wonderful Ad-*

ventures of Mrs. Seacole in Many Lands, which was reprinted in 1984. The memorial service is now held annually and is a fitting honor for a significant leader in nursing's history.

The Nightingale Philosophy. Although early philosophy identified nursing strictly with the care of the sick, Florence Nightingale had a different conception of the word, pointing out that there were two major aspects of nursing—"health nursing and sick nursing." Nightingale continually spoke of health, not illness, described disease as a reparative process, and defined nursing not as the administration of medicines or medical regimens, but as the proper use of air, light, warmth, quiet, cleanliness and diet "at the least expense of vital power to the patient" (Nightingale, 1860, pp. 1-2). She set forth a clear, concise charge to nurses to adopt a broad definition of nursing—caring for, caring about, and caring for the whole person, thus advocating a holistic approach to patient care.

It is interesting to note that Miss Nightingale disliked the germ theory. She apparently thought that embracing a belief in germs would severely weaken the principles of sanitation in which she believed and which she supported so strongly. This was consistent with her tenet that when the environment is changed, the patient can be placed in the best conditions for nature to act. Thus, numerous factors had to be considered to create a favorable environment: food, water, light, noise control, room temperature, stimulation, and ventilation. Of these, ventilation was the most important, and an inherent part of the miasmic theory of disease, which held that diseases such as cholera and the Black Death were caused by a noxious form of "bad air." Nightingale wrote about miasmas in *Notes on Nursing*, believing that pockets of

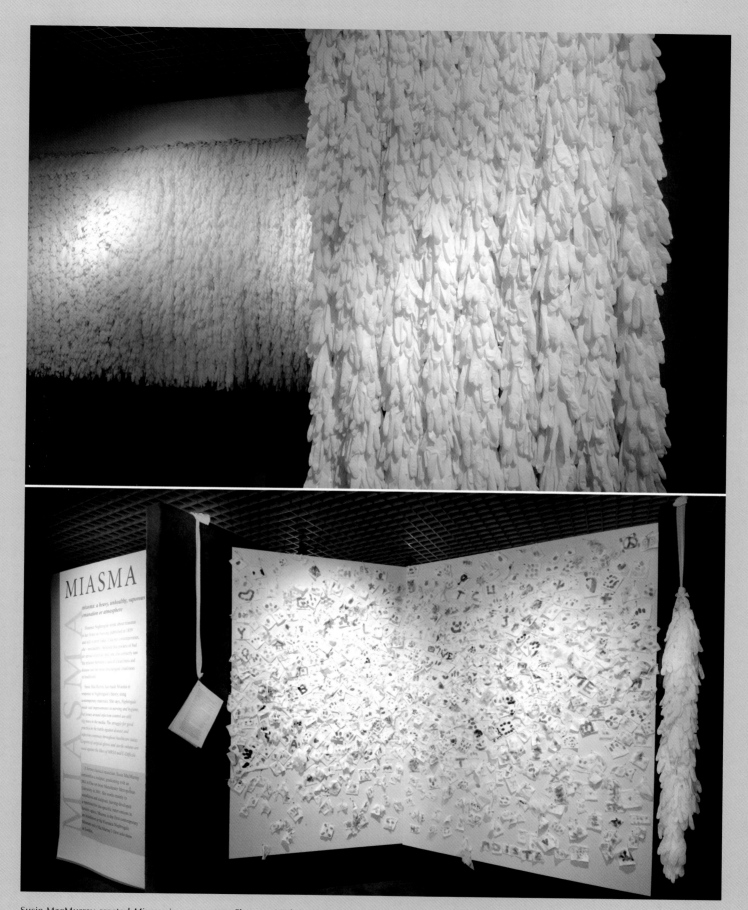

Susie MacMurray created *Miasma* in response to Florence Nightingale's miasma theory using contemporary materials. Thousands of disposable latex gloves hung from strips of crepe bandage and covered a wall over 12 meters long at its opening at the Nightingale Museum in London in July of 2008.

Susie MacMurray, *Miasma*. Courtesy of the Florence Nightingale Museum Trust, London.

bad air spread infection. Although the theory was disproven with the discovery of bacteria and viruses, it clearly identified the connection between dirt and disease, the association of poor sanitation and hygiene with disease. Nightingale's emphasis on cleanliness as a necessary element for disease prevention initiated vast improvements in hospitals, where cleanliness and fresh air became the standard for years to come.

The Nightingale School. Florence Nightingale developed the first organized program of training for nurses. The Nightingale Training School for Nurses opened in 1860 as an entirely independent educational institution financed by the Nightingale Fund. A council of distinguished persons had been appointed to administer the fund and negotiate the establishment of the school. The members investigated the existing London hospitals and chose St. Thomas's Hospital, where the resident medical officer, R. G. Whitfield, was sympathetic and the matron, Mrs. Wardroper, had made her mark by exhibiting an upright character, an unremitting devotion to her task, and success in reforming hospital abuses. An overwhelming majority of London physicians opposed the project. Of 100 physicians queried, only 4 favored the school. Strong opposition came from within St. Thomas's itself through John Flint South, a senior consulting surgeon. South vehemently opposed the school and published a pamphlet, *Facts Relating to Hospital Nurses* (1857), in which he asserted: "As regards the nurses or ward-maids, these are in much the same position as housemaids, and require little teaching beyond that of poultice-making." Nightingale's ill health prevented her from taking charge of the program, but she acted as a chief adviser for many years.

The aims of the Nightingale school were to train hospital nurses, to instruct nurses in the training of others, and to train district nurses for the sick poor. Consequently, students went into homes as well as into hospitals to care for and teach patients and families about the preservation and maintenance of health. The length of the program was one year, after which the nurses were drafted into the staff of a hospital for two years' further experience. A distinction was made between ordinary probationers and "lady nurses," which reflected British class consciousness. The former were drawn from relatively uneducated levels, and their expenses were paid by the Nightingale Fund; the latter were gentlewomen who paid their own way (tuition fees) and were expected to become future matrons. The graduates of this program were destined to become nursing leaders on an international scale. As soon as they were available, they were in demand at other hospitals.

The Nightingale school was extremely important to nursing. It served as a model for other schools, sent graduates to foreign lands, and raised nursing from degradation and disgrace to the rank of a respectable occupation for women. The opening of the school was the opening of a new way of life for women. Gone forever, at least in England, was the reign of Sairey Gamp and Betsy Prig.

A small book of 77 pages written by Florence Nightingale, *Notes on Nursing* (1859), held special interest for nurses. It was used as a text in the Nightingale school and in many schools founded by the nurses who studied there. In 1860 the book was rewritten, enlarged, and translated into Italian, German, and French. Concern over the meager number of available copies prompted a reprinting in 1946. The fundamental principles that were set forth in this book remain as true today as they were when they were written. Their scope is described in the preface: "The following notes are by no means intended as a rule of thought by which nurses can teach themselves to nurse, still less as a manual to teach nurses to nurse. They are meant simply to give hints for thought to women who have personal charge of the health of others" (Nightingale, 1859, p. iii).

After the founding of the school, 50 years remained for Nightingale. She survived until the age of 90. This half-century was spent in constant, fruitful activity. She died in August 1910 and was buried in the family plot at East Wellow, near Romney, in Hampshire. A small cross with her initials and dates marks the site of the grave. The family refused burial in Westminster Abbey in respect for Nightingale's wishes. There are numerous monuments to her in various places in the world: in London, Derby, Milbank, Florence, and Calcutta and in St. Paul's Cathedral, St. Thomas's Hospital, the Royal Infirmary, and the Episcopal Cathedral in Washington, D.C. In this last structure is the famous and beautiful stained glass Nightingale Window, composed of six panels that depict the events in the life of Florence Nightingale.

One need not review all the causes to which Florence Nightingale gave of herself to appreciate her role as a creative social force. She was a living memorial to a new type of thought that would forever influence the direction of nursing.

> "The definite dividing-line between the old nursing and the new, is the demarcation between pre-Nightingale nursing and Nightingale nursing. In the sense that Hippocrates (460-370 BC) was the father of medicine, Florence Nightingale (1820-1910) was the founder of nursing: systematized medicine is thus an ancient art, while organized nursing is a recent art. Miss Nightingale hewed a new profession out of centuries of ignorance and superstition. The greatness and the goodness of Florence Nightingale combined to emancipate woman from the curse of not finding her work: Florence Nightingale gave to woman the blessed work of the trained nurse of the human race." (Robinson, 1946, p. 129)

THE BIRTH OF THE RED CROSS

A further stimulus for nursing reform culminated in the development of the International Red Cross organization. Its founder was J. Henri Dunant, an investment banker from Geneva, Switzerland. A humanitarian, Dunant had journeyed to Italy to secure a meeting with Napoleon III of France but found himself at Solferino, where he was a witness to the horrors of the bloodiest battle of the war between France and Austria. He was depressed by the lack of medical services; only two physicians were attending to nearly six thousand wounded men. Dunant enlisted local people to give whatever aid and nursing care was possible. He subsequently appealed to various European governments to set up an international organization that would provide volunteer nursing aid on battlefields.

Dunant repeatedly referred to Florence Nightingale and her work in the Crimea as the inspiration behind his crucial trip to Italy. Her work had also fortified his belief in the feasibility of such an organization. In 1862 he published the

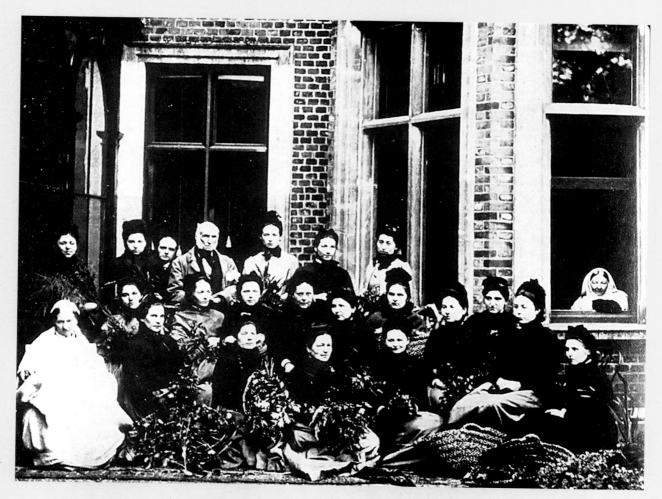

Florence Nightingale with Nurses from the Nightingale School, 1887, photograph.

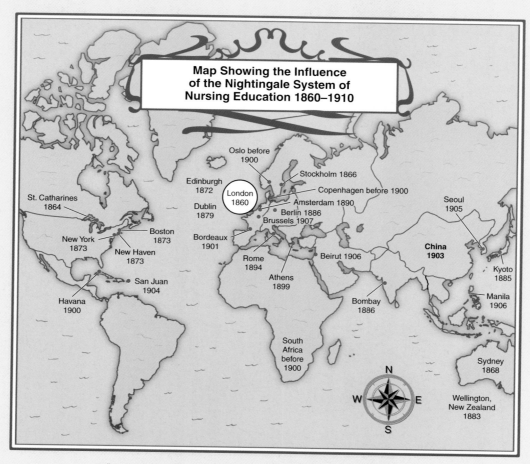

Influence of the Nightingale System of Nursing Education 1860-1910, map, Mosby.

123

famous *Recollections of Solferino (Un Souvenir de Solferino)*, which contained the idea for the birth of the Red Cross. He first presented his plan to the Society of Public Utility in Geneva (1863). After 5 years of hard work, Henri Dunant observed the gathering of a national congress in Geneva to consider the ways and means of accruing volunteers to serve in the event of another war. On August 22, 1864, 12 governments signed what is now known as the Treaty of Geneva. It contained principles to govern and protect those wounded in war, the supplies needed for their care, and the personnel attending the wounded through the use of a single specific emblem. The design chosen for the common flag of the organization was that of the flag of Switzerland with its colors reversed—a red cross on a white background.

(The Red Cross societies of Muslim nations use a red crescent on a white background for their flag. Iran has a red lion and sun, which for many years has been the Persian national symbol.) Each government agreed to honor Red Cross nurses as noncombatants and to respect their hospitals and other facilities. In addition, societies in neutral countries would be permitted to render humanitarian services to both sides.

National Red Cross societies were built up in many countries, and some older groups that had carried on relief work in the earlier wars of the 19th century became affiliated with it. The Geneva treaty was signed by England in 1870. The United States refrained from confirming it until 1882; it was confirmed only after Clara Barton, with rugged determination, paved the way for Congress to ratify it.

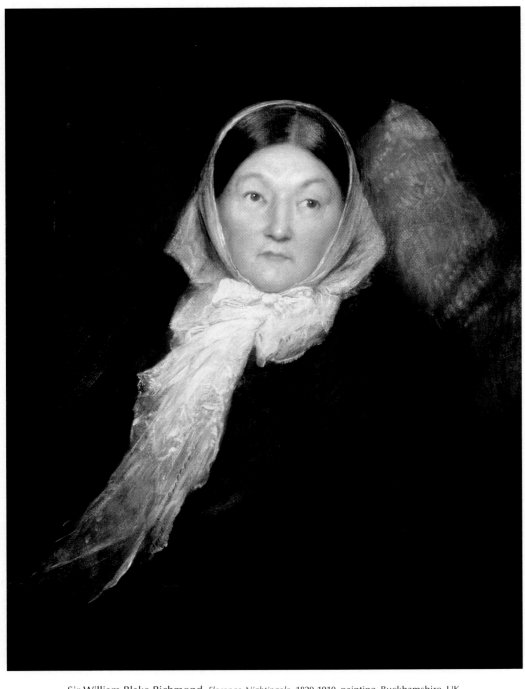

Sir William Blake Richmond, *Florence Nightingale*, 1820-1910, painting, Buckhamshire, UK.

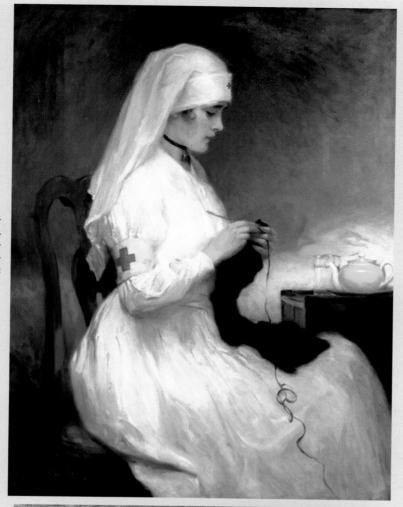

Gabriel Emile Niscolet (1856-1921), *Portrait of Nurse—Red Cross*, painting, Colnaghi & Co. Ltd., London, UK; The Bridgeman Art Library; Nationality/copyright status: French/out of copyright.

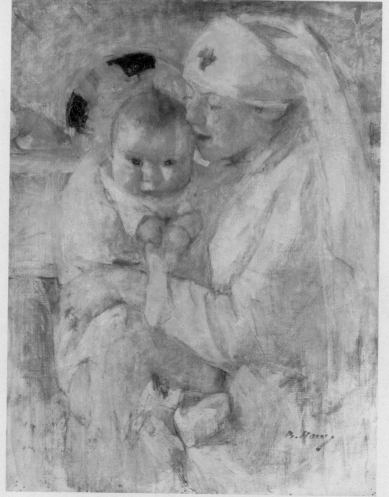

Beatrice Howe, *L'Infirmiere (The Nurse)*, c1914-1918, painting, 654 × 470 mm, The Tate Gallery London/Great Britian. Copyright Tate, London, 2009.

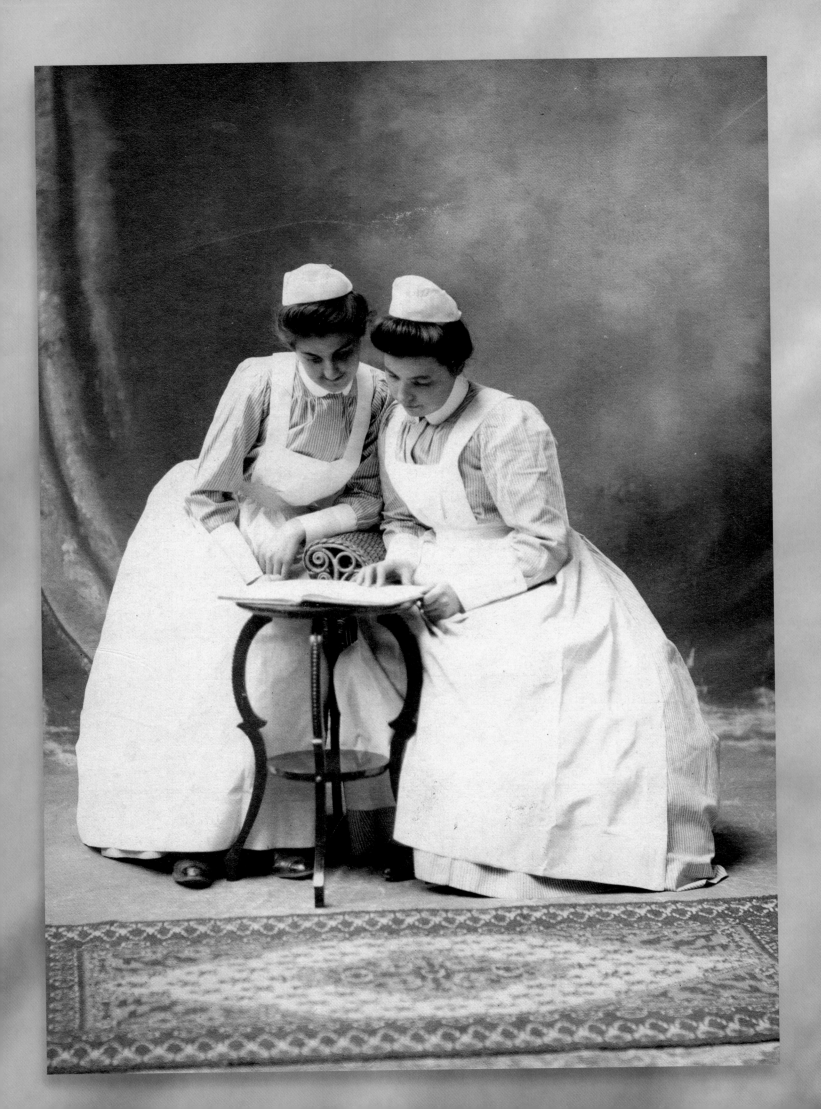

UNIT Four

The Development of Nursing in America

n the early nineteenth century, the status of nursing in the United States was not unlike that in England prior to the influence of Florence Nightingale. Large city hospitals were in existence and nurses were haphazardly trained in the hospital. There were few trained nurses and no formal training programs. The Civil War, much like the Crimean War in the case of England, brought the need for skilled nurses to the attention of government agencies, and brought about the first major reforms in nursing in this country. In the latter half of the century, the growing sense of social responsibility for health, the improved status of women in society, and the influence of the Nightingale concept all contributed to the development of nursing education and improved nursing practice. The United States produced many women who greatly influenced nursing during the same period that Florence Nightingale made her reforms, and later.

— GLORIA M. GRIPPANDO

Early State University of Iowa nursing students studying.

University of Iowa, *Cover of History of Nursing,* photograph, University of Iowa, College of Nursing.

The Development of Nursing in America

	1500	1600	1700	1800
Nursing		**1606-1673** Jeanne Mance, one of the most romantic figures in Canadian nursing **1617** Maria Hubow, first woman to nurse in North America **1639** Three Augustinian Sisters staff Hôtel Dieu at Quebec **1657** Three hospital nuns of Society of St Joseph de la Flèche staff Hôtel Dieu in Montreal	**1727** Ursuline Sisters arrive from France to nurse at L'Hôspital des Pauvres de la Charite in New Orleans **1739** Order of Grey Nuns becomes Canada's first district nurses **1774-1813** Mother Elizabeth Seton, first native-born American canonized for charitable work **1797-1881** Sojourner Truth, early feminist and volunteer Civil War nurse	**1817-1901** Mother Bickerdyke, volunteer Civil War nurse **1820-1913** Harriet Tubman, abolitionist and volunteer Civil War nurse **1821-1912** Clara Barton, volunteer Civil War nurse and founder of American Red Cross **1839** Nurses Society of Philadelphia organized for home maternity services
Medicine and Health Care	**1524** Cortez established first hospital on the American continent, built in the Tenochtitlan capital **1528** Hospital of Santa Fe built **1578** First medical school established at the University of Mexico	**c. 1600** Medical School at University of Lima established **1639** Hôtel Dieu at Quebec opens **1642** Hôtel Dieu at Montreal founded **1658** Bellevue Hospital precursor founded by the Dutch West India Company	**1731** Philadelphia Almshouse erected **1737** Charity Hospital of New Orleans founded **1745-1813** Benjamin Rush, most renowned physician of colonial times **1751** Pennsylvania Hospital designed solely for care of the sick **1765** Medical school established at College of Philadelphia **1783** Medical school at Harvard established **1786** Quakers establish Philadelphia Dispensary for home care of the sick **1791** New York Dispensary opens	**1810** Medical School established at Yale **1847** American Medical Association (AMA) established
Science and Technology	**1492** Leonardo da Vinci draws a flying machine **1525** Dürer compiles first German manual on geometry **1540** G.L. de Cardenas discovers the Grand Canyon **1547** First predictions of astrologer Nostradamus **1595** Mercator's Atlas published **1596** Galileo invents thermometer	**1631** William Oughtred proposes symbol "×" for multiplication **1656** Thomas Wharton describes anatomy of glands	**1714** D.G. Fahrenheit constructs mercury thermometer with temperature scale **1775** Priestly discovers hydrochloric and sulfuric acids	**1816** Laënnec invents the stethoscope
The Visual Arts		**1644** Last age of fine Chinese porcelain **1647** Dresden Academy of Arts founded **1656** Rembrandt declares bankruptcy **1662** André Le Nôtre designs park and gardens of Versailles	**1699–1779** Jean Chardin, French painter **1715** Early beginnings of Rococo **1738–1815** John Singleton Copley, American painter **1738–1820** Benjamin West, American painter **1793** The Louvre, Paris, becomes national art gallery	**1834** Statue of Liberty by F.A. Bartholdi, French sculptor **1836–1910** Winslow Homer, American painter **1844–1915** Thomas Eakins, American artist, illustrates scientific basis of patient care
Daily Life	**1492** Columbus lands in America **1519** Hernando Cortez conquers Mexico **1535** Jacques Cartier sails into the St. Lawrence River	**1605** First permanent French settlement at Port Royal in Nova Scotia **1607** First permanent English settlement in America at Jamestown **1620** Pilgrims land in Plymouth **1626** Dutch East India Company establishes "New Netherlands"	**1775–1781** America Revolution	

1862 Louisa May Alcott serves as a volunteer Civil War nurse

1862 Walt Whitman serves as a volunteer Civil War nurse in Washington DC

1873 Linda Richards becomes America's first trained nurse

1873 Bellevue, Connecticut, and Boston Training Schools established

1874 St. Catharine's, Ontario, begins nurse training school

1876-1901 Clara Maass, nurse who gave her life to conquer yellow fever

1879 Mary Eliza Mahoney becomes America's first black professional nurse

1886 Spelman Seminary in Atlanta establishes training for black nurses

1889 John Hopkins Hospital Training School opens

1899 Teachers College program for nurses established

1861 United States Sanitary Commission established

1869 Bellevue hospital establishes ambulance service

1871 Leprosy bacillus discovered

1878 Iodoform used as antiseptic

1887 Phenacetin, an analgesic drug, discovered

1889 Von Mehring and Minkowski prove that pancreas secretes insulin

1890 Rubber gloves used for first time in surgery at Johns Hopkins

1893 Medical School established at Johns Hopkins

1904 W.C. Gorgas eradicates yellow fever in Panama Canal Zone

1909 Ehrlich prepares salvarsan for cure of syphilis

1910 *Flexner Report* published

1921 Heart disease becomes leading cause of death in the U.S.

1927 Cancer becomes one of the top three causes of death

1928 Alexander Fleming discovers penicillin

1935 First blood bank set up at Mayo Clinic, Rochester, U.S.

1937 Insulin used to control diabetes

1939 Rh factor in blood discovered by Levine and Stetson

1948 First World Health Assembly meets in Geneva

1955 Salk develops polio vaccine

1871 Leprosy bacillus discovered

1873 Color photographs first developed

1878 Iodoform used as antiseptic

1887 Phenacetin, an analgesic drug, discovered

1889 Von Mehring and Minkowski prove that pancreas secretes insulin

1894 Röentgen discovers x-rays

1903 Electrocardiograph developed by Wilhelm Einthoven

1903 Wright brothers make first powered flight

1905 Albert Einstein, physicist, formulates specific theory of relativity

1906 Model T Ford produced

1906 Jansky classifies blood into four groups

1919 First experiments with short-wave radio

1920 James Smathers develops first electric typewriter

1922 Radio broadcasting begins

1922 Self winding watch invented

1927 Iron lung developed

1951 J. Andre-Thomas invents heart-lung machine

1853–1890 Vincent Van Gogh, Dutch painter

1863–1944 Edvard Munch, Norwegian painter

1874 First impressionist exhibition in Paris

1875 *Gross Clinic* painted

1881-1973 Pablo Picasso, Spanish painter

1889 *Agnew Clinic* painted

1889 Alexander Gustave Eiffel designs the Eiffel Tower

1895 Art Nouveau style predominates

1903 Gustav Klimt paints ceiling at Vienna University

1910 Frank Lloyd Wright becomes well-known architect

1926 Academy of Motion Picture Arts and Sciences founded

1942 Peggy Guggenheim opens the gallery Art of This Century in New York

---

1861–1865 American Civil War

1864 Geneva Convention establishes neutrality of battlefield medical facilities

1865 United States abolishes slavery

1876 Korea becomes an independent nation

1877 Edison invents the telephone

1878 Electric street lighting installed

1880 The game of Bingo is devised

1883 First skyscraper built in Chicago

1888 Yellow Fever epidemic in Florida

1889 Johnstown flood

1890 Global influenza epidemic

1893 World's Fair in Chicago

1898–1899 Spanish-American War

1900 First trial flight of the Zeppelin

1900 Cake Walk is most fashionable dance

1901 Oil drilling begins in Persia

1908 Fountain pens become popular

1911 Titanic sinks in North Atlantic

1918 Worldwide influenza epidemic strikes nearly 22 million people

1929 Term "apartheid" used for first time

1934 Refrigeration process for meat cargoes devised

1939 Nylon stocking introduced

1950s Beginning years of the "Cold War"

1957 Russian Sputnik launched

he social movements that had characterized several centuries in Europe had their American counterparts. The time of the Reformation, which had split European nations into Catholic and Protestant, was also a period of great discoveries and early emigration to America. Groups from the Old World migrated to various regions of the New World, bringing with them their customs, including those related to the care of the sick. The earliest evidence of nursing in the Western Hemisphere, however, occurred among the preliterate peoples who inhabited North, Central, and South America. Even before the Jesuit fathers of France had pioneered in medicine and the Catholic sisters had established mission hospitals, the American Indians had practiced crude methods of medical and surgical treatment. They had their own folk and magic medicines and could care for their sick without knowledge of medical science. The newcomers were often impressed by the native "medicine men," who served as doctors and herbwomen. (The latter assumed the functions of nurses.) According to Nutting and Dock (vol. 2, 1907), the Aztecs and the Incas had built their hospitals and taken care of their sick in the very dawn of history. In *Native Races of the Pacific States of North America,* Bancroft states that in all of the larger cities of ancient Mexico there were endowed hospitals attended by physicians, surgeons, and nurses and that the Mexicans had studied and practiced medicine from ancient times; women physicians were common and obstetricians were women. Shryock, however, makes the statement that "even the civilized Indians of Mexico and of Peru had developed nothing in the way of such institutions . . . of hospitals and of nurses there was no evidence" (Shryock, 1959, p. 170).

Although discoveries of land had been made in the New World before the time of Columbus, no lasting colonies had been established. A northwest passage to India was being sought by navigators and sailors. Thus Columbus named the natives he encountered in the Western world Indians because he thought they were on a land that was part of India. As new lands were discovered, they were generally bestowed on the sovereigns who had financed the expeditions. It was hoped by specific governments that the expeditions would lead to the attainment of wealth and trade from the new lands. Ultimately, kingdoms would be extended and empires created. Columbus, Vespucci, Balboa, Hudson, Cartier, Drake, and others were supported in their endeavors by their homelands. Other factors also compelled individuals to journey far from their native lands: freedom from religious persecution and the desire by missionaries to convert the so-called heathens to Christianity.

SETTLEMENTS OF THE NEW WORLD

The settlements of the New World were closely tied to the mother countries of Spain, France, and England. The new territories or colonies were thought to exist for the advantage of the homeland, and trade with them was organized from that perspective. Adventurers who were fascinated by tales of the strange new lands and the fabulous wealth that supposedly existed there left their homelands to explore and conquer. Many of the colonists also included members of religious orders who became the teachers, nurses, and physicians.

Need for additional provision for care of the sick was created when the first boatload of adventurers started out from Europe. Crude conditions of travel led to deadly outbreaks of scurvy, as well as of disease contracted before leaving the homeland. On his second trip, Columbus was careful to bring a physician. Explorers, conquerors, and conquered—all were exposed to infections for which they had no immunity. Unfortunately, it was almost simultaneous with this need that the period of depression in European nursing was being induced by the Renaissance and the Protestant Revolt—a depression to be prolonged by revolutions to establish religious freedom and the civil rights of man. A great era of discovery opened up and facilitated the spread of disease, at a time when opportunities for its control were becoming fewer and less adequate than ever.

— *JAMIESON AND SEWALL, 1950, P. 279*

The problems of medical care and nursing were met in different ways by the various colonists and were usually dependent upon the customs of the homelands. Spain was best prepared because Protestantism had not weakened her Church. Religious orders of the Catholic Church accompanied the Spaniards to America. In addition to protecting the public health, they explored and converted pagans to Christianity. Nursing was clearly a function of the religious, which included devoted service and the salvation of souls. As hospitals were erected, they were also controlled by the religious, who supported the institutions through gifts they had received. France also used the Dominicans, Franciscans, and Jesuits and, later, the nursing orders, but England had no comparable support. Organization was lacking, and individuals were given the responsibility for medicine and nursing. Eventually, in the colonies settled by Protestant countries, nursing was done by persons hired at low wages or supplied by inmates of houses of correction.

SPANISH AMERICA

Spain rapidly established colonies from Mexico to Peru during the 1500s. These colonies became a large, energetic realm nearly one hundred years before the first permanent settlements of other Europeans were established. In some areas, native peoples were able to mingle their culture with that of the conquerors. In others, particularly in the chief centers such as Lima and Mexico City, Spanish civilization followed the pattern of the homeland. The University of Mexico and the University of Lima were founded in 1551, and the various departments of theology, arts, rhetoric, grammar, scripture, canon law, civil law, and medicine were present. Here the medical science of the Renaissance was cultivated and the first medical schools appeared: the first at the University of Mexico in 1578, the second affiliated with the University of Lima before 1600.

In 1519, Hernando Cortés conquered what we now call Mexico. His conquest brought into Spanish possession the great wealth of the Aztecs, Toltecs, Mayas, and Incas. The well-meaning reigning chief of the Aztecs, Montezuma, had received Cortés into his palace. Montezuma had been taught to believe in a white god, who he thought had appeared in the form of Cortés. Montezuma was met, however, with cruelty. He was imprisoned and his capital of Tenochtitlán was seized. The Aztecs had risen to a high degree of culture; their temples and pyramids are thought to predate those of Egypt. They had acquired large amounts of gold, silver, and precious stones, which were seized and shipped back to Spain. The American Indians were cruelly treated and in some cases their tribes were nearly obliterated. Where they proved to be unfit for work in the mines, African slaves were introduced. Missionaries protested the inhumane treatment of the natives and slaves and tried to improve their situation.

The medicine of the Aztecs was highly developed. The Aztecs had hospices for the care of the sick; used minerals and plants as drugs (they had knowledge of three thousand plants) and soporifics to deaden pain; and had midwives for prenatal and postpartum instruction and for assistance at deliveries (Frank, 1953). The god of medicine was Tzapotlatean. So skilled were the Aztec surgeons and physicians that Cortés asked the Spanish government to refrain from sending medical practitioners from Spain; he preferred the American Indians because he believed they were superior. The Incas were not as advanced. They used purging, bloodletting, trephining, amputation, and potions made from a single herb. The Incas believed that the cure for a particular disease would be found in the area in which the disease was prominent; therefore quinine from the cinchona tree was found in the malaria-infested jungles.

Beautiful churches, buildings, bridges, roads, and aqueducts were built under Spanish rule. Gratitude to God for success found expression in the development of charitable institutions, frequently in the form of hospitals. Approximately thirty hospitals were erected between 1524 and 1802, and the majority of them were staffed by religious men and women. The first hospital on the American continent was built in the Tenochtitlán capital (later renamed Mexico City) by Cortés in 1524. According to legend, this hospital was built on the site where Cortés first met Montezuma. It was originally named the Hospital of the Immaculate Conception (Hospital de Nuestra Senorao Limpia Conception); it is now called the Hospital of Jesus of Nazareth (Hospital de Jesus Nazareno). This building is a reflection of the beauty and spaciousness of Spanish hospital architecture under Muslim influence. Cortés donated funds for the completion of the hospital and also built a convent and a seminary. In his will he left an endowment for the hospital to thank God for his successes and to expiate his sins. This institution was to care for rich and poor alike. In 1528, the hospital of Santa Fe (Holy Faith) was built in what is now New Mexico. In Lima, several institutions were built, including almshouses, hospitals, and lazarettos for those afflicted with contagious diseases. Hospital care, however, was reserved for the sick poor, and most of the nursing was done by the Sisters of Charity of St. Vincent de Paul.

THE FRENCH IN AMERICA

The first permanent settlement of the French was established in 1605 at Port Royal in Nova Scotia. The Canadian area of North America had been visited earlier: Norwegians had landed there in about 1000. John Cabot, a Venetian under King Henry VII, sighted land near the Gulf of the St. Lawrence; Frenchmen arrived in the area early in the 16th century. In 1534, Jacques Cartier, under Francis I, sailed for the North American continent. He returned to France after finding neither gold nor a northwest passage to the Orient. When Cartier returned a year later, he sailed into the St. Lawrence River, where he found established American Indian villages. According to Frank (1953), Cartier questioned the natives about the name of the country. Thinking that he

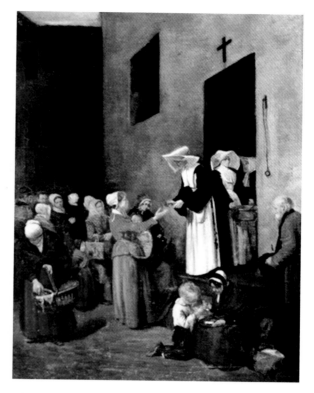

Francois Bonvin, *The Sisters of Charity*, 1851, oil on canvas, The Granger Collection, NY.

was referring to the village, they answered "Kanata," which meant *the place where we live*. Therefore, Cartier called the land Canada, its present-day name. This land has also been referred to as New France.

Cartier was followed to Canada by explorers, Franciscan friars, Jesuits, Dominicans, and other settlers. The French priests soon summoned help from the motherland for religious women to teach the children and care for the sick. The first woman to nurse in this new land, however, was Maria Hébart Hubou (the name of her second husband). She was the wife of the surgeon-apothecary Louis Hébart, whom Samuel de Champlain, the famous explorer, brought with him in 1617 (Gibbon and Mathewson, 1947). The Jesuits published reports of the need for aid in the *Jesuit Relations*. They sought to establish schools for American Indian children, build hospitals for the sick, and make general improvements in all social conditions. The Europeans had transmitted measles, smallpox, and tuberculosis to the natives, who blamed the white people for the destruction of their race. The priests found it almost impossible to combat the diseases in the prevailing conditions. They were thwarted in their attempts by dirt, cold, crowded living conditions, lice, and the savagery of the natives.

Great interest arose in the men and women of France through Jesuit publications and reports. The Duchesse d'Aiguillon, a niece of Cardinal Richelieu, was moved to action. She signed a contract in 1637 with the Augustinian Hospitallers of Dieppe for their services as hospital sisters and sent workers to lay the foundations for the first hospital in New France. The Hôtel Dieu in Quebec opened in 1639 and was staffed by three sisters of the Order of St. Augustine (Augustinian Sisters) upon their arrival on August 1, 1639. These Augustinian nuns belonged to a cloistered order and had been prepared to care for the sick. They wore white woolen dresses with black leather belts and black veils. All three were from good French families: Marie Guenet de St.

Ignace; Anne Lecointre de St. Bernard; and Marie Forestier de St. Bonaventure de Jésus. They encountered many hardships, and within 8 months one of the sisters had died.

> The Hospital Nuns arrived at Kebec on the first day of August of last year (1639). Scarcely had they disembarked before they found themselves overwhelmed with patients. The hall of the Hospital being too small, it was necessary to erect some cabins, fashioned like those of the savages, in their garden. Not having furniture for so many people, they had to cut in two or three pieces part of the blankets and sheets they had brought for these poor sick people. In a word, instead of taking a little rest and refreshing themselves after the great discomforts they had suffered upon the sea, they found themselves so burdened and occupied that we had fear of losing them and their hospital at its very birth. The sick came from all directions. . . . [T]heir stench was so insupportable, the heat so great, the fresh food so scarce and so poor. . . . In brief, from the first of August until the month of May, more than one hundred patients entered the hospital, and more than two hundred poor savages found relief there.
> — *KENTON, 1925, PP. 169-170*

The hospital in Quebec had a facility similar to that of an outpatient department that was used for the treatment of American Indians who were not sick enough to be hospitalized. Native American women were trained by the sisters to assist in the care of the sick, but their duties were chiefly domestic, such as cooking, cleaning, and preparing supplies. From 1640 to 1644 the Augustinians went to Sillery, the Jesuit mission not far from Quebec, to care for the native peoples, but they returned when the Iroquois became hostile.

The Ursuline Sisters accompanied the Augustinians on the voyage from France. They were an order of teaching nuns enlisted by Madame de la Peltrie, who had undertaken the establishment of a mission school for the American Indians. However, they were soon schooled in the care of the sick in order that they might assist during the epidemics. Smallpox broke out in the school, and the Ursuline dwelling was rapidly turned into housing for the infected. In this emergency hospital many American Indians died until the disease finally ran itself out. This short-term instruction in the care of the sick could be regarded as the earliest training and supervision of nurses in America. As soon as it was feasible, the Ursuline Sisters returned to the work for which they had been prepared initially.

A second settlement was founded about 200 miles farther up the St. Lawrence. Included in the original plans for Montreal were a school and a hospital, with the latter deemed to be an immediate necessity. The establishment of this hospital is the story of Jeanne Mance (1606-1673), a romantic figure in Canadian nursing who is considered to be the founder of the Hôtel Dieu of Montreal as well as the cofounder of Montreal itself (Gibbon and Mathewson, 1947). She was the daughter of wealthy French parents and had been educated at an Ursuline convent. From her earliest childhood, Jeanne Mance had demonstrated a religious inclination. She received instruction in nursing care while assisting the Ladies of Charity in 1638 during a severe epidemic. Upon her arrival in Canada, she was also permitted to enter the Augustinian cloister at Quebec, where she waited for completion of the construction of the fort at Ville Marie, the future Montreal. Here Jeanne Mance was pro-

vided an excellent opportunity to learn more about nursing and the administration of a hospital. She arrived in Montreal on May 17, 1642, under the financial sponsorship of a wealthy philanthropist, Madame de Bullion, who wanted her to erect a hospital there.

The inhabitants of the settlement lived in peace for about a year. The floods and then the warring Iroquois followed. More than half of the settlers met death at the hands of the Iroquois. In a tiny cottage hospital inside the fort, Mance tended to men wounded by arrows. She compounded her own medicines, treated chilblains and frostbite, practiced bloodletting, and cared for the Iroquois Indians as well as the colonists. By October 1644 a larger hospital had been established in a building that measured 60 by 24 feet; it was divided into 2 wards, servants' quarters, a kitchen, and a room for Mance. The hospital was surrounded by a palisade and protected by a moat because of the ever-threatening Iroquois. For almost 15 years Mance did all the nursing there, with the help of a few assistants. She earned the reputation of being the first lay nurse of Canada and of North America as well.

Mance returned to France in 1657 to seek financial support and recruit personnel. Three hospital nuns from the Society of St. Joseph de la Flèche (Hospitallers of St. Joseph) returned to Montreal to staff the Hôtel Dieu, with Mance as the administrator, a position she held until her death in 1673. The sisters suffered from a variety of misfortunes during the 1st century of the hospital's existence—American Indian attacks, severe poverty, fire, earthquake, and famine. They persevered and eventually experienced considerable prosperity and recognition for their good work. The next century saw all French developments at Montreal and Quebec pass into English control as a result of the Seven Years' War.

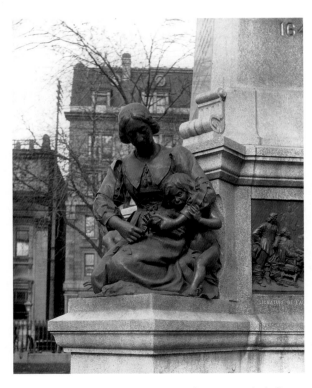

At the foot of the Maisonneuve Monument, four statues, including one of Jeanne Mance (who can be seen here caring for a young Native), recall individuals who played key roles in the founding of Montreal.

Louise-Philippe Hebert, *Maisonneuve Monument*, about 1896, sculpture, Place d'Armes, Montreal, Quebec, Canada. Copyright McCord Museum.

JEANNE MANCE
(1606-1673)

Jeanne Mance fonda ici l'Hôtel-Dieu de Montréal, un des plus anciens hôpitaux du pays. Arrivée à Ville-Marie avec Paul de Chomedey de Maisonneuve en 1642, elle en est la seule infirmière jusqu'à ce qu'elle fasse venir les Hospitalières de Saint-Joseph en 1659. À l'époque où les affrontements avec les Iroquois sont nombreux, elle soigne les blessés et les malades avec compassion et diligence, tout en multipliant ses efforts pour recruter de nouveaux colons. Première infirmière laïque au Canada, Jeanne Mance demeure toujours une source d'inspiration pour qui se destine à cette profession.

Hôtel Dieu historical site commemorative plate in Old Montreal. The plate is located on the pedestrian street of cours Le Royer.

Hotel Dieu Historical Site Commemorative Plate, photo of plaque, photographer: Gene Arboit, taken October 21, 2005, Montreal, Canada.

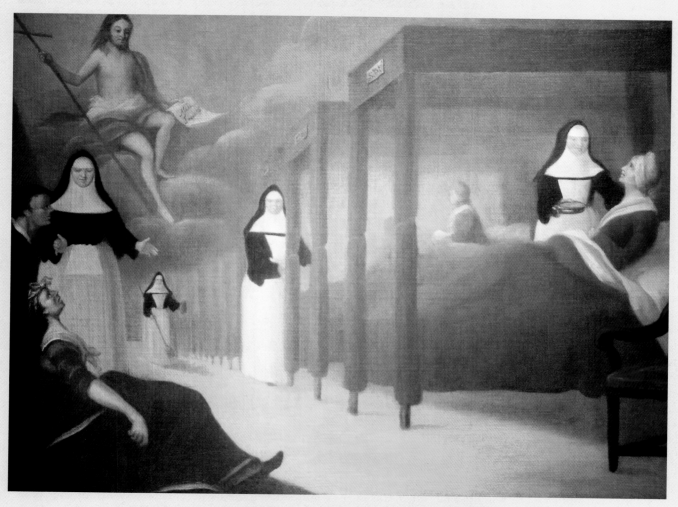

Hospitallers Hotel Dieu Montreal, 18th century, oil painting. Musée des Hospitalières de l'Hôtel-Dieu de Montréal.

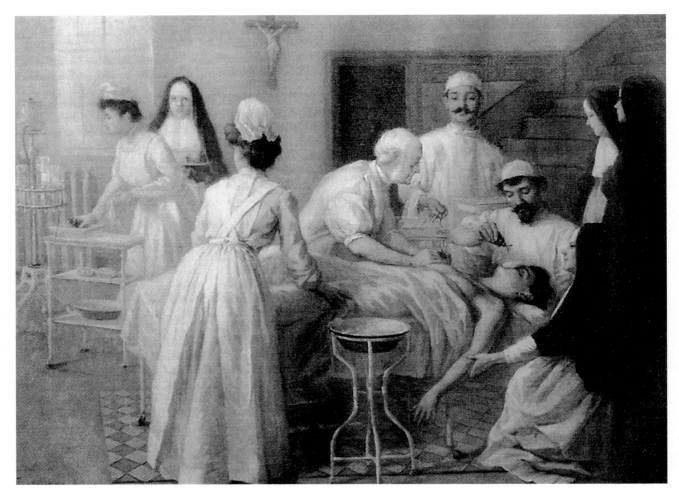

Religious and lay nurses assisting the physicians.

Joseph-Charles Franchere, *Dr. Hingston and the Operating Room*, 1905, painting. Musée des Hospitalières de l'Hôtel-Dieu de Montréal.

A number of other hospitals and orders were organized in Canada. One of particular note was the order of Grey Nuns established by Madame Marguerite Marie d'Youville in 1739. The members were not cloistered and were thus able to carry their work into the homes of the needy. The Grey Nuns were Canada's first district nurses. However, they were misunderstood because people were not comfortable with nuns walking freely on the streets.

Early nursing in Canada did not particularly affect the development of nursing in the country that later would become the United States. The French settlements of New Orleans and those farther up the Mississippi River, however, did have an influence on American nursing. This territory was called Louisiana in honor of France's king. It, too, was ravaged by epidemic diseases, particularly yellow fever and smallpox, in addition to the scourges common to a seaport. New Orleans desperately needed teachers and nurses. An almshouse had been built there and housed criminals, indigents, the mentally ill, and the sick poor. This inspired Jean Louis, a French sailor, to leave twelve thousand livres upon his death to "serve in perpetuity to the founding of a hospital for the care of the sick of the City of New Orleans . . . and to secure the necessary things to succor the sick" (Henrietta, 1939, p. 249). Ursuline Sisters arrived from France in 1727 to nurse in the new hospital, the first in the United States established through a private gift. The hospital, which was legally named l'Hôpital des Pauvres de la Charité, developed slowly and went through several name changes. It eventu-

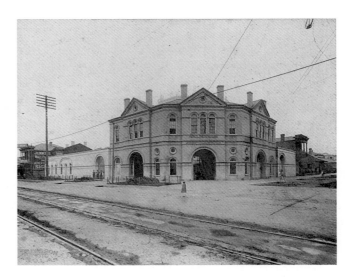

John Teunisson, *Charity Hospital*, 1900, photograph, 19 × 24 cm, Louisianna Sate Museum, New Orleans, LA.

ally became the great and famous Charity Hospital of New Orleans. The Ursuline Sisters were very active throughout Louisiana. They opened numerous hospitals and performed many heroic deeds that reached a peak with the nursing done during the Battle of New Orleans. In later years they restricted themselves to teaching, and their work was carried on by the Daughters of Charity.

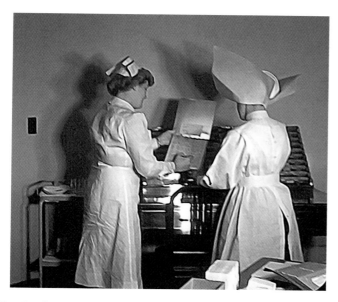

Two Carville, Louisiana Leprosarium staff nurses exchange information regarding their patients inside what was called the "chart room," where every patient's records were stored, making these records accessible to physicians and nurses. This image portrays a public health nurse consulting with a Sister of Charity.

Chart Room in the Infirmary, 1950, photograph, National Hansens Disease Museum, Baton Rouge, LA.

THE ENGLISH COLONIES

Europeans emigrated to the English colonies for a variety of reasons, including freedom from religious oppression, a spirit of adventure, and the chance to start again. It is said that approximately a quarter of a million came as indentured servants. They committed themselves to work for a number of years to pay for their passage. Many of them came from the jails and debtors' prisons, seeking an opportunity to begin a new and rewarding life.

England laid claim to the portion of the Atlantic coast that lay between the claims of Spain and France. Colonization was a private affair, in that the English government granted permission to an individual or a chartered company to establish a colony. Royalties were paid to the Crown; profits and losses were assumed by the proprietors. The first permanent English settlement in America was made in Jamestown in 1607 by the London Company. The area was named Virginia, after the virgin queen, Elizabeth. The colony faced many hardships and suffered American Indian massacres, illness, starvation, and heavy mortality. Medical care was lacking, and little of what could be called nursing was available. The first three years in the new colony were a period of human devastation. All but sixty of the original five hundred settlers died of malnutrition or dietary insufficiency. A shipload of women arrived in Jamestown in 1619 to be auctioned off as wives. During that same year the first slaves were brought from Africa.

A succession of colonies followed Jamestown. A group of Separatists, who were later known as Pilgrims, sailed on the *Mayflower* and landed at New Plymouth in 1620. This group was augmented by the Puritans, who were being persecuted in England. (The Plymouth Company was later incorporated as the Massachusetts Bay Company, which became identical with the Massachusetts colony.) In 1626 the Dutch East India Company established a colony called New Netherlands, which was located in what are now Staten Island, Manhattan, and Delaware. The principal town, called New Amster-

dam, was located on the island of Manhattan. Maryland was founded as a refuge for English Catholics in 1633 by Lord Baltimore, Cecil Calvert; a group of Jesuits; and three hundred carefully selected colonists. Connecticut and Rhode Island were founded as a result of grievances among members of the Massachusetts colony. Pennsylvania was given to William Penn by Charles II in payment of a debt to Penn's father. This Quaker colony was noted for tolerance and religious freedom. English colonization became a reality as other equally important settlements developed. There was, however, little similarity and unity among them. Each colony was self-governed, and there was no central power to coordinate them. They remained isolated and even antagonistic toward one another for almost a century and a half. Their differences were caused particularly by religious beliefs, although varying temperaments and the prevalence of bigotry played a role.

The Pilgrim Fathers brought a stern philosophy with them to the New World, and it was not conducive to the development of institutions for the care of the sick. They took it for granted that welfare work was a function of private charity or the state. It was assumed that families would look after their own unfortunates and therefore that public refuge was unnecessary. Early treatments of diseases consisted largely of prayer intermingled with much superstitious medical practice. Samuel Fuller, a deacon, acted as a physician in New England for thirteen years after his arrival on the *Mayflower*. Physicians did not need degrees; the educated individuals among the colonists (clergy, governors, and schoolteachers) were thought to be well-enough equipped to handle the role of physician. Ignorant quacks were in abundance. American Indian folklore soon became incorporated into the overall scheme. "Obviously this clerical and lay medicine would have to be very primitive. It was a peculiar mixture of religious medicine, folk-medicine, and scientific principle. One invoked the word of God, let blood, or prescribed drugs, to the best of one's understanding. We must not forget that at this period European medicine, even when practiced by physicians, was effective only in exceptional cases" (Sigerist, 1934, p. 37).

The English settlers lacked the organized service of the convent or the mission, the experience of nuns and priests. Consequently, hospitals developed slowly in the original thirteen colonies. Social welfare was considered the responsibility of the individual, the family, or the neighborhood. Relatives or friends supplied nursing care when needed. Otherwise, nursing fell to those persons who were inclined to do it. When the settlements reached a certain size, however, some sort of public refuge had to be provided. The colonists followed the pattern of the homeland and ultimately organized institutions for the sick and the poor. This was not done out of Christian charity as much as for social convenience. The poorhouse and the hospital were placed under one roof, and the conditions were similar to those found by Elizabeth Fry in Britain.

HOSPITAL DEVELOPMENT IN AMERICA

The growth of hospitals in colonial America was slow. In the 150 years before the American Revolution (1776-1784), approximately 5 hospitals were founded outside of Canada. The earliest were not hospitals in the true sense of the word. They were usually almshouses that included infirmaries where the sick poor were attended by inmates. Regarded by some as the first hospitals in the English colonies, they later evolved into separate municipal hospitals.

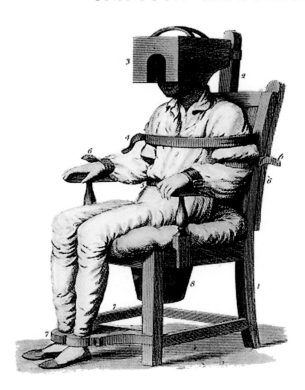

Tranquilizing Chair, engraving, The Granger Collection, NY.

Several hospitals claim to have been the first established in America. This discrepancy is directly related to the definition of *hospital* and the specific focus of the institution. As indicated previously, many of these early hospitals were developed as poorhouses; the care of the sick was incidental. However, the earliest hospital on record was established in New Amsterdam by the Dutch West India Company in 1658. Located on Manhattan Island, it cared for sick soldiers and slaves coming into port as cargo on company ships.

The Philadelphia Almshouse, erected in 1731, cared for the sick, the indigent, the insane, the infirm, prisoners, and orphans. (In 1919 the hospital was separated from the almshouse.) From 1835 to 1902 it was known as the Philadelphia Hospital; the name was changed to the Philadelphia General Hospital in 1902. Servants, criminals, and paupers cared for the sick. This institution is usually designated as "the oldest hospital in continuous service" and was affectionately known as Old Blockley. It offered the typical picture of the almshouse of the late 18th and early 19th centuries. The treatment of the insane was particularly disheartening. The female lunatics were under the supervision of a male keeper who was assisted by two male paupers. These men slept among the insane and entirely managed the violent cases, even bathing and dressing the women. "Some of the patients, even in their madness, shrunk from this rude handling and raved with increased fury at their indecent exposure. Revolting to decency as this practice was, it was not without difficulty, and only by degrees, abandoned" (Nutting and Dock, vol. 2, 1907, p. 333). In addition, it was the custom to permit the public to visit these insane wards to stare, laugh, and jeer at the inmates.

The nursing in this institution was as crude and indifferent as anything that had taken place in London. During a cholera outbreak in 1832, for example, the attendants were found to be continuously intoxicated. In their drunken state, they fought over the beds of the sick or lay in a stupor beside dead bodies.

Nurses became clamorous for an increase in wages, which was granted. Those between terror and want of moral sense were seized with a kind of mad infatuation. They drank the stimulants provided for the sick, and in one ward where the pestilence raged in its most fearful forms, and where between the dead and the dying the sight was most appalling, these furies were seen lying drunk upon or fighting over the dead victims of the disease. In this state of disorder, application was made to Bishop Kendrick for Sisters of Charity. The request was granted, and these devoted ministers of mercy at once entered upon their mission of danger, restoring order and diffusing hope by the calm and self-possessed manner with which they moved among the diseased. These Sisters remained at their post until the 20th of May 1833. The situation improved with the introduction of the Sisters of Charity of Emmitsburg, who undertook the task of reform. This transpired after investigations in 1793 and 1832, which brought the shocking conditions to light. After the sisters departed, unsatisfactory conditions returned and remained for a long time. Finally, Alice Fisher, a Nightingale nurse, arrived in 1884 and proceeded to upgrade the quality of nursing care.

— BUSH, 1890

Bellevue Hospital had its beginnings in the small hospital established by the West India Company in 1658. It was sold in 1680 and a better building was provided. In 1736 another new building was added to serve as a Publick Workhouse and House of Correction of New York. This building became the immediate predecessor of Bellevue and stood where New York's City Hall now stands. It was rebuilt and enlarged several times. Buildings changed according to societal needs, and the city eventually assumed a share of the expenses of charity. In time, the present Bellevue Hospital was concentrated on the bank of the East River. The building was originally (1794) used as a pesthouse to serve victims of yellow fever and for several years was used only when yellow fever broke out in the city. In 1811, more ground around the hospital was bought, and a new almshouse was built and dedicated on July 29, 1811. Officially opened in 1816, this institution contained the almshouse, a penitentiary, wards for the sick and the insane, and rooms for the resident physician, warden, and attendants. The sick were cared for by paupers or prisoners, political graft flourished, and epidemics were frequent. For many years Bellevue was a house of horrors. "Hospitals were as a rule in a disgraceful state of degradation. They were dirty and ill ventilated, they reeked with infection, so that patients who came in suffering from one disease, or from a wound, caught another disease or some virulent infection. The death rate was fearfully high, sometimes actually more than 50 percent. In the days before Lister, hospital surgery was extremely discouraging. The only nurses that could be obtained for hospitals were women who did the menial work besides caring for the patients" (Walsh, 1929).

A committee was designated in 1837 to investigate the deplorable state of the hospital. According to Carlisle (1893), the prevailing conditions cited by the committee included filth, no ventilation, overcrowded wards, no clothing or supplies, patients with high fever lying naked in bed, putrefaction, and vermin. In addition, it was stated that the resident physician—with his students, the matron, and the nurses—had left the building. As a result, the pesthouse, the prison, and later the psychiatric wards were removed to Blackwell's Island. A new era began with the creation of a medical board in 1847. The almshouse and hospital, however, remained

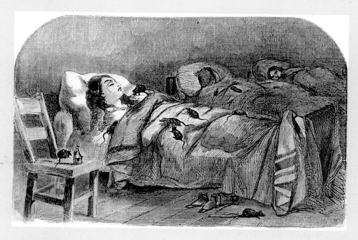

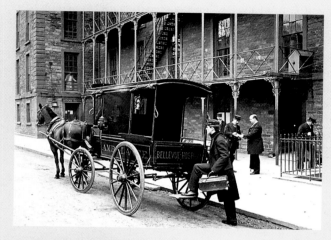

We give herewith a picture of the beds in Bellevue Hospital in this city, in one of which the newborn child of Mary Connor was eaten by rats on Monday morning, April 23… the building's swarming with rats, as many as 40 having been found in the bathtub one evening, and Mary Connor herself mentions that in her agony, she felt them running over her body.

Bellevue Hospital, 1860, color engraving, The Granger Collection, NY.

The Bellevue Hospital ambulance in New York.

Ambulance, 1895, photograph, The Granger Collection, NY.

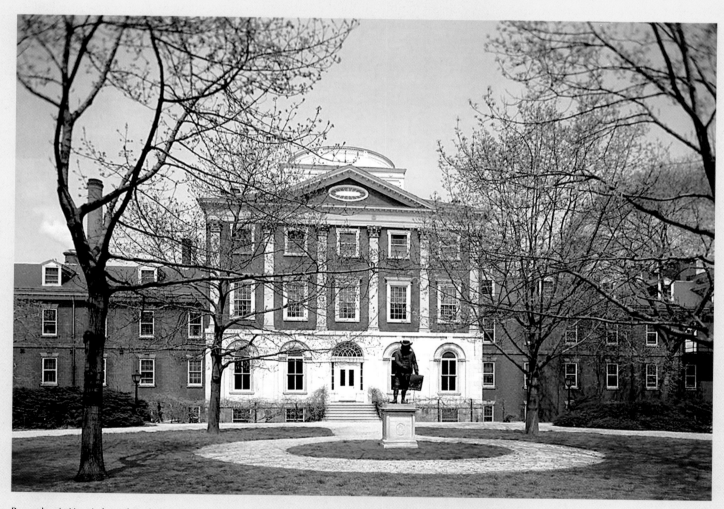

Pennsylvania Hospital was founded at the suggestion of Benjamin Franklin. It became the first hospital in the United States that was designed solely for the curative care of the sick. Its seal is that of the Good Samaritan: "Take care of him and I will repay thee." An inscription written by Benjamin Franklin appears on the cornerstone.

Pennsylvania Hospital, 1796, photograph, Arts of the United States Collection, University of Georgia.

together until 1848, when Bellevue began its ensuing career as a hospital.

Bellevue was probably the first institution to establish an ambulance service (1869). Provisions were made for emergency treatment: "Beneath the driver's seat was a box containing a quart flask of brandy, two tourniquets, a half-dozen bandages, a half-dozen small sponges, some splint material, pieces of old blankets for padding, strips of various lengths with buckles, and a two-ounce vial of persulphate of iron" (Kane, 1934, p. 332).

In 1751 the first hospital, in the truest sense of the word, was founded in Philadelphia through the efforts of Dr. Thomas Bond and other Philadelphia physicians. This group proposed that a general hospital be established there, and they worked to obtain contributions. With the assistance of Benjamin Franklin, they were able to secure funds from the Province (State) of Pennsylvania and from private donors. The Pennsylvania Hospital became the first hospital in the United States designed solely for the curative care of the sick.

After careful selection, servant-nurses were employed. The seal of this institution is that of the Good Samaritan: "Take care of him and I will repay thee." The most renowned physician of colonial times, Dr. Benjamin Rush (1745-1813), served the mentally ill in Pennsylvania Hospital. His most famous work, *Medical Inquiries and Observations Upon Diseases of the Mind,* was published in 1812 and contained a foresightful approach to care. A separate department for the mentally ill was developed in 1841, and it was referred to as Kirkbride, after Dr. Thomas Kirkbride, who was in charge of the service for 42 years. Before that time, lunatics had been caged in the basement of the general hospital.

The New York Hospital received its charter from King George III in 1771. According to Nutting and Dock (1907), it did not, however, receive patients until January 1791. The original building burned to the ground. The hospital was used by British and Hessian soldiers as barracks, and it suffered the disorganizations of war. It was backed by the most prominent and cultured citizens, and its attendants were probably superior to those of Bellevue and Blockley. The care offered to patients was also better than that given in the almshouses. Dr. Valentine Seaman gave the nurses a series of lectures that focused on anatomy, physiology, maternal nursing, and the care of children. The later lectures were published in *The Midwife's Monitor and Mother's Mirror* in 1800. Dr. Seaman regarded midwives as indispensable, and he believed that they should be thoroughly and carefully taught. He did not seem to make a clear differentiation between midwifery and nursing.

In addition to the Pennsylvania Hospital in Philadelphia and the New York Hospital, Massachusetts General Hospital (1807) was also located in a large city. All of these hospitals had excellent buildings (block-type) for the period and tended to follow the British models. Massachusetts General was a private enterprise and was established by a group of prominent physicians. It subsequently began to build pavilion wards with the idea that patients needed to be segregated and provided with increased light, air, and space. It eventually acquired a reputation for cleanliness and good nursing care.

Other hospitals that still carry on public service, along with several dispensaries, originated before 1860. The Quakers established the Philadelphia Dispensary in 1786 to care for the sick in their homes. It was independent of any hospi-

tal, and finances were taken care of through appeals to public sympathy. The concept that large numbers of people needing treatment were not sick enough to be hospitalized was a relatively new one. As a result of this idea, the expense of hospital care became unnecessary. Medical, surgical, and obstetrical services were offered under the supervision of Dr. Joseph Warrington. Physicians treated individuals without charge and made home visits when necessary. The dispensary was a success, and the idea spread to other cities. The New York Dispensary was opened in 1791; the Boston Dispensary, in 1796. The latter had the first dental, lung, and evening clinics for working people in the nation; in addition, it housed the first food clinic in the world. The dispensaries sank into neglect and almost obscurity when public and professional interests turned to hospitals. Services dwindled until first-aid service and the issuance of free medicines were the only remaining functions.

MEDICINE IN THE COLONIES

Medicine could offer little help against rampant disease and sickness in colonial America. Medieval methods were used in diagnosis, and treatments generally were not scientifically based. Emetics, purgatives, and bleeding continued to be the chief methods employed in the care of the sick. Brandy and whiskey became favorite remedies for febrile illnesses and continued to be so for a number of years. By the middle of the 19th century, however, the contributions to scientific knowledge made by Pasteur, Lister, Koch, and others began the modern era of medicine and surgery. The science of bacteriology provided the foundation. The introduction of ether and chloroform as general anesthetics facilitated surgical practice. These advances altered the course of medical history to the point where the concepts of illnesses, treatments, and hygienic practices at the end of the century bore little resemblance to the perceptions of them in the beginning. "Looking back, one may say that medicine was groping in the dark but was seeking light with growing anticipation. New concepts as well as further knowledge were essential if light was to be found" (Shryock, 1959, p. 195).

Serious health problems were brought to the New World with the migrants who left Europe. Scarlet fever, diphtheria, influenza, typhoid, typhus, tuberculosis, yellow fever, and other infectious diseases produced epidemics that were constant nightmares. Scurvy and pellagra were the prevalent nutrition-oriented diseases and indicated the lack of proper food, particularly among the poorer classes. One in five individuals was afflicted with smallpox, which proved to be a formidable and dreaded disease. Fear became so great that experiments with inoculation were undertaken. Nearly all physicians opposed it, but the prominent clergy supported it. The opposition arose apparently because of the risk factors involved in inoculation (occasionally, deaths followed). The process of inoculation represented the beginnings of preventive medicine or, more specifically, immunology. A modified form called vaccination replaced the use of smallpox inoculation. Developed and reported in 1798 by Edward Jenner, it employed the use of the cowpox "virus," which proved to be safer and equally effective.

The true nature of disease remained an enigma. In addition, few persons understood how the prevailing practices used in disease and illness worked. They were ignorant of the actions within the body that brought about the observed effects. In many instances it was enough just to know that it

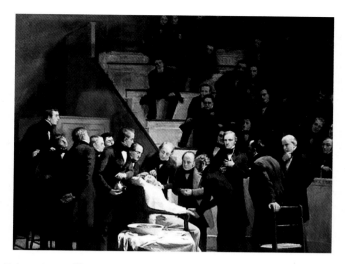

Robert C. Hinckley, *The First Operation Under Ether,* 1882-1894, oil on canvas. Boston Medical Library in the Francis A. Coutnway Library of Medicine.

worked. "Learned men" gave advice on care of the sick and surgical care. Many laypersons thus functioned as physicians without ever having received formal medical degrees. Colonial physicians were generally poorly educated. According to some sources, the title *doctor* was not even used in the colonies before 1769. It was an age of few doctors and of many profiteering quacks.

> Of medicine the Puritans knew little and practiced less. They swallowed doses of weird and repelling concoctions, wore charms and amulets, found comfort and relief in internal and external remedies that could have had no possible influence upon the cause of the trouble, and when all else failed they fell back upon the mercy and will of God. Surgery was a matter of tooth-pulling and bone-setting, and though post-mortems were performed, we have no knowledge of the skill of the practitioner. The healing art, as well as nursing and midwifery, was frequently in the hands of women. . . . The men who practiced physic were generally homebred, making the greater part of their living at farming or agriculture. Some were ministers as well as physicians. . . . There were a number of regularly trained doctors—though not a physician had more than a smattering of medicine.
> — *ANDREWS, 1918, VOL. 6, P. 82*

Individuals who could afford the expense went to Europe to study in the medical schools of Edinburgh or Vienna. Otherwise, young students of medicine were apprenticed to practicing physicians, to whom they paid a fee (usually one hundred dollars) and rendered services in the houses and stables. They were permitted to observe their masters treat patients and upon completing the duration of the apprenticeship would receive the textbooks and instruments essential for their practice. The learning techniques comprised observation, reading, and practice. The average time spent in this process was approximately one hundred and forty-four weeks, or close to three years. The preceptors ultimately became a powerful force that prevented progress in medical education and care.

As the colonies continued to develop, the issue of medical education increased in importance. Yet the medical departments did not find places in colleges or universities until Harvard, the first American university (founded in 1636), was more than one hundred years old. They were then orga-

nized rapidly and included the Medical College of Philadelphia in 1765 (later a part of the University of Pennsylvania); King's College in New York City in 1767; Harvard in 1783; and Dartmouth in 1798. Other programs developed in the next century and included those established at Yale in 1810 and at Johns Hopkins University in 1893.

> When the nineteenth century dawned, America had only four small medical schools to supply physicians for its burgeoning population, compelling most doctors to acquire their training by apprenticeship. In 1807 the University of Maryland Medical School was organized by a small group of Baltimore physicians as a private venture, and in succeeding years dozens of these proprietary medical schools came into existence. Three or four physicians would apply for a state charter, rent or buy a building, and begin advertising for students. The school year ordinarily lasted eight to fourteen weeks, and the course work consisted exclusively of listening to lectures. Many proprietary schools granted degrees after one academic year, although they usually required the student to have served a one- or two-year apprenticeship prior to admission. These schools were dependent upon student fees for income, so few applicants were ever turned down and even fewer failed to graduate.
> — *LYONS, 1978, P. 534*

Approximately 400 medical schools were established before 1860, and many of them graduated poorly educated physicians. The quality of instruction was inferior, libraries were inadequate, there were no laboratories, and dissection opportunities were limited. Little had been done to regulate these programs. The formation of the American Medical Association in 1847 finally led to the reform and advancement of medicine. This organization advocated the improvement of medical education, the establishment of a code of ethics, and the promotion of public health measures. The advent of this association moved American medicine toward professionalization. The American Medical Association created a permanent committee on education in 1904, and it became the American Medical Association Council on Medical Education in 1906. This council persuaded the Carnegie Foundation for the Advancement of Teaching to evaluate medical schools according to the ability of their graduates to pass licensing board examinations. Abraham Flexner was employed by the foundation to survey the field. His report, commonly referred to as the Flexner Report, was published in 1910 as *Medical Education in the United States and Canada.* It was a damning indictment of medical education and brought foundation money to the higher quality schools; the weaker schools were forced out of business. The council, in turn, classified the schools into A, B, and C categories, which played a primary role in the standardization of medical education.

The remarkable progress that was finally achieved in the scientific basis of patient care was illustrated by Thomas Eakins (1844-1916). This American artist left two paintings that vividly present before-and-after looks at the medical scene. His celebrated painting *The Gross Clinic* (1875) depicts grand rounds in which Dr. Samuel Gross explains to medical students the surgical operation being performed. It appears that he is totally unaware of the patient and oblivious to the horror of the patient's mother, who sits to his right. *The Agnew Clinic* (1889) depicts a distinct change and a striking contrast to the earlier work. The surgeons are wearing

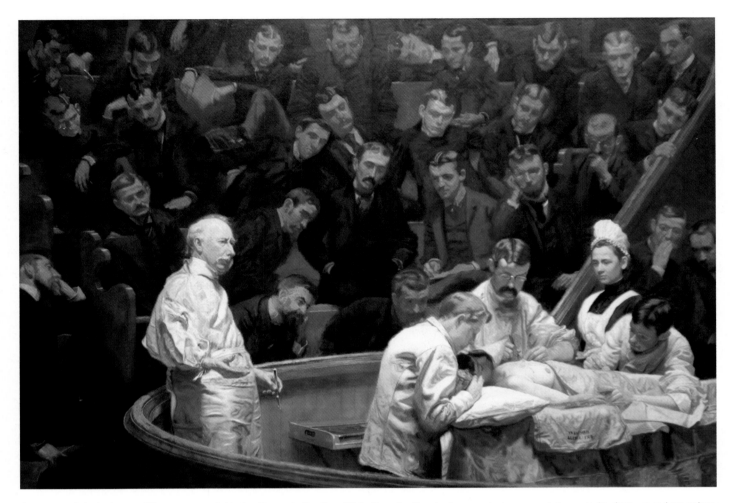

The Agnew Clinic depicts a striking contrast to Eakins' earlier work, *The Gross Clinic*. Here significant reforms and advancements in surgical techniques and procedures in the operating room are apparent. Surgeons wear gowns, instruments are sterilized, ether is used, and the patient is covered. An operating room nurse is a prominent member of the team.

Thomas Eakins, *The Agnew Clinic*, 1889, oil on canvas, 106" × 143". Courtesy of the University of Pennsylvania Art Collection, Philadelphia, PA.

gowns, instruments are sterilized, the patient is covered, and ether is being used. The operation being performed is a mastectomy for breast cancer. This painting also depicts an operating room nurse (nursing schools had finally opened) as a prominent member of the operating team. The needed reforms had begun to occur.

RELIGIOUS NURSING ORDERS IN AMERICA

Many priests and nuns came to America with the French and Spanish settlers and supplied at least a minimum of nursing care to the Catholic communities. The Augustinian Nuns, Ursuline Nuns, and Sisters of Charity are mentioned most commonly in the history of nursing service in the hospitals of North and South America. Religious orders of women also contributed greatly to nursing care during the Civil War. Their organization and motivation provided distinct advantages over the so-called lay nurses of the day. The members of these orders had some education and had been carefully instructed. Those recruited to these orders were usually refined, intelligent women with sincere interest in the care of the sick.

Among the earliest religious communities that took part in the care of the sick in hospitals and homes in the United States were the Sisters of Charity of Emmitsburg, Maryland. This order was founded by Mother Seton (1774-1821) in 1809. Elizabeth Ann Bayley Seton became the first native-born North American to be canonized (in 1976) for her charitable

works. Her original community was known as the Sisters of Charity of St. Joseph's, but in 1850 the members united with the worldwide community of the Daughters of Charity of St. Vincent de Paul. A habit of blue with a large linen headdress (cornette) was chosen at that time in lieu of the original dress of the community. Eventually numerous orders and different branches of orders in the Roman Catholic Church bore the name Sisters of Charity: the Sisters of Charity of New York (Black Cap Sisters of Charity); the Sisters of Charity of Greensburg, Pennsylvania; of New Jersey; of Cincinnati; of Halifax, Nova Scotia; and of Nazareth, Kentucky. The last community was founded by Mother Catherine Spalding; its members used horses to travel to the homes of patients. These various orders were also called by other names: Grey Sisters or Grey Nuns, Daughters of Charity, and Sisters of St. Vincent de Paul. Opportunities were provided in nursing education, the delivery of nursing service, and parochial education.

Elizabeth Seton was the daughter of Richard Bayley, an eminent American physician who was the first professor of anatomy at King's College (now Columbia University). Elizabeth Seton and other society matrons established the Society for Relief of Poor Widows with Small Children (1797) in New York to raise money for poor widows, to visit them in their homes, and to nurse and comfort them. Upon her husband's early death in 1803, she was left with five children and no financial support. Her conversion to Catholicism alienated friends who otherwise might have assisted her.

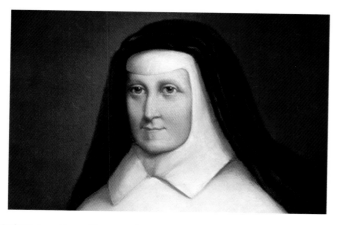

Catherine and two of her associates entered the Convent of the Presentation Sisters in Dublin on Sept. 8, 1830 to begin formal preparation for founding the Sisters of Mercy. Fifteen months later, the trio pronounced vows of poverty, chastity, and obedience, and to persevere until death in "the Congregation of the Sisters of Mercy." Thus the new community was founded on December 12, 1831.

Catherine McAuley, portrait. Image courtesy of Sisters of Mercy.

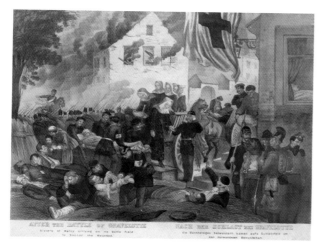

The first Sisters of Mercy arrived in Pittsburgh in the United States from Dublin, Ireland in 1843. Their energy in ministering to the sick and economically poor attracted many new members. By 1854, sisters had come from Ireland to settle in New York and San Francisco, and they continued to spread throughout the country, establishing schools and hospitals.

After the Battle of Gravelotte. Sisters of Mercy Arriving on the Battle Field to Succor the Wounded, 1870 or 1871, lithograph. Bridgeman Art Library.

She turned to teaching and opened a school for girls in Baltimore. A piece of land in Emmitsburg was chosen for the school, and it was not long before other young women joined her and became sisters in this teaching order. This event was the beginning of parochial education in the United States.

These Sisters of Charity became well known for their remarkable work in hospital nursing and in nursing during epidemics. They were asked to manage a number of hospitals, including the Baltimore Infirmary, the Mullanphy Hospital in St. Louis, Missouri, and the Charity Hospital of New Orleans. Nursing thus became an important branch of their work. The members were also instrumental in founding several hospitals and mental and foundling asylums.

Demands for nursing care by the religious orders increased as the settlements of the new country progressed. The various Catholic nursing orders responded rapidly and developed extensive networks throughout the country. The Sisters of Mercy, the Sisters of the Holy Cross, the Irish Sisters of Mercy (who came to America in 1843), the Domini-

cans, the Sisters of the Poor of St. Francis, and other communities worked in hospitals and homes and in all types of settings. The majority of them also nursed under fire on the battlefields. They founded hospitals everywhere and provided the highest standards of nursing of the times. Many of the first hospitals in America were named Mercy Hospitals, such as those in Pittsburgh, Chicago, and San Francisco. These were the better hospitals that were available at the time of the Civil War.

Sisterhoods of the Protestant church also contributed to the nursing effort in America. The Episcopal Sisterhood of the Holy Communion was founded in New York in 1845 by Pastor Muhlenberg at what is currently St. Luke's Hospital. The work of the English Lutheran Church began with four deaconesses who were brought to Passavant's Hospital in Pittsburgh by Pastor Fliednor in 1849. In Baltimore there was a branch of the English All Saints Sisters. The English Sisterhood of St. Margaret's (Episcopal) was brought to Boston in about 1869, the beginning of its 40-some years of service to the Children's Hospital of that city. Many deaconess hospitals were established, particularly in the Midwest. Protestant religious nursing groups also gave nursing care to the sick and the wounded during the time of the Civil War.

THE EVOLUTION OF SCHOOLS OF NURSING

The experiences of the Civil War emphasized the inadequate preparation of the majority of nurses who participated. Public interest in nursing was thus aroused, and awareness of the need to develop training programs for nurses increased. This movement was assisted by the large number of women from socially prominent families who had served. Their involvement and support lent a certain measure of respectability to the image of nursing. Two specific documents clearly indicated this rising interest in the potential development of nursing education. The first was written by a group of physicians; the second appeared as an editorial in a prominent women's magazine.

In 1868, Samuel D. Gross (1804-1884), president of the American Medical Association, voiced support for the training of nurses:

> I am not aware that the education of nurses has received any attention from this body; a circumstance the more surprising when we consider the great importance of the subject. It seems to me to be just as necessary to have well trained, well instructed nurses as to have intelligent and skillful physicians. I have long been of the opinion that there ought to be in all the principal towns and cities of the Union institutions for the education of men and women whose duty it is to take care of the sick and to carry out the injunctions of the medical attendant. There is hardly one nurse, of either sex, in twenty who has a perfect appreciation of the requirements of the sick room, or who is capable of affording the aid and comfort so necessary to a patient when oppressed by disease or injury. It does not matter what may be the skill of the medical practitioner, how assiduous or faithful he may be in the discharge of his functions as guardian of health and life, his efforts can be of comparatively little avail unless they are seconded by an intelligent and devoted nurse. Myriads of human beings perish annually in the so called civilized world for the want of good nursing.
>
> — *COMMITTEE ON THE TRAINING OF NURSES, AMERICAN MEDICAL ASSOCIATION, 1869*

The following year at the New Orleans meeting of the American Medical Association (1869), Samuel Gross, chairman of the Committee on the Training of Nurses, presented a report. This committee had been appointed to investigate the best possible method of organizing and managing institutions for the training of nurses. The strange neglect of nursing in the United States was identified and the need for good nursing emphasized. Early American efforts toward hospital reform were mentioned, and the vast extent of volunteer nursing in the Civil War was stressed. The committee made the following proposals:

> I. That every large and well-organised hospital should have a school for the training of nurses, not only for the supply of its own necessities, but for private families; the teaching to be furnished by its own medical staff, assisted by the resident physicians.
>
> II. That, while it is not at all essential to combine religious exercises with nursing, it is believed that such a union would be eminently conducive to the welfare of the sick in all public institutions, and the committee therefore earnestly recommend the establishment of nurses' homes, to be placed under the immediate supervision and direction of Deaconesses or lady superintendents.
>
> III. That, in order to give thorough scope and efficiency to this scheme, district schools should be formed and placed under the guardianship of the county medical societies of every State and Territory in the Union, the members of which should make it their business to impart instruction in the art and science of nursing.
>
> — PROCEEDINGS OF THE AMERICAN MEDICAL ASSOCIATION, 1869, PP. 339, 351

Further suggestions related to the importance of forming societies of nurses, the qualities necessary for the nurse to possess, and the sending of copies of the report to medical societies all over the country. It is particularly interesting that in November of that same year, Rudolf Virchow presented similar recommendations to a women's association in Berlin, Germany.

The *Godey's Lady's Book and Magazine,* popular in the late 19th century, strongly influenced women's fashions and manners. It had been founded by Louis A. Godey, who appointed Sarah Josepha Hale as editor in 1837. Hale's interest in the education of nurses was illustrated by an editorial titled "Lady Nurses," which appeared in the February 1871 issue:

> Much has been lately said of the benefits that would follow if the calling of sick nurse were elevated to a profession which an educated lady might adopt without a sense of degradation, either on her own part or in the estimation of others. . . . There can be no doubt that the duties of sick nurse, to be properly performed, require an education and training little, if at all, inferior to those possessed by members of the medical profession. To leave these duties to untaught and ill-trained persons is as great a mistake as it was to allow the office of surgeon to be held by one whose proper calling was that of a mechanic of the humblest class. The manner in which a reform may be effected is easily pointed out. Every medical college should have a course of study and training especially adapted for ladies who desire to qualify themselves for the profession of nurse; and those who had gone through the course, and passed the requisite examination,

should receive a degree and a diploma, which would at once establish their position in society. The "graduate nurse" would in general estimation be as much above the ordinary nurse of the present day as the professional surgeon of our times is above the barber-surgeon of the last century.

> — HALE, 1871, PP. 188-189

The need for nurses was great. According to Hale, however, this need also involved a well-planned educational program that would generate "professional nurses." Training schools for nurses were eventually established, and they proliferated.

FIRST INSTRUCTION FOR NURSES

Until the inception of the first formal training schools for nurses, individuals who were involved with the care of the sick, as well as midwives, received intermittent lectures from physicians in the eastern cities of the United States. This was in no way, however, an organized course of instruction. Most information was gleaned simply by doing nursing, such as it was. The only organized preparation available was offered in Catholic sisterhoods, and it was restricted to members of the order.

It is difficult to determine who should receive the distinction of having the first trained nurses in America. There were a number of individuals whose foresight led them to appreciate the need for the training of nurses. These pioneers attempted to rectify the situation. Valentine Seaman, a medical chief at the New York Hospital, is usually credited with initiating the first system of instruction for nurses on the North American continent. Below his portrait in the original hospital building is an inscription that praises his achievement: "In 1798 he organized in the New York Hospital the first regular training school for nurses, from which other schools have since been established and extended their blessings throughout the Community" (Nutting and Dock, vol. 2, 1907, p. 339).

Almost a generation later, the next attempt was made to train women for obstetrical nursing. This movement was initiated by Joseph Warrington, a physician in obstetrics to the Philadelphia Dispensary for the Medical Relief of the Poor. (He formed another institution in 1832, the Philadelphia Lying-in Charity for Attending Indigent Females in Their Own Homes.) As a result of his efforts, the Nurse Society of

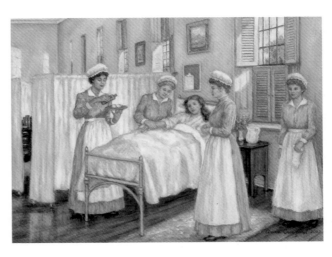

Anne Crawford, *Nurses,* circa 1883, painting, Historical Med Arts.

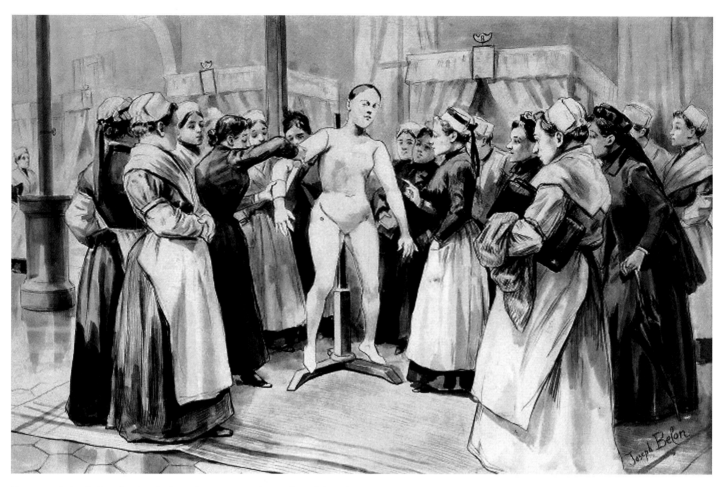

Nurses are being lectured on bandaging using a mannequin on a hospital ward.

Joseph Belon, *La Laicisation des Hopitaux Ecole des Infirmieres*, 1900-1927, charcoal with pen and ink, with wash and heightening, 33.1 × 48.6 cm. Wellcome Libarary.

Philadelphia was formed on March 5, 1839. The women followed a plan of instruction that included lectures given by Warrington, demonstrations, and practice on a mannequin. They received certificates and were eligible for calls after satisfactorily serving six cases. Accepted candidates, who were referred to as probationers, had been thoroughly screened. Early reports refer to this structure as the First Nurse Training School founded in America and the First School in America established to Train Women as Nurses. In 1897 the plan of instruction was extended to one year.

Woman's Hospital of Philadelphia opened a training school in 1861. It progressed slowly until 1872, when it received an endowment permitting it to be called the first endowed school of nursing in America. This school was organized and conducted by two women physicians, Ann Preston and Emmelin Horton Cleveland. It was unique in the sense that it had been planned specifically with the education of student nurses, rather than the care of patients, as its primary objective. In 1863, Preston wrote a pamphlet, *Nursing the Sick and the Training of Nurses,* which described the ideal nurse as having "the patience of hope [and] the faith of love. The good nurse is an artist!" The course of instruction lasted 6 months and covered content concerning surgery, medicine, obstetrics, poultice and plaster preparation, dietetic principles, and methods of cooking.

Similar developments were transpiring in Boston. As early as 1860, the *New England Hospital for Women and Children* had attempted the teaching of nurses. This institution, staffed by women physicians, took the first step toward the

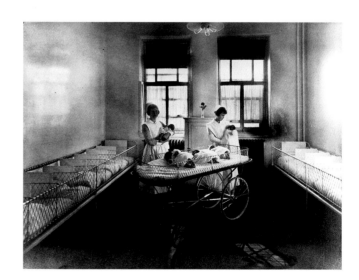

About 1900, most babies were born at home under the care of a midwife or doctor. As the 20th century progressed, rapid advances in modern medicine and the arrival of sophisticated scientific and technical equipment in hospitals occurred. Doctors stressed that it was safer for women to give birth in a modern hospital where chances for survival were higher. Increasing numbers of women decided to give birth in a hospital. By the 1960s it was rare for women to give birth at home.

Montreal Maternity Hospital, *Nurses, Cribs, and Baby Trolley,* 1925-1926, photograph, 19 × 24 cm, McCord Museum, gift of Miss Caroline Barrett.

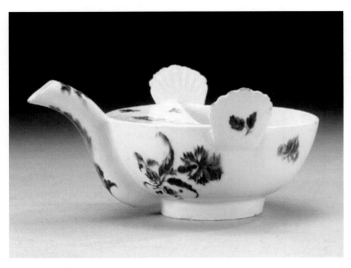

Ceramic cup with handle and wide spout, used to feed convalescing patients.

Feeding Cup.

development of a school of nursing with the arrival of Dr. Marie Zakrzewska in 1859. Upon her advice, the hospital charter issued in 1863 included a nursing school. Students were required to attend the entire 6-month course, which included practice at the bedsides of patients. The first month was a probationary period. Few women applied, and only 6 were trained over the next 2 years. In 1872 the hospital moved to new quarters in Roxbury, Massachusetts, and admitted a class of 5 students to its newly formed training school. The specific plan of the school has been described in the following way:

> Young women of suitable requirements and character will be admitted to the Hospital as school nurses, for one year. This year will be divided into four periods; three months will be given respectively to the practical study of nursing in the Medical, Surgical, and Maternity Wards, and night nursing. Here the pupil will aid the head nurse in all the care and work of the wards under the direction of the Attending and Resident Physicians and Medical Students.
> In order to enable women entirely dependent upon their work for support to obtain a thorough training, the nurses will be paid for their work from one to four dollars per week after the first fortnight, according to the actual value of their service to the Hospital.
> A course of lectures will be given to nurses at the Hospital by the physicians connected with the Institution beginning January 21. . . . Certificates will be given to such nurses as have satisfactorily passed a year in practical training in the Hospital.
>
> — MUNSON, 1948, P. 552

This school was under the direction of Dr. Susan Dimock. The students worked from 5:30 AM until 9:00 PM and slept in rooms near the ward in order that they might be immediately available if necessary. Their uniforms consisted of simple calico dresses and felt slippers. Dr. Zakrzewska taught the simple details of nursing. There were no head nurses and no superintendent. The growth of the school continued, and in 1882 the course was extended to 16 months. By that time the school had 2 head nurses and a superintendent of the training school. The program was lengthened to 2 years in 1893 and finally, in 1901, to 3 years.

One student graduated at the end of the first year, on October 1, 1873. Melinda Ann (Linda) Richards (1841-1930) received her certificate and became known as the "first trained nurse in the United States" or "America's first trained nurse." She was overwhelmed with job offers upon her graduation but finally decided to accept the position of night superintendent at Bellevue Hospital. A variety of experiences awaited her there, some of which were particularly appalling. During her stay at Bellevue, Richards made three significant contributions: she insisted on light at night (the gas had been turned so low that a lighted candle was necessary, but only two candles per week were allowed to each ward); she instituted written case histories instead of verbal reports; and she exposed the mortality rate resulting from puerperal fever, which thus led to the removal of mothers to Blackwell's Island (Robinson, 1946). After a year, Richards went to the Boston Training School (Massachusetts General Hospital) as its superintendent. There she gave actual patient care as well as performing the required administrative duties.

In 1877, Linda Richards went to England to study nursing methods and there became acquainted with Florence Nightingale. From 1885 to 1890 she was in Japan, where she organized the earliest training school in the islands of the Orient. Richards eventually returned to her alma mater and became the superintendent of the New England Hospital for Women and Children. Her later efforts, in collaboration with Edward Cowles, were directed toward the nursing of the insane. It is to her credit that for more than half a century she was an avid, active supporter of adequate education for nurses.

Mary Eliza Mahoney (1845-1926) completed the sixteen-month course of training at the New England Hospital for Women and Children on August 1, 1879. She is considered to be America's first black professional nurse, the first to graduate from a school of nursing. Throughout her life, she engaged primarily in private-duty nursing and worked for the acceptance of blacks in nursing. (As in most Northern schools, racial quotas had been established at the New England Hospital; the charter of the nursing school allowed for only *one* Negro and *one* Jewish student to be accepted each year.) Mahoney gave the welcoming address in 1909 at the first convention of the National Association of Colored Graduate Nurses. After her death, the association established an award in her honor that was presented for the first time in 1936. The Mary Mahoney Medal is presented at the American Nurses' Association convention to an individual who has been instrumental in promoting equal opportunities to minority persons in nursing.

Separate schools for educating black nurses eventually arose. They became a necessity in order that blacks, who were banned from many schools, could receive training in nursing. The first of these was established at Spelman Seminary in Atlanta, Georgia, in 1886. Two similar institutions began in 1891: Hampton Institute in Virginia and Provident Hospital in Chicago. A school of nursing was also started at Tuskegee Institute in Alabama in 1892 but was developed primarily to provide service rather than education. These schools experienced difficulties similar to those of the early white schools, but they also suffered from societal prejudice toward blacks.

Work was also begun in Canada to provide training for nurses. Around 1864 the community of St. Catharine's, Ontario, started a hospital with a little house, one nurse, a

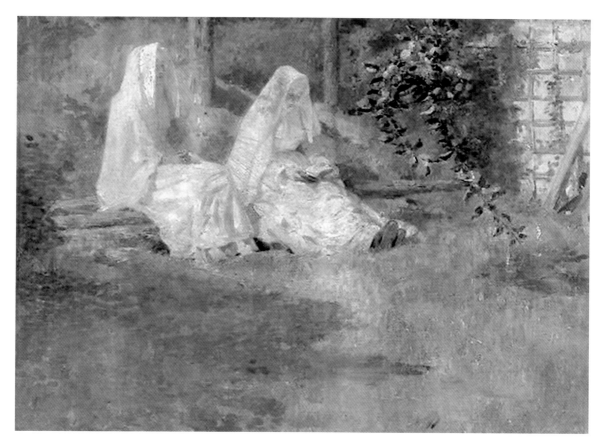

Alfred de Richemont, *La Lecture,* 19th century, painting, 46 × 55 cm. Photo courtesy of artnet.

steward, and ideas for the teaching of nurses. Under the direction of Theophilus Mack, a physician at the hospital and president of the board, the hospital grew steadily and definite teaching for nurses emerged in 1873. He was certain that the prejudice of many sick people against going into public hospitals would be overcome by a profession of trained lay nurses. At Mack's direction, a woman named Money was sent to England to bring back two trained nurses and five or six probationers. A system of training was in effect by 1874. The hospital was named St. Catharine's General and Marine Hospital. The nurses were required to stay for three years, during which time they were probationers without pay for the first 6 months. They then received a stipend, board, and uniforms. The first annual report, dated July 1, 1875, illustrated the value of trained nurses:

> The vocation of nursing goes hand in hand with that of the physician and surgeon, and they are absolutely indispensable one to the other. Incompetency on the part of a nurse renders negatory the best efforts of the doctor in the most critical moments, and has frequently resulted in loss of life. All the most brilliant achievements of modern surgery are dependent, to a great extent, upon careful and intelligent nursing, and the obstetrician knows only too well how fearful may be the consequences of ignorance and negligence on the part of attendants in the chamber of accouchement. The skilled nurse, by minutely watching the temperature, conditions of skin, pulse, respiration, and the various functions of all the organs, and reporting faithfully to the attending physician, must increase the chances of recovery twofold.

— *GIBBON AND MATHEWSON, 1947, P. 145*

THE NIGHTINGALE PLAN IN AMERICAN SCHOOLS

Improvement in the care of the sick in both hospitals and homes rested with the development of a system for training nurses. The time was finally ripe for the organization of schools of nursing. Following the Civil War, interest in nursing education was high and culminated in the almost simultaneous appearance of three important schools. In 1873 the famous trio of schools that encouraged the steady progress of nursing evolved: the Bellevue Training School in New York City on May 1, the Connecticut Training School in New Haven on October 1, and the Boston Training School (later the Massachusetts General Hospital Training School for Nurses) on November 1. Initially, these schools were based

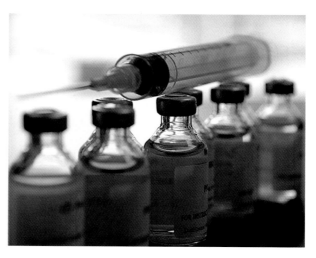

Nanette Bedway, *Vigilance,* photograph, Nannette Bedway Studio, Cleveland, OH.

145

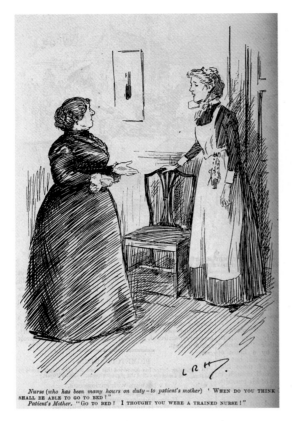

Nurse (who has been many hours on duty—to patient's mother) ' WHEN DO YOU THINK I SHALL BE ABLE TO GO TO BED !'
Patient's Mother. "GO TO BED ! I THOUGHT YOU WERE A TRAINED NURSE !"

Leonard Raven-Hill, *Exhausted Nurse,* wood engraving, Wellcome Library.

on the Nightingale model, but they were soon forced to deviate and follow a somewhat different path. The alterations that occurred greatly influenced the direction of nursing in America.

The earliest schools were created independent of hospitals by committees or boards that had the power to develop the schools. They were soon absorbed into the hospitals to which they were attached because of lack of endowment. This factor proved to be the greatest weakness in the system because many hospitals soon discovered that schools could be created to serve their needs, and a valuable source of almost free labor could be obtained.

> In the absence of public or private support, the schools from the time of their inception faced financial problems of major proportions. An agreement by the school to give nursing service for the hospitals providing clinical experience was the primary means of overcoming this difficulty. This type of apprenticeship agreement was the factor promoting hospitals to establish schools on their own initiative. Having a school of nursing became accepted as the most popular and least expensive means of providing nursing care. The hospital was the master and the student nurse was the apprentice, with the latter giving free labor to the former in return for informal training in the traditional manner.
> — ASHLEY, 1976, P. 9

Nursing care became the major product dispensed by hospitals. The real function of the school of nursing became not education, but service. In addition, no policy for the control of the numbers of nursing schools or for the standards of admission and graduation was established or accepted. Consequently, a proliferation of nursing schools occurred, and they became known as "diploma schools of nursing." The first decade of the 20th century demonstrated a period of phenomenal growth, with the establishment of close to seven hundred new schools. All school functions were ultimately placed under the control and general direction of hospital authorities, particularly physicians and hospital administrators.

Bellevue Hospital Training School. Women involved in the reform movement after the Civil War turned their endeavors toward the improvement of hospitals. Louisa Lee Schuyler and other women who had been prominent during the war effort and the U.S. Sanitary Commission founded the New York State Charities Aid Association in 1872. This voluntary body was concerned with the care of paupers, orphans, and the sick and regularly visited charitable institutions. Their intent was to evaluate the need for reforms. Some very prominent women—Mrs. Joseph Hobson, Mrs. William H. Osborn, Julia Gould, and Euphemia and B. Van Rensselaer—constituted one of its committees (Kalisch and Kalisch, 1995). This particular committee, with Mrs. Joseph Hobson as its chair, inspected Bellevue Hospital and found it in a deplorable state of affairs. The nursing care was given primarily by women who were ex-convicts; fees were collected from the patients for the inadequate services they received; drunkenness and foul language were prominent; supplies such as soap, linens, and dishes were unavailable; and conditions were particularly bad at night, when three night watchmen made periodic rounds of the wards. On the basis of the shocking report that was presented to the association, it was determined that the improvement of nursing must be one of the essential ingredients of hospital reform.

A resolution passed in April 1872 and addressed to the Commissioners of Charity begged this group to consider a plan for establishing a training school for nurses. The commissioners, in turn, referred the plan to the medical board, which remained silent on the subject for a time. However, Dr. Gill Wylie of the hospital staff voluntarily visited England to study schools established under Florence Nightingale, who had identified the essentials of a good training school. The following is a sample of some of those essentials:

> A year's practical and technical training in hospital wards, under trained head-nurses who themselves have been trained to train.
> The training of probationers should be as much a part of the duty of the head-nurse as directing the under-nurses or seeing to the patients.
> To tell the training, you require weekly records . . . kept by the head-nurses of the progress of each probationer in her ward-work, and in the moral qualities necessary in her ward-work; a monthly record by the matron of the results of the weekly records; and a quarterly statement by her as to how each head-nurse has performed her duty to each probationer. The whole to be examined periodically by the governing body.
> Clinical lectures from the hospital professors . . . elementary instruction in chemistry . . . physiology . . . and general instruction on medical and surgical topics; examinations, written and oral, at least four of each in the year, all adapted to nurses; as also lectures and demonstrations with anatomical, chemical and other illustrations, adapted especially to nurses. . . .
> A good nurses' library of professional books, not for the probationers to skip and dip in at random, but to be made careful use of, under the medical instructor and class-mistress. . . .
> The authority and discipline over all the women of a trained lady-superintendent . . . who is herself the best nurse in the hospital, the example and leader of her nurses in all that she wishes her nurses to be. . . .

An organization not only to give this training systematically, and to test it by current tests and examinations, but also to give the probationers, by proper help in the wards, time to do their work as pupils as well as assistant-nurses, and above all to make it a real moral as well as nursing probation—for nursing is a probation as well as a mission. Accommodation for sleeping, classes, and meals; arrangements for time and teaching and work; surroundings of a moral and religious, and hard-working and sober, yet cheerful tone and atmosphere, such as to make the training-school and hospital a "home" which no good young woman of any class need fear by entering to lose anything of health of body or mind; with moral and spiritual helps, and an elevating and motherly influence over all, such as to make the whole place which will train really good women, who can withstand temptation and do real work, and neither be "romantic" nor "menial."

— *Florence Nightingale, 1883, pp. 1039-1041*

Although Wylie was unable to confer with Nightingale personally, he received a letter from her upon his return home. This letter offered support and encouragement along with valuable information regarding the mechanics of a nursing school. In addition, it reiterated Nightingale's position that the nurse and the physician have different aspects of service and render different kinds of care. Finally, opposition was overcome, although somewhat reluctantly, and the commissioners agreed to the use of six wards in Bellevue for the training of nurses. Funds were raised and a house was rented for the nurses' home. The purpose of the program was "to train nurses for the care of the sick in order that women shall find a school for their education and the public shall reap the advantage of skilled and educated labor" (Dock, 1901, p. 90). Sister Helen Bowden of the Sisterhood of All Saints was selected to direct the program because she was familiar with the Nightingale system. She adopted a system similar to that of St. Thomas's School. The Nightingale system became known in America as the Bellevue System because it was introduced in that institution.

The Bellevue Hospital Training School for Nurses was founded in May 1873, and five students enrolled in the first class. The program was to last for 1 year, but students were required to remain in service for a second year. The students received only occasional lectures; the majority of time was spent in practical work through which they gained experience. They received 10 dollars per month after completing a probationary period of 1 month. Initially the students wore no uniforms, but after the first year, the training school committee decided that a standard uniform should be adopted. (No nurse in America had ever before worn a uniform.) This created a stir among the nurses, who were reluctant to wear uniforms. The committee astutely granted Euphemia Van Rensselaer—one of the students with a distinctive family name, social position, and personal beauty—a 2-day leave of absence from Bellevue. She returned in a uniform, apron, and cap that had been made especially for her. Her tailored uniform consisted of a long blue seersucker dress with a white apron, collar and cuffs, and a white cap. Within a week, every nurse was wearing the uniform, which eventually became the mark of a Bellevue nurse. A pin designed by Tiffany and Company in 1880 also distinguished its graduates.

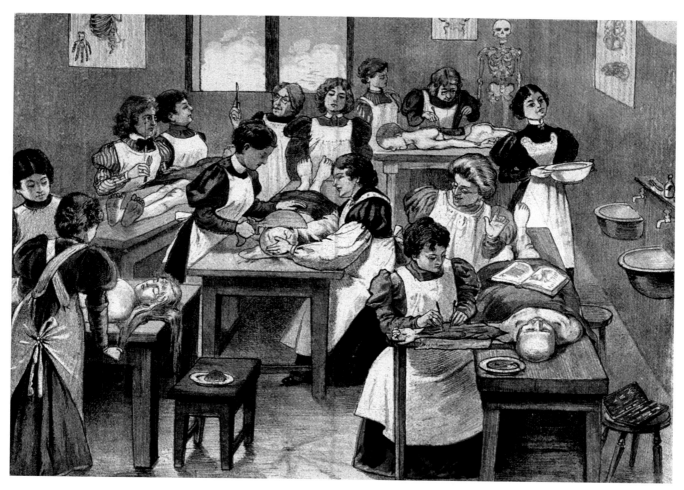

Dissection Lesson, 1897, lithograph, The Granger Collection, NY.

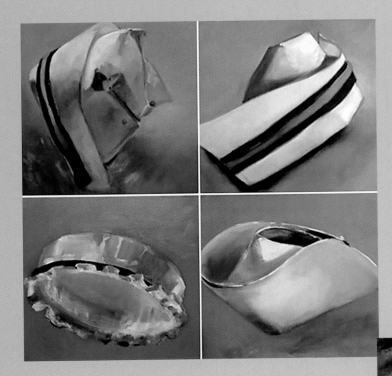

"Capping" was one of the most important milestones of progressing through the rigor of nursing school. It was derived from the nun's habit and over time became a symbol of hard work, loyalty, and service to mankind and a nearly universally recognized symbol of nursing. It was originally designed to cover the very long hair of women but eventually was replaced by a small cap that was representative of the nurse's alma mater. The use of nurses' caps in the United States (as well as many other nations) all but disappeared by the late 1980s since they no longer served any purpose. They are still worn in many developing nations.

Therese Cipiti Herron, *Colleagues Nursing Cap Portraits*, 2007, oil, each cap 12" × 12", Artists Collection. Published in *American Journal of Nursing*, January 2008.

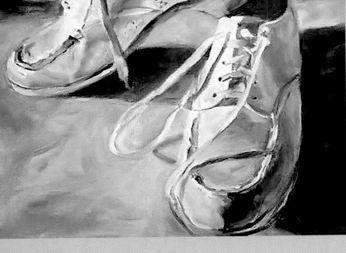

For many years, the Clinic shoe was the classic shoe worn by nurses, conveying a distinct professional look. Although long out of fashion, the Clinic shoe was renowned for its comfort and practicality.

Therese Cipiti Herron, *The Clinic Shoe*, 2005, oil, 12" × 12".

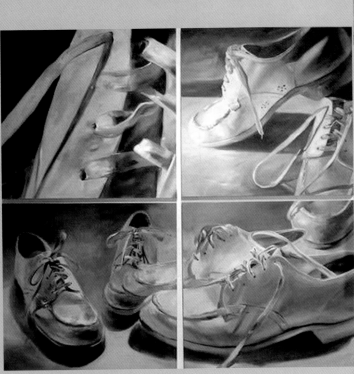

Therese Cipiti Herron, *Lost Soles*, 2005, oil on canvas, 72" × 72".

Connecticut Training School. The Connecticut Training School in New Haven was established through the efforts of Georgeanna Woolsey Bacon, her husband, Dr. Francis Bacon, and a wealthy philanthropist, Charles Thompson. Georgeanna Bacon and her two sisters had served as nurses in the Civil War and remained actively involved in nursing. The training school, established as an organization separate from the hospital, opened in October 1873 with four students. It was controlled by a board of directors who contracted an exchange with the hospital whereby nursing service would be provided for educational services. Physicians supported the school from the very beginning. Miss Bayard, who had been trained at the Women's Hospital of Philadelphia, became the head of the school, and it grew rapidly. By the end of the second year of operation, the first graduates were sent out to private families. By the fourth year the school was able to furnish superintendents of nursing to other hospitals. The school remained independent until 1906, when the hospital assumed control.

In 1879 the *New Haven Manual of Nursing*, created by a committee of both nurses and doctors, was published by the Connecticut Training School. It was a comprehensive text that found widespread acceptance among the nursing schools in the country. The school was one of the first to obtain a university affiliation (1924, Yale University) and an endowment of one million dollars from the Rockefeller Foundation. The Yale School of Nursing was the first in the world that was established as a separate university department with an independent budget and its own dean, Annie W. Goodrich.

Boston Training School. The Massachusetts General Hospital of Boston was the last of the three institutions to open a school for nurses. The idea was initiated by the Woman's Educational Association which called a meeting to consider the subject. A training-school committee was established to decide upon a plan, to ask for the cooperation of the physicians, to raise funds, and to seek permission from the trustees of Massachusetts General to develop a school in connection with that hospital. The school of nursing began operation as the Boston Training School and opened its doors in November 1873 with a superintendent, two head nurses, and six pupils to take charge of two wards. Mrs. Billings, who had experience as a hospital nurse in the Civil War, was the first superintendent.

From the very beginning, the medical staff had not favored or supported the school. Under the new arrangement the wards did not run smoothly, and the school was identified as the source of the difficulties. The training school committee was given another year's trial only after assuring the trustees that a graduate nurse would be placed in charge of the school; at the end of that time, a decision would be made to close or to continue the school. Linda Richards was placed in charge in November 1874, an event that marked a steady march of progress and success for the floundering program. She reorganized the school, conducted classes, and personally cared for patients. Because of the high quality of her nursing, Richards proved to be an excellent example for students to follow. The training committee administered the school until 1896 when, faced with financial problems, control reverted to Massachusetts General Hospital.

These early schools soon proved their value, and by 1879 there were eleven training schools in the United States. By the turn of the century there were no fewer than 432 schools, and most of them had expanded their programs to two or three years. The standards, however, varied greatly among the schools. Active renovation in hospitals and the creation of new ones occurred between 1873 and 1895. One of these was Johns Hopkins Hospital (Baltimore), whose training school opened in 1889 under Isabel Adams Hampton (Robb). The function of the hospitals slowly changed from being refuges for the destitute to being institutions for the care of the sick and injured. The value of trained nurses had finally been proven, and that resulted in a growing demand for trained nurses.

Canadian Schools

Canada had one of the earliest schools patterned after the Nightingale schools; it was located at the General and Marine Hospital in St. Catharine's (1874). The bylaws for nurses were laid down in the regulations for the training school (later called the Mack Training School) and were influenced by the Nightingale principles. Excerpts from *The First Annual Report of The St. Catharine Training School and Nurses' Home*, dated July 1, 1875, are particularly enlightening:

> Every possible opportunity is seized to impart instruction of a practical nature in the art of nursing, while teaching will be given in chemistry, sanitary science, popular physiology and anatomy, hygiene and all such branches of the healing art as a nurse ought to be familiarized with. . . . The vocation of nursing goes hand in hand with that of the physician and surgeon, and they are absolutely indispensable one to the other. . . . By observing the known principles of hygiene, she will co-operate intelligently with him, also in placing the sufferer from disease in the best relation to the ground he is above, the surrounding heat, light, air, aliments he is sustained by, and the liquids he drinks. She will, likewise, by the proper precautions well recognized in hygiene, avert the evils of contagion or infection, and the spread of disease by noxious miasma. . . . Finally, she will inspire confidence, allay terror, soothe anxiety, and often quiet the mental state while taking care of the physical, and prevent injurious interference from officious bystanders.
>
> — *Gibbon and Mathewson, 1947 p. 145*

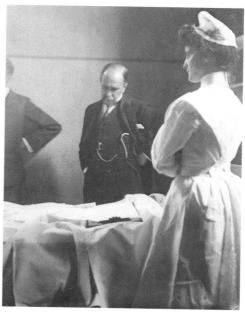

From the beginning, nursing students at Johns Hopkins benefited from the practice of teaching at the patient's bedside. Physician-in-Chief William Osler consulted his notes as Elizabeth Boley, 1903, focused her attention elsewhere on the ward.

Dr. William Osler & E. Boley, 1903, photograph, Johns Hopkins Nurses Alumni Association.

The second Canadian hospital to consider the idea of a training school for nurses was Montreal General (1821). In 1875 the hospital board sought the assistance of Florence Nightingale in establishing a school. Five nurses were sent from St. Thomas's Hospital, but they were appalled by the environment and eventually resigned; one of the original five died of typhoid fever. The conditions in the Montreal General Hospital were much like those of Bellevue. Filth was the primary feature, with armies of rats scurrying about the wards and sometimes attacking patients. Other attempts were made to start the school, but they also proved unsuccessful. Finally, Nora Gertrude Livingstone, a graduate of the New York Hospital, succeeded in establishing a school in 1890. Under her direction the nursing school had its real beginning.

The history of the Toronto General Hospital was similar to that of Montreal General. From 1877, attempts were made to establish a training school, but it was not until 1884 that the real fame of the school began. At this time Mary Agnes Snively, a graduate of Bellevue Hospital, became the superintendent. She reorganized the school and developed a modern plan of work and study. During her tenure the school became well known throughout the nursing world as embodying the highest ideals in nursing. Snively remained until 1910 and greatly elevated the standards of the Toronto school.

Other schools soon followed in Canada: the Children's Hospital at Toronto in 1886; the Winnipeg General (1887), which claims to have been the first hospital in western Canada to start a training school for nurses; St. Boniface General in Winnipeg (1890); the Royal Jubilee at Victoria (1890); Victoria General in Halifax (1892); and the Royal Victoria at Montreal (1894). Snively reported that by June 1909 there were 70 schools for nurses; of these, 10 offered a 2-year course, three had a program of 2.5 years; and 57 required a 3-year course (Gibbon and Mathewson, 1947). The introduction of training schools for nurses became almost automatic for progressive Canadian hospitals after 1890. Trained nurses began to emerge in Canada almost simultaneously with those in the United States.

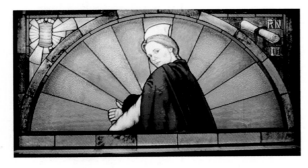

This stained glass window is over the main door of the Nurses' Association of New Brunswick. The central figure is a nurse; the scarlet cape lining symbolizes energy and vitality and Hygeia, goddess of health; the blue and white of the uniform are for spirituality. Light comes from Nightingale's lamp and a rolled diploma symbolizes the ongoing education of nursing practice.

Designer: Arlee Hoyt-McGee; artisans: Hugh MacKinnon and Ned Bowes, *Nurses Window*, June 2000, stained glass window, Nurses Association of New Brunswick, Fredericton, Province, New Brunswick, Canada. Copyright permission provided by the Nurses Association of New Brunswick (NANB). This photo may not be reproduced, in any form or by any means electronic, mechanical, photocopying or otherwise without permission of the publisher.

EDUCATIONAL ADVANCEMENT FOR GRADUATE NURSES

By the end of the 19th century, new educational opportunities became available for graduate nurses attending Teachers College, Columbia University. The Teachers College program was founded as a direct result of the efforts of the American Society of Superintendents of Training Schools for Nurses (renamed in 1912 the National League of Nursing Education and reorganized in 1952 under the present name, National League for Nursing). A special committee of the society, with Isabel Hampton Robb as its head, was created to investigate a better means of preparing nurses for leadership in schools of nursing. According to one source, "It was useless to look to our own institutions for the solution of this problem, and the ordinary normal school or college was equally incapable of adjusting its facilities to our peculiar needs" (Stewart, 1909, p. 1). Teachers College, which had opened ten years earlier for the training of teachers, seemed the logical choice. The program was originally designed to prepare administrators of nursing service and nursing education. It was established as an 8-month course in hospital economics in 1899.

> The original course for nurses in hospital economics at Teachers College was at first rather heavily weighted with technical subjects in the household arts with some recognition of the sciences also present. Pedagogical subjects such as psychology and the philosophy of education were soon identified as valuable in the study of the problems of nursing education and were incorporated within the program. Additional lectures by leaders in the Society shared nursing experiences gained through accumulated years of practical service in hospitals and training school work. In 1906, a new department of institutional administration was established in the college, the course in hospital economics becoming incorporated within its structure. From this time forward there was no longer any question as to the place of nursing in the general scheme of university education. The department continued to grow, broaden its educational program, emphasize the social and educational phases of the nurse's work, and include nursing specialties, such as teaching and supervision, public health nursing, school nursing, and other related branches. Eventually, the name was changed to the Department of Nursing Education.
>
> — DONAHUE, 1981, PP. 41-42

Mary Adelaide Nutting, former superintendent of nurses and principal of the Training School for Nurses at Johns Hopkins Hospital, came to Teachers College in 1907. She became the first nursing professor in the world and the first nurse to occupy a chair on a university faculty. Under her direction the department progressed and became a pioneer in education for nurses. The school became known as the "motherhouse" of collegiate education because it fostered the initial movements toward undergraduate and graduate degrees for nurses.

ADVANCING TOWARD NEW FRONTIERS

By the turn of the century, the trial period was over. The training school as well as the trained nurse were recognized and accepted by hospitals, medicine, and the general public. This revolution in nursing, combined with new developments in surgery and sanitary science, led to a tremendous expansion of hospitals. It was nursing that would ultimately make the application of these discoveries possible. Hospitals of all types sprang up, multiplied at an astonishing rate, and became independent entities because there was no regulating body of any type to set and enforce controls. It soon became apparent that a school of nursing was almost indispensable to the running of a hospital. Not only did nursing students improve the nursing service to patients, but also the cost of the improved service to the hospital was lower. The students worked long hours and did hard physical labor in payment for the training they received. Most hospitals, therefore, set up their own schools or assumed control over schools that had been developed on an independent basis. The right of the hospital to set up a school was not questioned, nor was there any interference with the manner in which the school was run. In some instances, hospitals had schools of nursing for the sole purpose of using the service contributed by students for the care of patients. The wide diversity among these schools and the exploitation of student nurses thus became important issues as the United States approached the 20th century.

New frontiers beckoned to women and to nursing in general. Greater numbers of women wished to be independent and free and to find the means of demonstrating their intelligence and capabilities and proving their value as citizens. They wanted to have widening opportunities to assume respectable positions in the social order of the times and envisioned nursing as an area in which this could be accomplished. However, a change in the system of nursing education and practice was necessary to achieve this goal. Nursing leaders began to organize for the control of their own educational standards and for the improvement of nursing practice. They were beginning to see that their educational difficulties could not be solved by isolated efforts, that the united energies of all nurses and all schools would be needed in any serious attempt to attack the chaos that had been created in educational standards and ideals. According to Stewart (1943, p. 129), "nursing leaders banded together to support educational standards, to set up some legal controls to prevent the spread of poor schools, and to prevent unlimited expansion."

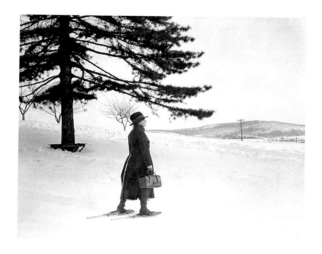

Lewis W. Hine, *Rural Health Nurse, Upstate New York*, photo, 7⅝" × 9 ½" [19.3 × 24.1 cm]. Photography collection, Miriam and Ira D. Wallach Division of Art, Prints and Photographs, The New York Public Library, Astor, Lenox and Tilden.

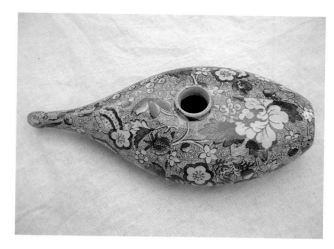

Late nineteenth century ceramic bottle with an off-center hole for filling and a fine spout extending at one end for feeding. The hole in the top was covered by the thumb to control the feeding rate. Bottle feeding was difficult due to problems with hygiene. Sterilization was not initiated before 1865, and bottle feeding often proved fatal for the infant.

Feeding Bottle.

THE TURN OF THE CENTURY

The 20th century has been referred to as the century of social consciousness. The beginnings of social endeavors in the 19th century finally became reality with the development of a variety of social agencies. The states had begun to assume at least partial responsibility for the relief of the poor early in the 19th century. In 1863, for example, Massachusetts had appointed a State Board of Charities that was charged with the care of the nonresident poor and with general supervision of state institutions. New York and Ohio created similar boards in 1867. By 1930, 41 states had created boards for the supervision of relief. This movement toward social reform brought about many changes that influenced health care and nursing.

Attention began to be focused on specific dependents, such as the blind and the aged, but the provisions were totally inadequate for their maintenance. Child health received particular emphasis with the initiation of the first White House Conference on Child Welfare in 1910. Within two years the Children's Bureau had been established (in 1912) by an act of Congress and placed under the auspices of the Department of Labor. Its function was to investigate and report all matters that pertained to the welfare of children and child life in all classes of people. Studies of infant mortality, care available to mothers and infants in rural communities, and methods of instruction in hygiene were undertaken by this agency. Finally, federal aid for the reduction of infant mortality was suggested by Julia Lathrop, chief of the Children's Bureau, in 1917. Her proposals were incorporated in the Sheppard-Towner Act of 1921, which authorized appropriations to provide grants-in-aid to states that would set up services for the welfare and hygiene of mothers and children.

Hundreds of nurses were employed to make home visits and supply mothers and infants with health education and health screenings. These monies continued for 7 years and stimulated the establishment of prenatal, infant, and preschool child health centers. By the time the act had expired, child health agencies had been established in 45 states and Hawaii. The impact of the Sheppard-Towner Act on the decrease in the infant death rate was well documented. Efforts were made to renew the Sheppard-Towner Act, but they were unsuccessful in the face of conservative forces. The continuation of this act was opposed by the American Medical Association: "Resolved that the House of Delegates condemns as unsound in policy, wasteful and extravagant, unproductive of results and tending to promote communism, the federal subsidy system established by the Sheppard-Towner Maternity and Infancy Act and protests against a renewal of the system in any form" (American Medical Association, 1930). Public health nurses, on the other hand, supported a renewal and watched with deep concern. When the federal aid ceased, the majority of the states continued to provide funds, although in decreased amounts.

The settlement house movement also became a popular cause. A settlement house commonly developed as a branch of a university, where intellectuals investigated the distressing conditions of the poor. The movement was started by the efforts of Arnold Toynbee, whose interest in the poor led him to establish university settlement projects. After his death, Oxford University students at Toynbee Hall (1875) in East London continued to study ways of alleviating community problems. Through their efforts the very poor had the opportunity to enrich their lives educationally, socially, and culturally. Every aspect of neighborhood and community welfare was aided by social workers who lived among the people they served. The primary purpose of settlement work was to teach and assist wage earners in developing their potential in order to provide their families with security and comfort. Philanthropists who lived among the lower classes thus became their role models.

The first American settlement house was developed on the Lower East Side of New York by Stanton Coit in 1886. Originally known as the Neighborhood Guild, it was later called the University Settlement. In 1889, Hull House was founded in Chicago by Jane Addams (1860-1935). This settlement house came to be typical of those that developed in other parts of America. In the beginning, Hull House was a big old structure that had been purchased by Jane Addams and a friend, Ellen Gates. The doors were opened to the neighborhood, which comprised representatives of more than thirty nationalities. Help of all types was offered for any situation. Addams's neighbors clung to their customs, yet they wanted education for their children and all the opportunities that America had to offer. Eventually, a day nursery, a kindergarten, and a library became essential components of Hull House. The community came to rely on Jane Addams, who also fought for women's suffrage and was the joint recipient of the 1931 Nobel Peace Prize (with Nicholas Murray Butler). By 1900 there were 103 settlement houses in the United States.

The Young Men's Christian Association (YMCA) was established in London in 1844 and in the United States in 1851. Its initial function was to deal with the spiritual, social, physical, and intellectual well-being of men, but it gradually expanded to include relief work, visiting the sick, and employment assistance. The YMCA also provided specialized services in wartime. Several branches joined to form the United States Christian Commission, which contributed to the welfare of soldiers during the Civil War. Later, this commission cared for prisoners and provided recreation for soldiers during World War I. In World War II it cooperated with other agencies to form the United Service Organization (USO), which planned recreational programs for members of the armed forces. Corresponding with the development of the YMCA was a movement among women that resulted in the formation of the Young Women's Christian Association (YWCA).

The Salvation Army (1878), founded by William Booth (1829-1912), was originally organized as a mission for the poor in London. Booth and his associates eventually became known as the Salvation Army and was set up in a military structure from that time on. By 1893 this agency had spread to a large portion of the world. It, too, was interested in the physical and spiritual welfare of the individual. Christian living was practiced by the giving of food, clothing, and shelter to the poor. Those who were miserable could find a certain amount of protection through the organization.

Social services had no boundaries, and missionaries helped to establish hospitals, schools of nursing, and dispensaries wherever they were needed. Nurses helped with these reforms by traveling to lands where people were in need of care. The work of Sir Wilfred Grenfell (1865-1940) is just one example of many remarkable achievements. Sir Wilfred was an English medical missionary who went to Labrador in 1892 and built a chain of hospital centers. Physicians, nurses, and college students volunteered at this mission, which ultimately developed into a complete health service that covered both physical and spiritual needs.

VISITING NURSING

The apostolic deaconesses are considered to be the ancestors of the current visiting nurses. Early nursing orders, too, particularly the Sisters of Charity, visited the sick in their homes and became well known for their efforts. During specific periods in history, home visits were the primary activity of nursing, until modern municipal hospitals were fully developed. The Protestant Sisters of Charity—organized by Elizabeth Fry—St. John's Home, the Order of St. Margaret, and other groups were initiated for this purpose. In addition, the deaconesses at Kaiserswerth received part of their nurses' training out in the community.

A formal structure for visiting nursing was established in

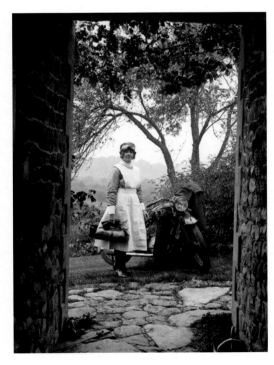

On September 28, 1931, Miss D. Swanx, the motorcycling nurse of Redford arrives at a patient's home on her bike.

Mobile Nurse, photograph, Redford. From Getty Images and Fox Photos.

Great Britain through the endeavors of William Rathbone, a wealthy citizen of Liverpool. His wife had died in 1859 after a long and painful illness during which she was cared for by a competent trained nurse. Rathbone pondered the fact that his wife, a woman who had had everything that money could buy, had received relief from skilled nursing care. He concluded that the poor, whose illnesses were compounded by the lack of wealth and by inadequate surroundings, would be helped even more. Nurses, therefore, should be sent to the homes of the needy sick. Rathbone employed Mary Robinson, the nurse who had cared for his wife, for a trial period of 3 months to give nursing care and comfort to the poor of Liverpool. His plan was opposed on the basis of the unsanitary conditions often found in the homes of the poor. According to Rathbone, a contemporary physician made this statement:

> It is evident that the essential conditions of rational and successful sick nursing such as good air, light, warmth, bedding, good food, etc., are altogether wanting in the homes of the poor. Of what use are the gratuitous supply and regular giving of medicines, if every necessity is wanting for ordinary healthy living? It is not that the nurse shrinks from the privations and injurious influences existing in the cottages and hovels, but it is the impossibility of being useful under such circumstances that renders home nursing unattainable for the poor. One can comfort them in their cottages, and give them food and medicine, but to nurse and heal them there with any prospect of success cannot be done.
>
> — RATHBONE, 1890, P. 7

The general feeling was that if the poor were seriously ill, they should go to a hospital. However, Rathbone disagreed on the basis that many patients with serious illnesses were refused admission to general hospitals, that there would never be enough hospitals to take care of all serious illnesses among the poor, and that care given by the visiting nurse was less costly than that offered in hospitals. He soon hired additional nurses and began to train them in the school he founded at the Liverpool Royal Infirmary. His persistence resulted in the firm establishment of visiting nursing in Liverpool, which grew into a powerful organization. This experiment was soon followed by the emergence of other visiting nurses societies.

Visiting nursing received a boost in 1887, when Queen Victoria celebrated her 50-year jubilee. Of the £76,000 raised by the women of England, the Queen donated £70,000 to the cause of visiting nurses. This sum was augmented by other sources to establish the Queen Victoria Jubilee Institute for Nurses, which received its royal charter in 1889. Nurses in this organization were called the Jubilee Institute Nurses, but they were also referred to as the Queen's Nurses. Their example was followed by similar groups: the King Edward VII Order in Canada, the Bush Nursing Association in South Africa, and the Plunket Nurses in New Zealand.

Although organized attempts to develop visiting nursing occurred quite early in the history of the United States, the momentum needed for its progression was slow in coming. The earliest visiting nurse services were connected with denominational groups participating in religious and charitable works. Nondenominational societies were established in 1877 in New York (the Women's Branch of the New York City Mission), in 1886 in Boston and Philadelphia, and in 1889 in Chicago. These visiting nurse associations, which employed trained nurses chiefly for the care of the sick in their homes, were often called Instructive District Nursing Associations. Teaching, as the name indicates, was also a vital function in the home care of the sick; principles of hygiene and sanitation were taught, in addition to specific aspects of health and illness. Isabel Hampton commented on the association's name in an address to the International Congress of Nurses in 1893: "In District Nursing we are confronted with conditions which require the highest order of work, but the actual nursing of the patient is the least part of what her work and influence should be among the class which the nurse will meet with. To this branch of nursing no more appropriate name can be given than Instructive Nursing, for educational in the best sense of the word it should be." The number of organizations continued to grow, and by 1890, visiting nursing was occurring in the United States through the efforts of 21 organizations.

THE HENRY STREET SETTLEMENT

The nursing settlement was one of the factors that assisted in the expansion of the scope of visiting nursing into the larger field of public health nursing. However, it approached social problems from the point of view of nursing. The work environment, low wages, the neighborhood environments, the cultures and customs of the people, and other variables were examined and evaluated for their particular influences on health. The first of these was the world-famous Henry Street Settlement, which was opened as a cooperative and partially self-supporting service in 1893. Its history is vividly described in two books authored by Lillian Wald, *The House on Henry Street* (1915) and *Windows on Henry Street* (1934).

Lillian D. Wald (1867-1940), a wealthy young woman of

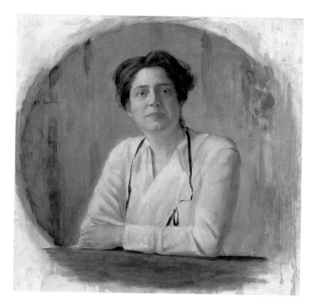

Those nurses requesting information about this portrait may be surprised to find Lillian Wald listed in the category of "Social Worker" by the National Portrait Gallery. This is understandable in view of the fact that her contributions to society included not only nursing but also those activities aligned with settlement houses. In addition, the activities of early nurses were frequently a combination of social work and nursing.

William Valentine Schevill (1864-1951), *Lillian D. Wald (1867-1940), Public Health Nurse, Social Worker,* gift of the Visiting Nurse Service of New York, 1919, oil on cardboard, 71.7 × 71.7 cm. Photo courtesy of National Portrait Gallery, Smithsonian Institution/Art Resource, NY.

high ideals, became interested in the need for nursing and social services among the poor soon after she graduated from the New York Hospital School of Nursing in 1891. Born in Cincinnati and raised in Rochester, New York, she was of Polish-German-Jewish stock. Lillian Wald was educated at Miss Crittenden's English and French Boarding and Day School for Young Ladies and Little Girls. Influenced by her physician relatives, however, she left to become a nurse. After her graduation she spent a year nursing at the New York Juvenile Asylum, but then she entered Woman's Medical College in New York. During her medical school days Wald was asked to go to New York's Lower East Side to instruct immigrant mothers in the care of the sick. She was profoundly shocked by what she found there when a child approached her for help as she was teaching a group of mothers. She described this turning point in her life in the following way:

> From the schoolroom where I had been giving a lesson in bed-making, a little girl led me one drizzling March morning. She had told me of her sick mother, and gathering from her incoherent account that a child had been born, I caught up the paraphernalia of the bed-making lesson and carried it with me.
>
> The child led me over broken roadways . . . between tall,

reeking houses . . . past odorous fish-stands for the streets were a market-place, unregulated, unsupervised, unclean, past evil-smelling, uncovered garbage cans, and perhaps worst of all, where so many little children played. . . . The child led me on through a tenement hallway, across a court where open and unscreened closets were promiscuously used by men and women, up into a rear tenement, by slimy steps whose accumulated dirt was augmented that day by the mud of the streets, and finally into the sickroom. All the maladjustments of our social and economic relations seemed epitomized in this brief journey and what was found at the end of it. The family to which the child led me was neither criminal nor vicious . . . and although the sick woman lay on a wretched, unclean bed, soiled with a hemorrhage two days old, they were not degraded human beings. . . .

That morning's experience was a baptism of fire. Deserted were the laboratory and the academic work of the college. I never returned to them. . . . To my inexperience it seemed certain that conditions such as these were allowed because people did not *know*, and for me there was a challenge to know and tell. When early morning found me still awake, my naive conviction remained that, if people knew things— and "things" meant everything implied in the condition of

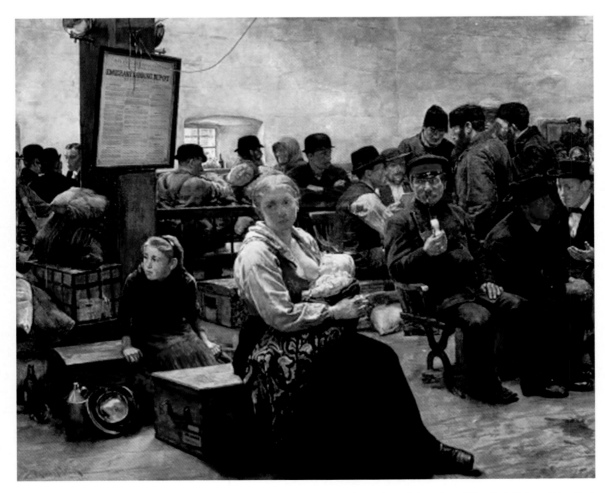

From 1855 to 1890, the Castle was America's first official immigration center, a pioneering collaboration of New York State and New York City. More than 8 million immigrants were welcomed here prior to its closure on April 18, 1890. Castle Garden was succeeded by Ellis Island in 1892.

Charles Ulrich, *In the Land of Promise—Castle Garden*, 1884, oil on canvas, The Granger Collection, NY.

this family—such horrors would cease to exist, and I rejoiced that I had a training in the care of the sick that in itself would give me an organic relationship to the neighborhood in which this awakening had come.

— WALD, 1915, PP. 4-8

In 1893, Wald persuaded a classmate, Mary Brewster, to go into the tenement district with her to live and work. The two nurses rented the top floor of a tenement house on Jefferson Street and began to carry on whatever nursing and social work fell their way. As their workload increased, the house at 265 Henry Street was acquired with the help of Jacob H. Schiff, a banker and philanthropist, and others. This House on Henry Street became the Henry Street Visiting Nurse Service and eventually encompassed nursing service, social work, and an organized program of social, cultural, and educational activities. The scope of the settlement went far beyond the care of the sick and the prevention of disease. It aimed at rectifying the causes that were responsible for the poverty and misery itself. In keeping with this aim, Lillian Wald battled for legislative reforms that would ensure

some measure of justice for the "unfortunates." Her initiative and skill in securing support for new ideas and new plans made her one of the most influential health workers of her day (Stewart and Austin, 1962).

Lillian Wald is regarded as the founder of what is now called public health or community nursing. She coined the phrase *public health nursing* and transformed the stereotyped visiting nursing of her time into the community movements that ultimately widened the horizons of modern nursing (Robinson, 1946). She created a system whereby patients had direct access to nurses, and nurses had direct access to patients. Wald insisted that the nurses be at the call of people who needed them, without the intervention of a medical man (Woolf, 1937). When warranted, however, a patient would be referred to a physician at one of the free dispensaries. No distinction was made between those who could pay and those who could not; services were available to all who sought them.

Lillian D. Wald's achievements and leadership were recognized through numerous citations and awards, including the degree of doctor of laws from Mount Holyoke College

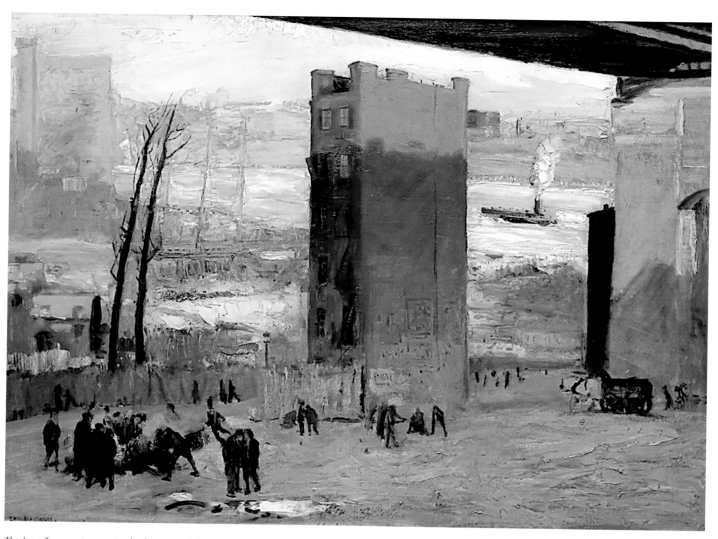

The Lone Tenement generates both a powerful image of urban dislocation and a poignant allegory of time's passage. The last remaining building underneath the approaches to the new Queensboro Bridge stands alone, everything else in the neighborhood having long since been razed. Transients huddled around a fire, a horse-drawn carriage, two lifeless tree trunks, a ship belching steam on the East River, and a factory smokestack are vital components of the composition.

George Bellows, *The Lone Tenement,* painting, National Gallery of Art, Washington, DC.

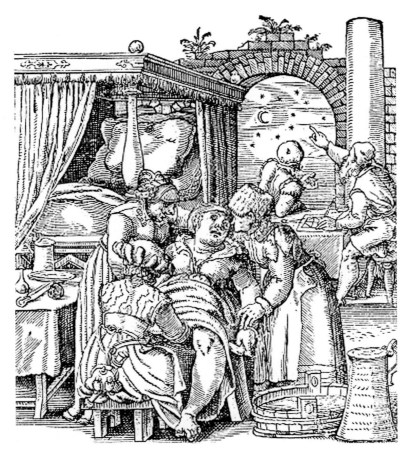

Midwives attend a childbirth while an astronomer casts a horoscope for the newborn.

Jost Amman, *Childbirth*, 1580, woodcut, The Granger Collection, NY.

(1912), the medal of the National Institute of Social Sciences (1913), and the Certificate for Distinguished Service to the City of New York (1937). She received one of the most esteemed awards when she was named to the Hall of Fame for Great Americans (1971). With the death of Lillian D. Wald, the nation had lost a unique citizen. Throughout her life she had opposed political and social corruption and supported measures that would improve the health, welfare, and happiness of humanity. The Henry Street Settlement had paved the way for the foundation of nursing settlements in other American cities. The earliest among them were in Richmond, Virginia (1900), San Francisco (1900), and Orange, New Jersey (1903).

THE FRONTIER NURSING SERVICE

There is a striking contrast between the development of midwifery in Europe and in the United States. Midwifery was always considered an important specialty in Europe, and a two-year course was usually required. Nearly all state-registered nurses in England were at one time registered midwives who had had 6 months or more of specialized training. Yet in the United States the training of nurses in the area of midwifery had been prevented primarily by the attitudes of physicians. The physicians held the view that every woman should be assisted in delivery by a physician, an attitude that continued to be prominent into the 1930s. This opposition, which was related to the belief that nurse-midwifery represented an intrusion into the field of medical practice, ignored the high maternal death rate. A large number of un-

trained, ignorant midwives were practicing; and thousands of women employed incompetent midwives.

The use of midwives was customary among the foreign-born in the cities, among those living in isolated communities, and among blacks, particularly those in the rural regions of the South. In many instances, medical care for these women was nonexistent. Approximately 30% of all deliveries in the United States were attended by midwives. Although many of the midwives had practical experience that was an asset in normal deliveries, injury or death to the mother or child (or both) often occurred with abnormal or difficult deliveries. Early in the 1900s studies were undertaken that began the long march to reform in the care of mothers and babies. In addition, some nurses began to advocate the training and use of nurse-midwives in America, particularly in areas where medical care was lacking. However, this movement lacked support from physicians, nurses, and the general public and therefore did not have a strong impact.

Several physicians aided the advances in training for women functioning in the area of midwifery. Joseph Warrington, while working as an obstetrician at the Philadelphia Dispensary for the Medical Relief of the Poor, became aware of the need for trained midwives to deliver the babies of poor women. In 1832 he formed the Philadelphia Lying-in Charity for Attending Indigent Females in Their Own Homes; no fee would be charged and the women would deliver in their homes. Warrington soon began to train nurses in the art of midwifery. Dr. Samuel Gregory of Boston facilitated another school for nurse-midwives in 1846. He firmly be-

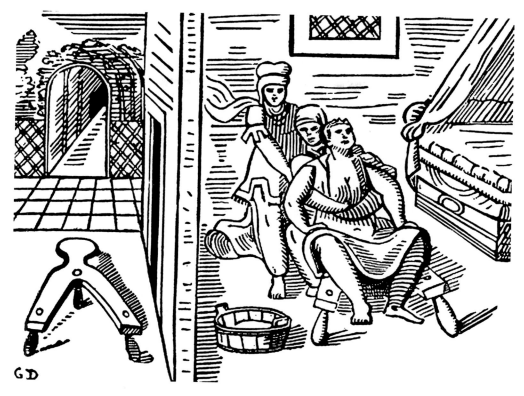

A woman giving birth with the aid of midwives and an obstetrical chair.

Obstetrical Chair, 15th century, woodcut, The Granger Collection, NY.

lieved that midwives should be able to acquire scientific knowledge upon which their practice would be based. To that end, he published several pamphlets stressing that more and better courses of instruction should be available.

A few schools for nurse-midwives were finally developed. In 1911, Bellevue Hospital established a school of midwifery that continued until 1935. This school was designed specifically to aid the 40,000 New York women who were being assisted in delivery by untrained women. It was discontinued when the majority of women entered hospitals for delivery. The founding of centers that offered courses and granted certificates in nurse-midwifery followed. Such institutions included the Maternity Center Association (which opened the first school for nurse-midwives in the United States) in connection with the Lobenstine Clinic in New York; the Tuskegee Institute in Alabama (a short-lived school for black nurse-midwives assisted by federal funds during the Civil war); the Frontier Nursing Service in Kentucky; and the Catholic Maternity Institute in New Mexico. Finally, certificates in nurse-midwifery were offered in conjunction with a master's degree at Yale University, Johns Hopkins University, New York Medical College, Catholic University, Columbia University, and the University of Utah (Dolan, Fitzpatrick, and Hermann, 1983).

The Frontier Nursing Service provided the first organized midwifery service in the United States. It was founded in 1925 by Mary Breckinridge, the daughter of a family distinguished in American history. Her only children, Breckie and Polly, died in infancy, and this was thought to be the catalyst for her interest and involvement in midwifery. Mary Breckinridge graduated from St. Luke's Hospital Training School in New York (1910) and later from the British Hospital for Mothers and Babies in Woolwich, London (1925), where she received her certificate in midwifery. For several years (1919 to 1923), she became occupied with public health activities

in devastated France and actually organized public health nursing there.

Mary Breckinridge recognized the need for a rural midwifery service in the Appalachian Mountains of Kentucky, where for centuries both nursing and midwifery had been practiced under almost medieval conditions by the "granny women." These "midwives" were generally illiterate, had no formal training in midwifery, knew little about prenatal or postnatal care, and were often superstitious. They rarely called a physician, even when faced with serious complications. Their practices ranged from the use of soot as a medication to the placing of an axe, blade side up, under the bed as a preventive measure.

The people who settled in these hills became isolated from the rest of the country because of their location. They maintained the old customs of early marriage and large families. The Appalachian area was part of the "cradle of the nation" and had one of the highest birth rates in the United States. Mary Breckinridge, who had witnessed midwifery services firsthand in England, New Zealand, and Australia, was determined to initiate a similar plan for the care of mothers, babies, and children in these foothills. To accomplish her goal she was forced for many years to use midwives trained in England because there were so few trained midwives in America.

The members of the Frontier Nursing Service worked in Leslie County, Kentucky, where the lack of highways necessitated travel by horse or mule. The area was divided into 8 districts of approximately 78 square miles each. Two nurses lived in the middle of each district and were responsible for the health of all who lived there. A primary form of health care was provided in which a family-centered approach was emphasized. Each of the "nurses on horseback" had certification as a nurse-midwife, and the nurses gave antepartal, intrapartal, and postpartal care to the women in their dis-

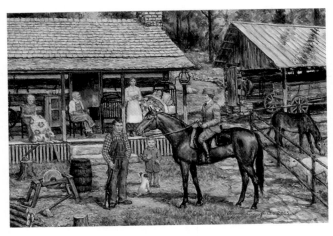

Anne Crawford, *Frontier Nursing Service*, painting, Historical Med Arts.

tricts. They performed normal deliveries but called a physician in the event of a complicated case. A study of the first 1000 cases showed that the proportion of complications during pregnancy and delivery was lower among patients cared for by the service than among the general population. Child-care services were also offered; babies under 1 year of age were seen twice a month, preschool children (1 to 6 years of age) once a month, and schoolchildren every 2 months. Mary Breckinridge and her staff had demonstrated the usefulness of such a service in areas where physicians were not readily accessible.

By 1935 a small, 12-bed general hospital, the Hyden Hospital and Health Center, had been founded and was functional. The medical director was responsible for the hospitalized patients and also responded to the nurses in the several districts. The advent of World War II prompted the establishment of a Graduate School of Midwivery when the British nurses wished to return home to care for their own people. This school was founded by the Frontier Nursing Service in 1939 at Hyden, Kentucky.

Growing numbers of nurses have recently begun to specialize in the practice of nurse-midwifery, which involves a definite return to or reintroduction of past techniques. For example, the practices of home delivery and natural childbirth, the use of the sitting position on obstetrical chairs or birthing chairs, and the employment of nurse-midwives are on the rise. In some respects this has been fostered by 3rd-party insurance reimbursement for midwifery services and the development of birthing centers in hospitals and freestanding maternity centers.

THE STATUS OF WOMEN

The development of nursing parallels and reflects the women's movement. For a long period in history, the position of women in society left much to be desired. The role of women remained passive, although statements about the equality of women with men were heard periodically. Throughout the centuries women were generally regarded as the property of men and had no legal rights or power. (Rare exceptions can be cited, such as the position of the Roman matron at the start of the Christian era.) For example, the Code of Hammurabi stated that women were the exclusive property of men. Ancient norms regarding women were enforced, particularly during the time of the Reformation. Yet some glimmers of potential for change began to surface as early as the beginning of the 17th century. A group of

courageous and persistent women emerged to champion the cause of their sex and earn the title of feminists. These women advocated equal rights for women that would include legal and academic privileges, marriage reform that would allow for preference rather than arrangement, and the right to vote, own property, and hold office. Although they met vehement opposition to their cause, they continued their struggle toward the emancipation of women. Through their efforts the position of women slowly began to improve.

Books, essays, and articles that dealt with women's rights began to appear. Works written by the early feminists included *The Excellencies of Women and the Errors of Men* by Lucretia Marinelli of Italy; *The Learned Maid* by Anna von Schurman of Holland; *A Serious Proposal to the Ladies* by the English feminist Mary Astell; and two volumes on *The Strictures on Female Education* by another Englishwoman, Hannah More. This movement owed much to Mary Wollstonecraft's epic book, *A Vindication of the Rights of Women,* written in 1792. The rights that were discussed in this work were simply human rights that should have been applied impartially to women. This author argued against the existing double standard of morality that was prevalent in the society. Mary Wollstonecraft was, indeed, a fitting example of her beliefs. She had acquired an education and entered the business world as a translator for a publisher in London. Supporters of her ideas turned those ideas into action.

Women became reformers, educators, and developers, making their voices heard in any way possible. They rallied to advance their right of suffrage when they discovered that social reforms could be achieved through the power of the vote. Prominent in the American women's movement was Susan B. Anthony (1820-1906). English women later began suffrage efforts and met with comparable resistance. Even Queen Victoria voiced her protest against "this mad, wicked folly of Woman's Rights, with all its attendant horrors. Lady— ought to get a *good whipping.* It is a subject which makes the Queen so furious she cannot contain herself" (Quoted in Robinson, 1946, p. 365). After nearly 75 years of frustration and struggle, the United States Constitution was amended in 1920 to allow women to vote.

Nursing leaders were involved in women's rights as well

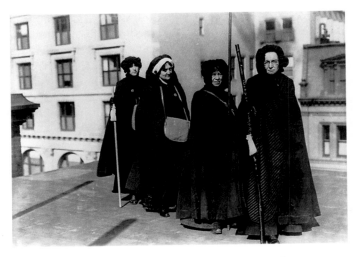

Lavinia Dock (third from left) holding a "Votes for Women" staff, 1913.

Lavinia Dock, 1913, photograph, from *Women of Protest: Photographs from the Records of the National Woman's Party,* Manuscript Division, Library of Congress, Washington, DC.

as in human rights. Nurses were found among the marchers in the pilgrimages of the suffragists. The most colorful and zealous suffragist was Lavinia Lloyd Dock (1858-1956), one of nursing's greatest leaders and a radical feminist. She was actively engaged in social protest, picketing and parading for women's rights and protesting against war; these were not regarded as "nurselike" or "ladylike" activities. She also voiced her opinions and concerns about social issues whenever an opportunity arose. At one point "Little Dockie" was to speak about the history of nursing in Europe to a group of nursing students at Teachers College. Nutting was away, and the incident was described by Isabel Stewart:

I was quite young and I'd never seen Miss Dock. . . . I was sure I'd know her when I met her, because she'd be tall and angular and intellectual looking. Who should turn up at the door but this small, short sort of roly-poly little person with curly hair. She'd just been at a suffrage meeting, and had "Votes for Women" across her hat and "Votes for Women" across her chest. She said, "Now what am I going to talk about?" I said, . . . "you were to talk about nursing on the Continent." "Oh," she said, "very bad. It'll not be any better till they get the suffrage. I'll talk about suffrage."

— STEWART, 1961, PP. 139-140

Stewart continued:
This suffrage thing—it was the whole thing for her; she wanted not only to work for it but really to suffer for it. She went over to Britain to work with Mrs. Pankhurst, and she wanted above all things to go to jail. Oh, she got there all right . . . that was during the war, at the beginning of the First World War. She was a member of the advanced wing of the Suffrage Party, and they were having a meeting in Washington at the time that Wilson was beginning to think of the possibility of war. They discussed it, and a friend of mine who was there at the time tells me that Lavinia got up and seized the flag which was there and said, "Youth to the Colors!" and on she marched, out of the door, and they followed her, and she went right to the White House, and they picketed the White House!

She is about this high, you know. . . . Anyway, they all went into the cooler for the night. I think it just pleased her no end.

— STEWART, 1961, P. 275

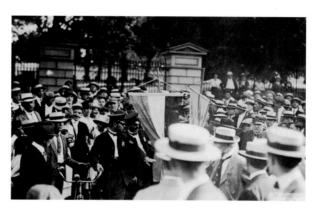

Police arresting pickets Edna Dixon and Lavinia Dock in a crowd in 1917.

Harris and Ewing, *Penn on the Picket Line,* 1917, photograph, Washington DC. *Women of Protest: Photographs from the Records of the National Woman's Party,* Manuscript Division, Library of Congress, Washington, DC.

Harris and Ewing, *Police Arresting Pickets,* 1917, photograph, Washington, DC. *Women of Protest: Photographs from the Records of the National Woman's Party,* Manuscript Division, Library of Congress, Washington, DC.

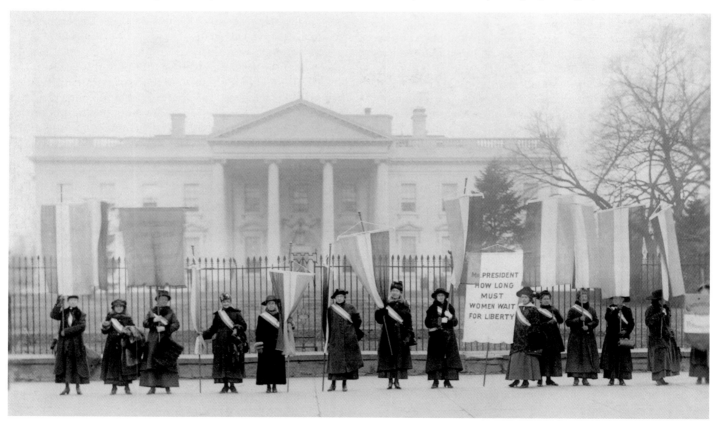

Lavinia L. Dock, one of six children of a cultured and affluent family, was born in Harrisburg, Pennsylvania. Both of her parents were well educated and insisted upon equal education for both their sons and their daughters. Lavinia was an accomplished organist and pianist, but she decided to enter Bellevue Hospital Training School for Nurses, from which she graduated in 1886. She became a night supervisor at Bellevue Hospital, where she wrote one of the first textbooks for nurses, *The Textbook on Materia Medica for Nurses* (1890). She was aware of the problems the students encountered in learning about drugs and solutions and wrote this book to aid them in the mastery of such content. The publisher was unwilling to make the original investment, so Lavinia's father advanced the necessary amount. According to Roberts (1956), this investment paid off handsomely; more than 100,000 copies of several editions were sold.

Lavinia Dock was concerned with the many problems that were plaguing nursing. She questioned the serious and long-term effects of women's subjugation to men. She believed that male dominance in the health field was the major problem confronting the nursing profession. In 1903, Dock spoke about the developments that would almost ensure male dominance and, in turn, have a major impact on the development of nursing. Her pleas for caution went unheeded, and nurses became accomplices in their own subordination. "Nursing leaders ignored all her warnings and in the second decade of the century actually became nonvoting members of the American Hospital Association. They worked with physicians and administrators on joint committees, expecting their oppressors to help them solve nursing problems. They sought approval from men, not liberation. As a result, from the first decade of the century onward, physicians and hospital administrators have remained in positions of dominance and control over nursing and health care" (Ashley, 1975, p. 1466).

The oppression of nurses was built into the law and the educational system through the legalization of paternalism and the institutionalization of apprenticeship. The threats became a reality as male domination progressed to a state of completion. A powerful combination of male domination and sexual discrimination surfaced and prevented the recognition of nurses as professional equals of physicians and as workers who had the right to practice independently. Even now, inequality in the health care field continues to be a serious impediment to the development of the highest potential of nursing.

Lavinia Dock served nursing in numerous elected capacities. Her keen and versatile mind was respected by her colleagues at home and abroad, and they looked to her for guidance. She conducted a study of professional-organization bylaws and was instrumental in the establishment of the American Society of Superintendents of Training Schools for Nurses. Dock became this organization's first secretary, as well as the first secretary of the International Council of Nurses (1899). She is regarded as the chief American influence on the organization of the nurses of the world and was active in the movement to effect passage of legislation for the control of nursing practice.

Outspoken on the then-taboo subject of venereal disease, Dock published a book in 1910, *Hygiene and Morality,* that shocked some people. The world of nursing profited by her numerous articles, which appeared in the early issues of the *American Journal of Nursing*. The four-volume *History of Nursing* (vols. 1 and 2, 1907; vols. 3 and 4, 1912), written in collaboration with M. Adelaide Nutting, became the classic text on nursing history. The condensed version, *A Short History of Nursing,* was coauthored with Isabel M. Stewart. The *History of American Red Cross Nursing* was a massive, comprehensive work. These studies made Dock one of the foremost of nursing historians, "a result achieved by the vitality of her style, knowledge of languages, command of facts, international outlook, an intelligence that would not compromise with stupidity, and a character that scorned to appease evil howsoever intrenched" (Robinson, 1946, p. 301).

At the turn of the century, some strides had indeed been made toward the achievement of equality and freedom for women. A particular milestone occurred with the readmission of women into the medical field. Elizabeth Blackwell (1821-1910) was the pioneer who was admitted to Geneva Medical College in Geneva, New York, in 1847. This occurred, however, only after she had been rejected by twelve other medical schools and after her Geneva application had been presented to the all-male student body for a vote. Her struggle to become a doctor took place during a time when options for women, although still limited, were gradually expanding. She was the first woman in America to graduate from medical school and be licensed as a physician. Unable to obtain a hospital staff appointment after graduation, she traveled to Europe, where she worked in hospitals in London and Paris. Eventually, Elizabeth and her sister Emily established the New York Infirmary for Women and Children in 1857. She was also responsible for the founding of the Women's Medical College of Geneva Medical College, where women physicians could get both training and clinical experience. Emily had also had difficulty in gaining admission to medical school. She was refused admission to Elizabeth's alma mater and to several other medical schools but finally was accepted by the Medical Department of Western Reserve University.

The women's movement continues today, and it experiences periodic defeats as well as intermittent successes. The ideal embodied in the efforts of these early nursing leaders has yet to be achieved. This is reflected in nursing's constant attempts to distance itself from anything having to do with the medical model and the fact that nurses have typically been characterized, along with women in general, as being passive, dependent, and emotional. The factors that keep nurses subservient, overworked, and underpaid endure today. Finally, nursing has not been valued intellectually or monetarily primarily because of its emphasis on altruism, caring, and nurturing.

THE RISE OF ORGANIZED NURSING

Modern nursing was still very young when a few farsighted leaders spurred the movement toward development in organization. These leaders realized that a group was stronger than an individual, that an organization could accomplish things an individual could not, and that from unity came strength. They believed nursing's real power and potential could be realized through the united efforts of individual members striving to promote common interests. Their commitment to organized nursing was fostered by serious conditions that jeopardized both the recipients and the providers of nursing care. The primary concern of these leaders was, therefore, twofold: the protection of the public from poorly trained nurses and the lack of standardization in nurse training. Indeed, the biggest problems facing nursing at the beginning of the 20th century were those dealing with the setting of standards. These conditions were depicted graphically in a history of nursing in Kansas:

> Lacking a model, the majority of the hospital founders conceived of the trained hospital nurse as a substitute for the competent mother or neighbor who cares for the sick in the home. Primarily she should be a "good housekeeper" of the neighborly type. Since the average housewife of Kansas was still scrubbing her own floors and doing the family washing, it was assumed that these and similar chores were part of the work of a nurse. Even after it became apparent that there was much waste in using educated women for such labors, hospitals continued to spend every available cent to add to their number of student nurses. . . . the students, promised an education, would work for little or for nothing except room and board. . . . Humanitarians, quite as much as the physicians who founded hospitals as money-making ventures, shared in the exploitation. . . . It simply did not occur to them that they were perpetuating one wrong in correcting another.
>
> — *KANSAS STATE NURSES ASSOCIATION*, 1942, P. 93

ORGANIZATIONS FOR NURSES

Conditions had reached a critical point by the end of the 19th century, and an organizational structure was viewed as the one mechanism whereby changes could be attained in nursing education and nursing practice. The first attempt to establish an organization of nurses took place in England. Mrs. Bedford Fenwick, an internationally prominent leader from London, began a campaign in 1887 for nurse registration. This idea was not well accepted, even though the quality of nursing care in Britain was inconsistent and frequently inferior. Mrs. Fenwick, however, was convinced that standards were necessary to improve nursing, and she founded the British Nurses' Association in 1888 to achieve legal sanction. This association was the first of its type anywhere in the world. It grew rapidly, and its members numbered a thousand by the end of one year. Membership was not limited to graduate nurses but also included some physicians. (A few were honorary officers!)

Although there was opposition to this organization, eventually it obtained a royal charter in 1892 under the title of The Royal British Nurses' Association. Similar societies developed in other countries as the advantages of such a united endeavor became clear. The overall aim of each of the organizations was similar—to improve the education and status of nurses and to secure for them state recognition.

The earliest nurses' association in America, on which there is scant information, was the Philomena Society. It was started in New York in 1886 but lasted only 1 year. As nursing schools developed, however, alumnae associations were formed to foster fellowship and mutual support and to provide economic assistance when necessary. These groups became convenient units for amalgamation, which later proved to be beneficial when the national organization emerged. The first alumnae associations were formed at Bellevue Hospital in New York (1889), Illinois Training School of Cook County Hospital in Chicago (1891), Johns Hopkins

Hospital in Baltimore (1892), Massachusetts General Hospital in Boston (1895), and Boston City Hospital (1896).

American Society of Superintendents of Training Schools for Nurses. The year 1893 marks the debut of American nursing and the beginning of a new era in nursing education. At the World's Fair in Chicago in that year, the International Congress of Charities, Corrections and Philanthropy was held. A part of this congress was devoted to hospitals and dispensaries. Through the encouragement of Mrs. Bedford Fenwick, Dr. John S. Billings, chairman of the congress, agreed that nursing should occupy a place on the program. The subsection on nursing was chaired by Isabel Adams Hampton, superintendent of nurses at Johns Hopkins Hospital. The meeting was attended by both American and Canadian nurses, and papers were read that reflected and frankly presented the major issues and concerns of nursing. In addition, the need for a national union was urged. Florence Nightingale sent an address that was read to the congress. In it she discussed the teaching of nursing and the training of nurses. She commented, "Training is to teach the nurse to help the patient to live. Nursing the sick is an art, and an art requiring an organized, practical, and scientific training, for nursing is the skilled servant of medicine, surgery and hygience." Isabel Hampton spoke about educational standards for nurses; Lavinia L. Dock discussed the relation of training schools to hospitals. The papers were eventually compiled in a publication, *Nursing of the Sick* (1893), and were viewed as a historical record of the progress made and the problems encountered in the 2 decades following the opening of the first training school of nurses.

The day after the program about nursing had taken place, Hampton arranged for a meeting with a small group to discuss the possibilities of establishing a nursing organization. This meeting was attended by directors of nursing schools and resulted in the formation of the American Society of Superintendents of Training Schools for Nurses as a binational organization. Membership was restricted to nurses associated with nurse training. In effect, it became an accrediting agency for schools of nursing in the United States and Canada (Stewart and Austin, 1962). The first official meeting of the society was attended by 44 superintendents in January 1894. The aim of the society was to develop high educational standards for schools of nursing through the establishment of universal requirements for admission, a sound program of theory and practice, and improved working conditions. A curriculum committee was promptly appointed, and a report was published 2 years later. In 1907, Canadian members formed their own independent organization, the Canadian Society of Superintendents of Training Schools, with Mary Agnes Snively as its first president. In 1912 the American society became known by a new name, the National League of Nursing Education, and still later as the National League for Nursing (1952).

The society was occupied for the first 2 years with the development of a national association of graduate nurses so the practice of all types of nursing could be represented. This effort was led by Isabel Hampton Robb, M. Adelaide Nutting, and Lavinia L. Dock, all of whom were at Johns Hopkins. Miss Dock carefully studied the laws under which professional organizations could operate and how they could be formulated. Her report to the society at the 1896 convention proposed that alumnae associations be the mode of entrance to the new organization; the development of local

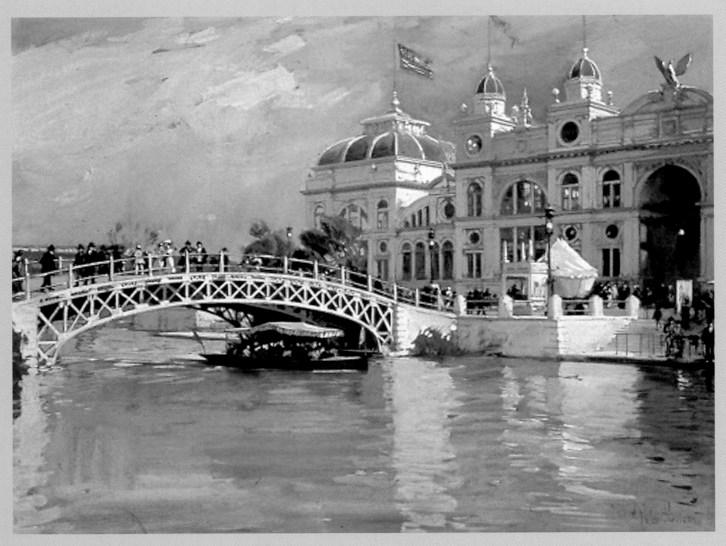

The International Congress of Charities, Corrections and Philanthropy was held in 1893 during the World's Fair held in Chicago. A part of the congress was devoted to hospitals and dispensaries. A subsection on nursing was chaired by Isabel Adams Hampton, and papers were read that reflected and presented the major issues and concerns of nursing.

Childe Hassam, *Columbian Exposition,* 1893, gouache, The Granger Collection, NY.

and state units would follow. A committee was appointed to prepare a constitution and bylaws for a national nurses' organization, and it was instructed to meet with a number of delegates from the oldest alumnae associations.

Nurses Associated Alumnae of the United States and Canada. The committee of the society and the delegates of the alumnae associations met in New York in September 1896. The following year the constitution and bylaws that had been prepared by this group were accepted, and a national nurses' association was established. This second organization, created for the rank and file in nursing, was called the Nurses Associated Alumnae of the United States and Canada. The original purposes of this association in 1897 were: "(1) To establish and maintain a code of ethics; (2) to elevate the standards of nursing education; (3) to promote the usefulness and honor, the financial and other interests of the nursing profession" (American Nurses Association, 1941, p. 2). A primary objective was to secure legislation to differentiate between the trained and the untrained nurse because the title *trained nurse* had come to refer to all grades of training and all grades of women.

When the Associated Alumnae sought to incorporate, it was found that New York law prohibited foreign membership, making it necessary to eliminate the words *and Canada* and barring further Canadian participation. Canadian nurses withdrew from the organization as early as 1900. In 1908 the Provisional Organization of the Canadian National Association of Trained Nurses was formed. The name was changed to the Canadian Nurses Association at the 1924 convention. In the early years of the Canadian association, "the recurring problems under discussion were education of student nurses, improvement of nursing care of patients, amelioration of conditions for nurses, and the need for state registration of nurses as a safeguard to the public" (Gibbon and Mathewson, 1947, p. 348). By the time the Associated Alumnae had been renamed the American Nurses Association in 1911 and chartered by the state of New York, Canadian membership had been discontinued.

The first president of the Nurses Associated Alumnae was Isabel Adams Hampton Robb (1859-1910). One author described her as "the radiant center of the magnetic force which brought the two national organizations into existence before 1900" (Roberts, 1954, p. 26). Another has called her the "architect of American nursing organizations" (Fitzpatrick, 1983). Whatever titles are used to describe her, Robb was undoubtedly one of the greatest early leaders in American nursing and perhaps the best loved. She was a forceful and farsighted individual, yet she demonstrated a gentle power that was considered a main characteristic of her leadership.

Isabel Adams Hampton was born in Canada (Welland, Ontario). She attended the Collegiate Institute of St. Catharine's, Ontario, after which she taught at the Merriton School for approximately 3 years. In 1881, she was admitted to the Bellevue Hospital Training School for Nurses and she graduated in 1883. For a brief period Hampton served as a relief supervisor at Women's Hospital in New York, followed by 2 years as a staff nurse at St. Paul's Hospice in Rome. Upon her return to the United States, she became superintendent of nurses at Illinois Training School in Chicago, where she introduced several innovations of educational import. Hampton implemented a graded system of theory and practice,

terminated the practice of students' doing private duty as part of their education (she believed this practice to be an exploitation of the students because the hospital received the fees), and originated the concept of affiliation, whereby students could gain necessary experience not available in their home institutions. These innovations were undoubtedly influenced by her experience as a teacher and by her grounding in educational theory.

Hampton was not yet 30 when she was chosen to organize the school of nursing of Johns Hopkins Hospital. It is said that she created quite a sensation upon her arrival because of her serenity and beauty. William Osler, a fellow Canadian, supposedly stated that she entered Hopkins like "an animated Greek statue." She was likened to Venus by both men and women. Lavinia Dock expressed the overall sentiment:

> I thought I had never seen a more beautiful or majestic figure except on the pedestal of some classic sculpture. Miss Hampton's color was rich and fresh, her eyes the clearest blue, unusually large and beautifully set and opened; her voice was one of her greatest charms, being very sweet and quiet, yet with a certain thrill in it when she was in earnest. Her hands were also extremely beautiful, displaying her character and power of organization. They were perfect enough to have been modeled.
>
> — *QUOTED IN ROBINSON, 1946, P. 173*

More innovations were attempted. Hampton became a "principal" rather than a "superintendent," and policies were established for a 12-hour day that included time for meals, recreation, rest, and study periods. She also recognized the

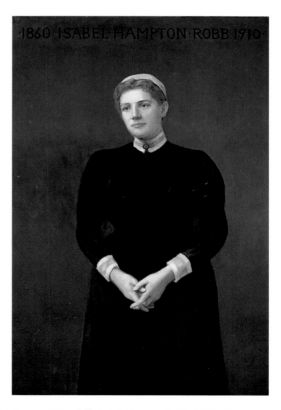

William Sergeant Kendall, *Isabel Hampton Robb*, 1909, oil on canvas, 60" × 40". Courtesy of The Alan Mason Chesney Medical Archives of The Johns Hopkins Medical Institutions, photograph by Aaron Levin.

need for nursing publications and wrote three influential books: *Nursing: Its Principles and Practice for Hospital and Private Use* (1894), *Nursing Ethics* (1900), and *Educational Standards for Nurses* (1907). It was at Johns Hopkins that Hampton met Hunter Robb, who had been a resident in gynecology. They were married at St. Margaret's, Westminster, London, on July 12, 1894, with the bride carrying flowers sent by Florence Nightingale. Robb was not well liked by Hampton's colleagues because they believed that he was not an equal match for her in intellectual ability or physical appearance. However, the Robbs settled in Cleveland, where they eventually had two sons. Unfortunately, she died prematurely in a traffic accident on April 15, 1910, in Cleveland Ohio.

Mary Adelaide Nutting (1858-1948) was a nursing leader who was greatly influenced by Isabel Hampton Robb and, in fact, became her successor at Johns Hopkins. Nutting, too, was born in Canada (Quebec) and received special instruction in music and art in private schools in Montreal, Boston, and Ottawa. An alumna of the first graduating class of Johns Hopkins, Nutting translated Hampton's dreams of a 3-year course and an 8-hour day into reality. However, Adelaide Nutting was an innovator in her own right. According to Christy (1969b), she was second only to Florence Nightingale in overall contributions to nursing. "Her influence as an educational experimenter and a creative thinker went far beyond the two institutions in which her main work was done, the second being Teachers College, Columbia University" (Stewart, 1943, p. 143).

During her tenure in Baltimore, Nutting initiated and developed the preliminary course, tuition fees, and scholarships at Johns Hopkins. She helped with the organization of the Maryland State Nurses Association, served as its first president, and facilitated the efforts of the nurses in their quest for state registration. She also began collecting materials and books for a historical collection for the nursing school. These later became the basis for the first two volumes of the four-volume *A History of Nursing* (1907 and 1912), written with Lavinia Dock. Nutting wrote many articles, some of which were published as a collection in *A Sound Economic Basis for Schools of Nursing* (1926). She prepared two influential reports on nursing education that were issued through the United States Bureau of Education. Her letters, speeches, and published works demonstrated her belief in a broad education for nurses that would prepare them for great responsibilities in all life situations. Her lifelong dream was to see basic education for nurses firmly established in institutions of higher learning—in universities.

In 1907, M. Adelaide Nutting took charge of the hospital economics course at Teachers College and became the first professor of nursing in the world. Her original title was Professor of Domestic Administration, but it was changed to Professor of Nurses Education in 1910. She remained at Teachers College until her retirement in 1925. In addition to her administrative and educational responsibilities at this institution, Nutting participated in many nursing activities, including organizational work, committee work, government projects, the war effort, publications, and international endeavors. She was the prime instigator in the establishment of the Vassar Training Camp of 1918, a program that drew women who were college graduates into nursing. Nut-

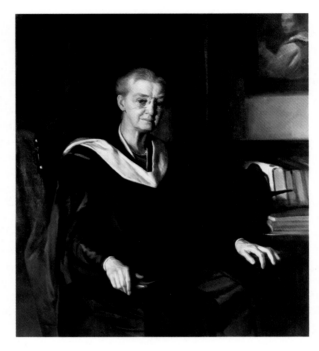

Cecilia Beaux, *M. Adelaide Nutting*, 1906, painting, Milbank Memorial Library, New York, NY.

ting received many awards in recognition of her deep and lasting commitment and service to nursing. Nutting died on October 3, 1948, after a long illness. She was a visionary whose words will long be remembered as being forever relevant: "We need to realize and to affirm anew that nursing is one of the most difficult of arts. Compassion may provide the motive, but knowledge is our only working power. Perhaps, too, we need to remember that growth in our work must be preceded by ideas, and that any conditions which suppress thought, must retard growth. Surely we will not be satisfied in perpetuating methods and traditions. Surely we shall wish to be more and more occupied with creating them" (Nutting, 1925).

American Nurses Association. The American Nurses Association (ANA) became the successor to the Nurses Associated Alumnae of the United States in 1911. The original federation of alumnae associations proved less workable as nurses became more mobile and began to move from state to state. A national organization with participation through state associations or through individual membership seemed more feasible, particularly because by 1912, thirty-nine state nurses' associations had been organized. The original body remained a federation of alumnae associations until the convention of 1916, when it was decided to establish membership through the state associations. State associations would eventually provide the means for achieving legal regulation. Unity of nurses within specific states, therefore, was essential to the passage of any licensing laws.

The ANA is *the* professional organization for registered nurses in the United States and as such, it holds membership in the International Council of Nurses. In the early years of the organization, state registration was a major concern. The purposes of the ANA have always been to create and maintain a code of ethics, foster high standards of nursing practice, promote the welfare of nurses, and improve the general working conditions of nurses. The association

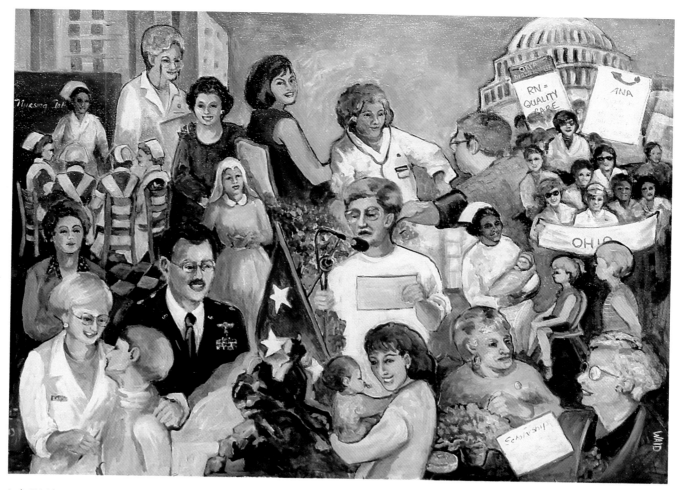

Judy Waid, RN, member of District Three, Ohio Nurses Association, District Three, ONA, *Faces of Caring*, unveiled May 5, 2005 as a prelude to National Nurses Week, acrylic on canvas, 40″ × 29 ¾″, District 3, Ohio Nurses Association, Youngstown, OH.

has functioned as a collective voice for registered nurses and a means of influencing health policy at all levels.

Currently, the American Nurses Association represents the nation's 2.9 million registered nurses through its 54 constituent member associations. Over the years, however, there has been controversy regarding the association's position on policies, which has resulted in the establishment of more than 70 national nursing organizations that represent specific nursing interest groups.

International Council of Nurses. The International Council of Nurses, established in 1899, is the oldest of all international organizations for professional workers. It was founded by Mrs. Bedford Fenwick in cooperation with nursing leaders from many countries. In 1900 the council's constitution was adopted, and the first meeting was held at the World Exposition in Buffalo, New York, in 1901. During this first meeting, Mrs. Fenwick proposed a resolution in favor of state registration:

> Whereas the nursing of the sick is a matter closely affecting all classes of the community in every land;
> Whereas to be efficient workers, nurses should be carefully educated in the important duties which are now allotted to them;
> Whereas at the present time there is no generally accepted term or standard of training nor system of education nor examination for nurses in any country;

> Whereas there is no method, except in South Africa, of enabling the public to discriminate easily between trained nurses and ignorant persons who assume that title; and
> Whereas this is a fruitful source of injury to the sick and of discredit to the nursing profession, it is the opinion of this international congress of nurses, in general meeting assembled, that it is the duty of the nursing profession of every country to work for suitable legislative enactment regulating the education of nurses and protecting the interests of the public, by securing State examinations and public registration, with the proper penalties for enforcing the same.
> — *Lavinia L. Dock, 1901, pp. 233*

Membership in the International Council of Nurses was open to self-governing national nurses' associations rather than to individuals. (As such, it was an association of associations.) Its established purposes were to provide a means of communication among the nurses of all nations and to offer opportunities for nurses from all parts of the world to meet and confer on questions relating to patient welfare and the nursing profession. The International Council of Nurses stands for the full development of the human being and citizen in every nurse and ever higher standards of education, professional ethics, public usefulness, and civic spirit.

National Association of Colored Graduate Nurses. Although the nursing organizations never expressed any racial prejudice, black nurses could secure membership in the American Nurses Association after 1916 only through membership in the state nurses' associations. They were thus denied membership in 16 southern states and the District of Columbia. Black nurses also realized they had problems of their own that would be best served by a separate organization. They needed to break down discriminatory practices that occurred because of the hue of their skin as opposed to their nursing proficiency.

The National Association of Colored Graduate Nurses (NACGN) was established in 1908. Its founding was the direct result of the vision, wisdom, and initiative of Martha Minerva Franklin (1870-1968), a graduate of the school of the Woman's Hospital Training School for Nurses in Philadelphia. Franklin had conducted a study of the status of black nurses before sending out letters to explore interest in the formation of a national organization. A meeting was held in August 1908 in New York under the sponsorship of the alumnae of Lincoln School for Nurses and its president, Adah Belle Samuels Thoms (1870-1943). By the end of this meeting the association had been formed and its objectives determined: to achieve higher professional standards; to break down discriminatory practices facing Negro nurses in schools, in jobs, and in organizational activities; and to develop Negro nurse leadership. Franklin was named the first president of this association.

Several leaders did, indeed, emerge and make significant achievements. Adah Thoms led the campaign for the acceptance of black nurses in the Red Cross. These nurses served with the Army Nurse Corps in World War I. Thoms also founded a registry for black nurses in New York (1918) and wrote the first book about the history of the black nursing profession, *Pathfinders,* in 1929. Estelle Massey Riddle Osborne (1901-1981) was the first black nurse to serve on the ANA board of directors, was awarded the NACGN scholarship for advanced study, and was the first black nurse to earn a master of arts degree with a major in nursing from Teachers College, Columbia University. Mabel Keaton Staupers (1898-1989) served as executive officer of the NACGN from 1934 to 1949, was elected the last president of the association, and chronicled the history of the organization in *No Time for Prejudice* (1961).

The NACGN continued to make valuable contributions to nursing. It brought the concerns of blacks in America to the attention of both nurses and the general public. In 1949 the organization believed it had accomplished its purpose and voted for dissolution. The program was phased out gradually over the next 2 years; a press release announcing its dissolution was issued on January 26, 1951. In 1950 the ANA had committed itself to assuming responsibility for the functions of the NACGN by virtue of a platform adopted by the ANA house of delegates. The platform supported "full participation of minority groups in association activities . . . and the elimination of discrimination in job opportunities, salaries, and other working conditions" (American Nurses Association, 1950). Some 20 years later, however, some black nurses would come to feel that the dissolution of the NACGN had been premature, and they established a new organization in 1971, the National Black Nurses Association.

National League of Nursing Education. With the change of membership and scope of functions, the American Society of Superintendents of Training Schools was renamed the National League of Nursing Education (NLNE) in 1912. The membership was expanded to include individuals whose greatest interest and training were in the field of nursing education, directors of public health nursing, members of state boards of nurse examiners, and those directly concerned with teaching and supervising in nursing schools. The goal of uniform standards was then seen to be impractical because the minimum requirements for state registration varied from state to state. The league decided to assist schools of nursing in achieving professional status comparable to that of similar professional groups, so special attention was given to increased financial support for nursing schools, sounder educational programs, and closer associations with institutions of higher learning. In 1932 the league became the Department of Education of the ANA, as voted upon by both organizations. Therefore, it was necessary to hold membership in the ANA in order to be a member of the NLNE. The NLNE was the organization most active in shaping educational thinking and practice in nursing for many years, and its annual reports became a major asset to nursing.

The National Organization for Public Health Nursing. The third national nursing association, the National Organization for Public Health Nursing (NOPHN), was established in 1912. By that time, district and visiting nursing had expanded rapidly to keep pace with the growth of new social services. National standards were urgently needed for one of the most promising movements of modern society. In addition, the care given by the nurse in the community differed from that given by the nurse in the hospital. A joint committee of the two national organizations, with Lillian D. Wald as chair and Mary S. Gardner as secretary, was appointed. The committee arranged for representatives of agencies employing visiting nurses to attend a meeting to be held in conjunction with the ANA and NLNE convention in Chicago in 1912. As a result, this organization came into being, but it was different in the makeup of its membership: "The name was selected with the utmost care to emphasize the fact that the new organization was not composed solely of nurses and that it would be concerned with the development of *nursing*" (Roberts, 1954, p. 88).

Lillian D. Wald was destined to become the first president of the new organization. Her social vision, excellent facility in public relations, and extraordinary gift for friendship were definite assets in the overall public health movement. Wald led the members in the enormous task of establishing standards for public health nurses, arranging courses to prepare them for their work, increasing the number of public health nurses, and building up organized voluntary and official agencies for home and community visiting nurse services. Two other officers were equally prominent: Mary S. Gardner, a pioneer in visiting nursing and the author of a book on public health nursing; and Ella Phillips Crandall, director of the first public health nursing program at Teachers College. *Public Health Nursing* was the official journal of the organization. Although the three major organizations had somewhat different functions, they also had common purposes and interests and worked closely together.

Sigma Theta Tau. Sigma Theta Tau was founded in 1922 at Indiana University through the creativity of six students who espoused excellence in scholarship and in practice. Their goal was to promote high standards for nursing care and to foster individual development. As the original national honor society of nursing, this organization promoted nursing research and leadership. Today, it supports these values through its numerous professional-development products and services that focus on the core areas of education, leadership, career development, evidence-based practice, research, and scholarship. Its members, who are selected on

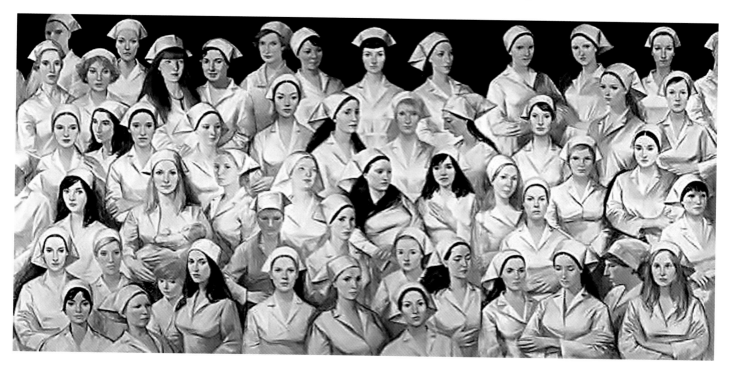

Natacha Ivanova, *Nurses*, 2008, oil on canvas, 195 × 390 cm, Cueto Project.

the basis of scholarly achievement and professional leadership, include students with baccalaureate degrees, graduate students in nursing programs, and community nursing leaders. Membership and chapters have increased steadily throughout the years. The honor society became incorporated in 1985 as Sigma Theta Tau International, Inc., and has thus embraced chapter development worldwide. This is consistent with the organization's vision of creating a global community of nurses that will enhance the health of all people and improve nursing care worldwide.

The Association of Collegiate Schools of Nursing. The Association of Collegiate Schools of Nursing (ACSN) was organized in 1933 to represent schools or departments of nursing associated with universities. In 1932 a decision had been made by representatives of more than 20 schools in San Antonio, Texas, to proceed with such an organization. The following January a conference was held at Teachers College, and it was decided to form the association. The standards or purposes adopted in 1935 were:

1. To develop nursing education on a professional and collegiate level.
2. To promote and strengthen relationships between schools of nursing and institutions of higher learning.
3. To promote study and experimentation in nursing service and nursing education.

— ACSN, 1943, p. 30

Membership standards were established, and membership was extended to schools that met specific criteria. The association did not originally consider itself an accrediting agency, but it visited and evaluated schools that applied for membership and thus was regarded by many as an accrediting body.

The ACSN was engaged in many activities related to higher education during its existence. It constantly emphasized the need for research in nursing and the preparation of nurse researchers. Both would be mandatory if nursing were ever to qualify on an equal basis with other departments in colleges and universities. In 1950 the association's Committee on Research recommended that the American Journal of Nursing Company be asked to publish a periodical that would focus on research in nursing. This was the first step toward the publication of *Nursing Research*. When changes in organized nursing ultimately occurred, the decision was made that the responsibilities of the ACSN would be assumed by the Department of Baccalaureate and Higher Degrees of the new National League for Nursing. The association had, indeed, proven its value to nursing and nursing education in a very short time.

A NEW LOOK FOR ORGANIZED NURSING

The numerous changes that had been occurring in nursing service and education mandated changes for organized nursing. The particular challenges of the Depression and World War I had forced some modification of organized nursing's structure and activities. Increased numbers of nurses were needed to meet the World War II effort, yet no one nursing association could speak or act for nursing as a whole. A commission representing all nursing interests was thus established to facilitate the efforts of both nursing and the national defense. Originally called the Nursing Council on National Defense, it was reorganized in late 1940 and renamed the National Nursing Council for War Service. The initial voting members of the council included the ANA, NLNE, NOPHN, ACSN, NACGN, and Red Cross Nursing Service. As soon as the American Association of Industrial Nurses (AAIN) organized in 1942, it gained membership. In addition, representatives of the Army and Navy Nurse Corps, United States Public Health Service (USPHS), Veterans Administration, Children's Bureau, Office of Indian Affairs, American Hospital Association, and the Canadian Nurses Association were ex officio members.

The representatives of these prestigious agencies were able to secure access to important sources of advice and information that greatly assisted the program. The council's preliminary work was financed by nursing. Later, beginning in 1942, the W.K. Kellogg Foundation became the council's principal source of income and contributed more than $300,000. (Allocations for special projects were received from other foundations and private sources.) For the duration of the war, state nurses' associations carried most of the local expenses of council-sponsored projects. The council was responsible for developing nursing programs to meet wartime needs.

When the war ended, the council decided to continue functioning until such time as another body replaced it or another method was recommended for continued coordination among the nursing associations. Esther Lucille Brown was engaged "to direct a study of the organization, administration, and support of professional and practical nursing as a basis for influencing the quality of nursing for the public" (Fitzpatrick, 1983, p. 169). The council also appointed a committee to plan for an accrediting agency for nursing education, and the National Nursing Accrediting Service was established in 1948. The council dissolved in that same year.

The accomplishments of the council during the war and several years after it proved that unified planning could be done by nursing and that cooperative efforts could and did improve the efficiency of organized nursing. The leaders of the associations were convinced that a permanent measure was necessary to ensure continued collaboration. A special committee, the Promoting Committee for the Structure of National Professional Nursing Organizations, began its study under Amelia Grant in 1945. This resulted in *Report on the Structure of Organized Nursing*, which was delivered at the biennial convention in 1946. It was determined that the six organizations in the study—the ANA, NLNE, NACGN, NOPHN, ACSN, and AAIN—were divided on three main points: nonnurse membership, special interests, and program emphasis. Considering the import of these issues, two alternative plans for organized nursing were proposed. The first suggested a single organization, the ANA, composed of five types of membership—professional nurses, public members, allied professionals, nursing schools and service agencies, and nonnursing organizations. The second plan was a two-organization system. One organization, the ANA, would accept only nurses. The other would be a national organization for nursing service composed of nurses, lay persons, allied professionals, and agency members. Cooperation would evolve through a joint commission for common concerns and a national nursing center that would include representatives from both organizations on its board.

After long months of deliberation by all concerned associations and individuals, more committee work, and the development of other plans, the ANA House of Delegates cast a majority vote for a two-organization plan at the 1950 Biennial Convention. The structure called for two distinct organizations: first, a somewhat reorganized American Nurses Association (ANA), composed entirely of nurses and able to speak for the profession and, second, the National League for Nursing (NLN), composed of nurses and non-nurses as well as individual and corporate members; it would represent those responsible for the sound development of and support for nursing services and nursing schools. The new structure was adopted at the Biennial Convention in Atlantic City, New Jersey, June 15-20, 1952. The two associations, under the direction of their newly elected presidents, Elizabeth K. Porter (ANA) and Ruth Sleeper (NLN), immediately initiated steps for the reorganization of state associations and the establishment of headquarters in New York. Several organizations were absorbed by the NLN: the National League of Nursing Education, National Organization for Public Health Nursing, Association of Collegiate Schools of Nursing, Joint Committee on Practical Nurses and Auxiliary Workers in Nursing Services, Joint Committee on Careers in Nursing, National Committee for the Improvement of Nursing Services, and National Nursing Accrediting Service.

THE CAMPAIGN FOR LEGISLATION AND REGISTRATION

The first published words regarding licensure for nurses came from a physician, Sir Henry W. Acland, in 1860. A regius professor of medicine at Oxford University, he wrote that nurses should be centrally registered, should follow a recognized curriculum of study, and should be able to meet a minimum standard of proficiency (Mollett, 1888). British nurses, however, did not begin to organize for state regulation of nursing practice until 1887. The first registration or licensing law for nurses was actually passed in Cape Colony, South Africa, in 1891. Although it was not a distinct nursing law but was incorporated as part of a medical and pharmacy act, it nonetheless gave hope to the British nurses who were having a difficult campaign. It was not until 1919, after a struggle commonly referred to as the Thirty Years' War, that these nurses were able to succeed in their efforts. In 1901, New Zealand passed a Nurses' Registration Act, which was the first true nursing act. Similar laws were adopted in five other countries, including Canadian provinces, by 1914. Meanwhile, American nurses had begun a campaign of their own for a proposed program of legislation. They believed that the protection of the public and the welfare of the individual nurse were primary issues of concern.

The need for professional controls that would protect nursing standards was made evident by the proliferation of schools of nursing. The maintenance of these standards, however, was not purely a nursing problem because public safety and welfare were involved. The continued development of poorly qualified schools jeopardized the public by the perpetuation of unqualified or improperly trained nurses. The newly formed nursing associations focused attention on acquiring a mechanism that would secure legal recognition for graduate nurses. Legislation that would distinguish between graduate and nongraduate personnel was desired. The control of education and professional practice in America came under the auspices of the states rather than the federal government. Therefore, state organizations were being formed to carry on what proved to be a long and bitter fight for nurse registration. The force of opposition came from outside groups who were financially interested in preventing nurses from achieving state recognition.

In 1898, a public statement concerning nurse licensure was made by Sophia Palmer before the New York State Federation of Women's Clubs. The idea was endorsed by the federation in the form of a resolution, and the campaign for legislation and registration was actively begun. This work was carried on for many years by the associations and the leaders in nursing. Finally, in a span of less than 2 months, the states of North Carolina, New Jersey, New York, and Virginia achieved licensure laws in 1903. North Carolina and New York had strong graduate nurses' associations that pushed to gain passage of legislation. An *American Journal of Nursing* editorial published in November 1903, presumably

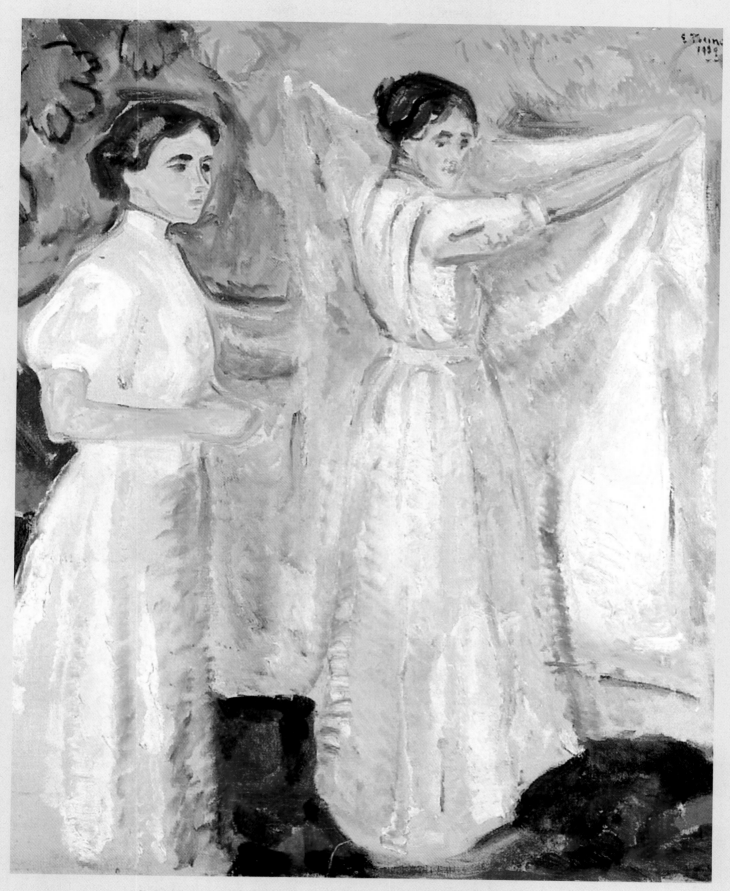

Sir Francis Bernard Disksee, *Two Nurses*, 1909, painting, 110 × 94 cm. Image courtesy of the Athenaeum.

written by Sophia Palmer, clearly and succinctly defined the issue and the nature of this push for registration.

Twenty years later, legislation regulating nurses' training was implemented in forty-eight states, Hawaii, and the District of Columbia. It provided for the licensing of nurses after examination and for nurse representation on examining boards. Boards of nurse examiners in the respective states were authorized by law to judge the competency of nurses applying for registration and licensing. Although the state laws were similar, they varied in their requirements and the power behind them. They were permissive, not mandatory; they denied the untrained the use of the title of registered nurse (RN); and they specified a time period during which qualified trained nurses were eligible for registration without examination. The conditions of the early nurse licensure laws, the first nurse practice acts, were weak and left much to be desired. Yet registration had positive results, such as accreditation and a movement toward uniformity in nursing schools. In addition, the campaign and struggle for state laws did much to strengthen and unite the whole of nursing.

State board examinations for nurses were developed but were generally inferior and unreliable during the 1930s. With the outbreak of World War II, pressure forced a look at the necessity of licensing individuals as soon as they had completed the nursing program. State examinations were not adequate; national norms needed to be considered. The Subcommittee on Tests of the Committee on State Board Problems of the NLNE met in 1942 and proposed that the league work closely with states to adopt machine-scored examination questions. The intent was the development of state board examinations that would be valid and reliable.

Individual state boards were asked to submit sample questions, which were evaluated by the Committee on Nursing Tests. Within 1 year after the examinations had been set up, the State Board Test Pool was operative and was being used by 15 states. The original examination contained 13 tests: anatomy and physiology, chemistry, microbiology, nutrition and diet therapy, pharmacology and therapeutics, nursing arts, communicable disease nursing, medical nursing, nursing of children, obstetrical and gynecological nursing, psychiatric nursing, surgical nursing, and social foundations of nursing. Six tests—medical nursing, surgical nursing, communicable disease nursing, psychiatric nursing, obstetrical nursing, and nursing of children—had become the norm by 1949. Ultimately, nursing became the first professional group to use the same licensing examination throughout the United States, Hawaii, and the Canadian provinces of British Columbia and Alberta.

In 1978 the National Council of State Boards of Nursing (NCSBN) was formed as a decision-making body composed of delegates from each state. The council contracts with agencies regarding all aspects of the licensure exam and in 1981 the first National Council Licensure Examination (NCLEX) was administered. Since 1994, the test has been administered using a Computer Adaptive Testing format. The NCLEX exam has gone through numerous changes since its implementation. Most are related to passing scores, redesign of content to reflect contemporary nursing practice, and innovative test items that allow for alternative formats, such as fill-in-the-blanks and the inclusion of pictures, tables, graphs, and calculations (Eason, 2004).

EDUCATIONAL TRENDS AND DEVELOPMENTS

After 1900 the increasing complexity of nursing services meant that there was continual pressure for the improvement of nursing schools. Most schools continued under hospital control; most operated on subprofessional levels. Nursing organizations, nurses, foundations, committees, agencies, and hospital groups began to conduct surveys and studies of nurses and nursing. Consequently, recommendations began to be made for educational standards and practices. The influence of newer educational viewpoints surfaced in experiments and innovations. Continued support for upgrading nursing education was being demonstrated. In *A Sound Economic Basis for Schools of Nursing,* M. Adelaide Nutting emphasized the subordination of the educational program: "Heavy demands of the wards made it impossible for all students to attend their weekly lecture and it was always arranged that some students would choose to take very full notes and read them later to the assembled group of less fortunate. Lectures came under the category of privileges like 'hours off duty' to be granted 'hospital duties permitting' " (Nutting, 1926, pp. 339-340).

What must be remembered is that the progressive development in educational reforms in schools of nursing was intertwined with aspects of life in the United States at the turn of the century.

> With the frontier gone, the continent subdued, and the nation now proud of its designation as a world power, a new era of mature consolidation was at hand. The democratic political foundations upon which the nation had been established remained intact, indeed were broadened by the termination of Negro slavery. Tens of millions of Europeans of many races and peoples had been absorbed without any serious social consequences and population had been established to seventy-six million. The national wealth in the last half of the nineteenth century had increased from seven to eighty-eight million dollars, and the standard of living for the common man was better than almost anywhere in the world. Great strides had been made in agriculture and industry, through the utilization of limited government assistance, cheap labor, plentiful natural resources, and "clever Yankee inventions." These factors made possible the rise . . . and the upgrading of the nursing profession which accompanied it in the new era now opening.
>
> — CHRISTY, 1969A, PP. 3-4

Some improvements were being made, particularly in the better schools of nursing. An early preparatory course was started in Scotland at the Glasgow Infirmary in 1893. Rebecca Strong, then superintendent, with the assistance of Dr. McEwen, who was one of Lister's students, succeeded in having nursing students enter St. Mungo's College for a short course of theoretical instruction followed by practical training in the hospital. This was the first connection of any kind that nursing students had with an institution of higher learning. The inception of preparatory or preliminary courses made these programs more like those of educational institutions rather than a strict apprenticeship system. The first such course in America was developed in 1901 through the efforts of Nutting at Johns Hopkins. This preparatory course was 6 months long and offered basic sciences as well as nursing principles and practice, the latter experience taking place in the hospital wards. The primary difference in this instance was that the clinical experience was for the purpose of education, not service. Within 10 years, approximately 86 schools had preparatory courses that averaged 3 to 4 months in length.

Other improvements and changes were also occurring. The terminology used to describe an individual in a nursing program was altered from *pupil nurse* to *student nurse*. This change was significant because the word *pupil* implies intellectual immaturity and guardianship, whereas *student* describes a more mature, independent, self-directed learner. The title of Principal of the School of Nursing was being adopted to portray the nursing program as educational. Teachers and lecturers were being referred to as nursing school faculty. A greater interest in pedagogical methods was observed. Efforts were also being made to introduce student government as a way of toning down the militaristic discipline, of treating students as adults. Other educational experiments begun at Johns Hopkins and later adopted at other schools were payment of tuition fees by pupils, payment of lecturers from university staffs, the 3-year course, full-time instructors, separate nursing school announcements outlining a fully organized course of study, high school graduation as a requirement for admission, the use of scholarships, and the 8-hour day (adopted by Johns Hopkins in 1895). It is clear that nurses were beginning to broaden their concept of the meaning and responsibility of the title *profession*, as pointed out by Nutting in 1905:

> "We claim, and I think justly, the status of a profession; we have schools and teachers, tuition fees and scholarships, systems of instruction from preparatory to postgraduate; we are allied with technical schools on one hand and here and there a university on the other; we have libraries, a literature, and fast-growing numbers of periodicals owned, edited, and published by nurses; we have societies and laws. If therefore we claim to receive the appurtenances, privileges, and standing of a profession, we must recognize professional responsibilities and obligations which we are in honor bound to respect and uphold"
>
> —NUTTING, 1905, PP. 654-655

Nursing literature was expanding in several ways. A great increase in the number of texts and reference books, as well as other types of nursing literature, had occurred. Nurses themselves had begun to produce a large portion of this material, either individually or through their organizations. When the schools of nursing were established, textbooks were urgently needed. Clara Weeks Shaw wrote the first American nursing text in 1885, *A Textbook of Nursing for the Use of Training Schools, Families and Private Students*. She was joined by other reputable authors, including Isabel Adams Hampton, author of *Nursing: Its Principles and Practice for Hospital and Private Use* (1893); Diana Kimber, who wrote *Anatomy and Physiology* (1893); and Lavinia Dock, author of *Textbook on Materia Medica for Nurses* (1890). By 1930 there were approximately seven hundred textbooks for nurses. Most of them had been written by nurses and published in the United States.

Journals also became necessary for establishing a means of communication among nurses in various locations. The first journal, *Nightingale,* was started in 1886; editing was done by a Bellevue graduate. *Trained Nurse and Hospital Review* (renamed *Nursing World*), established in 1888, was the

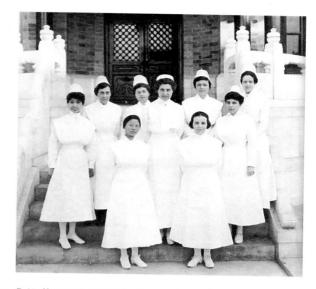

Anna D. Wolf (center), a 1915 Hopkins nursing graduate, served as the first Superintendent of Nurses and Dean of the School of Nursing at Peking Union Medical College, the first Western-style nursing and medical school in China.

John Hopkins and Peking, photograph, page 60 of *Johns Hopkins Nursing,* Spring 2008, vol. VI, issue 1. Courtesy of the Alan Mason Chesney Medical Archives of the Johns Hopkins Medical Institutions.

first national nursing and hospital journal. It was eventually combined with *Journal of Practical Nursing, Nightingale, Nurse, Nursing World,* and *Nursing Record.* One of the first activities of the Associated Alumnae was to consider and investigate the possibility of establishing a professional journal that would be its official magazine.

On October 1, 1900, the first issue of *American Journal of Nursing* appeared through the particular efforts of Mary E. P. Davis and Sophia E. Palmer. Individual nurses and alumnae associations had bought shares of stock to finance the original enterprise. By 1912 the ANA had become the sole owner of *Journal* stock; some of it had been donated, but the majority of it had been purchased. Palmer served as editor until her death in 1920, when she was succeeded by Mary M. Roberts. The first office of *American Journal of Nursing* was the home of Palmer, where a trunk held manuscripts and other materials related to the magazine. This publication became the official organ of the ANA and one of the leading professional journals in the country.

Mary Roberts was also committed to this journal's success, and she secured special preparation in journalism. Under her leadership the American Journal of Nursing Company was formed, and it slowly moved toward the expansion of publications. Roberts, a historian in her own right (author of *American Nursing: History and Interpretation* [1954]), fostered the story of nursing in the pages of the journal. Nell V. Beeby was appointed editor upon the retirement of Roberts in 1949. Under Beeby's administration two new journals went into production: *Nursing Outlook,* the official journal of the NLN, and *Nursing Research,* the vehicle of communication concerning all types of studies relating to nursing.

Affiliations among hospitals for the purpose of rounding out the students' clinical experience were also begun. They were often lengthy and were set as conditions for registration, particularly in the smaller and more specialized institutions. The first formal program of affiliation was developed at the Illinois Training School in Chicago; Bellevue in New York was also a recognized leader in this regard.

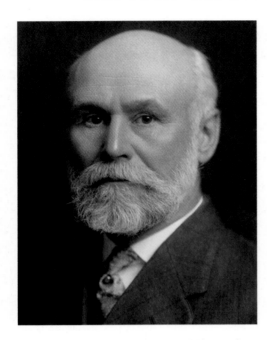

Dr. Richard Olding Beard, 1910s, portrait, 8.5" × 5.5". Photograph courtesy of the University of Minnesota Archives, University of Minnesota—Twin Cities.

A trend emerged in which university hospitals were established in various geographical locations in connection with medical departments. In a sense, nursing schools thus became parts of the general university system. In most instances, however, the education program was not classified as a university program, nor were the student nurses considered students of the university. An attempt was made to accomplish this in 1897, when the University of Texas assumed control over the John Sealy Hospital of Galveston and established it as a university hospital. The nursing school was recognized as a regular school of the medical department, and the superintendent of nurses occupied a place on the university committee of instruction. The school, however, was not required to meet the standards of the university.

In 1909, through the influence of Dr. Richard Olding Beard, the School of Nursing of the University of Minnesota became the first nursing school organized as an integral part of a university. Nursing students were admitted and registered as regular students of the university, with all university requirements and privileges. "It was not an independent unit, however, since both hospital and nursing school functioned under the college of medicine and surgery. Nor did it offer at that time a college degree" (Stewart, 1943, p. 175). Ten years of pioneering effort went into the upgrading of the school before it offered a degree-granting basic program (1919). Similar schools were established in the universities of Indiana and Cincinnati and later in several other colleges and universities.

In 1916, 2 5-year bachelor-degree programs were established at Teachers College, New York, in cooperation with Presbyterian Hospital and the University of Cincinnati's School of Nursing and Health. Within 7 years, similar programs had been instituted in thirteen universities and three colleges (Committee for the Study of Nursing Education, 1923). A combined academic and professional course of 5, or sometimes 4, years led to both a college degree and the nursing diploma. In general, an attempt was made to mix occupational preparation with a liberal arts education.

Another significant innovation in nursing education oc-

curred with the development of associate degree programs in community colleges. These schools exhibited phenomenal growth, but their nursing programs evoked a great deal of controversy. It was felt that this community college connection equated nursing education with vocational training at a time when professional status was being sought for nursing. This model of education was developed by Dr. Mildred Montag of Teachers College in 1949 as the result of planned research and eventual controlled experimentation. The original pilot project began in 1952 with seven junior and community colleges and one hospital in each of six regions of the United States. The program was administered by Teachers College, and Montag directed it. The product of this new type of program was to be the nurse technician, who operated somewhat below the level of professional nurse but above that of the practical nurse. The project concluded in 1957 and was followed by the rapid proliferation of community college nursing programs.

The first steps in the evolution of schools of nursing from hospitals to universities had occurred. As time went on, the superior educational opportunities afforded by a university or a college became abundantly clear. As an integral part of the university—with its liberal education, physical facilities, resources, and level of instruction—a school of nursing would be primarily an educational undertaking. "Hardly less valuable is the effect of the university atmosphere and surroundings on the student 'morale.' Ambition reacts to the atmosphere of intellectual competition; the student nurse is stimulated to do her best and take her place with credit among her fellow students of the various schools. She feels, too, a new sense of dignity and of the importance of her work through her recognition as a member of an educational institution" (Committee for the Study of Nursing Education, 1923, p. 483).

STUDIES OF NURSING AND NURSING EDUCATION

The first comprehensive and critical survey of schools of nursing in the United States was *The Educational Status of Nursing* (1912). It was sponsored by the Federal Bureau of Education and directed by M. Adelaide Nutting, who developed the questionnaire and interpreted the data. The majority of the eleven hundred schools that responded were classified as mediocre educationally and utilitarian in purpose. It was noted in the report that the "exceptional" schools had an adequate supply of applicants; the "poor" schools complained of a continual shortage of applicants. Several recommendations were offered: that the standards of nursing schools be raised; that schools of nursing secure financial independence; and that the schools become educational institutions in fact, not just in name. This study set a precedent for future investigations that soon followed.

The need for alterations in nursing and nursing education became apparent as the nation absorbed changes in its social, political, and economic structures. Rapid developments in medical science, technological advances in hospitals, and increased demands for health care highlighted this need. It was World War I, however, that particularly dramatized the indispensable role played by nursing and the need for more and better-prepared nurses. A pamphlet by Isabel M. Stewart, *Developments in Nursing Education Since 1918* (1921), summed up the impact of the war years on the nursing profession:

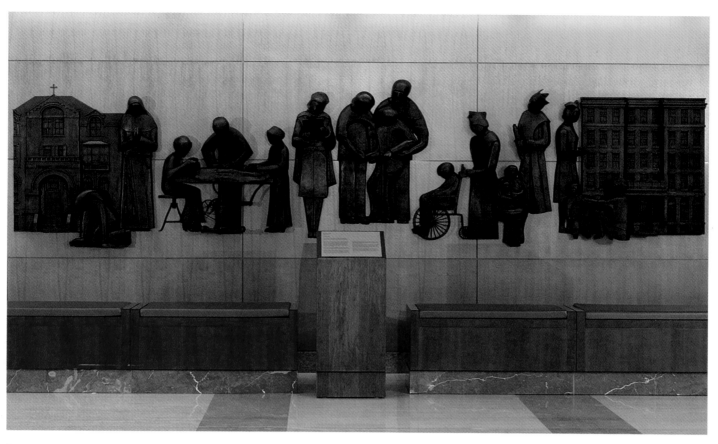

Forever Caring is a bronze panoramic sculpture. The left-most panel reflects the impact of the Sisters of St. Francis and their dedication and willingness to serve at all levels. The next scene features a nurse anesthetist monitoring a patient undergoing surgery. Next is a nurse assisting a man walking with the aid of a crutch, and the last set of panels advance to the diversity of services the field of nursing now encompasses. Pediatrics, geriatrics, orthopedics, and academia are some of the areas portrayed. The caps (hats) depicted reflect the styles worn by each generation of nurses throughout the history of Mayo.

Gloria Tew, *Forever Caring*, 2005, sculpture, Mayo Clinic, Rochester, MN.

Probably the greatest contribution of the war experience to nursing lies in the fact that the whole system of nursing education was shaken for a little while out of its well-worn ruts and brought out of its comparative seclusion into the light of public discussion and criticism. When so many lives hung on the supply of nurses, people were aroused to a new sense of their dependence on the products of nursing schools, and many of them learned for the first time of the hopelessly limited resources which nursing educators have had to work with in the training of these indispensable servants. Whatever the future may bring it is unlikely that nursing schools will willingly sink back again into their old isolation, or that they will accept unquestionably the financial status which the older system imposed on them.

— STEWART, 1921, P. 6

Stewart firmly believed that the educational status of nursing schools was in some ways better at the end of the war than it had been at the beginning. Numerous studies were initiated, but only a few exerted a profound influence on the development of nursing. These specific studies are briefly reviewed.

NURSING AND NURSING EDUCATION IN THE UNITED STATES (THE GOLDMARK REPORT OF 1923)

Following World War I, attention was focused as never before on the issues of public health. In 1919 the Rockefeller Foundation invited representative men and women to a conference to consider the status of public health nursing in the United States. The consensus was that the usual programs in basic schools of nursing did not adequately prepare nurses for community health practice. A committee was subsequently appointed and financed by the Rockefeller Foundation to study public health nursing education. Dr. C. A. Winslow, professor of public health at Yale, was appointed chair; Josephine Goldmark, a social worker and author, was appointed secretary and chief investigator. It soon became evident that the scope of the study was too narrow and that the subject of nursing and nursing education needed to be investigated as a whole. The work was expanded and the Committee for the Study of Nursing Education began "to survey the entire field occupied by the nurse and other workers of related type; to form a conception of the tasks to be performed and the qualifications necessary for their execution; and on the basis of such a study of function to establish sound minimum education standards for each type of nursing service for which there appears to be a vital need" (Committee for the Study of Nursing Education, 1923, p. 7).

Representatives of 23 schools of nursing and 49 public health agencies in various sections of the country were surveyed. After 3 years a preliminary report was released in 1922, followed by the final report in 1923, commonly known as the Goldmark Report but sometimes called the Winslow-Goldmark Survey. The conclusions clearly echoed the statements that had been made by the nursing leaders of the day.

A direct outcome of the study was the establishment of

the Yale University School of Nursing (1923), financed by the Rockefeller Foundation. Under the leadership of Annie W. Goodrich and her associate, Effie J. Taylor, who succeeded her, this school successfully demonstrated the importance of an independently endowed and professional school of nursing. Other endowed schools followed at Vanderbilt University, the University of Toronto, and Western Reserve University.

STUDIES BY THE COMMITTEE ON THE GRADING OF NURSING SCHOOLS

The Committee on the Grading of Nursing Schools was composed of representatives of nursing, medical, and hospital organizations, as well as a few educational and lay members. William Darrach, a well-known surgeon, was the chairman. Dr. May Ayres Burgess, an educator, psychologist, and statistician, directed the study. The committee was officially established in November 1925 to grade and classify schools of nursing, to study the work of nurses, and to define the duties within the scope of nursing. The study was partially financed by outside sources, but nurses themselves donated $115,000 over a 5-year period.

Nurses, Patients, and Pocketbooks (1928). The first report that focused on the supply and demand of nursing service, *Nurses, Patients, and Pocketbooks,* was published in 1928. The original purpose of the committee that wrote this report, the grading of nursing schools, was postponed because it was determined that grading ought to be based on and accompanied by careful inquiry into nursing education and employment. The committee thus decided on a 5-year program that would be divided into 3 separate projects: a study of the supply of and demand for nursing services, a job analysis of what nurses did and how they should be prepared to function, and the actual grading of nursing schools based on the facts of the other 2 projects.

The report covered a wide-ranging and interesting group of problems and vividly demonstrated the economic conflict between nurses and their employers and between student service and the objectives of schools of nursing. Specific findings included the following: educational requirements for entrance into nursing schools were minimal; most nursing schools were of poor educational quality; nursing schools existed merely to provide service to hospitals; a serious overproduction of graduate nurses had led to chronic unemployment; and salaries and working conditions were extremely poor. These findings were serious indictments of nursing education and showed its failure to meet existing social needs for nursing service. After the findings were published, the American Medical Association withdrew from the committee without expressing a clear reason for its action.

In general, the conclusions of this committee agreed with those of the Committee on Nursing and Nursing Education in the United States and with the comments and criticisms of nursing leaders. One immediate measure recommended was the replacement of student nurses in hospitals by graduate nurses. In addition, two important resolutions were unanimously adopted by the committee:

1. No hospital should be expected to bear the cost of nursing education out of funds collected for the care of the sick. The education of nurses is as much a public responsibility as is the education of physicians, public school teachers, librarians, ministers, lawyers, and other students planning to engage in professional public service, and the cost of such education should come, not out of a hospital budget, but from private or public funds.

2. The fact that a hospital is faced with serious financial difficulties should have no bearing; upon whether or not it will conduct a school of nursing. The need of a hospital for cheap labor should not be considered a legitimate argument for maintaining such a school. The decision as to whether or not a school of nursing should be conducted in cooperation with a given hospital should be based solely upon the kinds and amounts of educational experience which that hospital is prepared to offer.

— *COMMITTEE ON THE GRADING OF NURSING SCHOOLS, 1928, PP. 447-448*

Nursing Schools Today and Tomorrow (1934). In the final publication of the committee, *Nursing Schools Today and Tomorrow,* the essentials of a professional program of education were outlined. The publication contained the facts necessary for reform in schools of nursing and became a vehicle to influence public opinion in favor of nursing. Conditions that would not be tolerated in any nursing school were also specified. The weaknesses in nursing education were thus clearly described. The following recommendations on professional standards were emphasized and stressed: "a collegiate level of education; an enriched curriculum, with more and better theory and less and better practice; a better-prepared student body and faculty comparable with those in other professional schools; an organization better fitted to safeguard the professional status and freedom of the school, 'dominated by neither hospital nor treasury, nor nursing traditions'; and funds adequate to provide for such a school" (Stewart, 1943, pp. 214-215).

The recurring theme of adequate financial support was once again identified as the greatest problem in positioning nursing education at a higher level. Compared with other forms of professional education, the nurse stood alone, with training dependent on service in the hospital. In addition, faculty were grossly unqualified; the majority of teachers in schools of nursing had not completed a high school education.

An Activity Analysis of Nursing (1934). It is possible that this study was not recognized as part of the five-year program adopted by the Committee on the Grading of Nursing Schools. As activities developed, it became evident that this part of the program dealing with the teaching of nursing and an analytical study of nursing procedures, a job analysis, could not be completed by the office staff. At the committee's request it was turned over to Ethel Johns, a nurse, editor and consultant, and Blanche Pfefferkorn, a nurse and director of studies at the National League of Nursing Education. As a consequence, it is more commonly known as the Johns and Pfefferkorn Activity Analysis.

Essentially, two questions were addressed: What is good nursing? and How can it be taught? An attempt was made to document the exact functions of nurses in various occupational categories: hospital bedside nursing, private-duty nursing in the home, and nursing in the field of public health. In addition, personal activities that should be practiced by the professional nurse were described. Johns and Pfefferkorn contended that these activities "have to do with matters of personal efficiency and the maintenance of good professional standards and relationships" (p. 102). These activities are particularly interesting and in many instances still very relevant to the mission of nursing. Finally, the report included a clear and concise description of what the patient, the physician, the hospital, and the general public expected of nursing. As one scrutinizes this 1934 study, it is difficult to avoid drawing distinct similarities between this classification and the ongoing work on the Nursing Interventions Classification (NIC), originally led by Drs. Joanne McCloskey and Gloria Bulechek at The University of Iowa College of Nursing.

At the completion of the studies, it was once again clear that reform in nursing education was necessary. The findings of the grading committee provided specific data that could be used to reinforce the debate for reform. Finally, the grading committee strongly recommended that the National League of Nursing Education undertake the accreditation of nursing schools.

CURRICULUM STUDIES AND REPORTS

From 1914 to 1919, Isabel M. Stewart served as secretary of the Curriculum Committee of the League (originally called the Education Committee), and she was its chair from 1920 to 1937. Three important studies emerged from this committee. The first was the *Standard Curriculum for Schools of Nursing*, published in 1917. "The purpose of this study was to bring about greater uniformity in the programs of nursing schools and to help in improving the content and quality of the teaching as well as other conditions affecting the education of nurses" (Stewart, 1943, p. 211). The body of this study contained a systematic plan for the education of nurses and outlined specific courses, along with their objectives, content, and methods; lists of bibliographies, equipment, and schedules completed the scheme.

Within a few years the second study was begun, and resulted in the publication of *Curriculum for Schools of Nursing* in 1927. The word *standard* was dropped to avoid the notion that it was a requirement to be adopted by schools of nursing. This study was essentially a revision and expansion of the first. A job-analysis technique was used to outline the functions and qualifications of the nurse, which constituted the practical objectives of the nursing school curriculum. Nutting and Stewart did most of the writing of these volumes, although the actual studies were conducted by the entire committee.

In 1935, Isabel Stewart urged that another revision be made to meet the current trends in nursing education necessary to comply with community needs.

> She called for a cooperative research project that would encourage participation by many people. She hoped that, through widespread involvement, schools that had been too dependent on the League's curriculum outlines might learn to build their own curriculums by taking materials from the common stock and adapting them to their different situations and stages of development. She desired a serious analysis of the philosophy of nursing education, goals to be aimed for and values to be conserved, the kind of services nurses should be prepared to give to society, the kind of individuals nursing schools should select for preparation, and the kind of preparation needed to fit them for living and serving.
>
> — *CHRISTY, 1969c, p. 47*

The project proved to be one of the most far-reaching and ambitious efforts undertaken in this area. It included

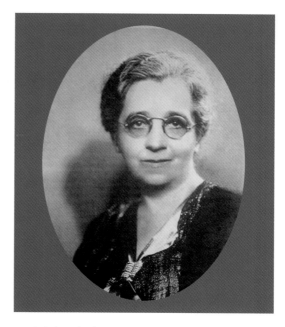

Isabel Maitland Stewart, painting, Donahue Collection.

the participation of representatives of all the professional organizations, the allied professions, and the community. The project called for a review and reevaluation, not only of existing curricula but of the traditional philosophies underlying them. Under the direction of Stewart, curriculum committees were organized in all of the state leagues of nursing education, with state subcommittees and local committees under them. Stewart prepared all the materials relevant to the various phases of the work for presentation to her central committee. They, in turn, were sent back to the state leagues, state subcommittees, and local committees. The project was a process of sharing in which participating individuals and groups were educated through their involvement. R. Louise McManus, Stewart's successor at Teachers College, emphasized the project's significance: "I have always thought of it as one of the first major, mass studies in nursing. But more than that, it was mass education, because many people who didn't know what a curriculum was before that, had an opportunity to participate in the construction of the curriculum—and learn what it was. It was 'operation bootstrap' for the profession and Miss Stewart did a masterly job. Through the materials that she prepared for the various committees she really educated the mass of nursing educators across the country" (McManus, cited in Christy, 1969c, p. 47). The report published by the league in 1937, *A Curriculum Guide for Schools of Nursing*, was the product of the scholarly mind and wise leadership of Isabel Stewart.

Isabel Maitland Stewart (1878-1963) was American nursing's most influential spokeswoman in the area of education for 45 years. It was Stewart who developed the first course dealing specifically with the teaching of nursing at Teachers College. Eventually this course was expanded and developed into an entire program for the preparation of teachers of nursing. Isabel Stewart's reputation as a curriculum expert became so well established that in later years she was known as "Miss Curriculum" (Stewart, 1961, p. 184).

Stewart was born in Fletcher, Ontario, a village near the city of Chatham. Her Canadian background is particularly significant in that she became part of a nucleus of three

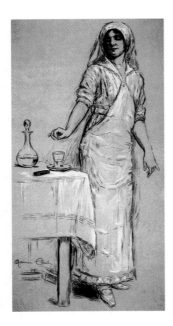

Maurice Clio, *Aspirine—Usines de Rhone,* 1910, color lithograph (poster), 58" × 78⅜" [147.3 × 199.1 cm], Philadelphia Museum of Art, The William H. Helfand Collection, 1981.

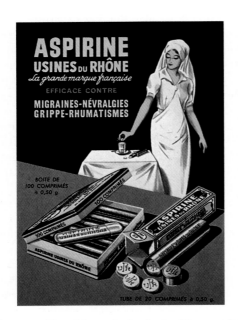

The emerging recognition of the professional role of the nurse led to the use of nurses in advertising. It is possible that this is one of the first advertising posters in which a nurse is used to promote a product.

French Aspirin, 1950, poster, The Granger Collection, NY.

Canadian nurses who helped to shape the destiny of nursing education:

> Many American nurses do not realize the debt we owe to our Canadian sisters. Three of our greatest leaders were born in Canada but spent most of their most productive years contributing to nursing and nursing education in the United States. The first, M. Adelaide Nutting . . . was born in Waterloo, Quebec; Isabel Hampton Robb . . . came from Welland, Ontario. The third, Isabel M. Stewart, was born in Ontario also, and one might speculate on what differences there might have been in the developments in both American and Canadian nursing had these three not migrated to the United States. . . . Isabel Stewart, particularly, following

in the footsteps of her mentor, M. Adelaide Nutting, had great impact on American nursing education.

— CHRISTY, 1969C, P. 44

Isabel Stewart was one of nine children, all of whom were encouraged to engage in educational pursuits. Beginning her career as a schoolteacher in Canada, she soon turned to nursing and graduated from Winnipeg General Hospital in 1903. Her pursuit of further education led her to Teachers College, where she earned several degrees. Stewart became an assistant to Professor M. Adelaide Nutting and eventually succeeded her as director of the college's Division of Nursing Education, a position she held for twenty-two years. Although best known for her accomplishments as chair of the Curriculum Committee of the League, Isabel Stewart was also an active research investigator who planned and implemented studies that led to a wealth of useful information for nursing education and practice. Until her death in 1963, she remained an active participant in nursing activities. Throughout her life she filled with distinction the roles of scholar, author, educator, researcher, administrator, and leader.

Isabel Stewart's interests were wide and varied. She was deeply interested in education in all aspects, particularly the education of women. Her study of history strengthened her belief that women could not rise to the full demands of any vocation or profession without education and knowledge of the social conditions and needs of their day. Thus the fullest development of nursing was not possible without emancipation from the conditions of subjection under which women and nurses had suffered for so many years.

Early in her professional career Stewart began her contributions to nursing organizations, which provided her with an essential vehicle for the improvement of professional training and curricula in schools of nursing throughout the country. She belonged to many nursing organizations, both national and international, in which she became a prominent figure. In these organizations she worked on a multitude of committees. A prolific writer, she published numerous works in which she interpreted modern trends in both general education and nursing education. Two of these publications stand out as being particularly important and were directly linked to her intense love of history: *A Short History of Nursing,* first published in 1920 and written with Lavinia L. Dock, and *The Education of Nurses* (1943). An examination of the latter work can lead to an important conclusion. It was written by an individual who had the outstanding ability to select significant facts and who had the rare vision, insight, and imagination to demonstrate relationships and interpret them to professional workers. *The Education of Nurses* was the closest thing to a philosophy of nursing education ever written.

As the years went by, Stewart feared for the loss of the humanitarian aspects that had long been a vital force in nursing. Recognizing that a definite decline in the study of this area was occurring, she commented:

> I feel very strongly these days that we are failing to develop the social and humanistic side of nursing—the spirit of nursing as we used to call it—and all that goes to the *balancing* of the scientific and technical aspects—it would mean a restudy of that whole area dealing with the philosophy and history of nursing and the social sciences, and the strengthening of our cultural roots, both in nursing schools (basic) and in the preparation of graduate nurses for developing this phase of nursing.

I am distressed to realize that we are doing less in this field today than we did a few years ago and there seems to be very little interest in it. Miss [Maude] Muse spoke of it the other day and she feels much as I do. It is a part of the sickness of our civilization that we have *overstressed* the scientific and technical side and have neglected the other aspects of our work and education.

— *LETTER FROM ISABEL M. STEWART TO LILLIAN A. HUDSON, C. 1940-1947*

NURSING FOR THE FUTURE (1948)

Nursing for the Future was initiated in connection with the postwar planning of the National Nursing Council. A grant of $28,000 was given to the council by the Carnegie Corporation in 1947 for the investigation of nursing practice and the preparation required for it. Esther Lucile Brown, a social anthropologist and director of the Department of Studies in the Professions at the Russell Sage Foundation, was authorized to conduct this study to determine the "needs of society" for nursing. Her data were obtained firsthand as she personally visited 50 geographically representative schools in the country, held 3 regional workshop conferences with nursing directors (representing 1250 schools), and met with individual nurses, physicians, hospital administrators, and others involved with nursing. A large number of far-reaching recommendations were published in this report, which is also known as *The Brown Report*. One of the strongest proposals was "that effort be directed to building basic schools of nursing in universities and colleges, comparable in number to existing medical schools, that are sound in organizational and financial structure, adequate in facilities and faculty, and well-distributed to serve the needs of the entire country" (Brown, 1948, p. 178). The report was endorsed in principle by the boards of directors of the six national nursing organizations in existence. However, many physicians and hospital administrators were openly hostile to its recommendations.

NURSING SCHOOLS AT THE MID-CENTURY (1950)

The Joint Committee on Implementing the Brown Report was established by the NLNE in 1948 (it was renamed the National Committee for the Improvement of Nursing Services in 1949). The early work of this committee consisted of the collection of factual information about nursing school programs and the interim classification of schools. This was to precede the development of a more comprehensive accreditation system and program. A questionnaire was used, and the hope was to obtain information from *all* schools of nursing (there was a 96% return rate in the United States). Each of the participating schools was evaluated according to criteria long accepted by the profession. The schools were classified according to a total score obtained by the weighting of the various criteria of administrative policies, financial organization, faculty, curriculum, clinical field, library, student selection and provisions for student welfare, and student performance on state board examinations. This classification of nursing schools was published in *American Journal of Nursing* in November 1949 as "Interim Classification of Schools of Nursing Offering Basic Programs." The publication of these data drew much criticism from the ranks of nurses. In 1950, the findings were published in *Nursing Schools at the Mid-Century* and provided a method for schools of nursing to evaluate their programs.

CANADIAN STUDIES

Through the initiative of the Canadian Nurses Association, a joint committee of this association and the Canadian Medical Association was established in 1929 to undertake a nationwide study of nursing education in Canada. The study was conducted by Dr. George M. Weir, a well-known educator and sociologist in the Department of Education of the University of British Columbia. *Survey of Nursing Education in Canada* (1932), also known as *The Weir Report*, pointed out serious weaknesses that existed in the hospital schools. Important reforms were recommended: higher educational standards, increased affiliations among schools, increased employment of graduate nurses, student tuition, and the employment of qualified instructors. The survey also recommended that "no hospital having fewer than 75 beds, exclusive of cots and bassinets, and a daily average of at least 50 patients, be recognized as competent to conduct an approved Training School" (Gibbon and Mathewson, 1947, p. 375).

Following the release of this report, the Canadian Nurses Association organized a National Curriculum Committee, which published *The Proposed Curriculum for Schools of Nursing in Canada* in 1936. This project was conducted by a special committee and chaired by Marion Lindeberg, director of the Department of Nursing Education at McGill University. The findings were similar to those in the United States and led to the closing of a number of smaller training schools. The study and the later *Supplement* became valuable guides that assisted in the establishment of a more sound educational foundation for nursing in Canada.

THE STATUS OF NURSING STUDIES

Studies of nursing education and practice have been initiated almost every five to ten years since 1923 (Ashley, 1976; Bridgman, 1953; Brown, 1948; Burgess, 1928; Committee for the Study of Nursing Education, 1923; Committee on the Grading of Nursing Schools, 1934; Department of Health, Education, & Welfare, 1963; Hughes, Hughes and Deutscher, 1958; Institute of Medicine, 1983; Johns and Pfefferkorn, 1934; National Commission on Nursing, 1983; National League of Nursing Education, 1917, 1927, 1937; West and Hawkins, 1950). There is no doubt that additional studies will be initiated to determine the possible need for the redesign of nursing education, the standardization of educational requirements, and a comprehensive view of how nurses practice and, more important, should practice. In making such investigations, it will be important to consider the common elements that have evolved from previous studies:

...several educational programs leading to entry into the same practice create consumer and employer confusion; the studies have not been conducted by nurses (groups such as government agencies, psychologists, historians, sociologists, allied health organizations, and private foundations became involved); the committees or commissions conducting the studies have not been dominated by nurses; study effects on nursing education and practice were varied; complaints of a shortage of hospital nurses were continual; and nursing experienced considerable difficulty in implementing the recommendations put forth for the education and practice of nursing.

— *DONAHUE, 2004, P. 14.*

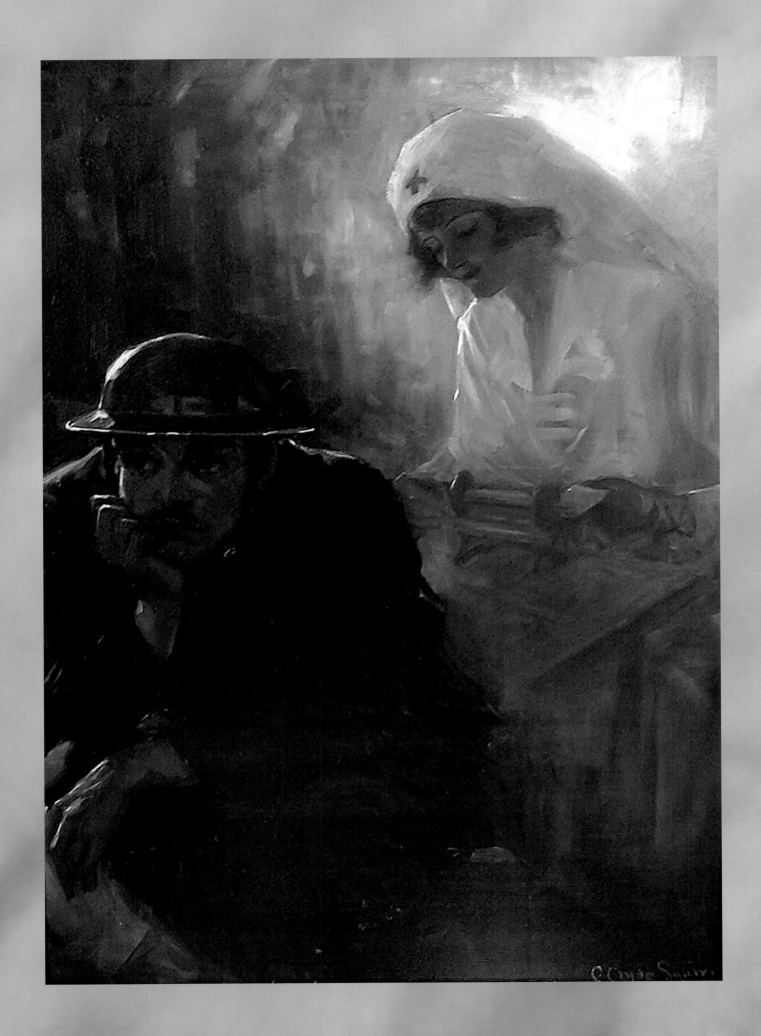

Nurses During War

Man's role in the grim business of war has been fully portrayed in art and literature. The exhausting strain, the danger, the suffering and the brutal death which are his portion, have all been given eloquent expression. . . . But the heroic part taken by women, in the terrible ordeal of war, is only faintly heard and little noted. The mute anguish transcending tears, the infinite sacrifice and the high courage which are theirs, are voiceless amid the full throated cannon's roar, nor do they inscribe a record by fire and sword. . . .

To only a few, among all the world's many gallant women, is reserved the solemn privilege of being a part of the great forces locked in battle, and of being numbered among those elect of earth who, as participants, directly govern the course of history. The nurse, because of her special training and the high calling to which her life is dedicated, brings to the battlefield indispensable attributes which she alone possesses. Voluntarily she comes in response to the utmost need of the men with shattered bodies whose cry is for the compassionate touch of a woman's hand. . . . She endures all of the ordeal borne by womanhood and in addition she shares with man his bitter lot upon the field of battle.

– JULIA O. FLIKKE

A stirring and patriotic World War I era original illustration.

C. Clyde Squires, *War: Meeting the Kind Nurse,* 1915, painting, 17″ × 24″, original use: Cover for *Womans Magazine,* July 4th edition. Photo courtesy of the Grapefruit Moon Gallery.

Nurses During War

	1900	1915	1930	1945
Nursing	**1901** Permanent Nurse Corps established as part of the U.S. Army Medical Department **1908** U.S. Navy Nurse Corps founded as part of the Navy **1910** Florence Nightingale dies **1910** Isabel Hampton Robb dies	**1915** Edith Cavell shot before a German firing squad **1918** Vassar Training Camp established in U.S. **1918** Army School of Nursing founded in U.S **1920** Members of U.S. Army Nurse Corps granted relative rank **1923** Goldmark report issued in U.S.	**1932** Wier Report issued in Canada **1940** Nursing Council for National Defense instituted in U.S. **1942** U.S. Army and Navy nurses taken POW in Philippines **1943** First class of Army flight nurses graduate **1943** United States Cadet Nurse Corps created	**1945** U.S. Army and Navy nurses released from Santo Tomas civilian prison camp **1945** Nurse POWs awarded Bronze Star **1947** Full commission rank established for nurses in U.S. military service **1949** U.S. Air Force Nurse Corps established
Medicine and Health Care	**1906** Term "allergy" introduced to medicine	**1922** Insulin first administered to a diabetic patient	**1930** National Institutes of Health (NIH) founded **1941** Penicillin first used **1941** Pap smear developed **1942** Streptomycin isolated **1942** Mobile Army Surgical Hospital (MASH) units appear	**1949** Philip Hench discovers cortisone
Science and Technology	**1907** Ross Harrison develops tissue culture techniques **1911** Roald Amundsen reaches South Pole	**1915** Henry Ford develops farm tractor **1929** James Doolittle pilots airplanes with instruments	**1930** Pluto discovered **1935** U235 identified **1936** Dr. Alexis Carrel develops artificial heart **1938** Nuclear fission discovered **1941** "Manhattan Project" of intensive atomic research begins	
The Visual Arts	**1908** First glass and steel building erected **1912** Peter Pan statue erected in Kensington Gardens **1913** First Charlie Chaplin films shown	**1919** Bauhaus revolutionizes teaching of painting, sculpture, architecture, and industrial arts in Germany **1928** Mary Cassatt dies	**1931** Empire State Building completed	
Daily Life	**1913** Income tax becomes U.S. law **1913** Foxtrot comes into fashion **1914-1918** World War I	**1917** America enters World War I **1920** League of Nations formed **1920** Nineteenth Amendment grants vote to women in U.S. **1928** Women participate in Olympic Games for the first time **1929** Stock market crashes	**1930** United Airlines begins hiring nurses as flight attendants **1933** Hitler becomes Chancellor of Germany **1937** Hindenburg explodes **1939-1945** World War II **1939** Commercial television introduced **1941** Japan bombs Pearl Harbor	

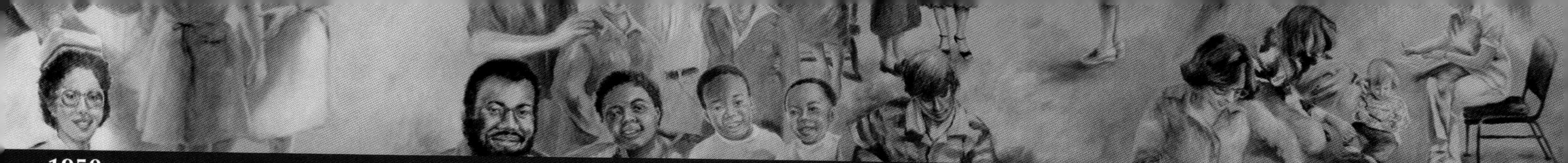

1952 NLNE, NOPHN, and AACSN combine to establish the National League for Nursing (NLN)

1954 Annie Goodrich, internationally known nurse, dies

1955 First men commissioned as nurses in U.S.

1966 Appointment of male nurses to regular Army, Navy, and Air Force Nurse Corps in U.S.

1953 Lung cancer linked with cigarette smoking

1958 Thalidomide linked with birth defects

1960 Artificial kidney introduced

1965 U.S. Congress passes law requiring label on cigarette packages: "Warning: Cigarette smoking may be hazardous to your health."

1953 DNA discovered

1960 First weather lab launched into space

1962 Boeing 727 makes first flight

1950 Matisse begins work on Venice Chapel

1962 Andy Warhol paints *Campbell's Soup Cans,* a key work of the Pop Art movement.

1965 "Op" art becomes the rage

1970 Environmental awareness spawns Earthworks, sculptural projects on the scale of the landscape itself

1982 Vietnam Veterans War Memorial dedicated in Washington, DC

1993 Vietnam Women's Memorial dedicated

1950-1953 Korean War

1951 Transcontinental dial telephone service begins

1952 TV dinners introduced

1961 Berlin Wall erected

1965-1975 Vietnam conflict

1969 Trousers become acceptable attire for women

1989 Berlin Wall dismantled

1991 Persian Gulf War

2003 Iraq War

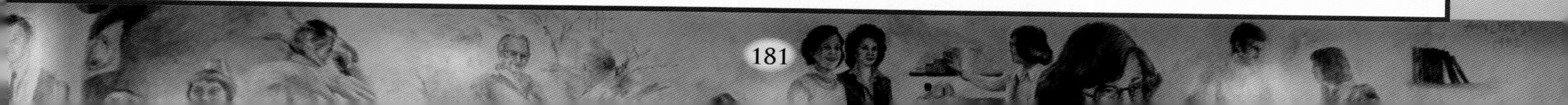

It has often been said that nursing has made its greatest advances and notable achievements in connection with wars. In general, this statement is probably true, particularly when viewed from a historical perspective. One might wonder, however, why this has been the case in that injury and illness have always existed side by side with humanity. It seems that the truth of the statement lies in the fact that nations tend to recognize, respect, and value nurses when faced with the human tragedies of war. The unique circumstances of war and the need for care of the wounded dramatically emphasize the value of nurses. Nurses are thus raised to a position of national stature.

NURSING DURING THE CIVIL WAR (1861-1865)

At the outbreak of the American Civil War, the Union had no army nurse corps, ambulance service, field hospital service, or organized medical corps. There was still no group of trained nurses in the country, but after the first battles, the need for nurses became a clear imperative. Many religious orders volunteered and offered their services, providing nursing care in their own hospitals, in army hospitals, and on the battlefield. Approximately 600 sisters from 12 orders participated during this critical period in history. They were given permission by President Abraham Lincoln to purchase any supplies needed for their work. Lincoln knew that most "good nursing" was being done by these religious sisterhoods, that they had helped in epidemics, were already organized, and were accustomed to discipline and obedience to authority. He therefore supported their efforts to the fullest. There were not, however, enough sisters to care for the large number of sick and wounded. Hundreds of other women and men, with and without experience, simply appeared in the camps and offered their services. They as-

sisted with nursing care in whatever ways they could. The majority were volunteers, although some received compensation. It is estimated that between 2000 and 10,000 women or more were engaged in nursing and hospital administration during the Civil War. (The large range is a result of the variance in citations in reference materials.) The most famous of these were Dorothea Lynde Dix, Clara Barton, Louisa May Alcott, Mary Ann "Mother" Bickerdyke, and Walt Whitman.

The total number of men lost as the result of battle injuries or disease during the American Civil War was 618,000. Of that number, 360,000 men were Union soldiers and 258,000 were Confederates. Many of them died on the battlefield. Those with less serious wounds faced inadequate sanitary conditions and a generally awkward and unorganized medical corps. Septicemia, erysipelas, gangrene, and tetanus were common complications in the wounded. Almost any type of building became a military hospital; base hospitals were located in hotels, churches, warehouses, schools, farmhouses, and other public buildings. In addition, structures were hastily erected or tents were pitched. Even the Capitol was used, with 400 soldiers being nursed in the Senate and House chambers and 300 in the Rotunda. Ward masters and orderlies were available in many of the hospitals to do as much nursing as possible. Women nurses gave medicines, tended to diets, and dressed wounds.

The sick and injured were originally removed from the battlefield in hand-carried litters. Later, a medical transport service was organized, and horse-drawn covered wagons were used as ambulances. These springless wagons often inflicted much pain on the wounded as they bumped for hours over badly kept roads. Hospital trains were furnished by the railroads. Vessels along the eastern seaboard and the Mississippi water route were used to evacuate patients and

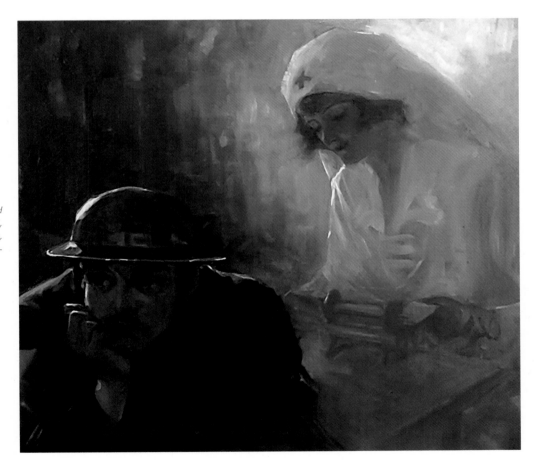

C. Clyde Squires, *War: Meeting the Kind Nurse* (detail), 1915, painting, 17" × 24", original use: Cover for *Womans Magazine*, July 4th edition. Photo courtesy of the Grapefruit Moon Gallery.

as floating hospitals. The first navy hospital ship, the steamer *Red Rover*, was put into service. Captured from the Confederates, this steamer was converted into a floating hospital and then added to the federal fleet of ships. The Catholic Sisters of Mercy volunteered to do the nursing on board and might be considered the first navy nurses.

UNITED STATES SANITARY COMMISSION

Within a month after Lincoln's initial request for soldiers, Elizabeth Blackwell, America's first woman physician, organized the Women's Central Association for Relief in New York City. Louisa Lee Schuyler was elected president.

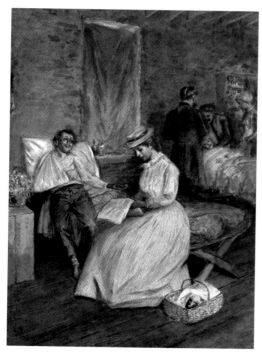

Volunteer nurses in military hospitals during the American Civil War sought tradition and direct involvement in the national struggle. They experienced at first hand the grim happenings of war—amputated limbs, mutilated bodies, disease, and death—and provided invaluable aid to the sick and wounded soldiers and medical authorities on either side.

William Ludwell Sheppard, *In the Hospital: Angels of the Battlefield*, 1861, watercolor, William Ludwell Sheppard. The Museum of the Confederacy, Richmond, VA. Copy photography by Katherine Wetzel.

Through the efforts of this group and similar ones, the Rev. Dr. Henry W. Bellows and four physicians were persuaded to go to Washington to plead for the establishment of a sanitary commission. This commission would act as advisor to the medical department of the army and would investigate the health conditions of the Union army. After both governmental and military opposition was overcome, the United States Sanitary Commission was established by order of President Lincoln on June 3, 1861. Its aim was stated as "a simple desire and resolute determination to secure for the men who have enlisted in this war, that care which it is the duty of the nation to give them" (Boardman, 1915, p. 53). About 5 million dollars in cash and 15 million dollars' worth of supplies were collected. This organization has been called the forerunner of the American Red Cross.

The Women's Central Association for Relief became a branch of the Sanitary Commission. Where branches did not exist, it stimulated the formation of new ones. It coordinated all the relief organizations throughout the country and sent nurses to the areas where they were needed most. Preparatory programs were planned for the nurses at New York Hospital, Bellevue Hospital, and several Boston hospitals. The nurses received 1 month's observation and work experience. The Western Sanitary Commission was distinct from the eastern commission but cooperated with it. It operated hospital steamers on the Ohio and Mississippi Rivers in addition to a hospital train. The Confederacy had no such organization, but a number of women's groups rendered valuable service to the cause of the war.

The Sanitary Commission wished to secure the most healthful conditions in the military camps and hospitals and on transports. It first inspected the army camps in the vicinity of Washington and found them to be lacking in a variety of areas, including sanitation and hygiene, rations, and space. The report revealed that 15% of the Northern regiment physicians were poorly qualified or totally incompetent. Soon after that, the Northern forces suffered defeat at the Battle of Bull Run, and an inquiry showed that the defeat lay in the conditions identified by the commission. In general, the soldiers had entered battle in unfit condition.

M. Fuller, *Red Rover*, circa 1900, sepia drawing, Naval Historical Foundation Washington Navy Yard, Washington, DC.

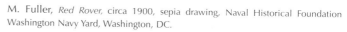

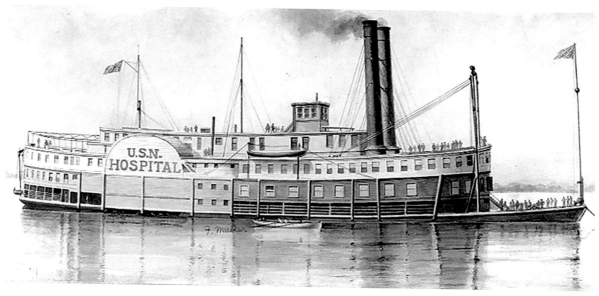

After the first battles of the war, the wounded had practically no care. 'Common soldiers, untrained, lazy, and indifferent or brutal, were cooks and nurses for the war hospitals, the largest of which had 40 beds. There were no medicines, no stores, nor ambulances. The camps were dirty and unsanitary.' When they (the Sanitary Commission) first offered supplies and service, the Government Medical Bureau looked upon the proposal with suspicion; but its dire need soon forced it to accept. The Commission collected and distributed supplies of all sorts, planned camps and attended to their sanitation, tended the wounded on the field and in hospitals; in short, undertook a large share of the health work for the army. It provided such things as green vegetables, given by the farmers for the soldiers, thus preventing scurvy, the great army scourge.

— *Goodnow, 1942, pp. 190-191*

Dorothea Lynde Dix

On June 10, 1861, Dorothea Lynde Dix was appointed Superintendent of the Female Nurses of the Union Army by the Secretary of War, Simon Cameron. This action provided for a corps of volunteer women nurses to be organized under her direction. Dix was given the power to organize hospitals for the care of all wounded and sick soldiers, to appoint nurses, and to oversee and regulate specially donated supplies for distribution to the troops. Dix was past the age of 60 when she received her appointment. She was not granted military rank, nor were the members of her corps. Although she did not have preparation in nursing, she possessed the necessary organizational skills as the result of her previous humanitarian efforts in the area of mental health. Circular No. 7 of the surgeon general's office in the War Department read: "In order to give greater utility to the acts of Miss Dorothy L. Dix as superintendent of women nurses in general hospitals, and to make the employment of such nurses conform more closely to existing laws . . . Miss Dix has been entrusted by the War Department with the duty of selecting women nurses and assigning them to general or permanent military hospitals. Women nurses are not to be employed in such hospitals without her sanction and approval except in case of urgent need. . . . Women wishing employment as nurses must apply to Miss Dix or to her authorised agents. Army regulations allow one nurse to every ten patients (beds)."

Dix's requirements for candidates were specified in Circular No. 8, dated July 24, 1862. No candidate for a nurse position would be considered unless she was between the ages of 35 and 50. Matronly and plain-looking persons of experience, of strong health, of superior education, of good character, and of serious disposition were to have preference. Compensation was stipulated as 40 cents per day and subsistence, along with transportation to and from the place of service. Many women who were unable to meet the requirements ignored them and nursed during the war without official recognition or compensation. At the close of hostilities, the office of the superintendent was abolished, and Dorothea Dix returned to her civilian life of reformative work in public institutions.

Mary A. Livermore (1820-1905) served as a nurse with the United States Sanitary Commission. She believed that the more accomplished and refined a volunteer was, the better nurse she would be. After the Civil War she became a leader in the suffrage movement and advocated for education for women. She would later address the sixth annual convention of the Nurses' Associated Alumnae in 1903 and acknowledge nursing as a new profession, which had arisen in part from the Civil War experiences.

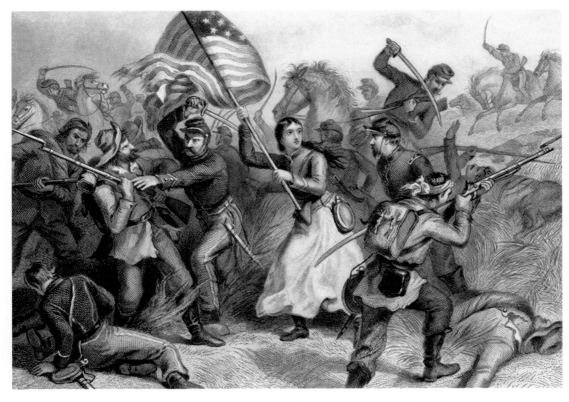

Union army nurse Bridget Diver, known as Michigan Bridget, waves a flag from a raging battlefield during the U.S. Civil War.

Michigan Bridget Keeps the Flag Aloft, January 1, 1863, 9.5" × 14.99". Stock Montage/Getty Images.

Clara Barton

During the Civil War, Clara Barton (1821-1912) became known as the "little lone lady in black silk." Nearly all war nurses were under the supervision of Dorothea Dix; the relief workers were associated with relief or aid societies, the Sanitary Commission, or religious organizations. Clara Barton, however, could not take orders or share authority and relied on her own initiative. She independently operated a large-scale war relief operation in which she arranged for huge quantities of supplies to be furnished to the army and the hospitals. She also personally nursed in federal hospitals, tended to members of the army on the battlefield, and cared for wounded Confederate soldiers. Her impartiality was expressed in the nursing care she extended to both whites and blacks, Northerners and Southerners. She frequently used her own resources to furnish such necessities as medical supplies, proper clothing, food, and bedding. On more than one occasion, bullets made holes in her dress, and the men she was nursing were shot in her arms. Barton eventually became one of the most prominent figures among the lay nurses of the Civil War. Her work embodied the ideals now characteristic of the Red Cross and became the foundation for her later success in the development of the American Red Cross.

Clara Barton (Clarissa Harlowe) was born in North Oxford, Massachusetts. A former New England schoolteacher, she was appointed to a clerkship in the Patent Office in Washington, D.C., in 1854. This may have been the first time a woman held a government position. Barton was, however, dismissed from this position because of her outspoken opinions on slavery. She seemed to have a flair for being the first to arrive on a scene and the first to leave when others appeared. She was already in Washington giving aid to the Sixth Massachusetts Regiment when Dorothea Dix arrived. When peace was finally made, Clara Barton conducted a prolonged search, at her own expense, for eighty thousand missing men of the army. She also delivered three hundred lectures about the battlefields of the Civil War and established the first national cemetery on the Andersonville grounds. Barton was overcome by nervous prostration, a condition that had surfaced earlier, and was directed by physicians to go to Europe, where she remained for 4 years. A month after arriving in Europe, she learned about the International Red Cross.

Clara Barton served with the Red Cross in 1870 during the Franco-Prussian War. On the battlefields and in the ravaged cities of France, she repeated her American Civil War performance. She also observed the systematic organization and remarkable effectiveness of the Red Cross and promised that America would join. She was subsequently decorated with the Iron Cross by the kaiser. After a four-year absence, Barton returned to the United States and began her crusade for the establishment of the American Red Cross. A Red Cross Committee was finally formed in 1881, but it took until 1882 for the U.S. government to ratify the Geneva Convention and give the committee official standing. Clara Barton became its first president and held this office until 1904. Her home in Glen Echo, Maryland, served as the national headquarters. According to the official charter, the Red Cross was dedicated "to continue and carry on a system of national and international relief in time of peace and to apply the same in mitigating the sufferings caused by pestilence, famine, fire, floods, and other national calamities, and to devise and carry measure for preventing the same" (Pitcher, 1907).

Assistance was first given in the United States during a yellow fever epidemic in Florida in 1888 and during the Johnstown, Pennsylvania, flood of 1889. Red Cross nurses thereafter rendered service in numerous disasters that included tornadoes, hurricanes, cyclones, floods, and fires. In 1909 the American Red Cross was reorganized under Jane Delano. At that time plans were made for a Red Cross Nursing Service to be staffed by a reserve corps of graduate nurses with specified qualifications. This pool of nurses acted as a supplement to the regular army and navy nurses, as the occasion warranted.

Volunteer Nurses

A large number of laymen and laywomen volunteered as nurses during the Civil War. Many of them emerged as leaders and greatly influenced nursing during the period. All of them gave devoted service to the soldiers in their time of need, brought hope to the abandoned, and gave faith to those who despaired. They nursed the sick and the wounded and comforted the dying. Most were amateurs, but their efforts had a positive effect on the troops. Robinson highly praised their efforts: "The Civil War is America's greatest tragedy, whose wounds have not healed with the balm of a century, yet it is a tragedy brightened by noble names in the North and in the South. America will lose a precious heritage if ever it permits these names to be forgotten. New ways and new names claim our attention, crowding out the old. From time to time, green leaves should be entwined with the sear laurels of the nurses of the Civil War" (1946, p. 207).

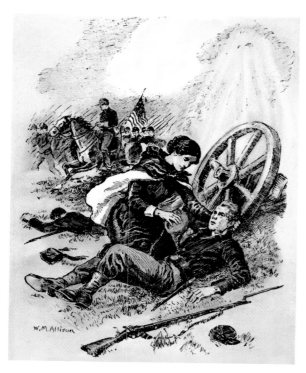

Clara Barton coordinated relief work during all types of natural disasters, including floods, famine, and epidemics. She is remembered for her contributions as a teacher, nurse, social and political reformist, journalist, and humanitarian. Here she is depicted nursing a wounded Union soldier during the Civil War.

Clara Barton, The Granger Collection, NY.

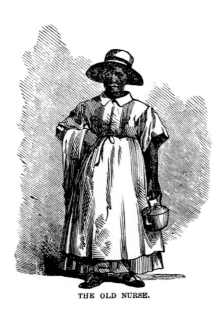

THE OLD NURSE.

HOSPITAL FOR FREEDMEN FOUNDED.

This print appeared in the *Brief* report of the services rendered by the freed people to the United States Army in North Carolina in the spring of 1862 after the battle of Newbern.

Vincent Colyer, *The Old Nurse,* 1864, print, 24 cm, Manuscripts, Archives and Rare Books Division, Schomburg Center for Research in Black Culture, The New York Public Library, Astor, Lenox and Tilden Foundations.

Mother Bickerdyke (Mary Ann Ball, 1817-1901) belonged to this saga of America. Her blanket-shawl, calico dress, and Shaker bonnet were indicative of her pioneer ways, which have passed with that period of American history. She was given the name Mother by the soldiers as an affectionate term that expressed their gratitude. Mother Bickerdyke was a widow from Galesburg, Illinois, who had been moderately educated and had two small sons when she answered the call to help with the war effort. Her minister, Henry Ward Beecher, had issued a plea for some women of his congregation to proceed to government hospitals and battlefields to care for the sick and the wounded. Her experience with wellness and illness included a short course in homeopathy with Dr. Samuel Hahnemann and the degree of doctor of botanic medicine (Baker, 1952).

Mother Bickerdyke served under fire in nineteen battles, from Fort Donelson in Tennessee to Savannah, Georgia. She organized diet kitchens, laundries, and an ambulance service. She supervised the nursing staff and distributed supplies. At night she often walked through the abandoned battlefields, afraid that someone who was still alive would be left. She became known as one of the greatest nurse heroines of the Civil War, and numerous tales were told about her exploits. "Looking from his tent at midnight, an officer observed a faint light flitting hither and thither on the abandoned battlefield, and, after puzzling over it for some time, sent his servant to ascertain the cause. It was Mother Bickerdyke, with a lantern. Stooping down (among the dead) and turning their cold faces towards her, she scrutinized them searchingly; uneasy lest some might be left to die uncared for. She could not rest while she thought any were overlooked who were yet living" (Baker, 1952, p. 11).

Mary Ann Bickerdyke was indeed the soldier's friend. She fought particularly hard for the rights and comforts of the common soldier. General Ulysses S. Grant and General William T. Sherman were among her powerful friends

(Davis, 1886). Her accomplishments were recognized by the government at the launching of the hospital ship, the *SS Mary A. Bickerdyke,* in 1943 at Richmond, California.

Louisa May Alcott (1832-1888) longed for a wider field of activity than that permitted a New England minister's daughter. She was a prominent advocate of women's rights, which at times got in the way of her ambitions. Alcott is best known for her books *Little Women* and *Little Men,* and her poems and short stories were published in *Atlantic Monthly.* This American novelist and writer of children's books served as a nurse at the Union Hospital at Georgetown (Washington, D.C.) for six weeks from 1862 to 1863 (Austin, 1957). This improvised hospital accommodated approximately 300 patients who were in various stages of injury and disease. Alcott was placed in charge of a 40-bed ward, where she performed a variety of functions in her role of nurse. She dressed wounds, read novels to soldiers, wrote letters, made night rounds, and gave medicines. Her daily schedule was hectic, as portrayed in her journal:

Up at six, dress by gaslight, run through my ward and throw up the windows, though the men grumble and shiver. But the air is bad enough to breed a pestilence, and as no notice is taken of our frequent appeals for better ventilation, I must do what I can, . . . for a more perfect pestilence box than this house I never saw—cold, damp, dirty, full of vile odors from wounds, kitchens, washrooms, stables. Till noon I trot, trot, trot, giving out rations, cutting up food for helpless "boys," washing faces, teaching my attendants how beds are made or floors are swept, dressing wounds, dusting tables, sewing bandages, keeping my tray tidy, rushing up and down after pillows, bed linens, sponges, and directions until it seems as if I would joyfully pay down all I possess for fifteen minutes rest. At twelve comes dinner for the patients and afterward there is letter writing for them or reading aloud. Supper at five sets everyone running that can run . . . evening amusements . . . then, for such as need them, the final doses for the night.

— *Alcott, 1863, p. 74.*

Alcott described the work done by the volunteer nurses in Civil War hospitals in letters that were published in 1863

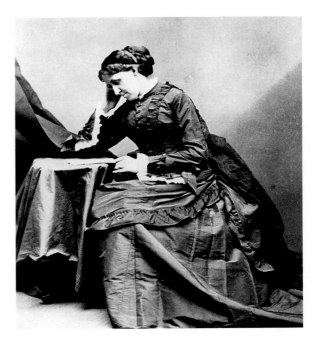

Louisa May Alcott, photograph, The Granger Collection, NY.

in a book titled *Hospital Sketches*, which is considered to be her first famous work. This small book of little more than a hundred pages is narrated by Nurse Tribulation Periwinkle, who vividly and at times humorously recounts the nursing experiences of these volunteers.

Another writer, Walt Whitman (1819-1892), left a record of his experiences while caring for the sick during the Civil War. It was a collection of poems, *Drum-Taps,* and a diary, *Specimen Days and Collect*. They describe his life as a hospital nurse in Washington. Whitman was described by the Danish scholar Frederick Schyberg as a "natural and inevitable product of the tendencies, the struggles, the crises of America in 1860." Accounts of his ministrations to the wounded and his varied responses to the war were dispersed in dozens of notebooks, newspaper dispatches, letters, and other types of published and unpublished works. They were compiled, edited, and then published for the first time in *Walt Whitman's Civil War* in 1960. Whitman carefully recorded each wounded soldier's simple request, noted his patients' names and addresses, wrote letters for soldiers who could not write, and drew a cross by the name of each patient who died. (In January 1995, four notebooks that contained these details and had been missing from the Library of Congress were discovered by Sotheby's auction house in New York while making an evaluation for a client).

Whitman was self-educated and learned the printer's trade in his boyhood. He subsequently worked at various jobs and was the editor of a number of newspapers. In 1862 he left his odd jobs to visit the Civil War front. Upon his return to Washington, he spent the rest of the war period as a volunteer nurse and companion to wounded soldiers. He did this while earning a modest living as a government clerk, a position from which he was fired in 1865 because of official disapproval of the sexual terminology in *Leaves of Grass*. Whitman spent his final years of life (1873-1892) as an invalid in Camden, New Jersey. Of all his Civil War poetry, Whitman's perceptions of the sufferings of the men and his efforts on their behalf are best described in "The Wound-Dresser":

Bearing the bandages, water and sponge,
Straight and swift to my wounded I go,
Where they lie on the ground after the battle brought in,
Where their priceless blood reddens the grass, the ground,
Or to the rows of the hospital tent, or under the roof's hospital,
To the long rows of cots up and down each side I return,
To each and all one after another I draw near, not one do I miss,
An attendant follows holding a tray, he carries a refuse pail,
Soon to be fill'd with clotted rags and blood, emptied, and fill'd again.

I onward go, I stop,
With hinged knees and steady hand to dress wounds,
I am firm with each, the pangs are sharp yet unavoidable,
One turns to me his appealing eyes—poor boy! I never knew you,
Yet I think I could not refuse this moment to die for you, if that would save you.

On, on I go, (open doors of time! open hospital doors!)
The crush'd head I dress, (poor crazed hand tear not the bandage away,)
The neck of the cavalry-man with the bullet through and through I examine,

Hard the breathing rattles, quite glazed already the eye, yet life struggles hard,
(Come sweet death! be persuaded O beautiful death! In mercy come quickly.)

From the stump of the arm, the amputated hand,
I undo the clotted lint, remove the slough,
wash off the matter and blood,
Back on his pillow the soldier bends with
curv'd neck and side falling head,
His eyes are closed, his face is pale, he
dares not look on the bloody stump,
And has not yet look'd on it.

— *Whitman, 1961, pp. 44-45*

Walt Whitman did not approve of respectable women nursing in military hospitals. Although his views were liberal, he did not believe that it was a proper activity for respectable women. Yet many of the women who served as nurses in the Civil War were women from socially prestigious families who possessed strong political beliefs and educational backgrounds. Among them were the Woolsey sisters (Jane Stuart, Georgeanna, Eliza Howland), Margaret Breckinridge, Harriet Foote Hawley, Ella Louise Wolcott, and Louisa Lee Schuyler.

The women of the Confederacy also gave heroic service during the Civil War. Religious sisters and lay women volunteered to function as nurses. They opened their homes to sick and wounded soldiers, and those homes became hospitals and convalescent centers. Some, as in the North, followed their husbands to war and to the battlefield, where they

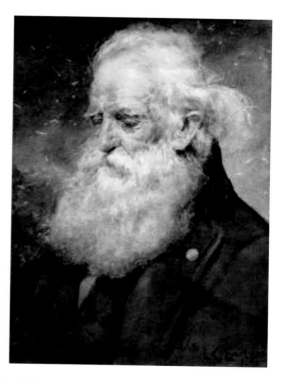

During the Civil War, Walt Whitman worked as a volunteer hospital nurse in Washington, DC, where he penned poetry about the conflict and wrote two of his most famous poems about President Abraham Lincoln, "When Lilacs Last in the Dooryard Bloom'd" and "O Captain! My Captain!" He was a volunteer nurse in the truest sense of the word. He cared for wounded soldiers in various hospitals; he talked to them, read to them, wrote letters, and gave them gifts. A number of his poems reflect his thoughts and feelings during his service in the Civil War.

Lawrence C Earle, *Walt Whitman,* 1898, painting.

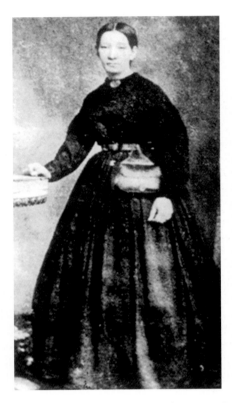

Captain Sally Louisa Tompkins, philanthropist and Civil War nurse, founded a Confederate hospital and was the only woman to receive an officer's commission in the Confederate Army.

Sally Tompkins, photograph, The Granger Collection, NY.

assisted in every way possible. The list includes Kate Cumming, Ella King Newsom, Annie Johns, Betsy Sullivan, and a host of others. However, one individual in particular stands out. The Confederate army did not appoint a director of nursing, but President Jefferson Davis granted the rank of captain to Sally Louisa Tompkins (1833-1916). She was the only woman to hold a commission in the army of the Confederacy.

Miss Tompkins was the daughter of a wealthy Virginian and had been active in the charitable works of her church. She established a private hospital in Richmond and maintained it entirely at her own expense. Tompkins needed the rank in order to requisition supplies, but she refused to accept compensation for her work. The most serious and critical cases were brought to her independent institution because of its reputation, and the mortality rate was low: only 73 of 1333 patients died.

Kate Cumming (1828-1909) chronicled her work as a volunteer nurse in a diary, *Journal of Hospital Life in the Confederate Army of Tennessee from the Battle of Shiloh to the End of the War: With Sketches of Life and Character and Brief Notices of Current Events during That Period* (1866). She described the care and lack of care of the sick and wounded in hospitals and battlefields. She identified numerous problems that occurred relative to food, transportation, clothing, and so forth, as well as diseases that were fatal. Although not prepared for nursing work, she volunteered her services, stating that "I had never been inside of a hospital, and was wholly ignorant of what I should be called upon to do, but I knew that what one woman (Florence Nightingale) had done another could." Her valor and that of other Southern women is revealed in the writings in her journal.

Black women also made significant contributions to Civil War nursing. Some were volunteers; others were employed under the general orders of the War Department at a salary

of 10 dollars per month. Until the past several years, however, a paucity of published works relating to the specific and general contributions of blacks in nursing made it difficult to render a fair and comprehensive portrayal of their work. Several of them competently cared for wounded soldiers in the Union army.

Harriet Tubman (1820-1913) was called the Moses of her people (Bradford, 1961) and is credited with making nineteen trips to the South to assist more than three hundred slaves in their quest for freedom (Miller, 1968). She was an abolitionist who became active with the Underground Railroad movement after her own escape to the North. At the onset of the Civil War, Harriet Tubman turned her energies to the care of those who needed her ministrations. She rendered her services in the Sea Islands off the coast of South Carolina (Hine, 1989). She was a highly respected, fearless, and courageous individual who served the sick and suffering of her own race. According to Bradford (1961), Tubman held the position of nurse, or matron, at the Colored Hospital in Fort Monroe, Virginia.

Sojourner Truth (1797-1881) could be regarded as an early feminist. She was an ardent supporter of the women's movement and actively participated in the cause. She was one of the first women to expose the similarity between the problems of blacks and the problems of women. She, too, competently assisted with the care of wounded soldiers for the Union army as an unpaid volunteer in Washington, D.C. After the Civil War she lectured and published her autobiography. In addition, she helped newly freed slaves to find jobs.

Susie King (1848-1912) was the wife of Sergeant Edward King of the 33rd W.S. Colored Infantry. She was a volunteer nurse during the Civil War for more than 4 years. Susie King was welcomed and respected by both physicians and soldiers and frequently accompanied Clara Barton on her rounds (Elmore, 1976). Her care went beyond the physical aspects; she read letters to the soldiers, offered comfort in whatever ways possible, and even began to teach some of the soldiers to read and write. Her knowledge of the curative properties of various flora served her well when she was treating black soldiers in Camp Saxton, South Carolina (Hine, 1989).

Large numbers of men and women served as nurses in a variety of capacities during the Civil War. They were volunteers, members of the army, persons from religious nursing orders, members of relief societies, or independent individuals who took it upon themselves to assist with the care for the sick and the wounded. These nurses represented all levels of society and constituted much intelligence, diplomacy, daring, and experience. Overall, they demonstrated a courageous spirit. "The ordeal of the Civil War matured America; by that time America had made many contributions of first rank in medicine and surgery, but not a single contribution to nursing. . . . A century elapsed from the date of the Boston Tea Party (1773) to the opening of America's first Nightingale school for nurses (1873), and many believed that, of the two experiments, the latter was the more daring" (Robinson, 1946, pp. 145-146).

Although many individuals devoted themselves to the care of the sick during the Civil War, only a few have been identified in this discussion. They were, however, unusual individuals who had the vision, great courage, perseverance, and compassion that facilitated the initiation of a foundation upon which nursing would be built. There is little doubt that the events of the Civil War forced attention to the need for nurses prepared by adequate educational systems. Yet it would take another 8 years after the war's end for the first formal nursing schools to be established.

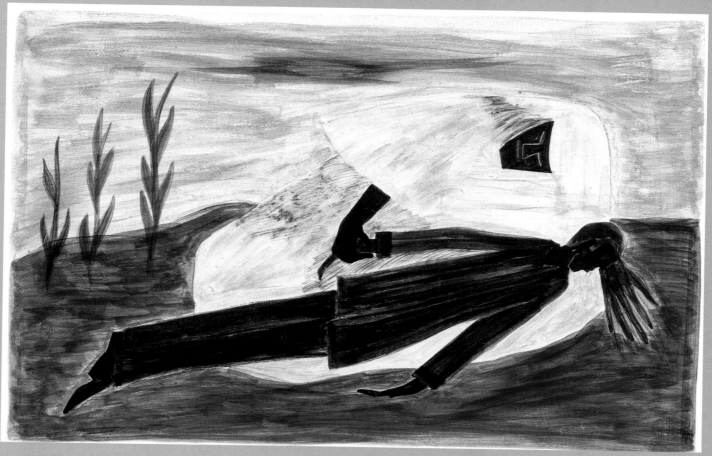

Harriet Tubman was called the "Moses of her people." After her own escape to the North, she became active with the Underground Railroad and assisted more than 300 slaves in their quest for freedom. During the Civil War, she held the position of "nurse" or "matron" at the Colored Hospital in Fort Monroe, Virginia, where she cared for those who needed her ministrations. When the soldiers were dying of some horrible disease, she extracted a healing draught from roots and herbs that grew near the source of the disease, thereby allaying the fever and restoring soldiers to health.

Jacob Lawrence, *The Life of Harriet Tubman*, 1940, painting, 12" × 17⁷⁄₈", Hampton University Museum.

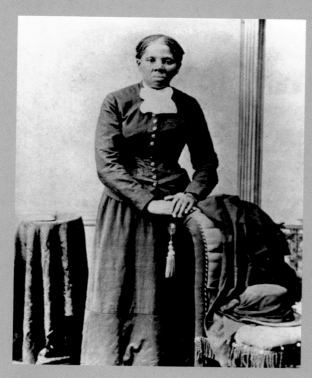

Harriet Tubman, 1911, photograph, Library of Congress.

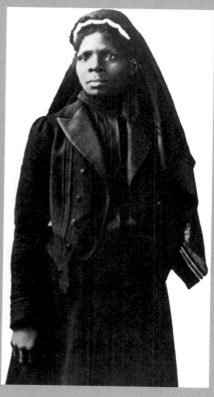

Susie Baker King Taylor, The Granger Collection, NY.

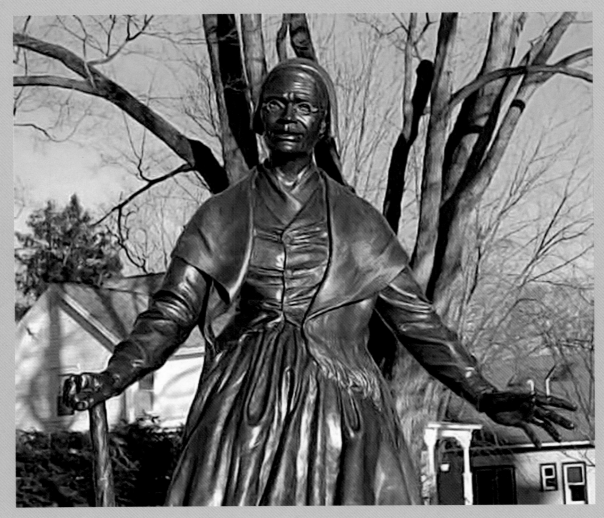

Sojourner Truth, a former slave who lived in Florence, MA, in the mid-1800s, was a nationally known advocate for equality and justice. A group of citizens came together to create a memorial statue and site honoring her life and work.

Thomas Jay Warren, *Sojourner Truth Memorial*, 2002, sculpture, Florence, MA.

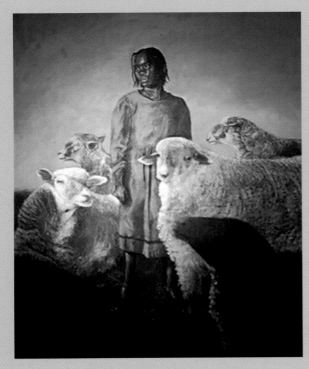

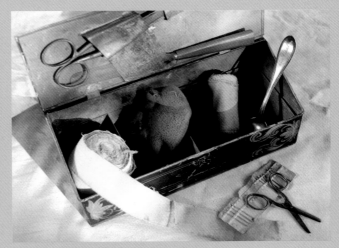

Civil War Nurses Kit, photograph. Courtesy of jupiterimages.

Sojourner Truth was taken away from her family and auctioned off when she was 9 or 10 years old. Because of weak bidding, sheep were thrown in with Sojourner to sweeten the deal.

Ed Wong-Ligda, *Six Sheep*, 1997, painting, 72" × 50", Sojourner Truth Institute, Battle Creek, MI.

NURSING DURING THE SPANISH-AMERICAN WAR

The war with Spain provided many American nurses with their first experience in army nursing. The Spanish-American War also graphically illustrated American deficiencies, such as the lack of a Red Cross nursing service, the need for an army nurse corps, and the lack of emergency reserves. The U.S. Army Medical Department was made up of 983 members, but it had very little prestige. Certainly, the number of members was not adequate to care for the twenty-eight thousand members of the regular army. American battle casualties were small during this war, but hastily constructed army camps were devastated by typhoid fever, malaria, dysentery, and food poisoning. Epidemic diseases caused ten times more deaths than did bullets. Nurses were desperately needed. The Nurses' Associated Alumnae of the United States and Canada (renamed the American Nurses' Association in 1911) offered assistance, but the army rejected it. The primary objection to the organization was that it had been in existence for a relatively short time and was not recognized as the representative body of nurses. Also, the offer had come one day too late. The Daughters of the American Revolution had already volunteered, and Anita Newcomb McGee (1864-1940), their vice-president and a physician with no previous administrative experience, had been placed in charge of the Army Nursing Service. McGee was given the position of acting assistant surgeon in the U.S. Army.

Congress authorized the employment of women nurses on a contract basis, which provided thirty dollars per month plus room and meals. The contract, however, did not provide for personal care if the nurses became ill. McGee preferred graduate nurses with proper endorsements from their schools and suggested that all applicants be examined and cleared through the Daughters of the American Revolution. Nearly 8000 volunteer nurses were placed under contract and, in essence, represented the beginning of the current Army Nursing Corps. Nearly 1600 graduate nurses served; members of Catholic orders also served in large numbers, particularly the Daughters of Charity. The first nurses were appointed in May 1898, and they were stationed in army hospitals in the United States, Puerto Rico, Cuba, Hawaii, and the Philippine Islands. In addition, they served on the hospital ship the *USS Relief*. This ship carried supplies of medicines and dressings and enough equipment to outfit a 750-bed hospital for 6 months. Six women nurses were aboard when it left Tampa harbor.

The army hospitals had been tended by hospital corpsmen who lacked training and experience. These men were recruits who were often the dregs of the units and were totally unqualified to care for the sick. They were guilty of unsanitary practices, such as using the same bucket for food and excrement, which helped spread disease throughout the camps. Consequently, conditions of the worst type met the nurses when they arrived. The nurses often worked day and night with inadequate supplies and shelter. They eventually won respect and recognition, not only from the servicemen but also from the surgeons, who initially had been prejudiced against them. Thirteen nurses died while rendering nursing care during this war.

The army was continually exposed to typhoid and yellow fever during the Spanish-American conflict. A committee

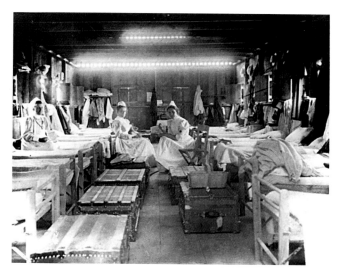

Dormitory C in Sternberg General Hospital, 1898, photograph.

headed by Major Walter Reed investigated and determined that flies and unclean practices were the obvious sources of the illness. Yellow fever had also been particularly virulent and the cause of many fatalities. A team of physicians, including James Carroll, Aristides Agramonte, Jesse W. Lazear, and Major Walter Reed, was sent to Cuba by the U.S. government to find some method of controlling this problem. Reed and Agramonte consulted with Carlos Finlay, a physician in Havana, regarding his theory (which he'd held for 19 years) that yellow fever was caused by a common house mosquito. They then proceeded to conduct experiments requiring that human volunteers be bitten by mosquitoes under controlled conditions so that reactions could be studied. The first volunteers were physicians; some survived, others died. These experiments proved that the mosquito now called *Aedes aegypti* was the yellow fever carrier, and that led the way to the conquest of the disease. The last person to be used for the yellow fever experiment was Clara Maass, a nurse who gave her life. She was remembered by the medical officer in charge of the hospital where her death occurred:

> On many occasions during the Spanish-American War the nurses showed heroism and devotion to duty equal to that of any soldier or sailor in battle. The majority of those with me at Las Animos Hospital, Havana, had not had yellow fever, yet they all unflinchingly nursed the malignant cases of that disease, staying by those who died, to the very last, trying to alleviate the suffering and save life, their clothing, hands, and sometimes their faces smeared with blood and black vomit. One of those Las Animos [sic] nurses, Miss Clara Maass, gave up her young life from a high sense of duty. She thought she would be more useful in Cuba as a nurse after having had yellow fever, and requested to be bitten by infected mosquitos in order to contract the disease and become immune. I tried to dissuade her from the step, telling her that her life was too valuable to be exposed to such great risk. . . . Nevertheless, she insisted, and the fatal mosquitos were applied to her arm. Three or four days later, she developed a malignant, hemorrhagic case of yellow fever, from which she died in about a week.
>
> — *QUOTED IN FRANK, 1953, P. 259*

Clara Louise Maass (1876-1901) graduated in 1895 from the Christina Trefz Training School for Nurses of the Newark

German Hospital, since renamed the Clara Maass Memorial Hospital, in Newark, New Jersey. Maass was one of the first five students to graduate from the 2-year program. She remained on the staff and 3 years later became a head nurse. She volunteered to become a contract nurse with the U.S. Army during the Spanish-American War and served in Florida, Georgia, Cuba, and the Philippines. After her term of service was complete, Maass volunteered in response to Major William C. Gorgas's call for nurses in Havana, where experiments in yellow fever were being conducted. She nursed the victims of this disease through the spring of 1901. On June 4, 1901, she allowed herself to be bitten by a mosquito. She suffered a mild attack of yellow fever, recovered, and was bitten again on August 14. She had seriously doubted that the slight fever had given her immunity to the disease. The second attack proved fatal, and she died 10 days later at the age of 25.

Maass was the only American and the only woman to die during the experiments. After her death the experiments were discontinued, but the disease was ultimately conquered. Maass's body was sent to Fairmount Cemetery in Newark for burial with full military honors. In 1951, a commemorative stamp was issued in her honor by Cuba. In 1976 the United States issued a commemorative stamp in honor of her service to humanity; it was the first U.S. stamp to honor an individual nurse. In addition, a special medal commemorating the 100th anniversary of Clara Maass's birth was struck by the Franklin Mint.

The war experience definitely proved the superiority of the trained nurse over the untrained volunteer and led to the initiation of a permanent nurse corps. Immediately following the war, both the Associated Alumnae, with the backing of influential citizens, and Anita McGee proposed bills that would establish a nursing corps that would have the sanction and permanence of law. These bills were not passed. Finally, in 1900, after a number of surgeons had spoken positively to Congress about the work done by the nurses, the Army Reorganization Bill was presented. It provided a permanent Nurse Corps as part of the Medical Department of the army; the corps would be composed of fully trained nurses (hospital school graduates) under an able director. An amendment stating that the superintendent of the Nurse Corps had to be a hospital school graduate was added before the bill was passed on February 2, 1901. The bill stated that the U.S. Army nurse's salary would be $40 per month for duty in the United States and $50 per month for duty elsewhere. In 1918, the name was changed to the Army Nurse Corps (ANC). Its motto has been "Where go the United States troops, there go the Army Nurses."

Because she was not a nurse, Anita McGee was forced to resign when the Army Nurse Corps was established. She was succeeded by Dita H. Kinney, head nurse of the United States Army Hospital at Fort Baynard, New Mexico. The status of the army nurse has shown slow but consistent improvement. Several events have assisted this process: army nurses were accorded relative rank in 1920; they became eligible for retirement benefits in 1926; in 1947, army nurses became part of the regular army with full commission, pay, and other benefits as granted to male officers. A succession of leaders served in the position of superintendent, including Jane Delano, Isabel McIssac, and Dora Thompson, the first to have served in the military. In 1908 the U.S. Navy Nurse Corps was founded as an integral unit of the Navy.

WARS OF THE 20TH CENTURY

Federal support of nursing and nursing education in the United States has been observed with each of the major wars, particularly World War II. This support has been demonstrated financially as well as by other means. In addition, the military has had a profound influence on nursing, the effects of which are still evident. Nursing, in turn, has affected the military. Its military members have shared a tradition of service; they have played an important role in the care of military personnel and their families, both in times of peace and in times of war. Frequently they have assisted with the development of new techniques and innovations that have benefited medical and nursing care for both soldiers and civilians. (For example, it was Air Force nurses who solved the problem of the placement of food trays for patients on litters.)

War brought a sharpened awareness of the nation's dependence on nurses and the urgent need to prepare them to meet the emergency. The speeding-up of military and industrial defenses mandated adjustments in the number of nurses in schools of nursing and in nursing services. New programs were needed to expedite nursing preparedness, funds were needed for educational expansion, and intensified programs of publicity were necessary to increase the supply of applicants for nursing schools and to recruit nurses for military and other defense services. War placed heavy demands on nurses and nursing to meet the overall crises at home and abroad. Faced with almost insurmountable tasks in times of war, nurses have always risen valiantly to the occasion. Particularly remarkable was the fact that during World War II a higher percentage of nurses volunteered for military service than did any other skilled or professional group, with the possible exception of physicians. Of 274,405 active graduate registered nurses, 75,000 applied for service (Editorial, *The Saturday Evening Post*, 1945). This was one of the outstanding voluntary achievements of this war, and it spoke well for the spirit of nursing. That nurses voluntarily went overseas was acknowledged by hundreds of soldiers:

> To all Army nurses overseas: We men were not given the choice of working in the battlefield or the home front. We cannot take any credit for being here. We are here because we have to be. You are here because you felt you were needed. So, when an injured man opens his eyes to see one of you . . . concerned with his welfare, he can't but be overcome by the very thought that you are doing it because you want to . . . you endure whatever hardships you must to be where you can do us the most good. . . .
>
> — QUOTED IN SHIELDS, EDITOR, 1981, P. 27

WORLD WAR I

A shot fired on June 28, 1914, in Sarajevo, Serbia, killed the archduke of Austria and his wife. This assassination was the precipitating factor of a series of events that ultimately forced the entrance of almost all of Europe and the world into a long and terrible war. A month later, Austria declared war on Serbia, and a chain reaction followed. On August 1, Germany declared war on Russia and then on France; England declared war on Germany, and declarations of war by nations all over the world were rapidly issued and continued

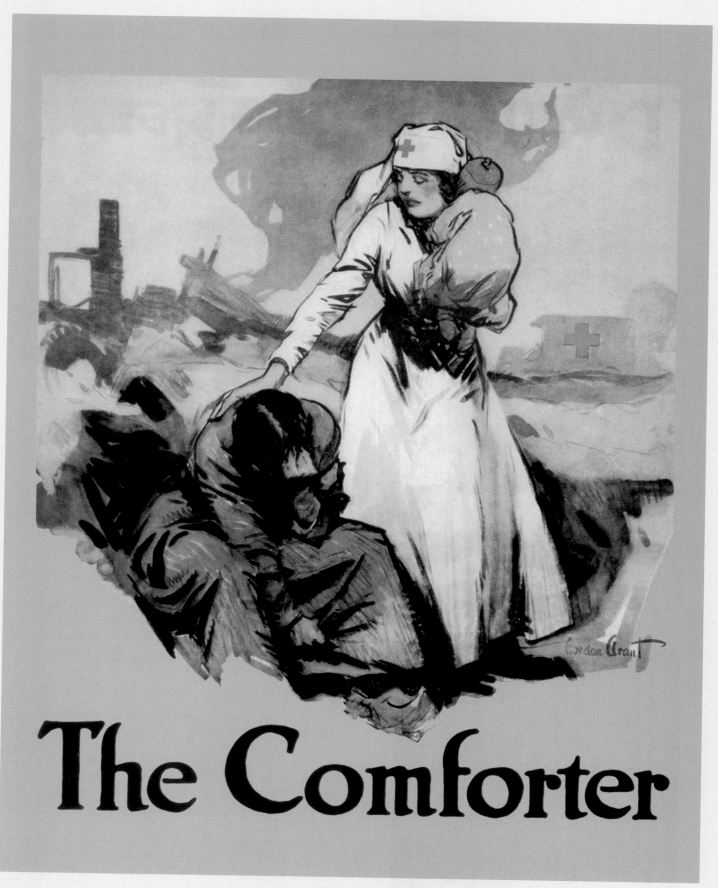

The Comforter

Gordon Grant, *The Comforter*, 1918, poster.

through June 1918. In 1914 no one believed that the war would last longer than a few months, nor was anyone prepared for the cost in human lives or the vast expenditure of resources.

World War I created a large demand for nurses and taxed the medical and nursing resources of the entire world. The warring countries rapidly faced extreme shortages of physicians, nurses, medical supplies, and other resources necessary for adequate health care. At the outbreak of the war the American Red Cross sent units of physicians and nurses to assist in France, England, Germany, Austria, Serbia, and Russia. However, when America finally entered the war in 1917, the American Red Cross Nursing Service became the reserve of the Army and the Navy. Under the able direction of Jane Delano, it served as a procurement and recruitment agency and equipped nurses assigned to overseas duty. Through this agency, approximately 20,000 nurses were assigned to military service. Many of these Red Cross nurses remained in Europe and Asia after the war to assist with the relief programs in the stricken nations.

After a long struggle to maintain neutrality, the United States declared war on Germany on April 6, 1917, and many agencies were caught unprepared. Confusion and conflict arose, particularly in regard to the use of nurses' aides for service abroad. This issue was resolved by government authorities, who mandated that only trained nurses be sent to France with the Army (Stewart and Austin, 1963). As the war progressed, it became apparent that the supply of nurses was insufficient to meet both civilian and military needs. Therefore, it was strongly recommended by prominent medical, hospital, and lay spokespersons that the admission and graduation requirements of schools of nursing be drastically cut and that legal requirements be waived. To counteract these proposals and other problems that might ensue, M. Adelaide Nutting, Annie Goodrich, and Lillian Wald met on June 24, 1917, and formed the National Emergency Committee on Nursing. Jane Delano, chairman of the American Red Cross Nursing Service; Lillian Clayton, president of the National League of Nursing Education; Dora Thompson, superintendent of the Army Nurse Corps; and Dr. Winford H. Smith, president of the American Hospital Association were among the members of the committee. The stated purpose of this committee was to develop "the wisest methods of meeting the present problems connected with the care of the sick and injured in hospitals and homes; the educational problems of nursing; and the extraordinary emergencies as they arise" (U.S. Council of National Defense, 1917, pp. 1-5).

In less than 2 months the National Emergency Committee on Nursing was officially appointed by the federal government and became known as the Committee on Nursing of the General Medical Board of the Council of National Defense. Although office space and secretarial services were provided by the government, funding was obtained through private contributions. One of the most formidable tasks facing the Committee was the need to increase the existent supply of student nurses, and that resulted in a recruiting campaign in which a variety of techniques were used. Publicity in the form of pamphlets, posters, and even motion pictures was created and dispersed. Speeches were given, and newspaper and magazine articles were written and published, all with the intent of enticing young women into service by entering schools of nursing. Typical of such activity was a *Ladies' Home Journal* editorial:

> Have you felt that you could best answer the war's appeal to you by entering the nursing service? Then this is the day of your opportunity, provided you are in earnest and wish to set your patriotic impulses free in the place where they will do the most good.
>
> That place is in a regular nurses' training school, such as is conducted in nearly every hospital in America. Many women, untrained in nursing, have been disappointed to learn that their services were not wanted on the field of battle, nor even in a base hospital.
>
> It is the professional nurse only who has been called and accepted, and more than a thousand of her [sic] are now in active service. More thousands will follow soon. They are the finest of their profession, and they go gladly; but do you realize that each one is leaving behind her important work in civil life, which must now be done by someone else?
>
> We have no right to expect—though we may hope for—a short war. We must put away makeshift methods and think of a year from now, two years, perhaps even three years. The woman who enters training today is the woman who a little later will be prepared to take the place at home of the nurse who has gone, or even to follow her to the Front.
>
> The Red Cross earnestly hopes that many young women, particularly those with the advantages of a good education, will let their desire to be of service take a most practical form and prepare to enter a profession which has been called upon to do so noble a work.
>
> — *TAFT, 1917, P. 5*

The Committee also asked existing nursing schools to do their part by requesting that schools enlarge their facilities, including dormitories and clinical facilities. More instructors were to be acquired to handle increasing student numbers; working hours were to be shortened to attract greater numbers. These methods proved to be successful, and the numbers of students entering nursing schools increased dramatically.

VASSAR TRAINING CAMP

The Committee on Nursing was also interested in attracting women with better educations into nursing. A plan evolved for a 3-month intensive theoretical training program for college graduates who wished to enter nursing schools. The original concept was proposed by Mrs. Minnie Comnock

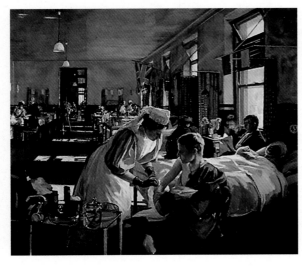

John Lavery, *The First Wounded*, 1914, painting, 176 × 201 cm, The McManus: Dundee's Art Gallery and Museum, Albert Square, Meadowside, Dundee, DD1 1DA. With permission from Felix Rosenstiel's Widow & Son Ltd.

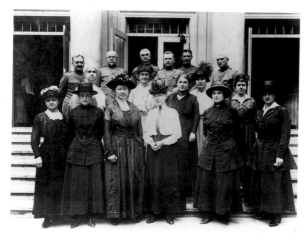

Represented in this photograph are some of the most prominent figures in the history of nursing: S. Lillian Clayton, President, National League of Nursing Education; Anna W. Goodrich, Dean, Army School of Nursing; M. Adelaide Nutting, Chairman, Committee on Nursing, Council of National Defense; Mrs. Lena S. Higbee, Supt., Navy Nurse Corps; and Dora Thompson, Supt., Army Nurse Corps.

National Emergency Committee on Nursing, August 18, 1918, photograph, Milbank Memorial Library, New York, NY.

Blodgett, a trustee of Vassar, who partially financed the project. This program, known as the Vassar Training Camp of 1918, was soon under way at Vassar College under the chairmanship of Isabel M. Stewart. It was in actuality a 3-month preparatory course for college graduates seeking admission to schools of nursing. More than 400 college graduates participated in the program. At the completion of the intensive course, the college graduates entered some 33 affiliated schools of nursing for a period of 2 years and 3 months. The nursing schools had committed themselves to accepting a specified number of these students. The students wore the uniforms of the affiliated schools, so they became known as Vassar's Rainbow Division. Five other universities (Western Reserve University in Cleveland, University of Cincinnati, University of Iowa, University of Colorado, and University of California) offered similar programs. This cooperative effort among universities and schools of nursing provided a higher standard of teaching and the advantages of an institution of higher learning. The far-reaching contributions of the camp were reiterated by Katherine Densford Dreves, a member of this program who became an influential leader in nursing:

> First, the camp brought college recognition to nursing . . . the fact that prestigious Vassar College chose the camp for its major war effort helped (1) to bring nursing out of its hospital cloister into higher education and (2) to challenge colleges increasingly to accept responsibility for nurse preparation. Then, the camp helped immeasurably to interest college women in nursing. The camp brought into nursing the first very large group of well-educated, versatile women, almost half of whom went on to complete the entire nursing course. Also, the camp enlisted national recognition of nursing by the public and of the need for public and private support of nursing.
>
> — DREVES, 1975, P. 2002

THE ARMY SCHOOL OF NURSING

In May 1918 the secretary of war authorized the establishment of the Army School of Nursing (also known as the Army Training School) at Walter Reed Hospital, Washington, D.C., with branches in other military hospitals across the country. The proponents of this school had presented the plan, prepared largely by the school's first dean, Annie W. Goodrich, before the twenty-fourth annual convention of the National League of Nursing Education (NLNE). Goodrich had been appointed chief inspecting nurse of the Army hospitals at home and abroad and was charged with the evaluation of the quality of nursing services in military hospitals. Her unfavorable report was accompanied by the proposal for an Army School of Nursing. Viable arguments for the establishment of the school were presented:

> It would attract a high type of young women who would appreciate the opportunity to acquire a professional education while giving patriotic service; since the service of student nurses was an acceptable method of providing civilian hospitals with nursing service it could be assumed that such service could provide equally satisfactory care for military patients; because affiliations would be required for experience not available in military installations some civilian hospitals could anticipate sharing the service of the Army school students; the graduates of the school, whether they remained in the ANC or not, would constitute an important addition to the nursing resources of the nation.
>
> — ROBERTS, 1954, PP. 138-139

The convention voted its support, and a budget was approved in June 1918. The chief distinction of the Army School of Nursing was that it was a separate educational unit with an independent federally fund budget that was specifically for educational purposes (Stewart, 1943). The course, based on the new *Standard Curriculum for Schools of Nursing* (1917), covered 3 years and gave 9 months' credit to college graduates. No tuition was required; board, lodging, laundry, and required textbooks were provided. The majority of clinical experiences were provided in military hospitals, and clinical experience in pediatrics, obstetrics, gynecology, and public health were obtained through affiliations. Applications were received from thousands of enthusiastic women. The first graduating class (1921) numbered 500 students, probably the largest class of nurses ever graduated at one time. A total of 937 women completed the course before the school officially closed its doors in January 1933.

Annie Warburton Goodrich (1866-1954) was the driving force behind many significant events in nursing. She was described as a crusader, statesman, dean of American nurses, most beloved of American nurses, and militant angel (Christy, 1970). Goodrich was known nationally and internationally for her leadership ability, which facilitated the promotion of nursing to professional status. She received many honors and served as president of the International Council of Nurses (1912-1915); the American Nurses Association (1916-1918); and the Association of Collegiate Schools of Nursing (1934-1936). Goodrich (1932) rendered the most esthetically pleasing and inspiring comments on the interrelationship of thought and action that pervades nursing's history:

> To the nurse, working in the different levels of the social structure, in touch with the fundamentals of human experience, is given a unique opportunity to relate the adventure of thought to the adventure of action—this to the end that the new social order to which we are committed by our forefathers may be realized. To effectively interpret the truly

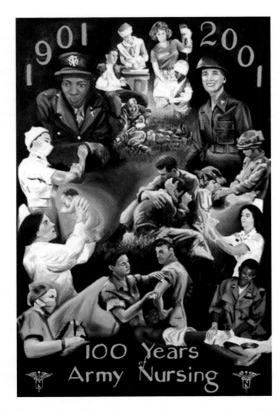

Carl Snyder, *100 Years of Army Nursing*, 1996, watercolor, Office of Medical History. Courtesy of the Office of the Surgeon General, Office of Medical History, United States Army.

> great role that has been assigned her, neither a liberal education nor a high degree of technical skill will suffice. She must also be master of two tongues, the tongue of science and that of the people.
>
> — *Christy, 1970, p. 14*

Annie Goodrich was designated as the third member of a group referred to as "the triumvirate" by Mary M. Roberts. M. Adelaide Nutting was the leader and sat at the tip of the pyramid; she was the educator who originated most of the ideas concerning developments in nursing schools. Lillian D. Wald, who occupied the second point in the triangle, was the practitioner and accepted founder of modern public health nursing. Annie W. Goodrich was the last of the trio, the skillful implementer who combined the ideas and desires of the other two (Christy, 1970). Goodrich worked closely with Wald while the latter was director of the Henry Street Settlement House in New York, and Goodrich simultaneously held the position of professor at Teachers College under Nutting.

Goodrich believed in collegiate nursing education and actively campaigned for that goal to be realized. Her positions as first dean of nursing at Yale University and at the Army School of Nursing epitomized this educational philosophy. "It is desirable that nursing education should find its place in the university, which is another way of saying that it belongs where all educational expressions have been increasingly placed, and for the reason that universal knowledge is here assembled and distributed in accordance with the needs of the students as future builders of the community" (Goodrich, 1932, p. 173). Her philosophy encompassed university preparation not only for teachers and administrators of nursing but also for practicing nurses. Throughout her life, Annie Goodrich fought the battle for educational standards for nursing along with other nursing leaders. Un-

doubtedly, her success at Yale University was the crowning achievement of her life. Her dream of university preparation for *all* nurses, however, has still not been realized. In her eyes, therefore, nursing is not functioning to its fullest capacity: "Our place has been found in the institutions of the sick, but we shall never render our full service to the community until our place is also found in the University" (Proceedings of the Eighteenth Annual Convention of the American Society of Superintendents of Training Schools, 1912, p. 43).

NURSING AT THE FRONT

Conditions of warfare had changed a great deal since the time of the Spanish-American War. Military nursing needed to be revised and modernized to account for such things as submarine warfare, air attacks, shrapnel lacerations and wounds, poison gas, and trench warfare. The nurses' powers of observation and technical skills were challenged by shock, hemorrhage, communicable diseases, infected wounds, and the inhalation of poison gas. World War I was also the first war in which nurses were exposed to the perils of actual battles. Nurses and the troops were constantly threatened by shelling, faced with the deaths of colleagues, forced to tolerate sordid living conditions, and exposed to communicable diseases. "Confronted with overwhelming suffering and awesome responsibility, nurses abandoned their customary obedience to authority and assumed independence in judgment" (Beeber, 1990, p. 39). Perhaps the most crucial aspect of this war was the idea that nurses were faced with the dilemma of caring for soldiers who would return to battle if they were able. How could they justify healing for destructive purposes? Reverence for all life against the violent destructiveness of war was indeed a contradiction. The effect of war upon these nurses' lives transformed their image of themselves in radical and irreversible ways (Donahue, 1995). Films about the war generally depicted nurses as melodramatic, sentimental, and romantically involved. The bravery and courage of the military nurses under dangerous conditions were never addressed (Kalisch and Kalisch, 1987).

Hospitalization was the largest and most difficult of the problems associated with medical care in the American Expeditionary Forces. Great effort and the efficient use of resources were required to care adequately for the numbers of sick and wounded requiring hospitalization. A plan of organization for use during battles that lasted for days had to be developed to care for the stream of sick and wounded. The American Army hospital service was divided into four stages. Advanced dressing stations (first-aid stations) were located at the front lines in somewhat protected areas near the fighting lines. They were usually staffed by physicians and orderlies. There, emergencies were treated and the wounded were prepared for transport to the field hospitals, located a little farther back. (No women nurses served at the front in first-aid stations, and only occasionally did they serve in the field hospitals.) The wounded were then transported to evacuation hospitals (clearing stations) approximately 10 miles back. Those wounded too seriously to travel farther remained here, where complete hospital services were available and care was given by nurses. Eventually, all wounded were sent to base hospitals, usually by the trainload. These hospitals were located safely away from the front.

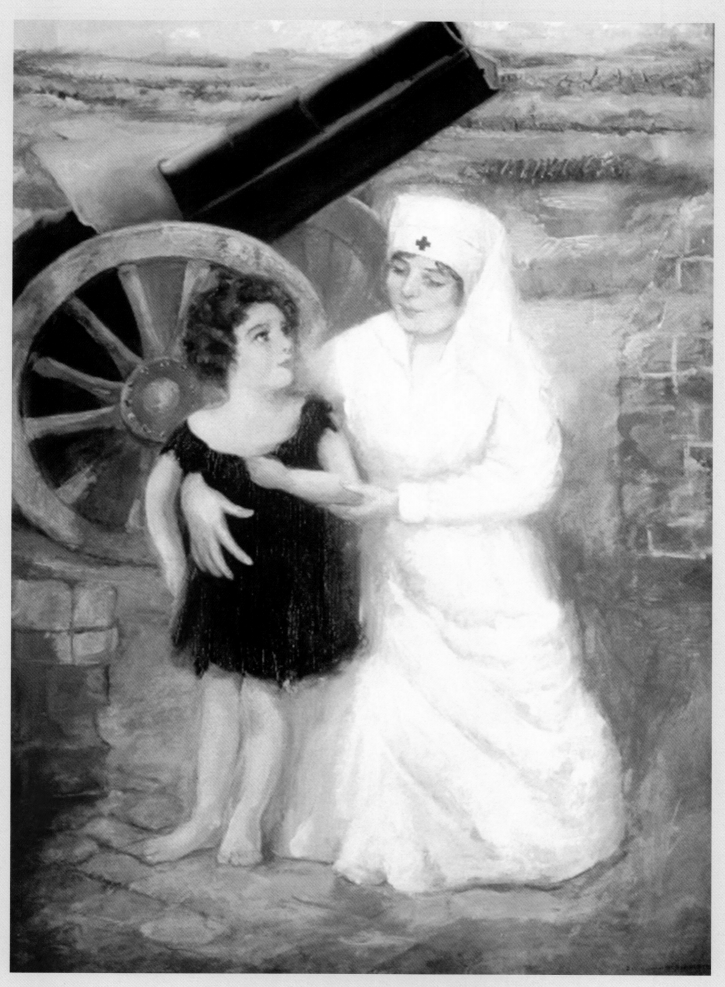

Besse Jeannette Howard, *War Orphan*, 1918, oil on canvas, 127.6 × 91.4 cm, Visual Resources Collections, Department of the History of Art, University of Michigan, Ann Arbor, MI.

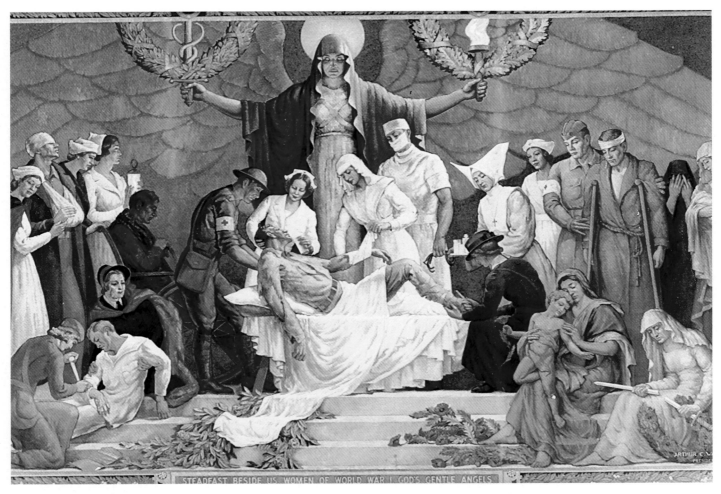

Mural honoring the doctors and nurses who saved lives during World War I. This painting is on the wall of Memory Hall at Liberty Memorial in Kansas City.

Daniel MacMorris, *Women in Service*, 1956, mural, 13' × 30', Liberty Memorial, Kansas City. Courtesy of the National World War I Museum.

The peak strength of the Army and Navy Nurse Corps during World War I was nearly 23,000 (Chow and colleagues, 1978). Of the nurses who served, 296 died in the line of duty; more than two thirds of the deaths were attributable to influenza and pneumonia. Two of three nurses wounded by enemy fire later died of their wounds. None, however, were killed in action.

> The nurses who returned from their baptism of blood, after their familiarity with death, looked deeper into life. But all did not return. Nurses in war service died all over the country, in camps, on the way to camps, in hospital trains, base hospitals, and general hospitals. Several died in line-of-duty on foreign soil. The war-born pandemic of influenza took the lives of many nurses still in military service. A ship that reaches port with White Caps home from war is a thrilling sight, but always there are some who do not come back. In the first World War, many nurses were cited and decorated, but for others the last decoration was the wooden cross of the soldier for those who gave up their lives like soldiers.
> — *ROBINSON, 1946, P. 327*

The Army was the largest single employer of nurses: 21,480 graduate nurses served in Army cantonments and hospitals; more than 10,000 served overseas (Vreeland, 1950). Awards presented to Army nurses included the Distinguished Service Cross (second only to the Medal of Honor, the highest combat decoration) to 3 nurses; the Distinguished Service Medal (highest noncombat decoration) to 23; the French Croix de Guerre to 28 nurses; the British Royal Red Cross to 69; and the British Military Medal to 2 nurses (Shields, 1981). It was World War I that afforded the Navy Nurse Corps the first real opportunity to demonstrate the importance of its role.

Navy nurses numbered 1224 in service in America and 327 who served abroad (Vreeland, 1950). The Navy Cross, the highest Navy decoration, was awarded to four Navy nurses during World War I, but an even greater honor was paid one of the four with the naming of a destroyer, the *USS Higbee* in January 1945. This was the first time a fighting ship had been named after a woman in the service. That woman was Lenah S. Higbee, the second superintendent of the corps from 1911 to 1923. In accordance with the requirements of naval service, the Navy Nurse Corps was reduced after the war. By 1935, with the Government Economy Act, the number in the corps had dropped to 332.

American nurses on active duty faced not only the horrors and dangers of war but other types of conflicts and frustrations as well. They arose primarily because the nurses had no military rank. Army and Navy nurses had not been designated by Congress as officers or enlisted personnel, although they had military status and were subject to military discipline. Consequently, the nurses could not assume the responsibilities of teaching and directing orderlies and corpsmen or of handling administrative problems when they were heads of wards and nursing services. After the war, with the help of legal and other advisers and the support of the Votes for Women Amendment (passed in 1920), nurses appealed to Congress. After a long, slow, and difficult battle, relative rank was granted to members of the Army Nurse Corps by amendment of the National Defense Act of June 4, 1920. At that time nurses were given officer status ranging from second lieutenant through major, but pay and allowances were not the same as they were for men. (In 1942, Navy nurses were accorded relative rank.) In 1944, nurses in both the Army and the Navy were given full military rank for the duration of World War II and 6 months longer. Finally, in 1947, full commissioned rank for nurses in the military services was established permanently. Florence A. Blanchfield became the first woman to be given the permanent commission of colonel in the regular Army. The Army-Navy Nurse Act of 1947 also provided for an Army Nurse Corps section in the Officers' Reserve Corps.

The first men were not commissioned as nurses until 1955—through the Bolton Amendment to the Army-Navy Nurse Act. Since that time, other legislative acts have improved the conditions of military nurses, including Public Law No. 90130, which removed most promotional restrictions on the careers of nurse officers in the Army, Navy, and Air Force. Numerous rank and privilege firsts have occurred in military nursing since then and will continue at a steady pace.

The story of World War I cannot be considered complete without the mention of one famous nurse heroine, Edith Cavell (1865-1915). She was an English nurse who founded a school of nursing in Brussels, Belgium, in 1909 and was its superintendent. Cavell remained at the school at the onset of the war and helped to organize an underground escape route for Allied soldiers. She also faithfully cared for sick Germans. Although she could have escaped and saved herself, she chose to remain at her post. Despite diplomatic efforts to obtain a reprieve for her, Edith Cavell was executed before a German firing squad on October 12, 1915. The charge was harboring British and French soldiers and assisting them with escape from Belgium. Cavell did not deny the charges and faced her death with tremendous courage. It is reported that the following were her last words: "I have no fear or shrinking; I have seen death so often that it is not strange or fearful to me. I thank God for this ten weeks' quiet before the end. Life has always been hurried and full

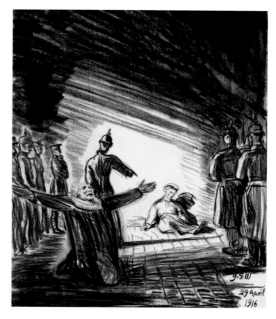

Jens Ferdinand Willumson (1863-1958), *Miss Edith Cavell's Martyrdom*, 1916, etching/engraving, 61.5 × 47 cm, Willumsen Museum. Photo taken by Anders Sune Berg.

of difficulty. This time of rest has been a great mercy. They have all been very kind to me here. But this I would say, standing as I do in view of God and eternity: I realize that patriotism is not enough. I must have no hatred or bitterness towards anyone" (Judson, 1941, p. 281). It should be noted here that some modern historians consider Cavell to have been romanticized and that her death was used by the British as propaganda against the Germans.

WORLD WAR II

The period between World War I and World War II was a time of great unrest because the defeated nations were dissatisfied with their lots. Depression on a worldwide scale led people to accept any type of leadership as long as it might restore them to prosperity. Bolshevism conquered Russia; Benito Mussolini and Fascism assumed control of Italy; Hitler and the National Socialist German Workers' Party (Nazis) steadily became more powerful in Germany; Spain underwent civil revolution; England and France were engaged in internal disagreements. It is no wonder that an era of dictatorship emerged and began to flourish in a number of nations. Major shifts in alignment also were observed as Italy and Japan, formerly in the Allied camp, joined with Germany in the so-called Axis, which opposed the United Nations.

The League of Nations had been established after World War I in an effort to preserve international peace. This organization was to act as a body of arbitration among nations. Members of the league would be committed to arbitrating all matters of dispute, and hostilities would be postponed for 3 months after a decision had been reached. The United States did not join this organization because of a traditional policy of remaining free from foreign entanglements. The league proved its value for a time but then began to weaken because it had no adequate means of enforcing its decisions.

During the late 1930s, as international relations slowly deteriorated, war broke out once again in Europe. From the time of the Treaty of Versailles, which had ended World War I, Germany had been denouncing the Polish Corridor. This

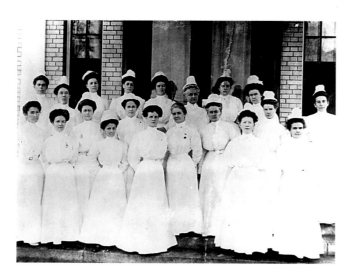

Group photograph of the first 20 Navy nurses, appointed in 1908.

U.S. Naval Historical Center, *The Sacred Twenty*, October 1908, photograph, 740 × 575 pixels, Department of the Navy; Naval Historical Center, 805 Kidder Breese SE, Washington Navy Yard, Washington, DC.

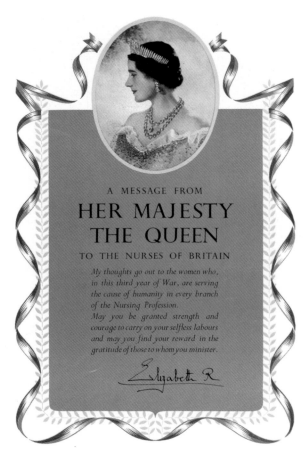

Elizabeth II, *A Message from Her Majesty the Queen to the Nurses of Britain,* 1939-1945, poster, 37 × 25 cm, University of Minnesota Libraries.

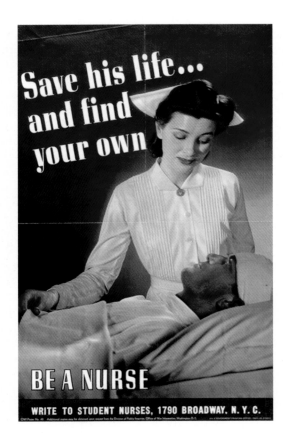

U.S. Office of War Information, *Save His Life . . . and Find Your Own,* 1943, poster, 56 × 36 cm, Minneapolis Public Library. Image courtesy of the University of Minnesota Libraries.

strip of land had been awarded to the newly formed state of Poland, and the German city of Danzig had been placed under the League of Nations. In 1939, Hitler demanded that Danzig be returned to the Reich and that Germany be allowed to build a road across the Polish Corridor. A series of events occurred that terminated in the invasion of Poland by Germany without a formal declaration of war. Two days later, Great Britain and France declared war on Germany. The United States had no desire to become involved in war. However, in 1940, anticipating the possibility that such a step might be unavoidable, it repealed the Neutrality Act of 1935. At this point the United States began to gear up for war. On December 7, 1941, the Japanese bombed Pearl Harbor, Hawaii, in a surprise air raid that ultimately changed the course of world events. On December 8, 1941, the United States declared war on Japan; two days later Germany and Italy retaliated and declared war on the United States. The world was immediately plunged into a terrifying conflict known as the "total war." Nursing and health care services were once again radically affected as every man, woman, and child of the belligerent countries became involved.

When war was again threatening the country in 1940, Isabel Stewart wanted nursing to be prepared, so as to avoid the mistakes and profit from the achievements of World War I. That summer, according to Stella Goostray, she wrote to the president of the National League of Nursing Education and emphasized:

> . . . the need of some official nursing committee or commission to think through the position that nursing should take with respect to national defense and the many adjustments that may be called for within the next few months. . . . I believe we should have such a commission or board that is representative of the nursing profession as a *whole* and that it should be at work *now,* and not wait until Miss Beard calls on us to do something in connection with the American Red Cross. . . . I do not want us to be stampeded into doing things we will be sorry for.
>
> — GOOSTRAY, 1954, P. 304

In July 1940, the Nursing Council for National Defense was instituted at Goostray's suggestion. The council included the six national nursing organizations (ANA, NLNE, National Organization of Public Health Nursing [NOPHN], ACSN, National Association of Colored Graduate Nurses [NACGN], and American Association of Industrial Nurses [AAIN]), the federal nursing services, and representatives from such organizations as the American Hospital Association. Major Julia Stimson of the Army Nurse Corps was chair of the council. With the declaration of war in 1942, the organization's name was changed to the National Nursing Council for War Service, and Stella Goostray became its head. Plans were formulated to promote a national inventory of registered nurses, determine the role of nurses and nursing in the defense program, expand facilities of existing accredited schools of nursing, and supply supplementary nursing services to hospitals and public health agencies.

As more and more graduate nurses withdrew from civilian agencies to enlist in the Army and Navy Nurse Corps, the council tackled the problem of recruiting students for schools of nursing. This work was assigned to the Committee on Education Policies and Resources. Isabel Stewart was appointed chair of this committee, the first one constructed under the egis of the council. The preliminary investigations of the committee indicated that financial aid to assist schools,

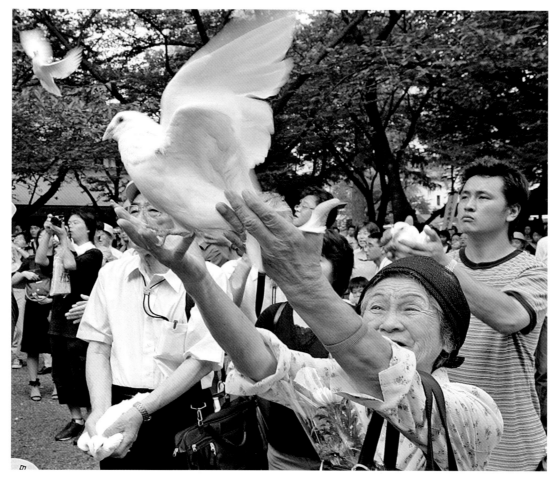

Eighty-six year old former military nurse Masako Ishikawa (front) along with others release doves during the commemoration of the end of World War II at the controversial Yasukuni shrine in Tokyo, August 15, 2005.

Yoshikazu Tsuno, *86-Year-Old Former Military Nurse Masako Ishikawwa Along with Others Release Doves During Commemoration of the End of WWII at the Yasukuni Shrine in Tokyo,* August 15, 2005, photograph, Tokyo, Japan.

to improve the preparation of faculty members, and to assist candidates who could not otherwise afford to enter nursing was a matter of primary importance.

THE UNITED STATES CADET NURSE CORPS

Convinced of the possibility of getting a federal appropriation for nursing education for defense needs, Isabel Stewart began to pursue avenues through which such a goal might be achieved. Commissioner Studebaker of the United States Office of Education was sympathetic to the cause and invited her to Washington to prepare a plan for a request of funds. This she did with the assistance of nine other committee members. The Proposal, as it came to be known, investigated the country's need for professional nursing services in both military and civilian situations, the plans necessary to meet that need, and the cost of such a program. It rapidly became apparent that nursing schools could not be expected to increase their enrollments and to increase instructional and housing facilities without financial assistance. The government had to be persuaded that federal aid for nursing education was a legitimate and imperative defense measure. The committee soon made these findings:

Uncle Sam was spending large sums in training his sons for national defense, but he had provided little or nothing for the preparation of his daughters who were to serve in the national forces. Apart from the experiment with the Army School of Nursing during the first World War, and the sti-

pends to nurses given through the Social Security Act, practically no federal funds had been appropriated for nursing education up to this time. . . . A plan was prepared and, after many vicissitudes, submitted in a lull to Congress. Finally, in June, 1941, with the assistance of friends of nursing education in Congress, a law was passed authorizing the expenditure of $1,200,000 for the current fiscal year to assist in the training of nurses for national defense. The administration of this fund was entrusted to the United States Public Health Service.

— *STEWART, 1943, P. 283*

The first support for nursing education by federal funds specifically appropriated for that purpose thus occurred. The Appropriations Act for 1942 (effective July 1, 1941) was passed with the inclusion of funds for nursing education through the efforts of Frances Payne Bolton, a Congresswoman from Ohio and a friend of nursing. In July 1942 this federal appropriation was increased to 3.5 million dollars. This major feat resulted largely from the leadership of Stewart, who served on the advisory committee for the initial project. The sum that was to be applied to refresher, postgraduate, and basic programs was inadequate for existing needs, but it paved the way for future financial assistance to nursing schools.

Subsequently a Nurse Training Act (Public Law No. 74, Seventy-Eighth Congress) was introduced into Congress in 1943 by Frances Payne Bolton. An appropriation of 60 million dollars was voted at this time to cover the cost of an accelerated

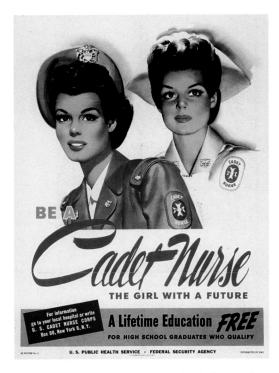

A recruitment poster emphasizing the wartime need and educational opportunities for those interested in nursing. This massive campaign to recruit people into nursing programs offered a free education. The only payback was a pledge to serve where needed for the duration of the war and 6 months after. President Roosevelt had signed the bill that created the Cadet Nurse Corps on June 15, 1943.

Cadet Nurse, 1941-1945, poster, National Archives, Washington, DC.

and expanded program of education for students entering approved schools of nursing, and later the amount was increased. The bill, commonly known as the Bolton Act, created the United States Cadet Nurse Corps. It provided for a 30-month basic program, free tuition and fees, free uniforms, monthly stipends for students in approved basic schools of nursing, and grants for postgraduate work.

The program of the Cadet Nurse Corps was administered by the United States Public Health Service, Division of Nursing Education, which was headed by Lucile Petry. (Petry was appointed Assistant Surgeon General of the United States Public Health Service in 1949. She was the first woman to hold this position.) This program proved to be a major incentive for the improvement of standards in nursing education because schools had to meet requirements developed by the NLNE to obtain the federal monies. Nursing schools were also required to admit all qualified applicants, regardless of race or religion. An intensive publicity and recruiting campaign was launched. The desirability of a student reserve with the benefits of an "attractive uniform," liberal scholarships, and subsistence grants was given wide press coverage. Students who entered pledged themselves to serve where needed (military or civilian agencies) for the duration of the war and 6 months thereafter. The potential overcrowding of available space resulting from the enormous influx of nursing students into this program was assuaged by the passage of the Lanham Act (1941), which provided funds for dormitories, libraries, classrooms, and other physical facilities that were needed.

Quotas based on national nursing needs were established for the Cadet Nurse Corps: 125,000 for the first 2 years, with 65,000 recruited during the first 12 months and 60,000 the following year. Both yearly quotas were exceeded,

and the total number who joined the corps was 179,000. The program was a unique experiment that achieved remarkable success. In addition, from the start the National Nursing Council had ensured the removal of all barriers resulting from various forms of discrimination. Some important racial barriers were therefore removed. The way was paved for the acceptance of black students into a greater number of nursing schools and for the enlistment of black nurses into the Army and Navy. A committee of the council, the Coordinating Committee on Negro Nursing, was set up to assist in the recruitment of well-qualified black students and the provision of better educational opportunities for these students. In 1944, the council also openly campaigned for racial equality in the military nursing services.

NURSING AT THE FRONT

The role of the nurse in war had been almost revolutionized since the time of Florence Nightingale in the Crimean War. By the time of World War II, nurses constituted an integral part of the military structure. Their contributions could no longer be ignored. Wherever American troops were stationed around the world, nurses could be found. They were accustomed to organization, had a working knowledge of war that had been gained through personal experiences, and were prepared to meet the demands of modern warfare. By the end of this war, the romance between the nurse and the American GI and soldiers worldwide would be real, built on mutual admiration and respect. The bravery of the nurses under the most rigorous and demanding situations was witnessed by many soldiers, who wrote of these experiences:

> They were 24 hours with plenty of things dropping all around—planes being shot down. Let me tell you they quickly learned to dig fox holes. I have seen them digging them with a spoon—two things they soon learn to do—wear helmets and dig foxholes. . . . They were pretty hard put for food. They had no water except in their canteens when unloaded. [When I arrived with the equipment] . . . they welcomed the "old man" with food and equipment. They had no tents. Each nurse was given one blanket in half shelter tent, their "B" and "C" ration and a musette bag. They were wearing fatigues and steel helmets. They used the ground for their bed—but they were there ready to go and waiting for us. . . .
> — *QUOTED IN AYNES, 1973, P. 245*

The global scope of World War II presented a sharp challenge to military nurses. By the end of the war, nurses had been stationed on the soil of approximately fifty nations scattered over the face of the globe. They worked and lived in the installations of the Army and the Navy, in hotels and other adapted structures, in cantonment barracks, in tent hospitals, and in Quonset and other prefabricated huts. Speed in rendering care was probably the biggest factor that kept the death rate below that of World War I. "The sulfonamides, the advent of penicillin, DDT, new developments in antimalarial therapy, and the ready availability of blood and blood derivatives, plus the heroism and ingenuity of the medical corpsmen, were among the factors which contributed to that favorable result" (Roberts, 1954, p. 344). Nursing care also contributed to the statistics and made a great difference in the recovery of sick and wounded soldiers.

The peak strength of the Army and Navy Nurse Corps was nearly 69,000 during World War II. These nurses gave care in front-line situations, field hospitals, evacuation hospitals,

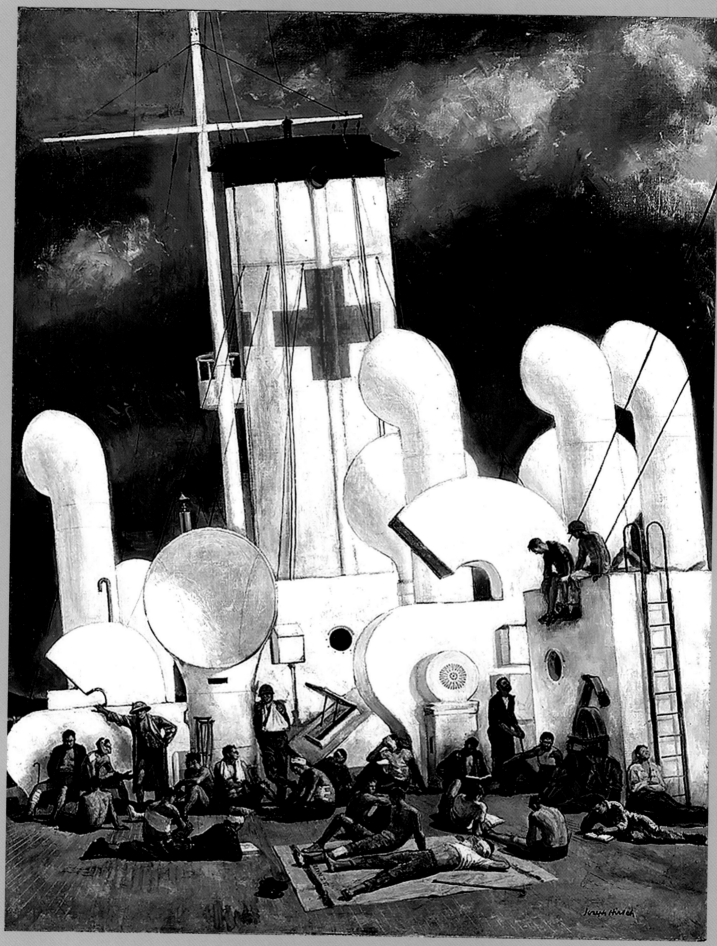

The Navy's hospital ships operate under the laws laid down by the Geneva Convention, being unarmed, fully illuminated at night, and painted white.

Joseph Hirsch, *Mercy Ship*, 1943, oil on canvas, 42" × 32", Navy Art Collection, Naval History and Heritage Command, Washington, DC.

base hospitals, hospital ships and trains, and in the air. Army nurses served at nine stations and 52 areas. Navy nurses served on 12 hospital ships and in more than 300 naval stations. Both served wherever the American soldier could be found. More than 1600 nurses were decorated for meritorious service and bravery under fire. They received honors that included the Distinguished Service Medal, Silver Star, Distinguished Flying Cross, Soldier's Medal, Bronze Star Medal, Air Medal, Legion of Merit, Army Commendation Medal, Purple Heart, and Gold Star. A total of 201 nurses died; 16 of these deaths were the result of enemy action. Throughout the war, nurses in both the Army and the Navy were held as prisoners by the Japanese in the Philippines at Santo Tomas civilian prison camp near Manila. They continued to give nursing care under terrific hardships until their release in 1945. Eleven Navy nurses were interned for a period of 37 months.

A new field of military nursing opened in World War II—flight nursing. Both the Army and the Navy instituted flight nurse programs for assistance with the extended use of air transport for the evacuation of wounded soldiers. Established through the Air Surgeon's Office in September 1942, this program prepared qualified nurses to convert transport planes (C-45 Commandos, C-47 Skytrains, and C-54 Skymasters) into flying ambulances rapidly. These transports had dual functions; they were used to transport cargo and troops to battle and then became ambulances for the return trip. They were not protected from enemy fighters because they were not marked with the Geneva Red Cross as noncombatants (Kalisch and Scobey, 1983). Flight nurses performed under great pressures and were instrumental in providing effective nursing care in frequently dangerous circumstances. The nurses were specially trained to give nursing care to the wounded on stretchers piled three tiers deep on either side of a cargo plane that had been converted into a rough ambulance. They were also taught to perform duties related to ground medical installations.

Admittance to the program began with application for commission in the Army Nurse Corps. That was followed by a

minimum of 6 months in the Army Air Force unit hospital. Application could then be made for admittance to the flight nursing school. Even after completion of these requirements, automatic designation of flight nurse was not granted. The nurse was then required to submit a request to the commanding general of the Army Air Forces for the designation. The first class of Army Nurse Corps flight nurses was graduated from the School of Air Evacuation at Bowman Field, Kentucky, on February 18, 1943. Many nurses desired entrance into the program because flight nurses represented the elite of the corps.

The final newcomer in the federal nursing services was the Air Force Nurse Corps, established within the Air Force Medical Service in July 1949. An Army Air Force regulation was published on June 8, 1949, that provided for the separation of certain Air Force activities that were formerly the responsibility of the Army Medical Department (Vreeland, 1950). The purpose of this enforcement was twofold: the complete separation of Army and Air Force medical activities and the establishment of the Air Force Nurse Corps. Procedures were developed whereby nurses in the Army who were on duty with the Air Force and nurses who were stationed at Army installations could request to be transferred to the Air Force Nurse Corps. Of Army nurses on active duty, 1199 transferred from the Army to the Air Force, becoming the nucleus for the Air Force Nurse Corps. A year later the corps prepared to assist with the air evacuation of battle casualties from Korea. This was to be a vital key to the survival of soldiers wounded in the Korean War.

THE NURSE DRAFT BILL

The large number of graduate nurses engaged in military service was still not enough, and voluntary enlistments were not meeting anticipated needs. During what were to become the closing months of World War II, steps began to be taken to draft nurses into military service. An article by the well-known columnist Walter Lippmann, which appeared on December 19, 1944, included a charge of gross neglect against the Army. Lippmann contended that the Army had not provided adequate numbers of nurses to care for wounded soldiers:

> The last thing our people will put up with is that sick and wounded American soldiers should suffer because the Army cannot find enough women to nurse them. Yet, I am reporting only the stark truth, which is well known to the Army and to the leaders of the medical profession, when I say that in military hospitals at home and abroad our men are not receiving the nursing care they must have, and that with casualties increasing in number and in seriousness, this will mean for many of the men brought in from the battlefields that their recovery is delayed, and even jeopardized.
> — LIPPMANN, 1944

It was not long before President Roosevelt, in his State of the Union message on January 6, 1945, came forth with an unprecedented request for a draft of women nurses. The ANA went on record as approving such a move provided that the Selective Service legislation include *all women*. The Nurse Draft Bill quickly passed the House of Representatives but became bogged down in the Senate. The threat of the draft initiated an overwhelming mass of applications from nurses for war service, and the result was an excess of nurses in the military. The conclusion of the war on the European front made the draft bill virtually unnecessary, and it was quietly withdrawn in May 1945.

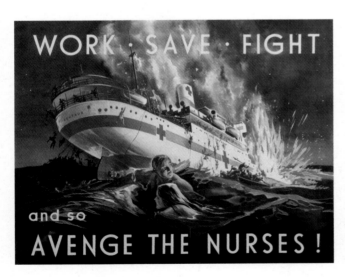

The hospital ship Centaur is being attacked by the Japanese off the coast of Queensland during World War II. In the water below the ship are a number of nurses and sailors from the ship. Approximately 286 lives were lost, including 11 out of the 12 nurses. The poster depicts moments after the ship was torpedoed; it later sank.

Centaur, 1943-1945, photolithograph, coloured inks on paper, 50.2 × 63 cm, Australian War Memorial.

THE KOREAN WAR

The Korean War broke out on June 25, 1950, and thrust nurses once again into service in combat areas. The nurses of the armed forces—Army, Navy, and Air Force Nurse Corps— were called upon as a result of the invasion of South Korea. Although this action was not officially designated as a war, the realities of casualties were nonetheless harsh. The United States was essentially forced to play a role in a situation created by the conflicting ideologies of the freedom-loving Western world and communism. Fears of an acute nursing shortage prompted the Joint Committee on Nursing in National Security, along with representatives of the six national nursing organizations, to recommend the following:

That all possible means be developed for recruiting more students for schools of nursing.

That as many practical nurses be trained and employed to help professional nurses as hospitals and other community agencies could utilize to good advantage.

That nurses be withdrawn systematically from the civilian services for military duty according to a plan that ensured their employment at the highest level of skill for which they were prepared.

That state and local advisory boards of nurses be organized and be given the authority by the government to review assignment of nurses to the armed forces and to civilian agencies.

That, if there was total mobilization, nurses be redistributed within the fields of nursing and within community agencies so that the most essential civilian needs would be taken care of first.

That major effort be directed to improving sound basic nursing education and to increase enrollment in schools of nursing that offered effective programs.

That selected nurses be encouraged to prepare for responsibilities as teachers, supervisors, and administrators, as well as for the special fields, in order to safeguard essential nursing service. That administration of nursing services be improved so that nursing skills would be used to the best advantage and their full value would reach more people.

That nursing service be stabilized as much as possible and turnover of staff held to a minimum through the adoption and application of sound personnel policies for nurses and allied workers.

— *JOINT COMMITTEE ON NURSING IN NATIONAL SECURITY, 1951, PP. 78-79*

During World War II the Army had experimented with and demonstrated the need for a new type of hospital that would be located as close to the front as was relatively safe, about 8 to 20 miles. This new unit first appeared in late November 1942 and was tried out under actual combat conditions in Korea. The Mobile Army Surgical Hospital (MASH) could be moved at a moment's notice. It was basically a 60-bed unit with the flexibility to expand five or six times beyond its standard bed capacity. Within a few hours several hundred patients could be admitted and treated. The hospital was usually staffed by 10 physicians, 12 nurses (2 were anesthetists), and 90 corpsmen. It could be set up in any type of location that was available—a barn, church, or schoolhouse, or in the tents that were carried with it (*American Journal of Nursing,* 1951, p. 387). An Army helicopter detachment was attached to each MASH unit to provide care as close to the front as possible and to provide for immediate evacuation for the critically ill.

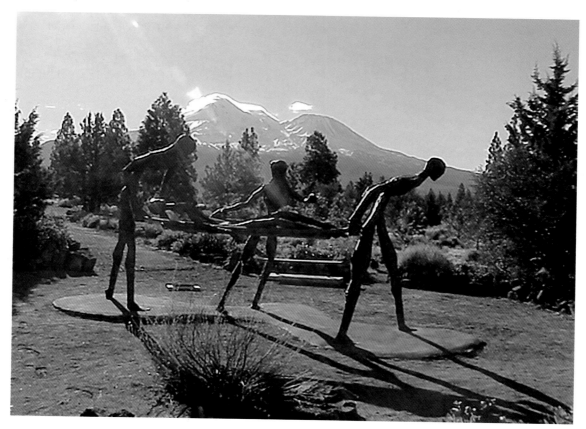

MASH unit nurses carry the wounded. The gardens are located just north of Weed, California.

Dennis Smith, *The Nurses,* circa 1986, sculpture, The Living Memorial Sculpture Garden, Weed, CA.

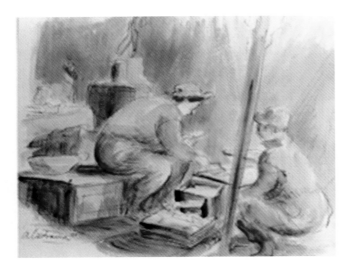

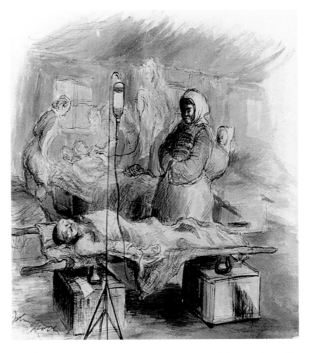

John Groth, *Nurses in Tent,* painting. Courtesy of the U.S. Army Center of Military History.

John Groth, *Nurse Giving Plasma,* painting. Courtesy of the U.S. Army Center of Military History.

The MASH unit became the first hospital to which the wounded were sent and was a great factor in maintaining morale. "The proximity of the unit to the front, its trained personnel, its adequate supply of whole blood, and its rapid helicopter and ambulance evacuation services all contributed greatly to the reduction of mortality rates in Korea as compared with those during World War II: the mortality rate among wounded soldiers who reached hospitals in Korea was half the corresponding rate during World War II" (Kalisch and Kalisch, 1978, p. 543). A pattern of action was followed as patients were admitted: pulse rates and blood pressures were taken and recorded on tags attached to each litter; infusion of whole blood was started; penicillin was given to everyone with an open wound; clothing was cut away and wounds exposed; critical cases were identified; and patients were sorted on the basis of treatment. Those designated as seriously wounded were transported either to southern Korea or to medical centers in Japan. The majority of cases involved chest, abdominal, or extremity injuries.

The fledging Air Force Nurse Corps faced its first major test during this war. The members' primary responsibility was the care of patients airlifted during the Korean conflict. The volume of patients was staggering. As many as 3925 patients were aeromedically evacuated on one day, December 5, 1950 (Chow and colleagues, 1978). The corps had mobilized its resources and accelerated training programs. By the end of the war, more than 350,000 patients had been evacuated by propeller-driven cargo aircraft. Rapid air evacuation in the Korean War served to virtually eliminate the hospital ship as the means of transporting the wounded. Although three hospital ships—*Consolation, Repose,* and *Haven*—were present in Korean waters during the conflict, they were used as floating hospitals; they transported patients only when en route to Japan for renovation. It had been proven that air transportation was the cheapest and most efficient method for transport of the wounded.

Throughout the ground fighting and during the prolonged peace negotiations that lasted for 2 years, until July 27, 1953, nurses served throughout the Korean peninsula. Fewer nurses served in Korea than in previous wars, but they had once again made tremendous contributions to advances in the delivery of care to the wounded.

THE VIETNAM WAR

The Vietnam War became the longest conflict in which American troops were committed in the history of the United States. It was a war like no other, and it evoked conflict and controversy at home. It was an extremely unpopular war; thousands of people marched in protest and hundreds were arrested trying to storm the Pentagon. Student unrest erupted on campuses across the country as the war dragged on and American casualties escalated. The futility of American intervention was felt, and it resulted in problems never before experienced by veterans of other wars. "There was widespread resistance to fighting, extensive drug usage, and racial conflict among American troops. Profound guilt, feelings of stasis, impotence, psychic numbness, and a deeply embedded antiestablishment anger were common" (Kalisch and Kalisch, 1978, pp. 634-635). Deep, lasting wounds occurred that were not always caused by enemy action. An appropriate name for this conflict could well be "the forgotten war" because there is a silence, and at times a mystique, that still pervades discussions of that war. This is consistent with published accounts in the nursing literature, which have increased but yet are fewer in number than those of either World War I or World War II.

Certainly the Vietnam War was a different war for a variety of reasons. Television sent images of the war to homes across the United States and the world, but reality was difficult to ascertain. Conscientious objectors fled to Canada, went underground, or were jailed. Minorities were drafted in disproportionate numbers. Many of their white counterparts, on the other hand, received either college or medical deferments or left the country in protest. Military minorities also bore the brunt of combat because they served primarily in the infantry, and they reported race and class oppression in concert with the horrors of battle. Even though it was not labeled as such, *it was a war*, and more than 58,000 Americans were killed, including 8 female and 2 male nurses who died of illness or injury sustained in Vietnam (Fischer, 1990;

Freedman and Rhoads, 1987; Lippard, 1990; Spelts, 1986; Walsh and Aulich, 1989). The Vietnam War was also a war of contrasts.

America's interest in Southeast Asia began in 1950. At that time, President Truman sent a 35-man military advisory team to assist the French in their fight against the North Vietnamese. In 1954, the French garrison at Dien Bien Phu fell to communist forces; this was followed by a subsequent agreement between France and North Vietnam to partition Vietnam. The agreement was, however, contingent on free reunification elections. South Vietnam believed that free elections were impossible in North Vietnam and refused to prepare for them. Other events occurred, including President Eisenhower's offer of economic aid and training for the South Vietnamese army. By 1960, North Vietnam had formed the National Liberation Front (Viet Cong) of South Vietnam. The number of American "military advisers" steadily grew in proportion to the increased terrorism in South Vietnam. The involvement of American military nurses did not begin until March 1962.

The first contingent to arrive in the Republic of Vietnam was a group of 13 Army nurses assigned to the Eighth Field Hospital, Nha Trang. Navy Nurse Corps officers were assigned to the Station Hospital, Headquarters Support Activity, in Saigon. By February 1966, 300 military nurses of the Army, Navy, and Air Force were serving. More than 200 were members of the Army; 37 (not including flight nurses assigned aboard medical air evacuation aircraft) were Air Force; and 39 were Navy, including the 29 serving aboard the hospital ship *Repose*. This ship was later joined by the *Sanctuary*. Both were equipped to give optimal medical and nursing care to the wounded. Between March 1962 and March 1973 more than 5000 nurses served in Vietnam (Shields, 1981). As with the Civil War, there are discrepancies in the reported numbers of women and nurses who served in Vietnam. There does not seem to be an accurate count. For example, the Department of Defense states that about 7500 American women served on active military duty in Vietnam; the Veterans' Administration indicates more than 11,000 (Hardaway, 1988; Norman, 1990; VVA, 1985).

The Vietnam nurses were not, however, prepared for the kinds of injuries they saw. The American napalm, white phosphorus, and antipersonnel bombs and small arms used by both sides inflicted massive, multiple injuries. Traumatic amputations, enormous blast wounds, and flesh burned down to the bone were common occurrences. The war was also a dirty war in which traumatic injuries were filled with dirt and debris. "Wounded men in an alien world thousands of miles from home were astonished and reassured at the sight of an American woman so close to the battlefield sharing this grotesque experience. The men seemed to gain a sense of security and comfort from the women's presence, a sense of a more normal way of life, a reminder of home" (Holm and Wells, 1993, p. 46). As in other wars, the presence of female nurses lent reassurance, comfort, and emotional support to a devastating experience.

Nurse casualties also occurred in Vietnam. The only nurse and only woman, however, to die as a result of hostile fire was First Lieutenant Sharon A. Lane of Canton, Ohio. Lieutenant Lane died of shrapnel wounds she received during an enemy rocket attack on June 8, 1969, while on duty at the 312th Evacuation Hospital, Chu Lai. Her memory and spirit will live along with those of the thousands of men killed in action in Vietnam and elsewhere.

The appointment of male nurses to the regular forces of the Army, Navy, and Air Force Nurse Corps was made possible by a congressional bill in 1966. Frances P. Bolton, representative from Ohio, had initially introduced the bill in 1961

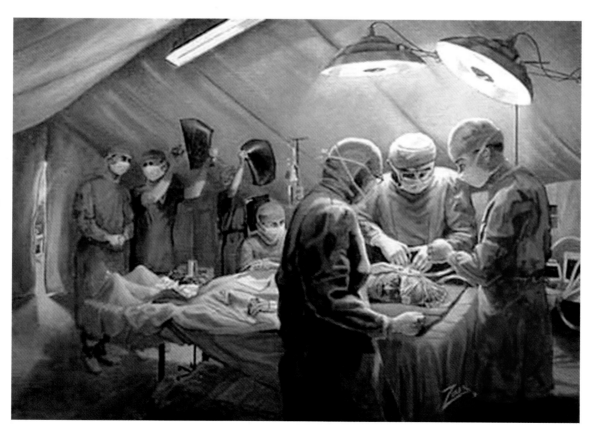

Edward Fenwick Zuber, *Gulf War—0500 Al Qaysumah,* painting. Canadian War Museum, Ontario, Canada. Image courtesy of Edward Zuber.

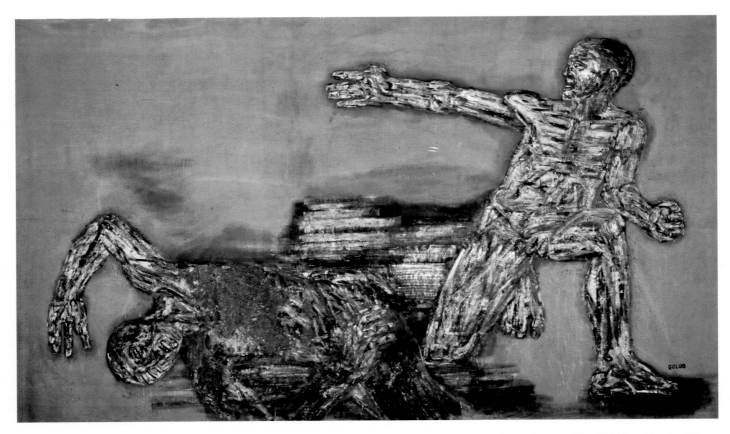

Leon Golub, *Napalm I,* 1969, acrylic on linen, 10' × 16', copyright Estate of Leon Golub/licensed by VAGA, New York, NY. Courtesy of Ronald Feldman Fine Arts Gallery.

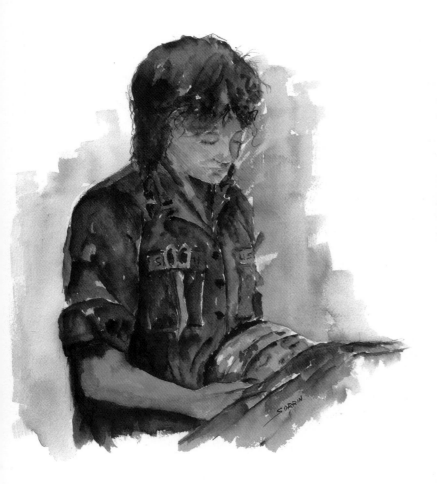

M'Lou Sorrin, *The Nurse,* watercolor, 12½" × 10", National Vietnam Veteran's Museum—Chicago, Hurley, NY.

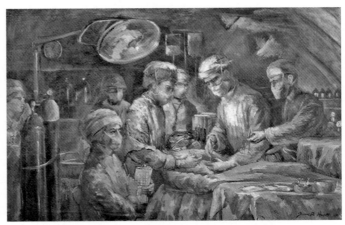

A portrait of doctors, nurses, and technicians in the operating room at the 25th Division Base Camp, Cu Chi.

12th Evac Cu Chi, RVN, 2004, painting, Army Medical corps Museum Fort Sam Houston, TX.

and resubmitted it in 1963. She again introduced legislation in January 1965, and it was followed by an identical bill submitted by Samuel S. Stratton, representative from New York, in May 1965. As a result, the number of male nurses in the services steadily rose. At one point all-male nursing units were established. They were dissolved as the presence of the female nurse was again recognized as an important morale booster.

No front lines in the traditional sense existed in Vietnam, nor were there secure road networks in combat areas. Therefore, the hospitals could not follow and support tactical operations, and ground evacuation was next to impossible. All hospitals became fixed installations, and helicopters became the primary means of evacuation. Inflatable rubber shelters known as Medical Unit, Self-contained, Transportable (MUST) hospitals became operational in Vietnam. They, too, were fixed but could have been moved under proper conditions. These semipermanent structures were equipped with integral electrical power, air conditioning, heating, hot and cold water, and waste disposal. Sophisticated medical equipment and facilities combined with quality nursing resulted in the best care ever available to those in combat.

A massive exodus of Vietnamese refugees took place at the end of the Vietnam War in April 1975. Military nurses worked diligently to provide nursing care to these homeless people in refugee camps and during air evacuation to the United States. They also contributed to the teaching of Vietnamese nurses and physicians while aiding in the health care of Vietnamese villagers.

AT WAR IN THE PERSIAN GULF

The Gulf War was in actuality the Second Gulf War. The original, or First Gulf War, was the conflict between Iran and Iraq that took place between September 1980 and August 1988. The Second Gulf War occurred between Iraq and the U.S.-led coalition and was precipitated by Iraq's invasion and occupation of Kuwait (Hiro, 1992). The genesis of this war can be traced to the history of the Middle East, but the more immediate cause was Iraq's need to increase the price of oil on the world market so as to meet its foreign debt. Saddam Hussein was deeply in debt as a result of his drive to create the most powerful armed forces in the Middle East and his 8-year war with Iran. According to his point of view, the Organization of Petroleum Exporting Countries (OPEC) was bowing to Western pressures to keep oil prices low. Oil sales were almost Iraq's entire source of funds, so Hussein had to do something to increase prices. He was also convinced that Kuwait was illegally pumping more than its share of oil from the Rumalia oil field, which stretches across the Iraq-Kuwait border, thereby keeping some of Iraq's income. In addition, Hussein did not accept the existing boundary between Iraq and Kuwait as binding because it had been imposed by old colonial powers. "In sum, seizing Kuwait would restore to Iraq what was rightfully its own—including whatever assets Kuwait possessed, such as the gold in its banks—and simultaneously enable Iraq to eliminate a $4 billion debt owed to Kuwait" (Blair, 1992, p. 11).

On August 2, 1990, Iraqi troops crossed the border into Kuwait. The main column, led by Soviet-designed T-72 tanks and supported by fighter aircraft and helicopter gunships, overwhelmed the Kuwaiti border guards and marched toward Kuwait City. The Iraqis were in control of the country by the end of the day. The United States immediately froze Kuwaiti and Iraqi assets and imposed a trade embargo on Iraq. Other countries such as Britain and France followed suit. At the instigation of President George Bush, the United Nations Security Council passed Resolution No. 660, which condemned the invasion and called upon Iraq to withdraw all troops from Kuwait. Further resolutions followed. Ultimately, Operation Desert Shield became a reality, with

Washington ordering military intervention (Hiro, 1992). Operation Desert Shield became Desert Storm (the code name of the air campaign of the U.S.-led coalition) on January 16 and 17, 1991. After 209 days of the Gulf crisis and warfare, a temporary ceasefire began on February 28, 1991, as the coalition forces suspended combat operations. "The armed force of the Coalition that defeated Iraq totaled 737,000 men and women in ground units, aboard 190 vessels, and flying or maintaining 1800 aircraft. While the United States provided the bulk of the Coalition forces—with 532,000 troops, 120 ships, and more than 1700 aircraft—34 other nations provided personnel and equipment in action or in support of Desert Storm" (Blair, 1992, p. 125).

One potential legacy of this conflict is that the Persian Gulf War and its popular support forced Americans to reexamine the Southeast Asian conflict and the way in which the country had treated its veterans. The Gulf War entered the daily lives of the citizens of the world through the media, which exposed them to the everyday happenings in the lives of those fighting for peace. Although Vietnam was the first televised war, there was no aspect of the Gulf War that was not directly affected by the mass communications media. The media helped to confirm not only the superiority of Western technology but also the courage of both allied servicemen and servicewomen and their willingness to participate, no matter what the risks. Perhaps more far-reaching is the fact that the Gulf War may well have become a historic turning point. A whole new level of international cooperation may have been achieved. But would it continue to progress?

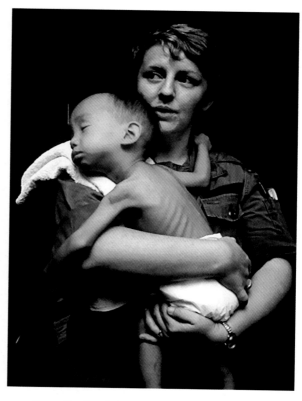

Army nurse Donna Hamilton holds a Vietnamese baby during her second tour of duty in the Vietnam War, Long Binh, Vietnam, 1968.

John Olson, *Portrait of Nurse Hamilton with Baby*, January 1, 1968, photograph, Time and Life Pictures/Getty Images.

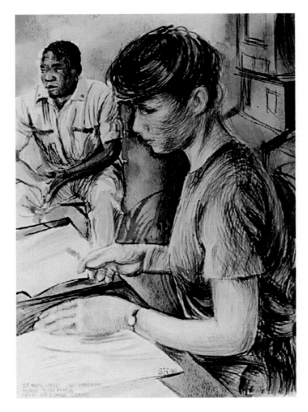

Sieger Hartgers, *Nurse, 5th MASH,* painting, US Army Center of Military History.

Several thousand nurses from the United States were deployed with Operation Desert Storm to provide nursing care for the 500,000 troops sent to Saudi Arabia and the Persian Gulf. They were sent to desert sites where troops were stationed. Nursing was also represented by other countries, as in the case of Great Britain. Nearly 6000 British medical personnel, including nurses, were part of the operations. Within a week of Iraq's invasion of Kuwait, nurses on active duty and in the reserves were in action in the Middle East. Both women and nurses were involved in the military conflict in crucial ways. About 32,000 women went to this war; women made up more than 10% of the U.S. military and staffed almost 40% of military medical units, the largest number in any specialty (David, 1991). There was a certain irony here, because Saudi Arabian women were not permitted to drive cars or even show their faces. Because of Saudia Arabian customs, American military women were not permitted to wear shorts, jog, or go shopping unless accompanied by a man. Yet they shared all duties except those on the front lines.

This war confirmed again the courage of military nurses and affirmed their willingness to care for the sick and the wounded. All branches of the military were represented. Although much has been written about the history, military aspects, and chronology of the Gulf War, information about the role of nurses is sparse. The reality is, however, that nurses, too, were faced with the threat of biological and chemical warfare and SCUD attacks, and they tolerated the brown, desolate Gulf landscape. "They put together 'hospitals' from tents to serve as super first-aid stations. In battle, crews of RNs and techs would work close to the scene of

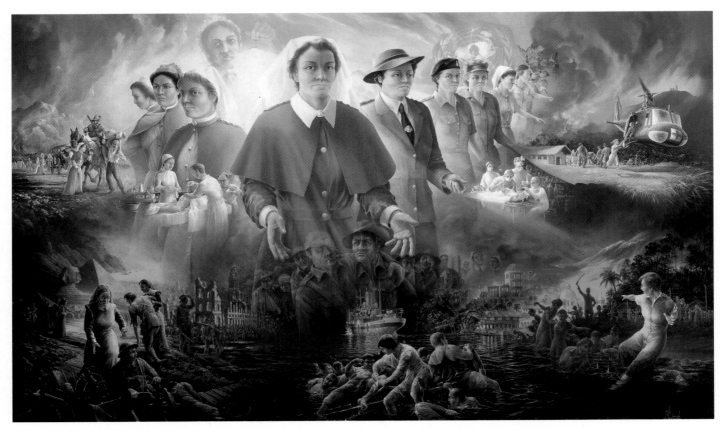

This print is dedicated to all Australian nurses who served their country in theaters of war, especially those nurses who lost their lives in the line of duty. The print depicts not the nurses' duties, but rather their environment and locals in which they were to serve.

Brian Wood, *Serving Humanity,* painting, Australia. Angels Twenty.

action, keeping men from bleeding to death and pushing oxygen and IV fluids. Once stabilized, the wounded would be transported to field hospitals, tended in flight by aerovac crews trained to deal with the impact of altitude on trauma patients" (*American Journal of Nursing*, 1990, p. 7).

Field hospitals were typically assembled by tunneling together eight or nine tents. Wounded were received as air evacuation teams delivered them. Navy nurses also functioned on the 1000-bed hospital ships, the *USNS Comfort* and the *USNS Mercy*, which were deployed to the Gulf. These ships were considered the world's largest trauma centers. Overall, nurses were equipped to handle at least 15,000 casualties daily (Kalisch and Kalisch, 1994).

As in previous wars, progress in health care occurred. Frozen blood was prepared for transfusion for the first time. Monoclonal antibody treatments were available for large wounds and multiple-system trauma; improved antichemical treatments were in place. The ensuing effects of this war on nurses remain to be seen, but it is possible that they too will suffer from the unknown and elusive disease (Persian Gulf syndrome) that is taking its toll on military personnel who served there. Posttraumatic stress disorder may also be experienced.

WAR AND CONFLICT ACROSS THE GLOBE

The new millennium began with much of the world consumed by armed conflict or cultivating an uncertain peace. At the turn of the 21st century, there were 41 conflicts in 35 countries. Eight major wars were under way by 2005, and as many as two dozen "lesser" conflicts were taking place in varying degrees of intensity. New wars have continued to emerge creating a less than peaceful world. The majority of these conflicts are considered to be civil or intrastate wars, but they are certainly no less significant. They are triggered by a variety of factors, including racial, ethnic, or religious animosities as well as ideological passion and enthusiasm. The most distinguishing factor of these modern conflicts is the fact that most victims are civilians (Project Ploughshares, 2008).

IRAQ: FIRST MAJOR WAR OF THE NEW MILLENNIUM

On September 11, 2001, the attacks on the twin towers of the World Trade Center in New York City and the Pentagon in Washington, D.C., and the demise of United Airlines flight 93 (its ultimate target thought to be either the United States Capitol or the White House) precipitated a series of catastrophic events that would forever change international relationships. The overwhelming majority of the 2974 people who died, excluding the 19 hijackers, were civilians from more than 90 countries. Additionally, 29 others were missing and presumed dead. The United States' reaction to the attacks was the initiation of the War on Terrorism; the invasion of Afghanistan to overthrow the Taliban, which had harbored al-Qaeda terrorists, and the call for an attack on Iraq.

Less than 2 years after 9/11, on March 19, 2003, American

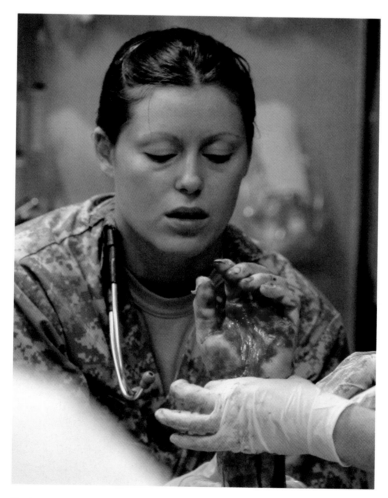

The Iraq war.

Thaier Al-Sudani, *Iraqi Hospitals*, October 30, 2006, photograph, Baghdad, Iraq. REUTERS.

and British forces, supported by smaller contingents from Australia, Denmark, Poland, and other nations, invaded Iraq. This preemptive action began a conflict that may become known as the Third Persian Gulf War, the Second Iraq War, or Operation Iraqi Freedom. The most provocative names that occur in current literature are the War of Imagination and the Forever War. Claims had been made that Iraq possessed weapons of mass destruction (nuclear, biological, and chemical) that posed a serious and imminent threat to Western national security and that Saddam Hussein was directing those weapons to al-Qaeda operatives. France, Russia, and Germany did not support this argument. Not only were these claims proven false following the invasion, but they had already been disputed in various agencies in the Pentagon and the American intelligence community (Banford, 2005; Murray and Scales, 2003). The more plausible reason for the invasion was to free the Iraqi people and end Hussein's brutality and crimes against humanity. Once the idea that weapons of mass destruction were present proved to be unfounded, President George W. Bush immediately declared that the invasion of Iraq was a step toward democracy in the Middle East. Unfortunately, neither peace nor democracy has yet taken hold in Iraq (Banford, 2005; Bodansky, 2004; Murray and Scales, 2003)

It is safe to say that the war in Iraq has created a great deal of controversy in the United States and worldwide. This was to be expected because nearly every aspect of America's conflict with Iraq has been misunderstood and was doomed from the start (Bodansky, 2004). It deeply divided and discouraged the American public and, contrary to what was originally expected, has not turned out to be quick and cheap. It may well be a seminal event in American history, and it is not yet over.

The Iraq War has closely resembled the Vietnam War in terms of cost, protests, duration, and the irregular nature of the combat. Differences exist in the type of weaponry used and the locations in which combat has occurred. American napalm, white phosphorus, and antipersonnel bombs and small arms were used in Vietnam. The signature weapon in Iraq has been the homemade bomb (the improvised explosive devices, or IEDs), although suicide bombers, land mines, AK-47 rifles, and rocket-propelled grenades have also been used. As a result, massive and multiple injuries such as traumatic amputations, enormous blast wounds, eyes pierced by shrapnel, and flesh burned down to the bone have been common occurrences in both wars. No front lines existed in Vietnam; the majority of fighting was in jungles. On the other hand, fighting in Iraq has centered primarily in cities and towns.

Nurses serving in Iraq have endured unbearable heat, frequent mortar attacks, medical supply shortages, and substandard facilities. They have been stunned by the numbers and types of trauma cases they have seen, and such cases create continual clinical, technical, and ethical challenges. They have witnessed courage in the face of injury and pain and loyalty in the face of grief, and they have provided comfort with the only thing left in many circumstances—human touch. First and foremost, they know they have made a difference, the difference sometimes being that between life and death. All have been irrevocably changed by their experiences. Most of the seriously injured soldiers (both American and coalition) and civilians are taken to the Combat Support Hospital (CSH) to be stabilized and treated after receiving their initial care from medics in the field. Most are then transferred to Landstuhl Army Medical Center in Germany and then to Walter Reed Army Medical Center in

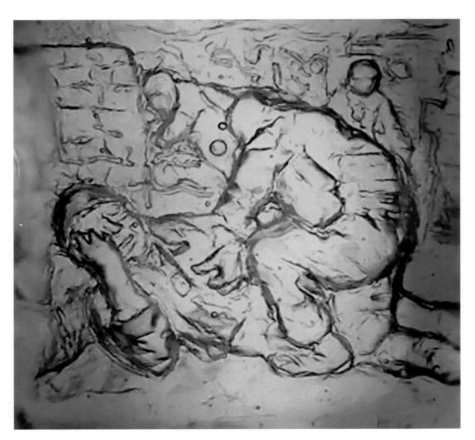

Administering care in Iraq.

Judi Charlson, *Giving Care to a Soldier in Iraq* (detail from the *Wall of the Journey of Life*), 2006, glass pane.

Washington, D.C. In the Army, the majority of the anesthesia care is given by certified registered nurse anesthetists (CRNAs), who are trained to function independently in the field. Although the nursing care is emotionally and physically trying, nurses remain dedicated to professional, competent, and compassionate care. On July 12, 2007, the first nurse died in Iraq. Maria Ortiz of Pennsauken, New Jersey, was killed by shrapnel when a mortar barrage struck in Baghdad, where she was treating injured Iraqis.

Many questions about the Iraq War remain unanswered: What has been gained? What has been lost? Is Iraq better off today than it was at the time of the invasion? Where and when will this war end? Is the war in Iraq really a "war of imagination?" One thing is certain—the Iraq War is now the longest military conflict to involve the United States, other than the Vietnam War. What is most tragic is the potential impact on the Americans that are serving and have served in this war. After Vietnam, military personnel returned dishonored and shamed, not even wanting to acknowledge their involvement in the war. With Iraq there seems to be an intense silence and secretiveness, even to the point of preventing the American public from seeing the rows and rows of coffins returning from Iraq. Indeed, the incidence of posttraumatic stress disorder (PTSD) among returning soldiers and nurses will greatly increase if preventive measures are not implemented. It was the Vietnam War that taught us that soldiers and nurses need to talk through their disturbing experiences to prevent PTSD and its debilitating symptoms.

Is it too much to hope that peace can be achieved in the future—that racial, ethnic, religious, and ideological differences can be understood and tolerated so harmony can be achieved throughout the world? With this hope, the United

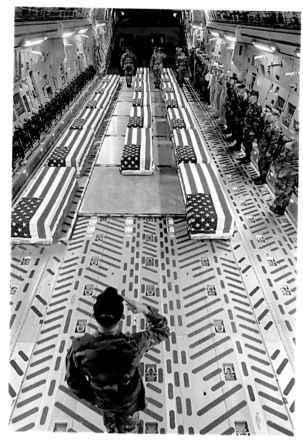

Flag Draped Coffins of U.S. Casualties of War, photograph. Courtesy of Russ Kick.

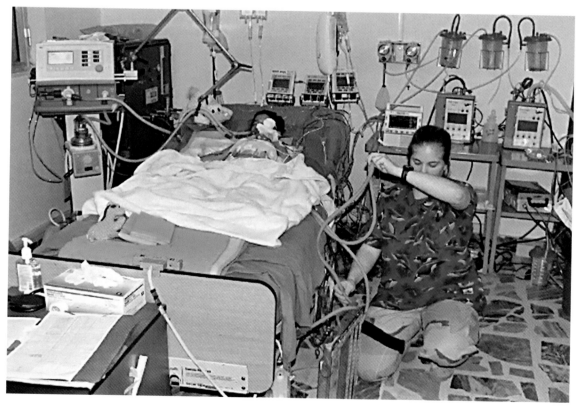

Peter Rimar, *U.S. Army Nurse at the Bedside of a Young Iraqi Boy*, April 2004, photograph, Sina Hospital, Baghdad, Iraq.

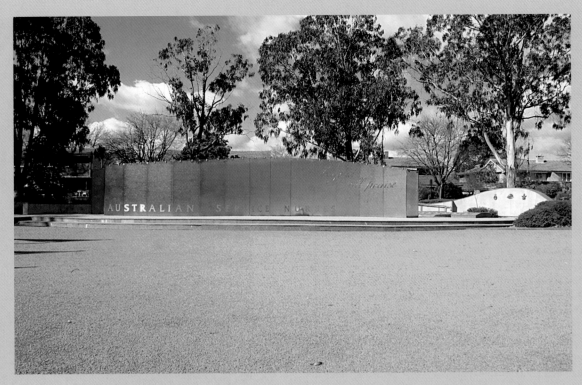

Nurses Memorial, 1999, sculpture, Canberra, Australia.

Frances Luther Rich, *Spirit of Nursing*, 1938, sculpture, Arlington National Cemetery.

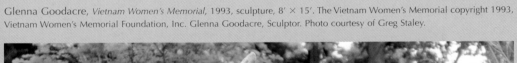

Glenna Goodacre, *Vietnam Women's Memorial*, 1993, sculpture, 8′ × 15′. The Vietnam Women's Memorial copyright 1993, Vietnam Women's Memorial Foundation, Inc. Glenna Goodacre, Sculptor. Photo courtesy of Greg Staley.

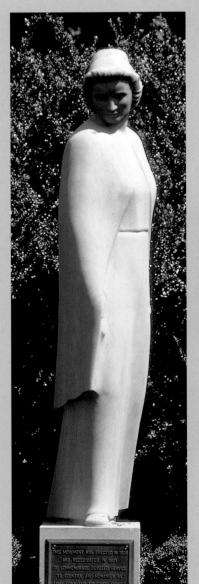

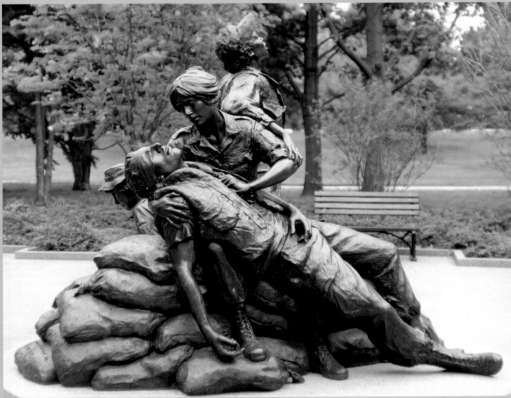

Nations "decided that, beginning in 2002, the International Day of Peace should be observed on 21 September each year. The Assembly declared in Resolution 55/282 that the Day be observed as a day of global ceasefire and non-violence, an invitation to all nations and peoples to honour a cessation of hostilities during the Day. It invited all Member States, organizations of the United Nations system, regional and non-governmental organizations and individuals to commemorate the Day in an appropriate manner, including through education and public awareness, and to cooperate with the United Nations in establishing a global ceasefire."

IN HONOR OF . . .

A considerable number of memorials have been dedicated to nurses and nursing worldwide. The majority can be categorized as ecclesiastical, military, or educational. Those related to military nursing bear testimony to the strong relationship between war and nursing. They represent a variety of methods of bestowing honor, such as statues, cornerstones, scholarships and loan funds, buildings, chapels, hospital ships, and stained-glass windows. A magnificent memorial was unveiled on October 2, 1999, to mark 100 years of military nursing in Canberra, Australia. It reflects the values of "human dignity and worth, dedication in bringing succour and care, commitment beyond self, courage, companionship and fortitude." The memorial consists of two curvilinear glass walls. Etched into the inner glass walls are a variety of images and events in a timeline sequence. A contemplative space surrounded by rosemary is particularly appealing and provides intimate moments for remembering.

Another impressive memorial is the Nurses' Monument in Arlington National Cemetery in Arlington, Virginia. This monument, which symbolizes the Spirit of Nursing, was dedicated to Army and Navy nurses. Carved by Frances Luther Rich, the daughter of actress Irene Rich, the monument is made of Tennessee marble. At the unveiling ceremonies on November 8, 1938, Julia C. Stimson, superintendent of the Army Nurse Corps (ret.) and current president of the ANA, made the dedication to "their tenderness and compassion, their competence, courage and human qualities . . . the spirit of nursing of the past, of today, and of the years to come" (*American Journal of Nursing,* 1939, p. 90). The Nurses' Monument, which overlooks the graves from the top of a hilly slope, was rededicated on March 11, 1971, by the chiefs of the Army, Navy, and Air Force.

A second imposing monument was erected to the memory of a single individual, Mary Ann Bickerdyke, of Galesburg, Illinois. Affectionately known as Mother Bickerdyke by sick, wounded, and dying soldiers, she served as a nurse under fire in 19 battles during the Civil War. This monument was erected on the public square in Galesburg in 1903, an event made possible by an appropriation of $5000 by the state of Illinois. On the 125th anniversary (1962) of Knox College in Galesburg, Mary Ann Bickerdyke was remembered by a commemorative cover that was franked with the 1950 U.S. 4-cent stamp honoring nursing.

Perhaps the erection of the Vietnam Women's Memorial will finally call attention to the great advances and notable achievements made by nurses during wartime. The service of these "forgotten veterans" is not well known and has received relatively little attention. However, on Veterans' Day in 1993, in Washington, DC, a dramatic event was witnessed by 35,000 people. On this day the Vietnam Women's Memo-

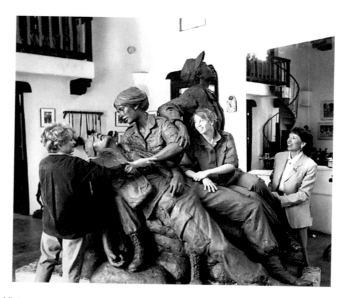

Vietnam veteran nurse/memorial advocate Diane Carlson Evans (R) looks on as artist Glenna Goodacre (L) uses model Sarah Gilman to work on the Vietnam Memorial sculpture of a nurse stroking the head of a fallen soldier as another woman scans the sky for evacuation assistance.

Dirck Halstead, *Sarah Gilman, Glenna Goodacre, Jane Carlson Evans,* April 27, 1993, photograph.

rial was dedicated to honor the strength, compassion, and service demonstrated by more than 250,000 women during the Vietnam War. Approximately 8000 nurses served in Vietnam. The dedication was the result of a decade-long struggle spearheaded by Diane Carlson Evans, a former Army nurse and Vietnam veteran. She had been a head nurse at a frontline Army unit in Pleiku, a village near the Cambodian border. This memorial project was not without controversy and rejection. However, with incredible tenacity, perseverance, and teamwork, obstacles were overcome and the project became a reality.

The memorial, a 7-foot bronze sculpture by artist Glenna Goodacre, beautifully and poignantly portrays four figures: a nurse tending to the chest wound of a soldier lying across her lap; a woman scanning the sky for a helicopter or assistance; and a kneeling woman staring at an empty helmet, bowing her head in grief and despair. The memorial is a symbol of healing that is set in a grove of trees 300 feet from the low black wall that is the Vietnam Veterans Memorial. At last—but only after exhausting years of convincing people of the need to honor female veterans, rallying financial support, lobbying Congress, and obtaining government support and permission—there is a visible symbol in the nation's capital that honors women's patriotic service.

In 1968, Americans did not want to hear about the suffering of soldiers in an unpopular war, did not want to hear from nurses who had served in Vietnam. Yet nurses have given undeniably beneficial service under extreme circumstances during every war in which they have served. Their legacy is profound, as is their legacy to society of the whole of nursing. Public recognition of their services, however, has been slow to evolve. Nurses have invested in the future of the world as they have diligently worked with tenderness, compassion, and expertise to comfort the suffering and save lives. It is time that they become *loudly heard and greatly noted* (Donahue, 1995).

IMAGINE A WAR, ANY WAR, WITHOUT NURSES

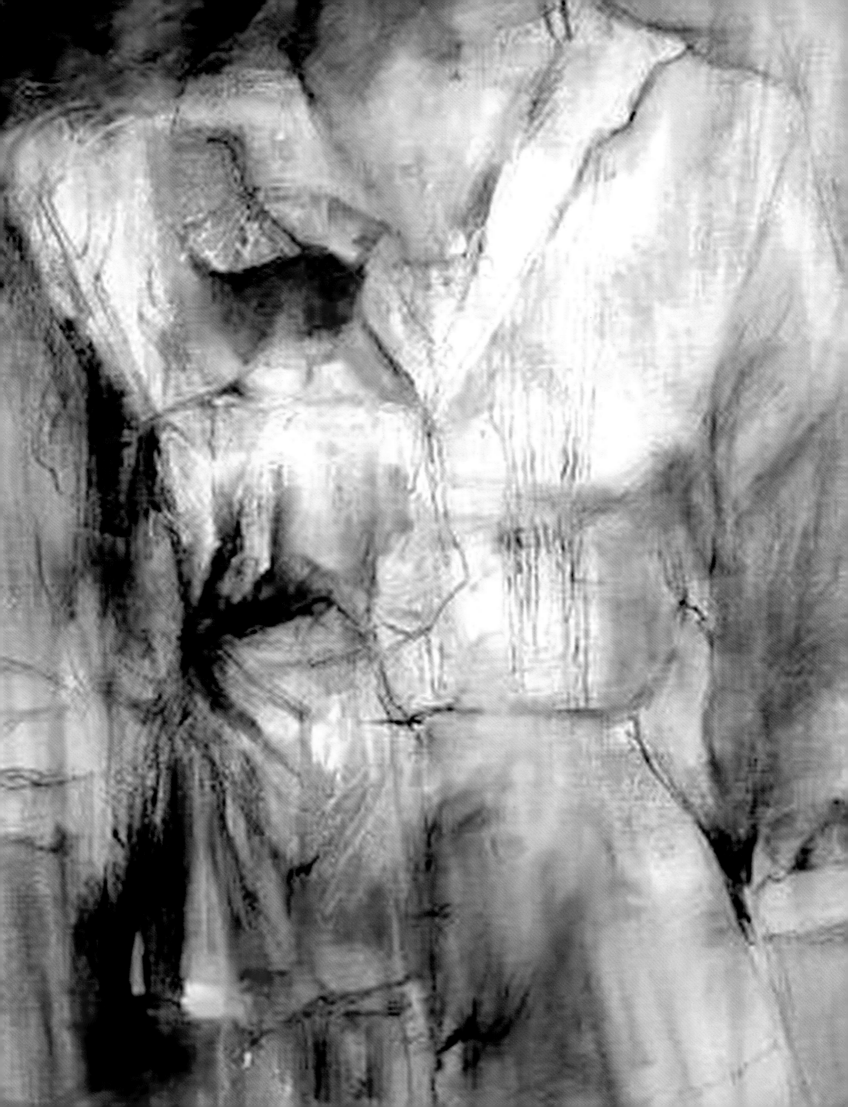

UNIT Six

$\mathcal{N}$ursing in an Era of Change and Challenge

In order to advance the discipline toward the future, the new tomorrow, nurses have to unite themselves in an effort to construct new organizational and legal structures and thus bring more clarity in their roles as professionals. They can no longer allow others to do the job for them. This has become even more important within the context of the 'Health for All' movement, that encourages nurses to redirect their attention from primarily hospital care to 'health for all,' the healthy and the sick in the community. Although this challenge has received a positive response from many nurse practitioners, the question is whether the discipline is ready to accept this challenge with competence and vision. Is nursing ready to take on a role as a pathfinder or trendsetter and engage in *anticipatory nursing* or are its members waiting directions given by other disciplines, who are often less well equipped to act as a liaison between the policy-makers and planners of care and the public at large?

— HANNEKE M. TH. VAN MAANEN

Therese Cipiti Herron, *The Way It Was,* 2005, oil on canvas, 72″ × 72″.

1920	1955	1971	1975

Nursing

1920s First doctoral program in nursing education (EdD) at Teachers College	**1955** American Nurses' Foundation established for research grants to graduate nurses	**1971** National Black Nurses Association established	**1975** ANA held formal ceremonies to honor first certified nurses
1934 New York University begins PhD and EdD programs in nursing	**1960s** Growth of specialization in nursing	**1971** M. Lucille Kinlein establishes herself as independent practitioner	**1975-1980** Community Nursing Center (CNC) movement begins
1950s "Progressive patient care" set into motion	**1963** Loeb Center for Nursing and Rehabilitation established at Montefiore Hospital	**1971** American Assembly for Men in Nursing organized	**1977** First undergraduate nursing informatics elective at University of Buffalo
1950s-1970s Emergence of nursing theoretical and conceptual frameworks	**1965** The "nurse practitioner" introduced at the University of Colorado	**1971** Florence Wald and associates found the U.S. hospice movement	**1977** Computers in nursing courses first emerged
1952 Dr. Hildegard Peplau publishes *Interpersonal Relations in Nursing*	**1965** American Nurses Association position paper on nursing education released	**1973** American Academy of Nursing established	**1978** International History of Nursing Society formed
1953 Team nursing introduced	**1969** American Association of Colleges of Nursing established	**1973** North American Nursing Diagnosis Association (NANDA) formed	
	1970s Advent of primary nursing		

Medicine and Health Care

1944 Quinine synthesized	**1956** Albert Sabin develops oral polio vaccine	**1976** Discovery of viral cause of multiple sclerosis	
1945 Vitamin A synthesized	**1966** Michael De Bakey implants plastic arteries leading to external artificial heart, providing bypass during valve replacement surgery	**1977** Last documented case of smallpox diagnosed in southern Somalia	
1950 Antihistamines become popular		**1977** World Health Assembly establishes goal of "Health for All by the Year 2000"	
	1970 Nuclear-powered heart pacemakers implanted in three patients in France and Britain	**1978** World Health Organization declares primary health care the strategy for achieving health for all	
		1978 First "test-tube baby" born in London	
		1979 World Health Organization declares smallpox eradicated	

Science and Technology

1941 Donald Bailey invents portable military bridge	**1957** U.S.S.R. launches first earth satellites	**1971** Three Russian cosmonauts die upon reentry into Earth's atmosphere	**1976** Discovery of viral cause of multiple sclerosis
1942 Enrico Fermi splits the atom	**1959** De Beers manufactures synthetic diamond	**1971** Human growth hormone synthesized in California	**1978** First ascent of Mt. Everest without artificial oxygen supply
1942 Bell Aircraft tests first U.S. jet plane	**1965** First flight around the world over both poles	**1972** Pocket calculator introduced	
1948 Long-playing record invented	**1970** First synthesis of gene announced in Wisconsin		**1978** Discovery of a moon orbiting Pluto

The Visual Arts

1940 Lascaux caves discovered with prehistoric wall paintings, France	**1959** Joan Miró creates murals for UNESCO building in Paris	**1971** Kennedy Center for Performing Arts opens in Washington, DC	**1975** Life-sized pottery figures (6000) from third century BC found in northwest China
1945 Trial of Hans van Meegeren, Dutch painter who forged great paintings	**1968** Sotheby's of London sells 400 impressionist and modern paintings in 3 days	**1972** Michelangelo's *Pieta* seriously damaged by hammer-wielding vandal	**1978** Norman Rockwell, American illustrator and painter, dies
1946 British Arts Council inaugurated	**1970** Henri Matisse exhibition in Paris	**1973** Pablo Picasso dies	
1951 Cinerama invented by Fred Waller			

Daily Life

1941 U.S. savings bonds and stamps go on sale	**1956** Andrea Doria sinks	**1971** Cigarette ads banned from U.S. television	**1974** Smallpox epidemic kills 10,000-20,000 in India
1945 "Bebop" comes into fashion	**1957** Words "beat" and "beatnik" come into vogue	**1971** Women granted vote in Switzerland	**1976** North and South Vietnam unite as one country after twenty-two years
1945 Atomic bombs dropped on Hiroshima and Nagasaki	**1961** Dag Hammarskjöld killed in air accident	**1971** Cigarette ads banned from United States television	**1977** Passenger service of Concorde supersonic transport begins
1948 Mohandas Gandhi assassinated	**1962** *The Sunday Times* issues first color supplement	**1971** India and Pakistan go to war	
1953 Queen Elizabeth II crowned	**1964** 300 spectators killed in soccer match riots in Lima, Peru	**1972** Death of eleven Israeli athletes at Olympics in Munich	
1954 Eurovision network founded	**1968** Mickey Mouse celebrates fortieth birthday	**1972** Tasadays, a tribe with Stone Age culture, discovered living in southern Philippine cave	
	1970 Television sets in use worldwide: 231 million		

Column 1 (1980)

1980 Nursing Case Management Model pioneered at New England Medical Center, Boston

1983 International Council of Nurses adopts statement on importance of human rights

1984 First AAHN Nursing History Conference

1985 Nursing Network on Violence Against Women, International founded

1985 Nursing Minimum Data Set (NMDS) developed

1986 National Center for Nursing Research (NCNR) founded

1987 First Arista STTI think tank meeting held

Column 2 (1988)

1988 University of Maryland, College Park opens first master's level program in nursing informatics

1988 Sigma Theta Tau becomes an international organization

1989 International Classification of Nursing Practice (ICNP) project starts

1990 Term "evidence based" first used by David Eddy

1990 Magnet Hospital Recognition Program for Excellence in Nursing Services approved by ANA Board of Directors

1990 Virginia Henderson International Nursing Library established by STTI

Column 3 (1991)

1991 Brig Gen. Clara Adams Ender becomes first black woman and nurse appointed commander general of a U.S. Army post

1991 First Nursing Informatics doctoral program at University of Maryland Baltimore

1992 International Nursing Center established by American Nurses Association

1992 *Nursing Interventions Classifications* (NIC) published

1992 State Senator Eddie Bernice Johnson elected to U.S. House of Representatives, the first nurse (black or white) elected to Congress

Column 4 (1993)

1993 NCNR receives status of institute: National Institute of Nursing Research

1994 Barbara Fassbinder, RN, infected with HIV in 1986, dies

1994 *The Online Journal of Knowledge Synthesis for Nursing* created

1995 Nursing resources developed for Virginia Henderson International Library moved to Internet

---

1981 Scientists identify acquired immune deficiency syndrome (AIDS)

1981 Valve inserted into skull of human fetus to prevent hydrocephalus

1981 Patricia Bath develops laser eye surgery for removing cataracts.

1981 WHO formulates strategy for health promotion, disease prevention, and curative and rehabilitative services

1982 First artificial heart implanted

1982 Combined heart-lung and kidney-pancreas transplant done

1984 AIDS virus isolated

1984 First frozen embryo baby born

1985 Lasers used to clean out clogged arteries

1990 Contemporary managed care movement begins in U.S.

1992 Term "evidence-based medicine" first appeared in medical literature

1995 Zaire suffers from outbreak of Ebola virus

1980 "Baby Fae" receives baboon heart transplant

1981 First successful space shuttle flight occurs

1981 IBM unveils its first personal computer

1983 Compact disc is launched

1984 Apple introduces Macintosh microcomputer with mouse

1984 Internet opened to public use

1986 Space shuttle *Challenger* explodes

1987 International scientists confirm ozone hole over Antarctica and postulate link with chlorofluorocarbon emissions

1990 Official start of the Human Genome Project

1994 HIV protease inhibitor invented

1995 eBay is founded in California

1995 Russian cosmonaut Valery Poliakov returns to earth after 439 days aboard the Mir space station, the longest stay in space

1995 DVD (digital versatile disc) invented

1985 Claude Monet's *Impression, Sun Rising,* the painting that gave the Impressionist movement its name, is stolen in Paris

1986 Film companies begin to colorize black-and-white films

1993 *Angels in America, Part One* on Broadway examines the history of HIV-AIDS epidemic

1995 The Metropolitan Opera installs screens on audience seats

1995 The Moving Collection (International artwork collection against Apartheid) shown in Zimbabwe at the All Africa Games

---

1980 Fifty nations boycott Olympics after Soviets invade Afghanistan

1984 Series of famines in Ethiopia

1985 World Bank organizes famine relief fund for Africa

1986 Chernobyl nuclear power plant accident occurs

1988 Famines in Ethiopia, Sudan, and Bangladesh

1989 Tienanmen Square Massacre in China

1989 Kenya calls for ban on ivory imports

1989 Fall of Communism in Eastern Europe

1990 English and French engineers meet under the sea as portions of English Channel tunnel linked together

1991 Collapse of USSR

1991 Internet revolutionizes access to information

1991 Apartheid ends in South Africa

1995 World Trade Organization created to promote economic development worldwide

2001 World Trade Center bombing

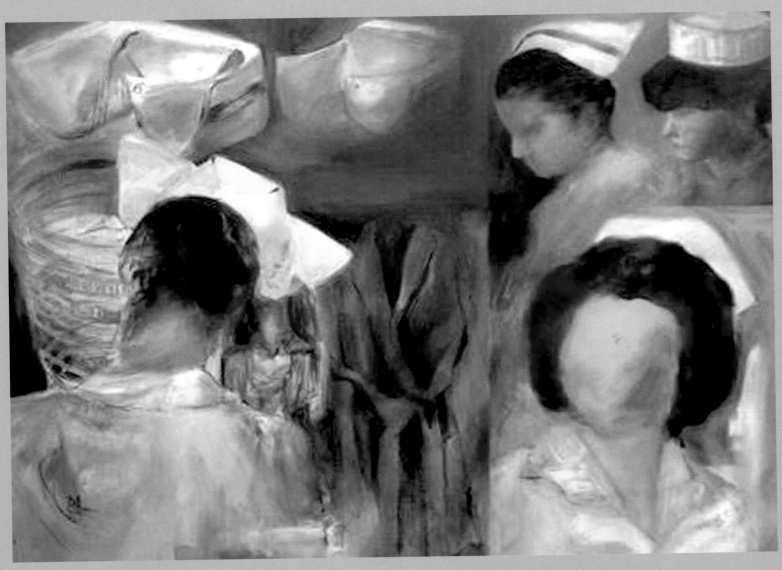

Therese Cipiti Herron, *Lost Image,* 2005, oil on Belgian linen, 32″ × 44″.

s the 20th century dawned, nursing stood poised between the past and the future. The question of what lay ahead was open to speculation because the state of nursing's art is ever changing and responsive to societal needs. The 20th century was marked by many changes in the healing arts; some were in striking contrast to those that had occurred during earlier epochs in history. Yet many of the extraordinary innovations were continuations of contributions from the past. These changes resulted from the interplay of numerous factors that arose in an increasingly technological age.

There is little doubt that nursing practice has been forced to make severe accommodations within this larger societal context as knowledge has continued to increase and attitudes and values have shifted. Nursing practice has expanded and extended in both horizontal and vertical directions. Some believe that this expansion has been too great and that professional growth comes by limiting functions rather than by extending them; they believe that the focus of concentration should be on the functions that are of a professional nature and integral to nursing. They argue that nursing has gone too far and that it has begun to encroach on the medical domain. Others believe that the expanded roles in nursing fulfill a vital need and provide health care services where none exist and where services are limited. In addition, the assumption of additional functions by nurses is viewed as necessary so that the best possible care can be rendered. Whatever the case, the changing environment has called for an education that keeps pace with the modern world. Yet the struggle for the inclusion of educational programs for nursing in institutions of higher learning still continues at a time when education is needed more than ever

to develop individuals who can deal with the problems of adjustment in modern life. Alfred North Whitehead, a scientist and philosopher, issued a warning in 1929 that is relevant to nursing's current educational situation: "In the conditions of modern life, the rule is absolute; the race which does not value trained intelligence is doomed. Not all your heroism, not all your social charm, not all your wit, not all your victories on land or at sea can move back the finger of fate. Today we maintain ourselves. Tomorrow science will have moved forward yet one more step, and there will be no appeal from the judgment which will then be pronounced on the uneducated" (Whitehead, 1929, p. 22). One thing is clear: the education of nurses for the future must provide for the society of the future. At the same time, the full potentialities of individual nurses and nursing at large must not be sacrificed.

The scientific, technological, and societal movements of the 20th century had a significant effect on the development of health care and on the direction of nursing services. A wide spectrum of change occurred and catapulted society from the horse-and-buggy era to the space age. Diseases such as smallpox, diphtheria, and cholera, which virtually devastated populations in the past, became rare or nonexistent.

Scientific advances made it possible for humans to prolong life. Sophisticated diagnostic methods permitted visualization of the most minute internal structures of the human body; anesthetic agents and improved asepsis enhanced surgical practice; grafts and transplants of healthy structures or even mechanical devices were used to replace diseased organs; miracle drugs wiped out formerly hopeless infections and bacterial diseases; the inner workings of the cell were open to scrutiny through physical and chemical means;

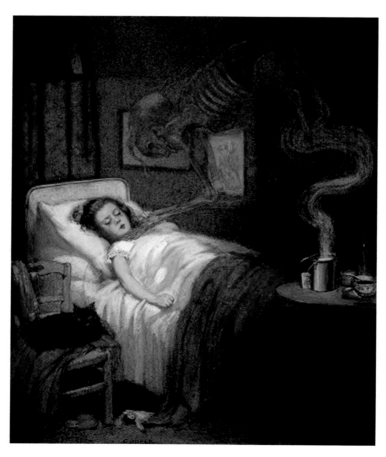

Richard Tennant Cooper, *Diphtheria Trying to Strangle a Child,* 1912, watercolor, Wellcome Library, London, England.

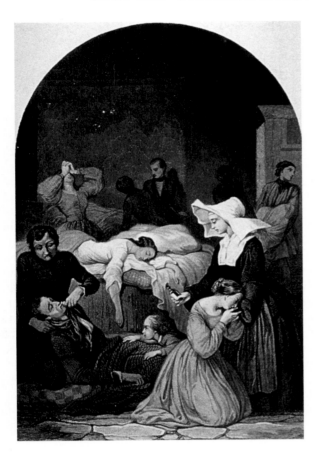

Interior view through a doorway showing cholera victims being treated.

J. Roze, *Le Cholera à Paris,* etching/engraving. Courtesy of the National Library of Medicine.

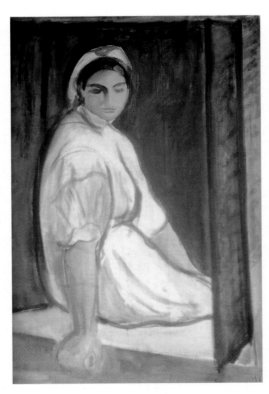

It is interesting to note that the artist did not paint his model in a hospital surrounded by beds and patients. This is perhaps because the painting is an infatuated artist's tribute to a woman in white. Still, he rendered a professional view of the nurse.

Helmuth Thomsen, *Sygeplejerske,* 1938, painting.

and the hospital moved from pest house to comprehensive health care center.

Other current events and social issues were also influencing, either directly or indirectly, the health care delivery system and the roles and functions of its providers. During the first 50 years of the 20th century many factors gave impetus to the progress of nursing: two world wars, self-organization of nurses, government and nursing legislation, problems of social welfare, support of health care fields by national foundations, and the complexities of medicine. In the latter part of the century other social movements profoundly influenced health care and nursing. They included the rise of consumerism (the increased awareness and expectations by the patient of high quality in health care delivery); changes in work and leisure patterns; the fight for civil rights; progress in public health; the development of voluntary and governmental health care organizations; and the struggle for equal rights for women. All these factors—combined with the internal forces in nursing of consciousness raising, role innovation, and the drive for professionalization—shaped the role of the nurse and of nursing (Reeder, 1978).

Industrialization transformed rural America into an urban society as the 20th century witnessed improvements in the general standard of living; significant progress in transportation, communications, and other areas; and the lengthening of the life span. The social scene was marked by increasing change and complexity in nearly every field of endeavor. Urban centers rapidly became overcrowded because of an unprecedented population expansion and the unrestricted immigration of millions of poor Europeans. Health problems were aggravated, and problems in the provision of adequate health care were intensified. Hospital services were broadened to provide for middle-class patients as well as the indigent and homeless. Consequently, the whole concept of nursing had to be reevaluated and changed to fit the needs of this age of reform.

The last 10 to 15 years of the 20th century might appropriately be called the decade of paradoxes in health care. A transformation had been taking place in the very core of society. Along with almost unimaginable technological advances came profound questions relative to life and death,

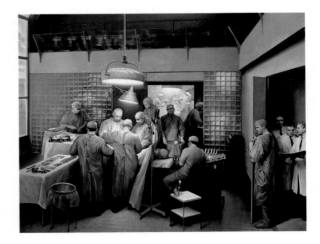

The first human kidney transplantation occurred on December 23, 1954 at the Peter Brent Brigham Hospital in Boston, Massachusetts. This historic surgery opened up the immense field of transplantation surgery.

Joel Babb, *The First Successful Kidney Transplantation,* 1996, painting, 70" × 88", Harvard Medical Library in Francis A. Countwy Library of Medicine.

which provoked serious doubts about the value of technology. Who will receive lifesaving organs when not all can?

Will the rich, the elderly, and the poor receive high-quality, if not equal, care? How and by whom will decisions be made in the face of limited resources? Will health care be available to all? Other issues in health care, such as those that concern diseases, in vitro fertilization, surrogate mothers, the elderly, access to care, financial resources, and governmental control can also be readily identified.

These paradoxes are interwoven with the strands of technology, bureaucracy, and healing. Bulger (1988) comprehensively discussed these three strands in relation to the American system of health care, but his statements can easily be applied to global societies without much alteration. Although his writing is several years old, it is still applicable to the current system. He pleads for a reintegration of technology, bureaucracy, and healing into a new, more humane, and more effective approach to health care. This "postmodern paradigm" would preserve ". . . liberty, freedom, hope, and a sense of human progress which incorporates suffering and death, all united through a sense of belonging and community" (pp. 86-87).

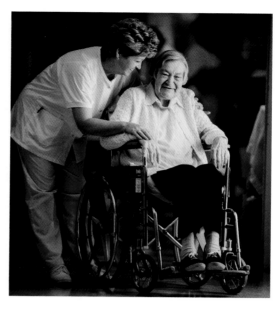

Lonnie Duka, *Nurse with Elderly Patient in Wheelchair,* photograph. Getty Images.

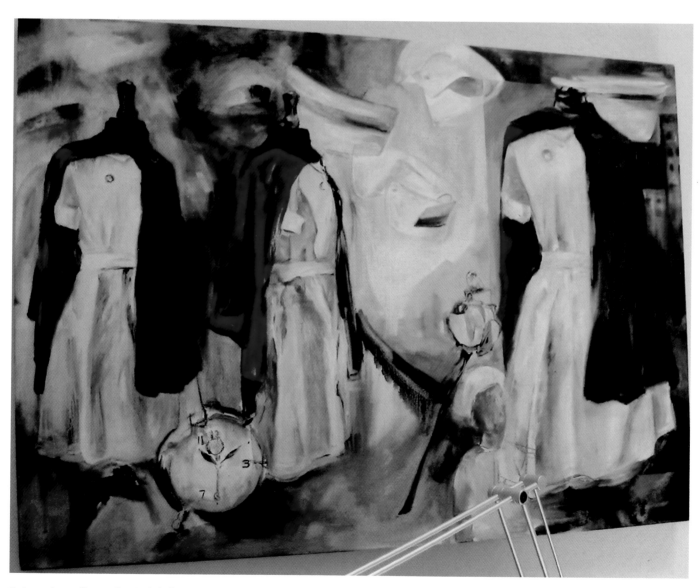

Early nursing uniforms often included a cape that was worn in place of a coat, particularly when students and graduate nurses hurried back and forth between the hospital and the nurses' residence. They varied in length and color according to the dictates of the nursing school. Some claimed that another purpose of the cape was to hide the body of the nurse. Capes were cherished by many nurses, as were caps and school pins.

Therese Cipiti Herron, *Vanishing Capes,* # 9 Nursing Series, 2007, oil/carbon on Belgian linen, 30" × 40".

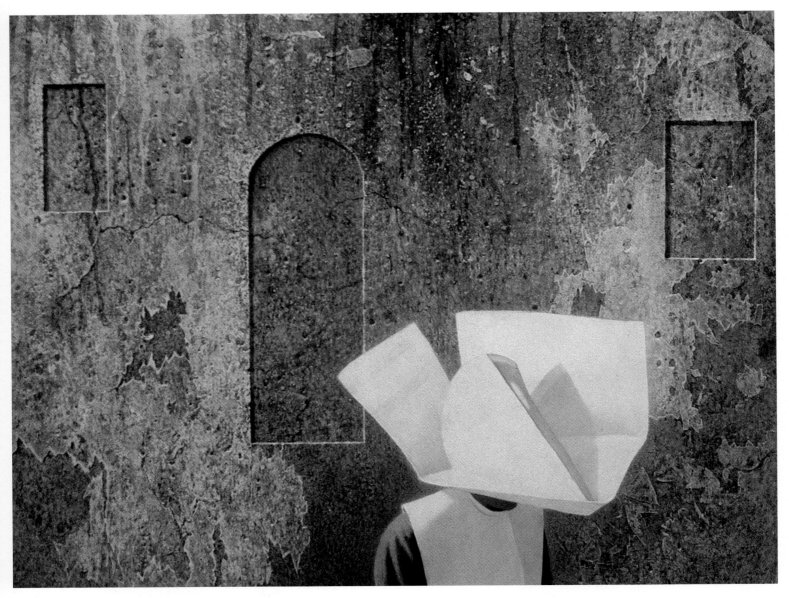

Robert Vickrey, *Nun,* painting. Copyright Robert Vickrey/licensed by VAGA, New York, NY.

As the 21st century rapidly approached, numerous questions were being raised in an attempt to guide health care policy toward greater social harmony, to alleviate social dilemmas created by competing sets of values, and to confront the realities of current health care economics. Instability, volatility, and incredible change were forcing a reexamination of societal values along with changing consumer expectations of health care. Those values of individualism, competition, cost containment, efficiency, and technology that were driving health care policy and health care systems were also influencing nursing's ability to provide quality care.

A look to the past demonstrates the evolving scene in nursing practice. In the 1960s and 1970s nurses were almost the exclusive providers of patient care. By the mid 1980s, diagnostic-related group reimbursement forced nurses to understand the necessity of cost containment and reduced the lengths of patient stay. Business and economics became the buzzwords as nursing care costs were coming under even closer scrutiny (Kalisch and Kalisch, 1995, 2004). As health care increasingly ran along business lines, competition occurred through mergers, acquisitions, and the expansion into new markets. What became clear was that quality of care was not the major focus of the competitiveness. Reduced revenues even led to a reduction in the registered nurse workforce as unlicensed assistive personnel were hired to reduce labor costs and act as nurse extenders. It became evident that new and creative approaches to health care and nursing care were needed.

THE HOSPITAL SCENE

A time of transition in health care institutions and health care in general was occurring. The issue of the allocation of scarce health-related resources had become almost paramount, leading to serious ramifications for institutions, health care personnel, and consumers around the globe. Ethical questions of the past had been related to affluence; the problems of today deal with scarcity. Yet efforts to control costs have been erratic, with various reasons given to explain high costs. Initially, the problem of rising hospital costs was attributed to poor management. Why was it that an individual could obtain better service in a hotel or in a restaurant at a lower cost? In the 1960s the rise of health care

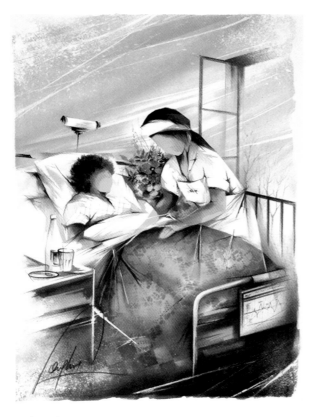

Raymond Poulet, *L'Infirmiere, (The Nurse)*, 1984, lithograph, 375 × 275 mm, France. Copyright Raymond Poulet, 1984. Reproduced by permission of the artist. Photograph courtesy of Idbury Prints Ltd.

costs was drastically influenced by what were referred to as thousands of "small-ticket" items, such as new laboratory tests and radiological examinations. The emergence and dissemination of "big-ticket" items, such as computerized axial tomography scans, lasers, transplantations, and nuclear magnetic resonance imaging devices accounted for increased costs in the 1970s and 1980s. More and more health care institutions were turning to business, industry, and the marketplace for the answers to managing costs. Debates about health care reform, decreasing revenues, and strategies for change continued throughout the world. But one thing remained clear: resultant changes in health care affected and will affect nurses financially, environmentally, and clinically, and they present one of the greatest challenges nurses have ever faced.

Historically and traditionally, the majority of sick and injured people were cared for by families. Eventually, early hospitals emerged that provided services for those who had no homes or families, including orphans, soldiers, travelers, the impoverished, nuns and monks (religious orders), and in some cases the insane. These early hospitals functioned in a variety of roles—as hostels, hotels, and hospitals in which care was primarily custodial and religiously motivated. Consequently, the caregivers were primarily men and women with religious callings.

During the time of the Reformation, another change in the hospital structure took place. As previously discussed and using England as an example, the religious orders were suppressed and the hospital became a secular institution. Other events occurred in the 18th century, such as the industrial revolution, the migration of populations to cities, and changes in the workplace environment and family structures, which necessitated further expansion of hospital systems to care primarily for the poor, but this time, the urban

poor. Even with the establishment of Nightingale's St. Thomas School of Nursing in the 19th century, hospitals were still sanctuaries for those devoid of family care, for the mentally ill, and for the poor (Bullough and Bullough, 1984). Hospitals were not numerous and were essentially insignificant because no "respectable" person entered them for treatment. In fact, a saying arose that stated that "people left the hospitals wearing only 'wooden pajamas,'" referring, of course, to wooden coffins. The wealthy continued to be cared for at home for a number of reasons, including available financial resources. In Rosenberg's analysis (1987) of the evolution of American hospitals, his description of the internal structure of hospitals during this time is enlightening:

> It (the hospital) was in its internal structure a very different institution from what we know in the late twentieth century. It was not directed by a bureaucracy of credentialed administrators; it was certainly not dominated by the medical profession and its needs. Lay trustees still felt it their duty to oversee every aspect of hospital routine. The hospital was very much a mirror of the society that populated and supported it, a society rooted in deference and hierarchy, a society in which traditional attitudes toward the responsibility of wealth were very much alive. Medical men needed and used the hospital; they could not control it (p. 5).

With the advent of the 20th century, major changes occurred and continued in hospitals throughout the century. Hospitals grew in size, spread widely, became more formal and bureaucratic, and began treating not only the indigent but also the wealthy and respectable. Increasingly, families began to rely on strangers for care during sickness and death. This occurred in part because the hospital environment had radically changed. Nursing had a significant part in this evolution. According to Rosenberg, "Perhaps the most important single

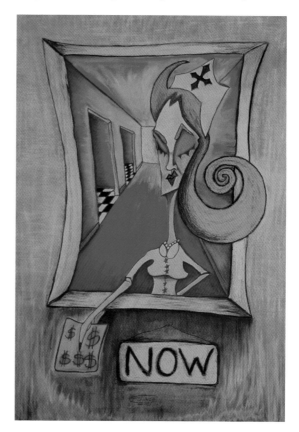

Jennifer Hlavach, *Got Insurance?*, 2005, painting, 24" × 36", artistrising.com.

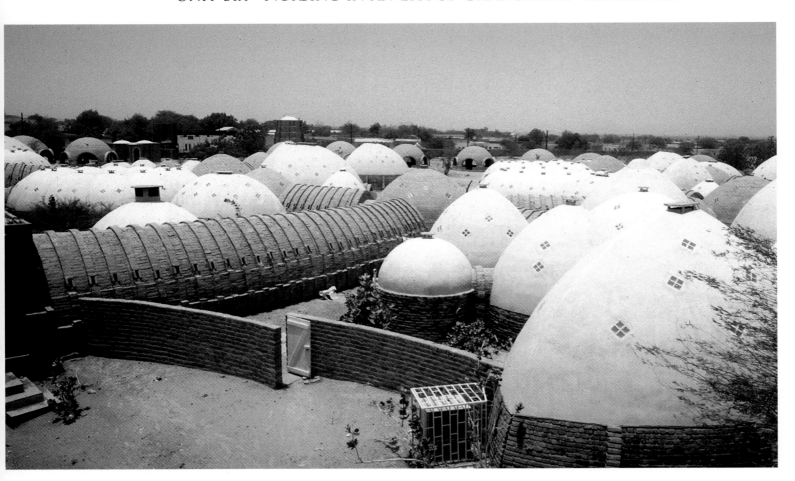

The Kaedi Regional Hospital is the largest health facility located near the border of Senegal, a remote sector in Mauritania and one known for its innovative architecture. It was built to provide health care facilities, especially for the rural people who suffered immensely due to lack of hospitals in their areas. The hospital involves the use of handfired, locally made brick and a design based on a sequence of simple and complex dome structures. The structure was made in such a way that the hospital remains naturally cool even with significant light from outdoors. The wards are donut shaped to provide ample cross ventilation; their petal-like corridors serve as isolation zones. The hospital is sophisticated but low-tech and won the Aga Khan Award for Architecture in 1995.

Kaedi Regional Hospital, 1989, photograph, Mauritania, image found on Archnet.org, Kamran Adle/Aga Khan Trust for Culture.

element in reshaping the day-to-day texture of hospital life was the professionalization of nursing. In 1800, as today, nurses were the most important single factor determining ward and room environment. Nursing, like professional hospital administration and changed modes of hospital financing, has played a key role in shaping the modern hospital" (1987, pp. 8-9). In addition, many decisions that shaped modern hospitals were directly related to medical ideas and values.

Events such as childbirth that had occurred in the home moved into the hospital; medical specialties emerged and escalated. Hospitals no longer remained charitable institutions; they often became profit-making institutions, particularly with the evolution of health insurance and government intervention. The hospital eventually became synonymous with high-level technology and bureaucracy; the alleviation of pain and suffering—and potentially cure—was rendered at enormous economic and emotional cost.

New organizational and administrative structures, job restructuring, shorter hospital stays, greater patient acuity, the rise of consumerism, and mergers were reshaping health care and hospitals. Hospital closures and downsizing (the negative connotation of the term *downsizing* is one factor that at one time led to the use of the term *rightsizing*) were occurring in the face of cost-containment pressures and a shrinking hospital industry, even in countries that had national health care systems. There was a trend toward privati-

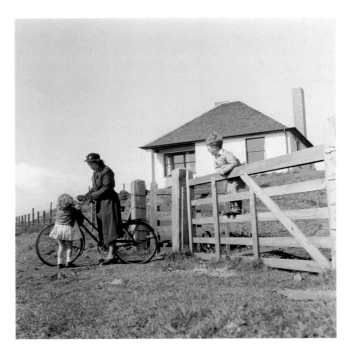

A district nurse, who works in the remote Scottish Highlands and outlaying islands, visits patients on her rounds, 1955.

Taconis, *Nurse of the Islands,* 1955, photograph.

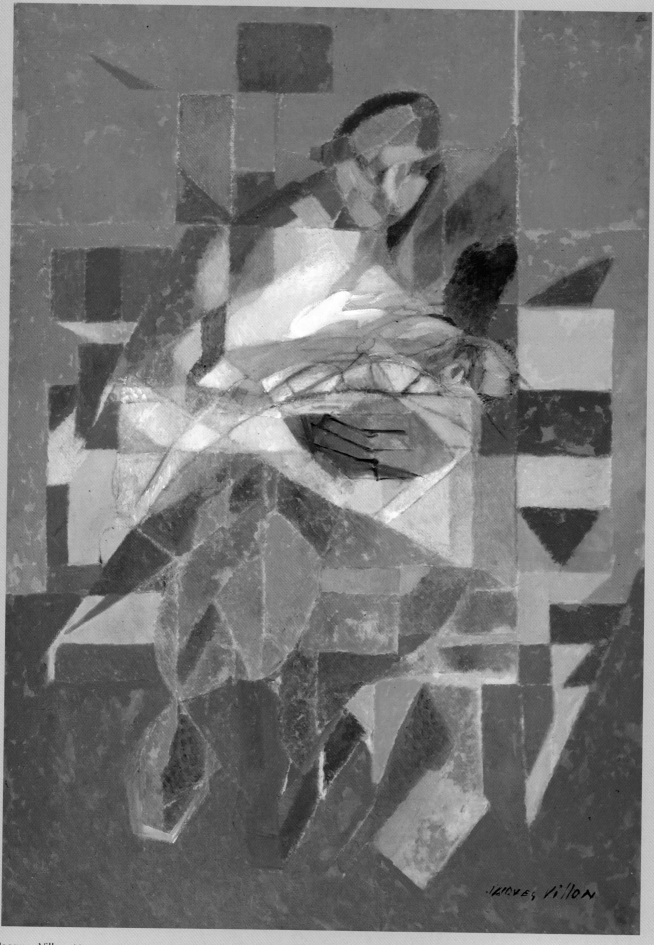

Jacques Villon, *Maternite*, 1948, oil on canvas, 146 × 96.5 cm, gift of Mr. and Mrs. Ira Haupt, collection of the Haggerty Museum of Art, Milwaukee, WI.

zation in Norway and the United Kingdom as a result of issues of efficiency and provision of services to low-income immigrant workers from developing countries. Canada was facing a major issue of hospital restructuring and closure in addition to the requirement of developing a more comprehensive primary health care service (Buchan, 1993). Regionalization occurred in New South Wales; the state was divided into 12 regions. Further subdivision occurred, leading to the establishment of 23 local health services under the Area Health Services Act of 1986 in which ". . . hospitals and other health care agencies within a defined geographical area are to be grouped together under one management board" (Duffield, 1988, p. 127). Integrated health care systems were on the rise.

The primary shift from inpatient to ambulatory care resulted in the need to develop new strategies for providing adequate, high-quality patient care. With the reduction in inpatient days, home-delivered medical and nursing services were becoming vital components of the system. Corresponding to that development, the nursing shortages of the 1980s gave way to a situation in which experienced nurses and new graduates were having difficulty finding employment.

THE MANAGED CARE REVOLUTION

The movement toward managed care as a method of solving the issue of high health care costs began in the early 1990s, although it was pioneered in the mid-1930s. In this early stage of its development, emphasis was not on cost containment. Managed care was seen as a system for organizing care and providing comprehensive coverage, not just as a strategy for financial control. The potential cost-saving aspect of the plan was to be the outcome of an efficiently run system that incorporated a full range of services, continuity of care, emphasis on prevention, and early intervention. The original Kaiser ship-building company initiated managed care in response to employee health care concerns during World War II. Kaiser developed a health care plan for his employees that provided a comprehensive range of services, from prevention to acute care. With this early approach, Kaiser's company ran its own hospitals and clinics and employed physicians, nurses, and other providers of care (Himali, 1995). This type of primary health care service was predicated on early entry into the system for the treatment of small problems before they became large ones. Enrollees were enticed by low monthly premiums and convenient, accessible medical centers.

The early Kaiser prototype of managed care is no longer the only model; various forms have emerged, and in many cases they minimally resemble the original concept. Few are currently operating according to the original principles and strategies of managed care. The following are familiar types:

- Health Maintenance Organization (HMO): Composed of hospitals and allied clinics; patients are enrolled as members for a fixed fee per year and receive all necessary health care services. They are usually organized in a specific geographical area.
- Preferred Provider Organization (PPO): Health care financing and delivery program comprising a group of providers, such as hospitals and physicians, under contract with a private indemnity insurance company for services on a fee-for-service basis. Customers use a select group of providers and pay less for services.

- Independent Practice Association (IPA): Similar to an HMO in which physicians who are not salaried employees of the plan contract to provide services at a discounted fee. Physicians share risks and profits through an incentive system designed to achieve high standards of quality and remain within the budget.
- Point of Service System: Similar to an HMO; members are permitted to go outside the system to physicians not in the plan's network. Depending on the system, however, a patient using an outside provider may pay a percentage of the medical bill with a potentially high deductible.

— *KALISCH AND KALISCH, 2004; STREEF, 1994*

These models of managed care have had a profound, rapid influence on both the private insurance market and governmental insurance programs (Medicare and Medicaid) in the United States. In fact, many areas of the country are now dominated by managed care, whereas other areas are attempting to follow suit. It will be interesting to observe the effect of managed care on other countries; will they begin to incorporate some of the principles into their own health care systems in the face of a significant number of pressures? Failure to manage health care effectively may lead to further crises and the collapse of systems. Organizational transformation appears to be the only solution and with it the challenge to nurses worldwide.

There is no doubt that the massive shift toward managed care had a major impact on nursing. The nursing profession and the practice field were being bombarded from all sides by global, geopolitical, social, demographic, epidemiological, technological, political, and industrial forces. Crosstraining of personnel, increased use of assistive personnel, and the emergence of new classes of workers were occurring at rapid rates (Styles, 1993). Yet most nurses would agree that managed care is good in principle and in practice if focused on high quality and primary health care services. But as hospital restructuring and downsizing escalated, managed care was being used as the rationale for employing fewer nurses for patient care and hence for layoffs and job losses. Was it only a few years earlier that hospitals had been

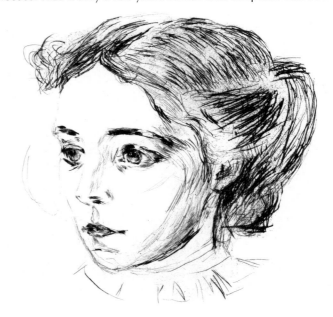

Edvard Munch, *The Nurse,* 1908-1909, drypoint on copperplate, 20.4 × 14.4 cm, Munch Museum, Oslo, Norway, Munch Museum/Munch Ellingsen Group/ARS 2009.

wooing nurses with cash and material bonuses? This was a bitter pill for nurses to swallow as they observed hospitals acquiring new equipment, continuing construction projects, and increasing the salaries of chief executive officers and increasing numbers of administrators. Even more alarming was the lack of emphasis on high-quality patient care.

In response to this dramatic reversal more than 25,000 registered nurses marched in protest in Washington, D.C., on March 31, 1995 (Himali, 1995; McCrary, 1995). This was the first-ever national demonstration by nurses. It was the brainchild of Laura Gasparis Vonfrolio, owner and publisher of *Revolution: The Journal of Nurse Empowerment,* and was co-sponsored by the American Nurses' Association (ANA). As the nurses marched down Pennsylvania Avenue, members of Congress met in the U.S. Capitol with approximately 200 nurses. Several state nurses' associations staged their own rallies in support of the march on Washington. The purpose of the demonstration was not only to cite job cuts but also to protest the erosion of care in health care institutions. A strong message was sent to the public and to Congress concerning measures that had reduced the number of registered nurses caring for patients and creating, in many instances, an unsafe environment.

In the face of adversity, nurses acted in the role of advocates, even though some jeopardized their professional careers to attend. A number of hospitals had sent out memos prohibiting their nurses from taking time off on the day of the rally. Using a variety of strategies, however, nurses engaged in activities that demonstrated the critical link between nurses at the bedside and safe, high-quality care. State rallies and walks, press conferences, position statements, collective bargaining, and political involvement were all being used to strengthen nursing's position in health care delivery and to assume a proactive stand.

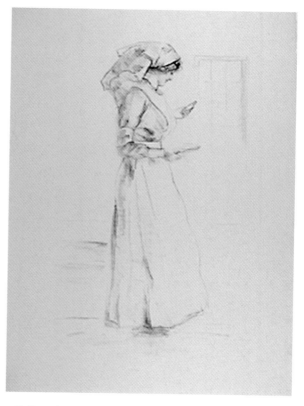

Albert Belleroche, *The Nurse,* 1877, lithograph, 24⁵⁄₁₆" × 17¹⁄₁₆", Harvard Art Museum, Fogg Art Museum, gift of George C. Kenney, M23018. Photo: Imaging Department, copyright President and Fellows of Harvard College.

CASE MANAGEMENT AND CRITICAL PATHS

The term *managed care* in and of itself can be confusing at times. The term is frequently used to indicate health care plans in concert with facilities that are designed to contain the costs of services while upholding the quality of care. Emphasis is on the achievement of specific patient outcomes within a fiscally responsible time frame. In other instances *managed care* is used to indicate a nursing model for patient care. In addition, *managed care* and *case management* are often used synonymously in the health care and nursing literature. Perhaps one of the more concise and comprehensible definitions of *managed care* is the following:

> Managed care is unit-based care that is organized to achieve specific patient outcomes within fiscally responsible time frames (length of stay) while utilizing resources that are appropriate in amount and sequence to the specific case type and to the individual patient. Outcomes are the patients' discharge conditions, stated in measurable terms, that result from the activities of nurses, physicians and other health care providers. The term *unit* refers to the geographic area in which the patient receives care. The focus of managed care is on redesigning tools and systems; the outcomes and processes of care are identified on a daily basis; hourly in areas such as the Emergency Room or the Operating Room; by visit in ambulatory settings. This facilitates identifying those patients who are deviating from the expected early enough to take corrective action.
>
> — BOWER, 1988, P. 1

It was clear that a new language had been created and that nurses, particularly those in advanced practice, needed to understand it. But even more crucial was the question of whether managed care had been a panacea for the ills of health care.

Managed care provided an even greater impetus for the increased use of case management as a mechanism for the coordination and sequencing of care. Case management is not a new phenomenon, but it emerged as a direct link to cost containment through the creation of an environment that attempts to control the quality and cost of patient care. Historically it has been used by a number of entities, including social service agencies, insurance companies, rehabilitation centers, and public health nursing as a means of community service coordination. Although psychiatric and mental health nurses had used it for a number of years, it took some time for it to be incorporated into the practice of nurses in inpatient settings, including emergency care settings.

Confusion about the term *case management* may occur because it is referred to by terms that are often used interchangeably: service management, care coordination, and care management. Some of the same arguments related to the use of *patient* as opposed to *client* have surfaced here. To some, the label *case management* is not appropriate because a patient is not a case but a person or client who needs care. *Case management* may be described as a system, process, service, role, and even as a technology. It may be defined in a variety of ways, depending on the focus of the particular agency or institution. It is, however, broader in scope than the term *primary nursing* and can decrease fragmentation of care by crossing all departments.

Case management may involve many professional disciplines, including nursing, social work, mental health, and medicine. In fact, depending upon program policies and client needs, it is often preferable to have an interdisciplinary team participate in the planning and delivery of care. However, even if a team approach is used, one member of the team is usually designated as the case manager for a specific client. The manager then collaborates in the delivery of care with other professionals as well as family members, the client, and others providing services.

— *ANA, 1988*

Case management is built on the foundation of managed care. Theoretically, any individual who possesses the appropriate knowledge and skills could be a case manager because direct patient care might not be part of the role. It stands to reason, however, that physicians and nurses would be the most fitting managers because of their clinical expertise. Each organization, however, may put case management to use differently according to the environment. The nature of the population to be served seems to be the primary factor behind the designation of the case manager. Be that as it may, nurses are in a prime position to provide case management in collaboration with physicians. The nurse's self-satisfaction and sense of autonomy could only be enhanced by such an approach.

Tools considered essential for managed care and case management were also evolving. Critical paths or their next generation, CareMaps (trademark and concept of The Center for Case Management, South Natick, MA), briefly and concisely map the sequence and timing of key tasks and technical aspects of the treatment plan and provide the framework for planning patient care. Originally developed at New England Medical Center in Boston, where the Nursing Case Management Model was pioneered in 1980, the critical paths specify daily events, tasks, and interventions that caregivers must provide (Zander, 1994). In other words, care is structured by critical pathways; care is achieved through collaboration of health care professionals. Processes and outcomes defined by expert physicians, nurses, and other interdisciplinary team members for the "usual" patient are generally reviewed by the patient and family members, thereby ensuring that all involved individuals are operating with the same time frame and process information. Variances can, of course, occur and they mandate a review of the existing plan and revision of strategies for resolving the problem.

There are numerous intricacies and ambiguities in managed care, case management, and the use of critical pathways. Whether managed care is here to stay remains to be seen, but the emphasis on cost control and resource management will not disappear. Health care providers will continue to be asked to do more with less. To succeed in doing so, they will have to be more collaborative than ever and to remember constantly that case management belongs to no one. This can be a disastrous time or a time of unique opportunity for nurses. As Ralph Waldo Emerson concluded, "This time, like all times, is a very good one, if we but know what to do with it."

THE CHANGING SCENE IN NURSING

Numerous changes occurred in nursing throughout the course of the 20th century. The advent of new drugs, new techniques, and new technologies placed new responsibilities on nurses and mandated radical changes in nursing care. The patient care of today is of necessity different from that given at the time of Florence Nightingale because nurses are now expected to perform many tasks formerly performed by physicians. Before the 1930s few graduate nurses were employed by hospitals because most nursing care was given by nursing students. At that time nursing included a variety of nonnursing tasks, such as scrubbing floors, carrying trays, and cleaning equipment, in addition to the so-called routine care of patients. The students were left with relatively little time to give adequate nursing care—let alone incorporate a holistic approach to that care.

By the 1940s many more tasks and procedures were being performed by nurses as a result of the introduction of innovations in health care. Nurses' functions then included blood pressure measurement, suctioning in a variety of conditions, transfusion assistance, oxygen administration, medication injection, and other more sophisticated techniques. Nurses were also assisting in operating rooms, delivery rooms, and outpatient facilities.

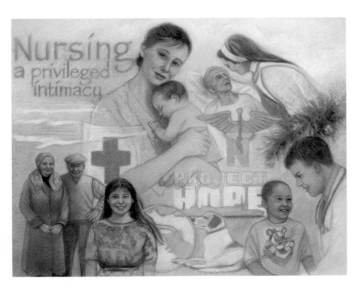

Mary Groth, *Nursing: A Privileged Intimacy,* 2008, pastel drawing, South Dakota Nurses Foundation.

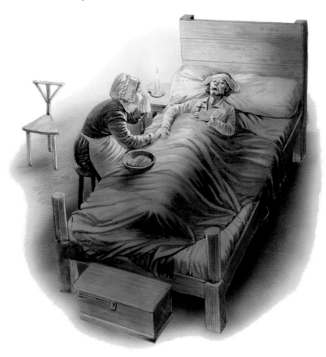

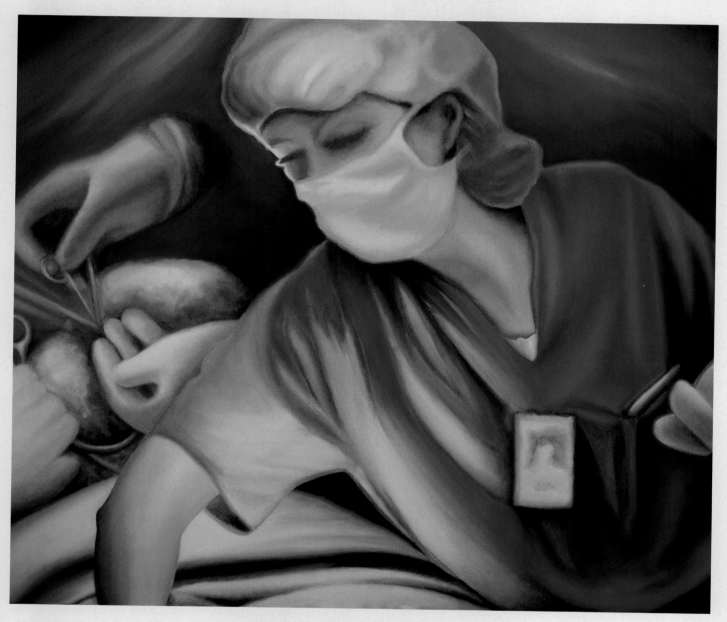

Hazel Mary Cope, *Scrub Nurse,* painting, www.arthives.com.

Facing page, A 17th-century woman sits in candlelight at the bedside of a sick man.

Peter Dennis, *Woman Nurses Sick Man.* Copyright Dorling Kindersley.

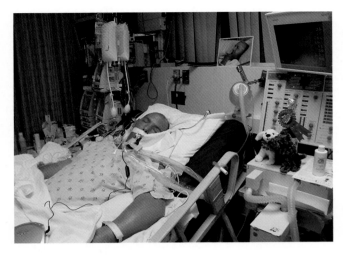

Chris Gregerson, *Marc in the ICU,* photograph.

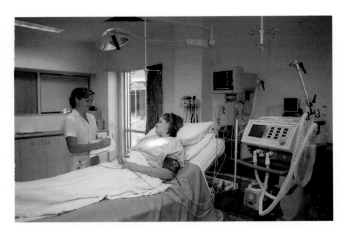

ICU, photograph. Courtesy of Bunbury Regional Hosptital, Western Australia.

More and more individuals were being admitted to hospitals for greater numbers of procedures as these institutions became safer and more efficient. This phenomenon was significantly enhanced by the advent of hospitalization insurance and prepayment plans for hospital care. In *Nursing for the Future,* Esther Lucile Brown reported that in one large teaching hospital more than 100 procedures (exclusive of surgical, obstetrical, and outpatient services) were being performed by nurses. This finding is substantiated by Dennison:

> [Nurses] managed the apparatus for Wangensteen suction, tidal irrigation, and bladder decompression. They irrigated eyes, cecostomies, colostomies, and draining wounds. They did artificial respiration, applied sterile compresses, and painted lesions. . . . They did catheterizations, sitz baths, and turpentine stupes. They gave insulin and taught the patient or his relatives to give the drug and examine urine. They administered approximately 1500 medications daily, by mouth or hypodermic. They assisted with lumbar punctures, thoracenteses . . . and phlebotomies.
>
> — DENNISON, 1942, P. 777

Nursing shortages occurred periodically throughout the 20th century. Even the belief that there would be an oversupply of nurses for civilian work after World War II was dashed. Many nurses stopped practicing to devote time to their family responsibilities. Many nurses did not return to practice, their answer to an authoritarian and paternalistic system in which they had no participation in the planning or decision making. Many refused to be involved in a work structure that offered few rewards, long hours, hard physical labor, and very low salaries.

Compounding this situation were other significant events that led to the gradual development of a new organizational pattern for hospital care. The demonstrated success of resuscitation stations on the front lines in World War II led to the emergence of special units for patient care. Postanesthesia and recovery rooms were established to prevent postoperative complications. Eventually this change was to transfer to a broader concept, the intensive care unit, after the use of Mobile Army Surgical Hospital units in the Korean conflict. The design of these units emphasized maximum efficiency and care delivery; they had "elevated, cen-

trally located nurses' desks to facilitate observation and one or two beds closed off by glazed partitions to provide quiet yet permit visual observation" (Haldemen and Abdellah, 1959, p. 40). By 1969 more than 50% of general hospitals had some type of intensive care unit (Stevens, 1989). Progression from the intensive care unit to the intermediate care, self care, long-term care, and home care units was thus possible. This concept of progressive patient care was set into motion and was in operation by the mid-1950s (Haldeman and Abdellah, 1959). However, the plan ultimately proved difficult to implement and financially challenging. There is no doubt that the development of specific types of units, although advantageous in many respects, created the need for specialized nursing skills and varying nurse-patient ratios in some areas, which contributed further to the nursing shortage.

As the ranks of nurses continued to diminish and new nursing demands increased, team nursing was introduced. This new and different method of assignment used fewer well-prepared personnel. It was designed to fit particular assignments to the background and expertise of the provider of service. In philosophic terms, team nursing was a system whereby different types of hospital nursing personnel could be placed into teams to provide high-quality nursing care for groups of patients. The professional nurse would directly supervise all patients and team members. In addition, team conferences would be held for planning and evaluation, nursing care plans would ensure continuity of care, and in-service education and on-the-job training would be provided as necessary (Lambertsen, 1953). However, the quality of nursing care and patient satisfaction diminished as fewer registered professional nurses were giving direct care to patients. The work was indeed coordinated, but the nursing care was fragmented. This was particularly disastrous as major advances in diagnostic and treatment procedures and the development of sophisticated technology continued. The 1950s and 1960s were a revolutionary time for health care:

> A sampling of major advances during the two decades includes the development of the heart-lung machine, openheart surgery, high-frequency implements for blood coagulation, and new vaccines, pharmaceuticals, and monitoring devices. The expanding field of medical science had made

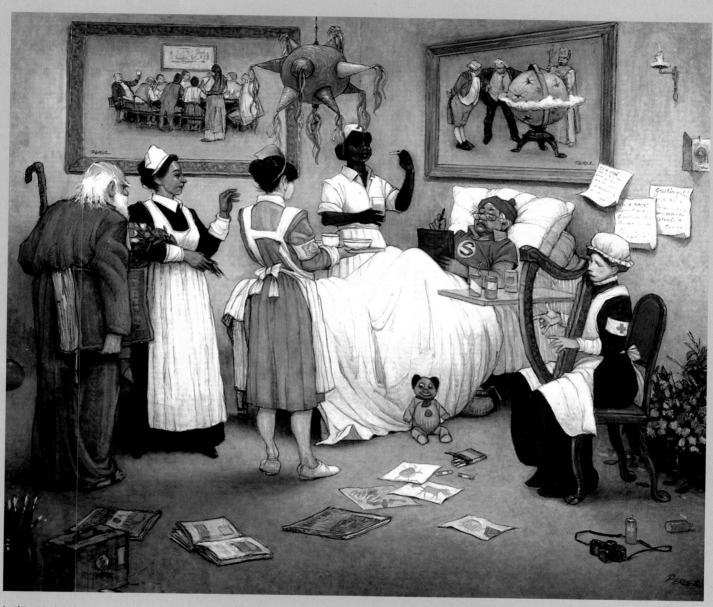

In this painting, Perez reinforces the notion that nursing is not merely a technique, but a process that incorporates the elements of soul, mind, and imagination. He has placed his nurses in a whimsical sickroom that symbolizes the child in all of us. Perez painted himself as the patient; the get-well card above the bed reads "Dear Jose."

Jose Perez, *The Nurse,* painting, WRS Group, Waco, TX.

nursing care increasingly more complex and had made demands of increasing gravity on nurses as well. To effectively give care, nurses needed to be able to identify very subtle changes in patients' status, learn new sophisticated treatment techniques, increase their ability to interpret laboratory data, recognize delicate physiological interrelationships, and closely monitor the efficacy of potent and sometimes experimental forms of drug therapy.

— *FITZPATRICK, 1983, PP. 34–35*

It became clear that a different approach to nursing care was needed, one that would provide both high quality and a holistic framework. A movement was begun in the 1960s to close the gap between the professional nurse and the patient. It was initiated as an important innovation in 1963 through the efforts of Lydia Hall, who was the inspiration behind the philosophy and work of the Loeb Center for Nursing and Rehabilitation at Montefiore Hospital in New York. The overall purpose of this center was to provide continuous, high-quality nursing care that emphasized the facilitation of healing, prevention of complications, promotion of health, and prevention of recurrences and new illnesses. Nursing care was given solely by professional nurses in a setting that enhanced the movement of the patient from the general hospital to home. The nurse was the primary factor in patient care and coordinated the combined efforts of the patient, the family, and the nurse in solving problems that might hinder ultimate recovery. Medicine and allied fields were viewed as ancillary treatment. In this structure the assumption was made that less medical care is needed; more professional nursing care and teaching were needed (Hall, 1963). Hall's philosophy that the nature of nursing promoted a therapeutic environment facilitating a patient's full recovery drove her model of Care (hands-on bodily care); Core (using the self in relationship to the pa-

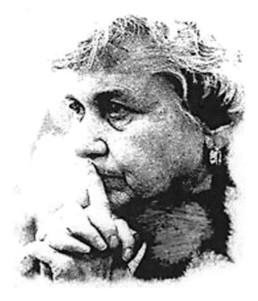

Ozzie Werner, adapted by Phillip Schwartzkopf, *Marie Manthey*, 2006, photograph, Creative Healthcare Management.

tient); and Cure (applying medical knowledge). Slowly, other such attempts were made by acute care hospitals under the guise of comprehensive, or total, nursing care. However, nurses were frustrated in their efforts by inadequate staffing, emphasis on efficiency, and lack of regard for patient orientation. In 1985, the focus of the Loeb Center was changed to the custodial care of a nursing home.

It was not until the 1970s that the combined goal of nursing care by professional nurses and total patient care (the holistic approach) began to be realized with the advent of primary nursing, a concept of Marie Manthey that was launched in 1969 (Manthey et al., 1970). The primary nurse was responsible for the patient's total care for the entire hospitalization period, 24 hours a day, 7 days a week. High-quality nursing care was promoted through this modality because the primary nurse assumed responsibility for the entire spectrum of functions, including teaching; consultation; comprehensive care with continuity, planning and evaluation of care; documentation of progress; discharge planning; and referrals to ancillary services or agencies (Marram, Barrett, and Bevis, 1979). When the primary nurse was not physically present, an associate nurse followed the plan of care. In this system nurses truly could be patients' advocates, they could be accountable for their own practice, and they could make decisions based on available data.

Although primary nursing had grown in popularity since its inception, its success depended on adequate staffing, administrative support, and technically and educationally prepared nurses. It was received favorably by patients, and it was hoped that it would gain total recognition and acceptance by health care delivery systems. Where it was tried, it succeeded and still has value in the delivery of care today. The best argument for its implementation was that it had the greatest potential for placing the patient in an environment conducive to the attainment of wellness. Primary nursing's greatest threat was the downsizing of hospital nursing staffs, which interfered with the nurse-patient association.

Some primary nurses began to engage in private practice or to share a private practice with a physician. One such independent practitioner, M. Lucille Kinlein, hung out her shingle in May 1971. Others engaged in various alternative

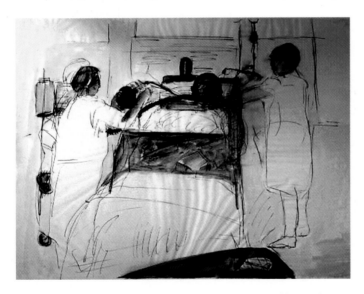

Two days later, the nurse on the Burn Intensive Care Ward told me, "The 75% burn patient, 36 years old, he's better than on Friday." I went to the twelfth floor where I had seen him last. Then I came down to the Emergency Room to get my drawing paper to draw the nurses bathing him. I hadn't taken my paper at first, as I did not expect to find him alive. The residents all thought that he would be gone by now, too, and were reassured by the news.
Red, raw tissue on his face and front and back, like a roasted pig! Even though they knew he would die, the nurses treated him so gently.
—*May Lesser*

May Lesser, Image from The Art of Caring.

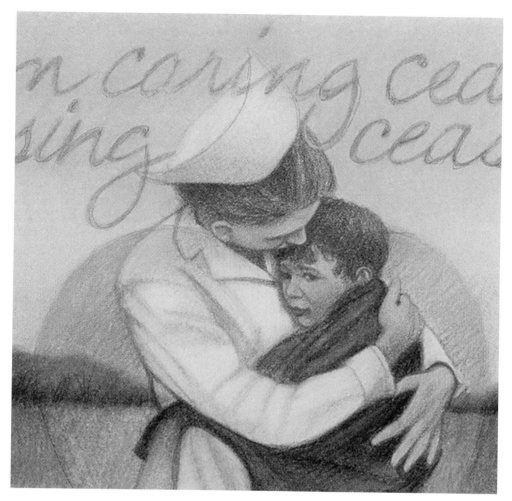

Mary Groth, *Caring to Heal: When Caring Ceases, Nursing Ceases*, 2000, pastel on paper.

methods of care. For example, Dr. Delores Krieger, a professor of nursing at New York University, repopularized the theory of therapeutic touch. She achieved national recognition for her expertise in this area and taught many nurses and other individuals to use this therapy.

Although great strides have been made in nursing, problems continue. Working conditions and environments are still sources of conflict. Nurses continue to voice their concerns regarding inadequate staffing; low wages; long hours; unsafe practices; nurses' inability to use their own knowledge, judgment, and decision-making abilities; and other circumstances that prohibit the rendering of high-quality nursing care. When all attempts at communication have failed, nurses have turned to organization through local units of the state professional organization or other types of bargaining units.

Nurses of today are expected to be many things to many people and to function in a variety of settings. They are to be excellent caregivers, adequate researchers, seekers of knowledge, and thinkers grounded in scientific and logical thought. Nurses are involved with scientific and technical advances and with all types of new roles that have broadened their opportunities but increased the scope of their responsibilities. They are slowly but steadily moving toward a goal of holistic treatment for all individuals in a structure that is not always supportive. Nurses will continue to meet the challenges of the future that were identified by Florence Nightingale:

No system can endure that does not march. Are we walking to the future or to the past? Are we progressing or are we stereotyping? We remember that we have scarcely crossed the threshold of uncivilized civilization in nursing; there is still so much to do. Don't let us stereotype mediocrity. We are still on the threshold of nursing.

In the future, which I shall not see, for I am old, may a better way be opened! May the methods by which every infant, every human being will have the best chance of health, the methods by which every sick person will have the best chance of recovery, be learned and practiced! Hospitals are only an intermediate state of civilization never intended, at all events, to take in the whole sick population.

— *NIGHTINGALE, 1860*

NURSING RESEARCH

Nursing research is new, yet old. Florence Nightingale is generally regarded by some as the first nurse researcher because her nursing reforms were based on careful investigation. Undoubtedly one of the first research reports ever written by a nurse was "Notes on Matters Affecting the Health, Efficiency and Hospital Administration of the British Army" by Nightingale. It was hurriedly prepared within a year of her return from the Crimea in 1856 and she printed it privately for distribution among influential government officials and friends. This report combined the techniques of both qualitative and quantitative research. In 1000 pages

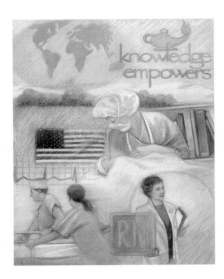

Mary Groth, *Knowledge Empowers,* 2008, pastel drawing, South Dakota Nurses Foundation.

she reported detailed observations of medicine and nursing in the Crimea and documented facts and figures with vital statistics.

In recognition of her great contribution to the field of social statistics, Nightingale was made a fellow in the Royal Statistical Society in 1858 and was granted an honorary membership in the American Statistical Society in 1874. Sir Francis Galton acknowledged her preeminence in statistics. Queen Victoria regretted that she could not have Nightingale, with her exceptional abilities, in the War Office. One author's comments illustrate her deep commitment to this field of endeavor:

> Miss Nightingale's attitude towards the application of statistics in the field of social dynamics was very similar to that of Thomas Buckle; they both deplored the fact that a wealth of data was available, but unapplied. Her typically practical philosophy demanded that if statistics were to be useful, they must be used. They must aid in the establishment of preventive measures. . . .
> Florence Nightingale was determined to make statistics an active reality which would influence the general welfare as well as the health of man. . . .
>
> — NEWTON, 1949, P. 33

Although the Nightingale tradition of education was transmitted to the United States, the approach to and use of research was not. The training schools in the United States were not conducive to the development of critical thinking or problem solving. Inquiring minds were not fostered by the prevailing atmosphere of rigid discipline and unquestioning obedience. These elements, which were strong influences in hospital nursing schools, reduced individualism, creativity, critical thinking, and assertiveness. They served to place students and graduate nurses in a subservient role, a position where they remained for many years. In some instances, even currently employed nurses believe that nursing is still held to a subservient role and that gains made to improve the situation are being consistently eroded.

The environment in which nursing operated was not conducive to nursing research, nor were nurses prepared with the skills to pursue it. Relatively few research studies in nursing were conducted in the United States before 1930. An exception was the work of Alice Magaw, who published

the first of her five research-based articles (1899, 1900, 1901, 1904, 1906) focusing on the effects of different anesthetics in 1899. Magaw had established herself as an exceptional nurse anesthetist, was renowned for administering 14,000 anesthetics without an anesthesia-related death, and was labeled the Mother of Anesthesia by Dr. Charles H. Mayo. Most remarkable for that time period was the fact that all of Magaw's articles reported specific anesthesia technique outcomes and were published in medical journals (Harris, 2006, p. 39).

In that era, nursing was helplessly swept along by rapid hospital expansion and the proliferation of hospital (diploma) training schools for nurses. These insistent demands pushed the need for studies into the background. It was also during this time that professional nursing organizations had their beginnings. It is no wonder that the early leaders were thus diverted from independent research and writing to the improvement in the training of nurses and organizational activities.

The need for nursing research was recognized by early nursing leaders, who were committed to the scientific method of collecting and interpreting data to generate new knowledge for the improvement of nursing care. Probably the earliest American research report was *The Educational Status of Nursing* (1912) written by M. Adelaide Nutting. A comprehensive analysis of nursing during this period, the report revealed the appalling practices and conditions under which student nurses functioned. Other reports followed during the first half of the 20th century, as did studies of nursing practice, nursing services, nursing education, nursing service administration, and virtually every field related to nursing. **The majority of these were done by individuals who were not nurses.**

Early leadership ability in the area of nursing research was demonstrated by Isabel M. Stewart. Although her activities and interests in this area were not widely known, they were nonetheless significant. Intrigued by time-and-motion studies related to the improvement of efficiency in industry and home economics, Stewart began to investigate the potential of this technique when applied to nursing. She visited Dr. and Mrs. Frank Gilbreth, who set up beds in the living room of their home in Providence, Rhode Island, for use as a laboratory.

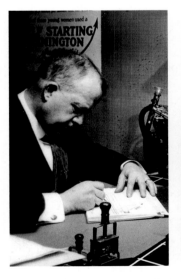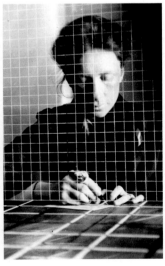

Frank Gilbreth, Sr., was a pioneer in the field of motion study and often used his family as guinea pigs (with amusing and sometimes embarrassing results).

Frank Bunker Gilbreth and *Lillian Moller Gilbreth*, photographs, Frank and Lillian Gilbreth Library of Management, Purdue University.

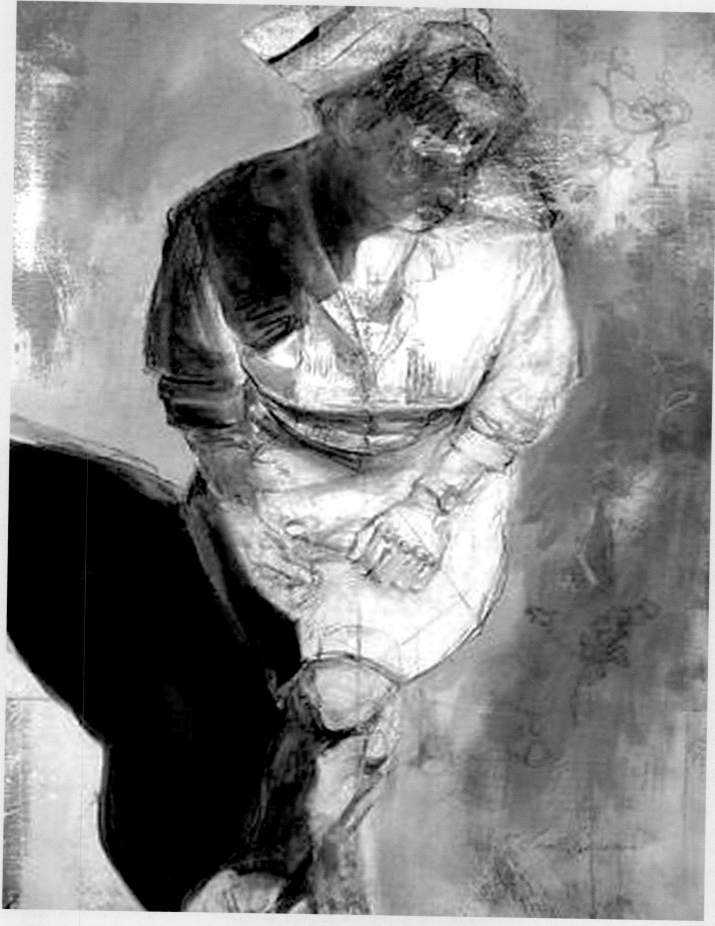

Therese Cipiti Herron, *Eclipse,* 2005, oil, 12″ × 12″.

This was the beginning of Isabel Stewart's attempt to set up an activity analysis of nursing that would differentiate between nursing and nonnursing functions. This minimal study still provides standards of nursing care that are useful in current nursing practice. From this meager beginning Stewart continued her pursuits and conducted research in nursing and nursing education. She studied philosophical, educational, and historical research methods and incorporated them into her books and other writings. Eventually she published the *Teachers College Nursing Education Bulletin*, possibly the first research journal in nursing. This was done in the face of opposition from other nurses, whose concept of research was limited to test-tube methods. In an editorial in 1929, Isabel Stewart explained her position:

> If nursing is ever to justify its name as an applied science, if it is ever to free itself from these old superficial, haphazard methods, some way must be found to submit all our practices as rapidly as possible to the most searching tests which modern science can devise. Not only bacteriological and physiological and chemical tests are needed, but economic and psychological and sociological measurements also, if they are appropriate and workable. There is not much use waiting for someone outside our own body to recognize our critical situation and to offer to do the work for us. Some help may be secured from physicians and from experts in other fields, but most of the experimentation that is done will have to be carried on in all probability by our own members. Nurses may not be prepared to make the more difficult studies at once, but if a few will prepare themselves to start in a small way and to show what can be done, others will undoubtedly become interested, and in time, resources will be found, if the results warrant them.
>
> — STEWART, 1929, P. 3

Stewart firmly believed that students should be oriented toward research, and she involved them in studies and projects that were needed or were under investigation. Thus she incorporated research training into the program of graduate study in nursing education. She recognized, however, that not all individuals were fit for investigation, so she proposed that a few minds could take a lead in such activities. With that goal in mind, Stewart consistently urged that graduate students have more advanced preparation in research. Student reaction was positive, as described by McManus: "Inspired, prodded and encouraged by Miss Stewart, an increasing number of students did undertake doctoral study. Without her interest, support, and patient understanding, I know I could and would not have persevered toward that goal; I am sure this is true of many others of her students. . . . Miss Stewart laid the firm foundation for nursing research and research preparation in the Division of Nursing Education at Teachers College" (McManus, 1962, p. 6). As a lasting tribute to Stewart's impact on nursing research, in 1961 Teachers College opened a fund with the goal of receiving $400,000 to establish the Isabel Maitland Stewart Research Professorship in Nursing and Nursing Education.

A series of events that eventually transpired led to a decided commitment to the incorporation of nursing research into the overall structure of nursing. Sigma Theta Tau initiated a research fund in the 1930s to develop awareness of the need for research. The Association of Collegiate Schools of Nursing sponsored a special forum on nursing research in 1941. The House of Delegates of the ANA approved a research pro-

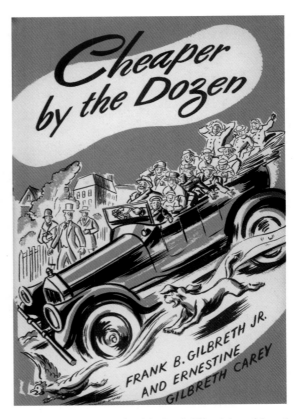

Cheaper by the Dozen is a 1948 book by Frank Gilbreth Jr. and Ernestine Gilbreth Carey that tells the story of time and motion study and efficiency expert Frank Bunker Gilbreth, his wife Lillian Moller Gilbreth, and their 12 children. It was adapted to film in 1950. The title comes from one of Gilbreth's favorite jokes that when he and his family were out driving and stopped at a red light, a pedestrian would ask "Hey, Mister! How come you got so many kids?" Gilbreth would pretend to ponder the question carefully, and then, just as the light turned green, would say "Well, they come cheaper by the dozen, you know," and drive off.

Donald McKay, *Cheaper by the Dozen,* book cover. Reprinted by permission of HarperCollins Publishers.

gram in 1950. This program was designed as a long-term research project to study (1) nursing functions in a variety of settings and geographical locations and (2) nurses' relationships with their coworkers and associates. Membership fees were used to fund these studies, which included interviews, activity classifications, and observational studies of nurses on the job. Teachers College established the Institute of Research and Service in Nursing Education during the early 1950s to provide a full-time mechanism for studying and developing nursing education through research.

The launching of the journal *Nursing Research* in 1952 was evidence of nursing's promotion of and communication of research and scholarly productivity. The first issue was sent to approximately 8000 subscribers across the United States and to 22 other countries. Increasing numbers of nursing researchers quickly adopted this journal as being necessary and basic reading. In 1955, the American Nurses Foundation was organized as a membership corporation of the ANA. The purposes of this foundation were to provide research grants to graduate nurses for scientific and educational projects; to conduct studies, surveys, and research; to provide grants to public and private nonprofit educational institutions; and to publish scientific, educational, and literary work. The ANA Board of Directors had donated $100,000 to the foundation specifically to be used during 1955 for studies of nursing functions. This donation was followed by the establishment of a Commission on Nursing Research

(1970) and a Council of Nurse Researchers (1972) by the ANA.

Government funds for nursing research began to be allocated at the end of World War II. Between 1940 and 1956, small grants were awarded to numerous individuals and institutions for various research projects through the Department of Health, Education and Welfare. An extramural grant program in nursing research was originated in the United States Public Health Service's Division of Nursing Resources in the fiscal year 1956. Monies were awarded to qualified researchers for projects in nursing. This was the first time grants from federal sources were made available for nursing research. Federal support of research training for nurses was also provided in a twofold approach: through special predoctoral fellowships established by the Division of Nursing Resources in 1954 and in 1962 through nurse-scientist graduate training grants to assist institutions with the development of nursing research competence and to provide stipends for graduate nursing students preparing for research. Finally, the integration of research into all nursing collegiate educational programs in the United States was accomplished in the 1970s.

The value of nursing research, which has already been demonstrated, will become even more important as nursing continues its march toward professional status and excellence in performance. Research has proven to be a mechanism for generating new nursing knowledge that will ultimately ensure the high quality of nursing care. A growing acceptance of nursing research as an effective method of cost containment has been recognized. The most efficient and effective modes of nursing can also be identified through nursing research. Overall, the recognition and acceptance of nursing research as significant to and valuable for the excellence of patient care and of health care in general has become internationally entrenched in the mission of nursing.

NURSING THEORY

Nursing has been one of several semiprofessions involved in extensive campaigns to achieve full professional status. One characteristic associated with established professions is the acquisition of a unique body of scientific knowledge through vigorous training. Discussions regarding the development of nursing theories that will assist in this generation of knowledge and assist in the definition and identification of the unique roles and functions of nursing have taken place since the middle 1960s and early 1970s. The origins of nursing theories, however, go back much further. Some individuals in nursing identify Florence Nightingale as the first nursing theorist. She, indeed, followed principles related to cleanliness, fresh air, good food, rest, sleep, and exercise. She was the first individual to define and describe nursing in her *Notes on Nursing: What It Is and What It Is Not.* She did have significant thoughts, ideas, and principles, although at times they were disjointed. Yet one must systematically analyze them according to defined criteria to establish whether they constitute a theory.

The struggle to identify clearly a unique knowledge base for nursing (nursing science) has been continuous, particularly in relation to defining and describing the functions of nursing. Definitions of these functions were published by the ANA in 1932, 1937, and 1955. However, they lacked specificity and prompted individual nurses to write their own.

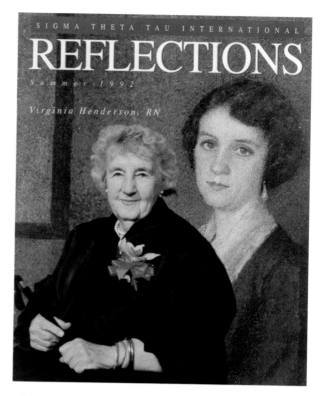

O. Y. Thomas, *Virginia Henderson,* photograph, Sigma Theta Tau International. Used with permission from the Honor Society of Nursing, Sigma Theta Tau International.

Two of the pioneers in this area were Virginia Henderson and Hildegard Peplau. Henderson's definition of nursing was first published in 1955 and revised in 1966: "The unique function of the nurse is to assist the individual (sick or well) in the performance of those activities contributing to health or its recovery (or to peaceful death) that he would perform unaided if he had the necessary strength, will, or knowledge. And to do this in such a way as to help him gain independence as rapidly as possible" (Henderson, 1966, p. 15).

In 1952, Peplau published *Interpersonal Relations in Nursing,* which described four phases of the nurse-client relationship and led to numerous studies in the communication area. She brought interpersonal theories from psychiatry into nursing as a basis for the analysis of these interactions in terms of therapeutic quality. It is possible that this work was one of the first proposed theoretical frameworks for nursing. Ida J. Orlando (1961) offered communications theory for the description of what she labeled "a deliberate nursing approach." Imogene M. King (1971) later began to explain the intricate transactional process between nurse and patient.

A significant catalyst in the movement for the development of nursing theory was Martha E. Rogers, whose work was a vivid testimony for nursing to be recognized as a science:

> The science of nursing is an emergent—a new product. The inevitability of its development is written in nursing's long commitment to human health and welfare. With today's rapid and unprecedented changes, new urgency has been added to the critical need for a body of scientific knowledge specific to nursing. Only as the science of nursing takes on form and substance can the art of nursing achieve new dimensions of artistry.
>
> The science of nursing aims to provide a body of abstract knowledge growing out of scientific research and logical analysis and capable of being translated into nursing practice.
>
> — *ROGERS, 1970, PP. 83, 86*

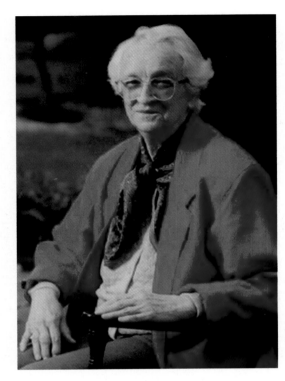

Hildegard Peplau, photograph.

The need for and development of nursing theories were prominent issues in the 1970s. The idea that a unique body of knowledge is an essential quality of a profession was embraced by scholars (Styles, 1982), giving credence to the issue of theory development. Several theories and conceptual frameworks emerged through the diligence of such individuals as Sister Callista Roy, Martha E. Rogers, Imogene M. King, Dorothea Orem, and Margaret A. Newman. There are numerous other nurses who have developed conceptual frameworks and theories that are equally important to nursing's knowledge development, but space limitations prohibit discussing all of them here. A question still posed by some in nursing, however, is whether any of these are indeed theories or whether they are all conceptual frameworks. Indeed, many of the nurses who fall into the category of theorist do not consider themselves theorists, nor did they intend to develop a theory. Tomey (1994) clustered the theorists into the following categories, which are particularly useful for the analysis and synthesis of their work: philosophies (analysis, reasoning, and logical argument used to identify nursing phenomena); conceptual models, or grand theories (broad in scope and usually requiring further specificity and distribution of theoretical statements for empirical testing and verification); and, nursing theories in the middle range (more precise than grand theories that focus on developing theoretical statements to answer questions about nursing).

Nursing is progressing in its quest to be recognized as a legitimate science, but a continuing momentum is necessary to achieve this goal. Early nursing theorists represent a phase in the development of nursing theory but clinical nursing and clinical nursing research may prove more important to the advancement of nursing, including its practice, education, and administration. The united efforts of nurse scholars and practitioners of nursing are needed to assist in the identification of a knowledge base for nursing and to formulate a theory or theories to validate professional practice. There is no doubt that differing conceptualizations of nursing will contribute to its ongoing evolution

and will enrich the discipline's knowledge of the environment, health, human beings, and nursing.

EDUCATIONAL ADVANCEMENT

The history of education in nursing at the master's level is rather vague because information about these programs was not available until the middle of the 20th century. What is known about the earlier programs is that they differed in organization and structure, varied in requirements, admitted students at differing times throughout the year, and used a variety of labels. Even more significant, initially all the postdiploma programs were considered postgraduate education and were identified as such. Therefore it was difficult to differentiate among some baccalaureate and master's level programs.

The growth of nursing education programs in universities sparked graduate study in nursing. The lack of nurses prepared for teaching and administrative positions was apparent, and the need to rectify this weakness was pressing. Master's degree programs were thus initiated and soon became viewed as the level for specialization in teaching and administration. Fitzpatrick (1983) described the following phases in this development that incorporate primary influences and changes.

Origins: 1939-1952. The phase of origins relates to the difficulty in tracing the development of nurse education programs. However, several important events were occurring. Baccalaureate programs of varying types were increasing in number. *Nursing for the Future* (1948) was published, and an accreditation system was established in 1949; both promoted the elucidation of the nature of collegiate education. An informal group of representatives from five New York schools was convened by R. Louise McManus. This group proposed baccalaureate education as the beginning level and master's level education as the specialized degree.

Transitional Stage: 1953-1964. It was during the 11 years of the transitional stage that the master's level was recognized as the advanced level of nursing education. A conference on graduate education was sponsored by the National League for Nursing (NLN) in 1954 and 1955. Guidelines were formulated for organization, administration, curriculum, and testing, and a Subcommittee on Graduate Education in Nursing (of the NLN) was created. The emphasis in content at the master's level vacillated and moved from clinical and functional role preparation in all programs for teachers, administrators, and clinical specialists to the elimination of double preparation in the late 1960s, as clinical specialization became extremely popular. A shift occurred once again in the 1980s, as the position in favor of double preparation gained momentum.

Regionalization. Regional planning in graduate education was begun in the 1950s with the development of two organizations: the Southern Regional Educational Board and the Western Interstate Commission on Higher Education. Both were committed to better nursing through strong master's degree programs to prepare faculty. The Western Interstate Commission for Higher Education in Nursing was begun in the western area of the country in 1955 to promote graduate and professional education in the health fields. These programs contributed greatly to graduate education that was research based.

Maturing of Education at the Master's Level: 1964-1975. Master's level education in nursing eventually matured and became an important credential for nurses in leadership

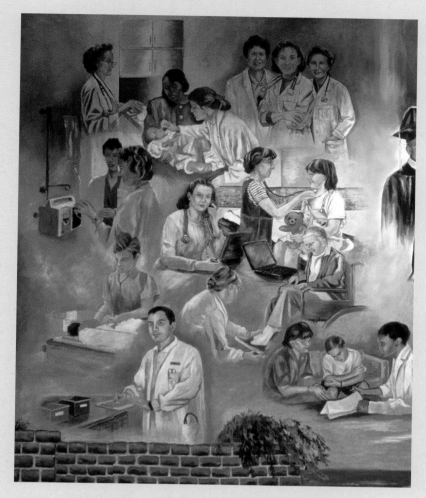

Ann Lyness, *Preparing Competent Graduates*, 2000, mural, 9′ × 25′, University of South Carolina College of Nursing.

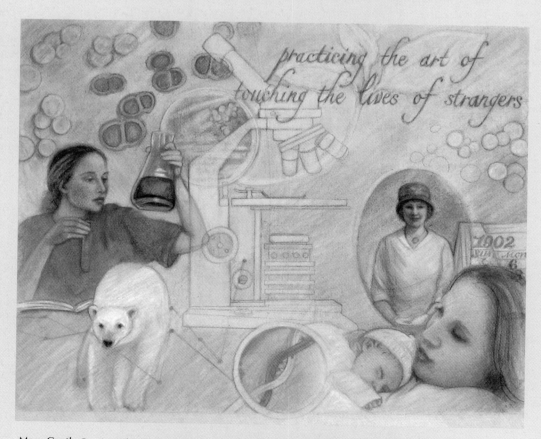

Mary Groth, *Practicing the Art of Touching the Lives of Others*, 2008, pastel drawing, South Dakota Nurses Foundation.

positions. Increased interest in research and an expanding number of graduate programs in clinical specialties occurred. The Nurse Training Act of 1964 (Title VIII of the Public Health Service Act, H.R. 10042) provided a comprehensive financial package for nursing school construction, faculty development, special projects grants, student loans, and merit scholarships. Between 1964 and 1971, sums exceeding $334 million were appropriated by Congress for nursing education.

Master's level graduate study became firmly entrenched in the structure of nursing education worldwide. Yet there were continuing discussions regarding both the purpose and the product of such an education. Consequently, the emphasis in content periodically shifts in relation to prevailing philosophies and theories, nursing care needs, social forces, technological advances, and health care reform. However, educational upgrading was apparent; the number of nurses attaining master's degrees rapidly increased.

Social forces that have affected the development of nursing have also influenced the development of doctoral education in nursing. Although the first graduate courses and graduate programs of study originated in 1899 at Teachers College, many years passed before a bona fide doctoral program came into being. The first doctoral program in nursing was initiated at Teachers College, Columbia University, in about 1920 and led to a doctorate in nursing education (Ed.D.). The evolution of additional programs was a slow process that was directly related to nursing's continuing struggle for respect, credibility, recognition, and power. One author has summarized the difficulty of this growth in the following way: "The evolution of the nursing profession has occurred within a political context that has placed many constraints upon the developmental process. Conflicts within administrative hierarchy, the effects of sexism, and circumscribed roles for women are but a few of the constraints. In this context, doctoral education for nurses and in nursing is but another step in the overall struggle for independence and recognition of worth" (Grace, 1978, p. 114).

Other factors inhibited rapid growth in doctoral preparation for nurses, including the following: nursing was perceived solely as a practice discipline; there was fear that nurses might become too knowledgeable and pose a threat to the medical hierarchy; a retarded growth in master's degree programs resulted in an inadequate pool of doctoral candidates until the 1960s; the nature, orientation, and direction of the nursing doctorate was not clearly defined; and a body of scientific knowledge was lacking.

In 1934, New York University followed Teachers College by offering doctorates in philosophy (Ph.D.) and education (Ed.D.) in nursing. In 1954, the University of Pittsburgh established a doctoral program in maternal-child nursing. The first doctorate in nursing science (D.N.S.) in psychiatric nursing was initiated at Boston University in 1960. Because there were so few doctoral programs in nursing before 1960, most nurses who sought doctoral preparation were forced to pursue degrees in other fields. Education was the most popular field; the natural, behavioral, and biological sciences were the other chosen areas of study. In 1964, the University of California-San Francisco established doctoral degrees in nursing science in several nursing specialties.

According to Styles (1977), the history of doctoral education divided itself into two logical components: the early years, which were dominated by doctoral education *for* nurses; and the current years, with their emphasis on doctoral education *in* nursing. This is consistent with Grace's discussion (1978) of the evolution of specific forms of doctoral programs in nursing. The first form was that of the functional specialty, with an emphasis on the methodologies and knowledge base necessary for teaching and administration. The second form involved preparation in basic scientific disciplines upon which the science and art of nursing rest. This movement was greatly enhanced by the nurse-scientist program of the federal government, in which grants were awarded to finance the education of nurses in closely related disciplines. The intent was for these graduates to return to faculty positions and provide input into basic science and research content in nursing. The third and current form is doctoral programs in nursing.

Two doctoral degree programs in nursing were offered: the Ph.D., or academic doctorate with emphasis on nursing research, and the D.N.S., or professional doctorate with emphasis on nursing practice. Disagreement continues as to which type best prepares a nurse to assume power and position and to exert influence in the health care system. Which better prepares a nurse for the generation and application of new knowledge? Which better enables a nurse to conduct and use nursing research? "Inasmuch as the problem also has plagued every other scholarly discipline and profession, the question of which is the appropriate doctoral degree for a nurse has never been found and continues to find little consensus" (Metarazzo and Abdellah, 1971, p. 404). Even more controversy would eventually occur as the nursing discipline ultimately contemplated a practice doctorate, the Doctor of Nursing Practice (DNP).

THE AGE OF SPECIALIZATION

The concept of nursing specialties was literally unheard of before the influence of Florence Nightingale and the advent of modern nursing. Each nurse was expected to provide for patients no matter what illness caused the need for nursing care. In hospitals, patients were not segregated according to disease until the early decades of the 20th century, when patients were placed in specific areas according to medical diagnoses. This change may have been the initiating factor in the movement toward specialization. Until World War II, most nurses worked as general staff nurses in hospitals, as public health nurses, and as private duty nurses, but the scientific and medical advances that were made during and after this war resulted in a vast body of knowledge that gave impetus to medical specialties. They were deemed necessary so that the knowledge could be used effectively and expanded.

Eventually the trend toward specialized care units gained momentum, and various nursing roles evolved. These roles became known as expanded roles and extended roles. Although the terms are frequently used interchangeably, there is a difference between the two. The term *extended role* refers to a physician extender with a cure orientation; the physician retains authority and decision-making power. The term *expanded role* is an expansion or broadening of care-oriented nursing in which the nurse collaborates with the physician when such collaboration is indicated in specific situations.

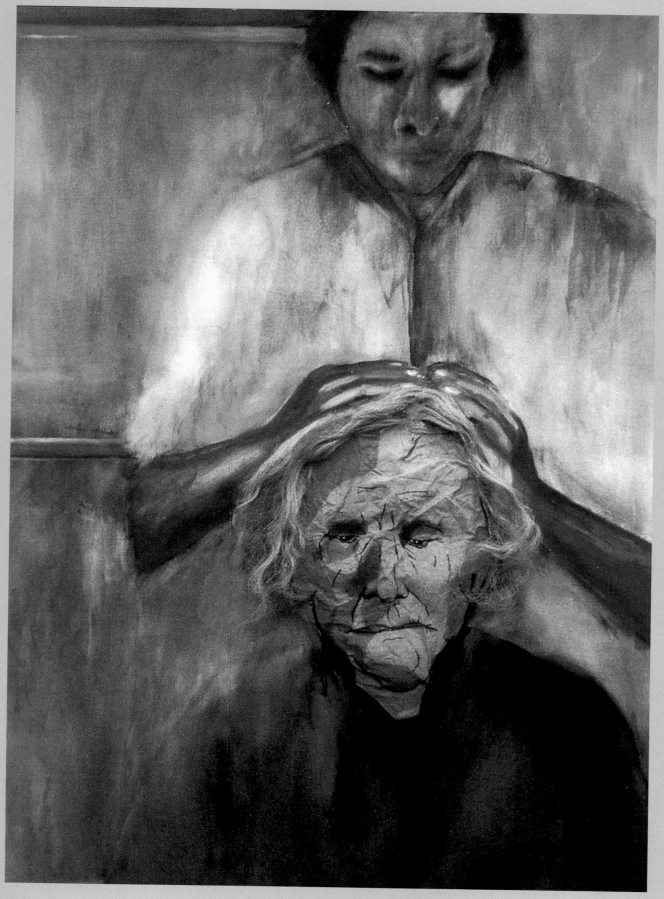

Painting celebrating Danish nurses.

Jorit Tellervo, *Untitled,* painting.

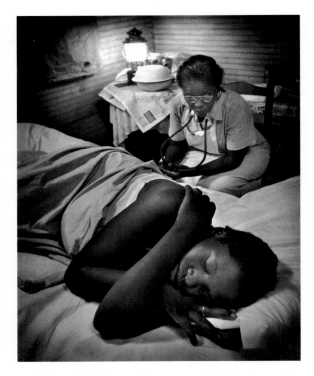

Nurse midwife Maude Callen attending to a woman in labor.

W. Eugene Smith, *Nurse/Midwife Maude Callen,* photograph.

Nursing specialists have existed since the late 19th and early 20th centuries: the nurse-midwife and the nurse-anesthetist. The training of nurse-midwives was a direct response to the need for improvement in mother-child care, the unregulated practice of untrained midwives, and the unavailability of obstetricians in poor rural areas. The role of nurse-anesthetist developed as part of the increasing sophistication in surgery in the early 1900s, when it was recognized that trained assistants were needed to administer anesthetics. No longer was it safe or satisfactory to have untrained medical students or attendants providing anesthesia. These early specialists were recruited from the available pool of trained nurses to meet very specific societal demands and needs. Opposition from particular specialty groups in medicine as well as legal barriers to practicing were among the specialists' greatest struggles. The same struggles continue to occur in the current circumstances of nursing specialization.

Although nurse anesthetists and nurse midwives were initially trained and supervised by physicians, the development of autonomous clinical specialization in nursing has not been well received by medical groups. Opposition to the training and clinical practice of nurse midwives and nurse anesthetists continues to be an issue . . . the nurse midwife and nurse anesthetist conflicts have resulted in underutilization and inappropriate use of these highly skilled nurse specialists. Debate and ambivalence regarding their role continues to confuse the American public. The resolution of territorial disputes between nursing and medicine is long overdue. However, it can be anticipated that debate and conflict will continue as long as highly skilled nurse specialists are perceived as a "threat to the other groups' social and/or financial status or its power or base of control."

— KRAMPITZ, 1981, P. 62

The need for legal restrictions of nursing practice and the placement of nursing practice under the direct supervision of doctors are concerns that have been heard consistently in discussions of specialization in nursing. This is not surprising because it has been historically documented that physicians have often tried to keep nursing under restraint. Now, as before, nurses must define and control their nursing practice and should heed the words of Lavinia Dock:

Nothing, I think dear Editor, is more trying to one's toleration than to see men—most of whom never did and never can comprehend what a woman's work really is, what its details are, or how it ought to be done—undertaking to instruct and train women in something so unquestionably her own special field as nursing. I do not limit this statement to men only, but will say that physicians, be they men or women, cannot teach nursing, any more than nurses can teach medicine. Medicine and nursing are not the same; and how-ever much we may learn from the physician about disease and its treatment, the whole field of nursing—as nursing is realized by the *patient* (the centre of the question)—is unknown to him. I agree that he can criticise nursing intelligently, but he cannot show how it ought to be done or do it himself, except in rare instances.

We need, then, to recognize those qualities and characteristics in our work which are superior to what men can teach us, and to hold firmly to them, refusing to give them up, and most unremittingly should we resist all attempts to take our right of teaching our own work out of our hands, putting nurses out of their true relation to their own calling, and bringing up a set of imperfect imitators of pseudoscientific men, mere satellites of the medical profession, who will be neither doctor nor nurse.

— DOCK, EDITORIAL, 1901

One other early nurse specialist bears mentioning—the industrial nurse. This specialty arose in response to the hazards and abnormal health conditions in shops, factories, and other fields of industry. Initially, little concern was given to the care of injuries. In its early stages, industrial nursing was a home visiting service; patient referrals were initiated by physicians. Ada Mayo Stewart was the first nurse in this specialty. She was hired by Fletcher D. Proctor in 1895 to act as a visiting nurse for the families of the employees of his Vermont Marble Company. The growth of industrial nursing was a slow one until the massive boom in the defense industry during World War II. Nurses were then rapidly employed in all types of manufacturing plants, a practice that in most instances was continued even after the war.

The 1960s witnessed another distinct growth period of specialization in nursing that has continued to the current time. All types of specialty areas—coronary care units, surgical intensive care units, medical intensive care units, burn units, dialysis units, oncology units—were developed in hospitals and necessitated changes in nursing roles. In addition, gaps identified in the health care system of the United States in this era led nursing to experiment with the role of clinical specialist or nurse clinician. This new concept allowed nurses to use their expertise, based on in-depth knowledge, for advanced nursing practice. Once again, nursing efforts were partially thwarted because hospital administrations commonly would not pay for such services

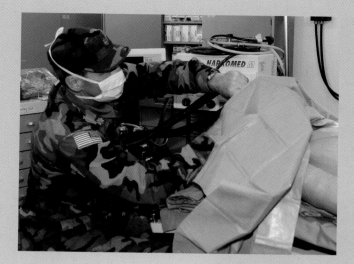

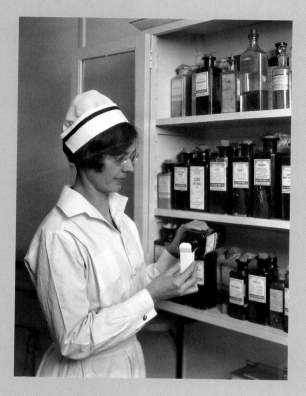

Rob Schuette, *Certified Registered Nurse Anesthetist Maj. Steve Hargens of the 452nd Combat Support Hospital Simulates Patient Care During an Exercise at Fort McCoy,* 2008, photograph, Fort McCoy, WI. Photo courtesy of U.S. Army Fort McCoy.

Lewis W. Hine, *Industrial Health Nurse,* 1909, photograph, George Eastman House, Rochester, NY. Courtesy of George Eastman House International Museum of Photography and Film.

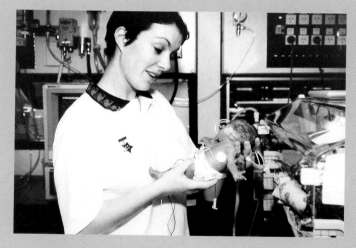

Sara McIntyre, *NNU Nurse,* photo, New Zealand Health Board.

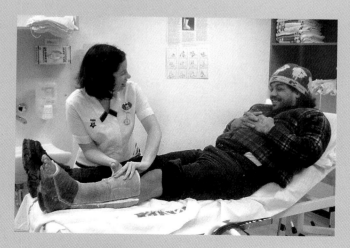

Sara McIntyre, *Ortho Poster,* photo, New Zealand Health Board.

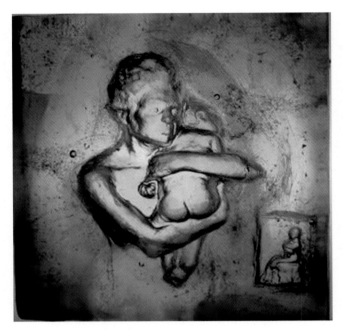

Judi Charlson, *Caring* (detail from the *Wall of the Journey of Life*), 2006, glass pane.

and would assign responsibilities to the specialist head nurse or staff nurse. The specialist was thus prevented from functioning in a clinician role. All obstacles to this role were never overcome, but clinical specialists currently function in a variety of settings, including hospitals and outpatient facilities, in conjunction with individual or groups of physicians, and in private or joint practice with other nurse specialists or physicians or both. In 1954, the first graduate level program to prepare clinical specialists was developed by Hildegard E. Peplau at Rutgers University; the specialty area of the program was psychiatric nursing.

The nurse practitioner was also introduced during this period as the result of a specific demonstration funded by the Commonwealth Foundation at the University of Colorado in 1965. Henry Silver, a pediatrician, and Loretta Ford, a public health nurse at the University of Colorado, collaborated in this venture. This demonstration project resulted in the establishment of the pediatric nurse practitioner program, which was designed to prepare nurses to give comprehensive well-child care in ambulatory settings. The nurses were further taught to make judgments about acute or chronic conditions in children and to perform as primary practitioners in childhood emergencies. One effect of these innovations was the development of numerous new titles in nursing, such as nurse clinician, clinical nurse specialist, and nurse practitioner. Each differed in meaning, in requirements for preparation, in levels of responsibility, and in expected performance. It is clear that standard titles are lacking, as is demonstrated by a significant list of differing titles for nurse practitioners. Numerous organizations now represent various types of specialized nursing practice, and the list continues to grow. The ANA, however, defined its position on the issue in a social policy statement:

The specialist in nursing practice is a nurse who, through study and supervised practice at the graduate level (master's or doctorate), has become expert in a defined area of knowledge and practice in a selected clinical area of nursing. Specialists in nursing practice are also generalists, in

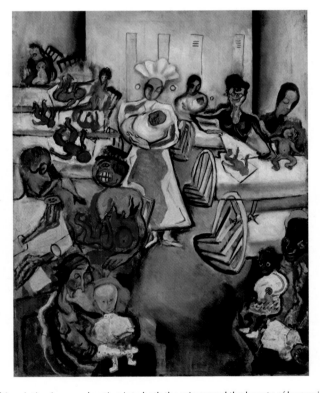

This painting is an exploration into both the misery and the beauty of humanity. The focus is the white-clad nurse who holds a baby in the center of the painting. Surrounding the "clean" nurse are adults and babies in less than desirable conditions.

Alice Neel, *Well Baby Clinic,* 1928-29, oil on canvas, 39" × 29". Copyright the Estate of Alice Neel. Courtesy of David Zwirner, NY.

that they hold a baccalaureate in nursing, and therefore are able to provide the full range of nursing care. In addition, upon completion of a graduate degree in a university graduate program with an emphasis on clinical specialization, the specialist in nursing practice should meet the criteria for specialty certification through nursing's professional society.
— *AMERICAN NURSES ASSOCIATION, 1980*

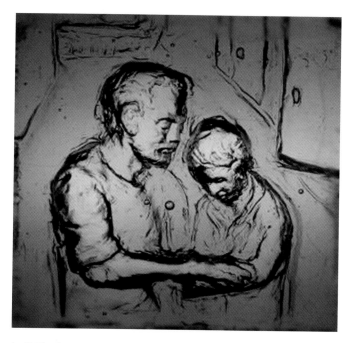

Judi Charlson, *Giving Care* (detail from the *Wall of the Journey of Life*), 2006, glass pane.

The role of the nurse is constantly changing, and nursing practice has become more sophisticated. New theories, techniques, skills, and tools are being used in practice to meet the current needs of a society that is highly technological, complex, and dynamic. Specialization has led to the development of revised or new curricula in basic educational programs and the establishment of new programs in graduate education to prepare nurses to acquire the knowledge, skills, and responsibilities consistent with this role. Distinct advantages to the creation of nurse specialists/ nurse practitioners have included the alleviation of extreme health care costs facing patients; a decrease in the gaps in health care; an increase in the level of responsibility of the registered nurse; the provision of appropriate opportunities for nurses to use their expertise fully; and transformed ambulatory settings staffed by nurse practitioners. The nurse practitioner movement slowly moved from a dubious experiment created as an alternative method of health care to one of far-reaching acceptance by patients, physicians, and nursing itself. As a result, programs for the development of various types of practitioners, such as family nurse practitioners, geriatric nurse practitioners, adult nurse practitioners, and rural nurse practitioners, were created and funded by federal and private agencies. These nursing roles would become even more important when the shortage of primary care physicians eventually occurred in the 1990s.

CONTINUED GROWTH OF ORGANIZATIONS

Nursing organizations with a variety of established purposes have proliferated around the world. They include organizations specific to countries such as the Japanese Nurses Association and global nursing specialty organizations such as the International Society of Nurses in Genetics, which are dedicated to fostering the scientific and professional growth of nurses worldwide. There is no doubt that the world as a whole and the world of nursing have become smaller and more closely intertwined. Yet at the same time, this phenomenon presents opportunities previously unimaginable for nurses everywhere to collaborate and cooperate, no matter where they are located.

The ANA and the NLN have continued to represent the interests of nursing in the United States since the restructuring process in 1952. Their combined achievements and contributions are many. Each has served to promote and improve conditions in nursing service, practice, education, research, and a number of related areas. Each has undergone some reorganization in programs in an attempt to keep pace with societal changes and demands. This period of change has resulted in advantages and disadvantages for both organizations.

The NLN adopted a new structure in 1967 to provide greater flexibility so that the national board of directors and the constituent leagues could enjoy a closer working relationship. The membership continued to include individuals and agencies in addition to the Assembly of Constituent Leagues for Nursing, which had six regional assemblies for the planning, coordination, and implementation of programs—the councils of Associate Degree Programs, Baccalaureate and Higher Degree Programs, Diploma Programs, Practical Nursing Programs, Hospital and Related Institutional Nursing Services, and Home Health Agencies and Community Health Services. Other changes also occurred, including those related to the administration of examinations for licensure. States had used the State Board Test Pool Exam until 1982, when the first National Council Licensure Examination was given. The National Council of State Boards of Nursing comprises members, executive secretaries, and directors of boards of nursing in the United States and territories. In 1992, the National Council voted to develop a Computerized Adaptive Test, which was implemented in 1994.

The various issues that arose in the organization were dealt with in the most feasible manner possible. One action that evoked a tremendous response from agency members was a historic statement titled "Nursing Roles—Scope and Preparation," issued by the NLN in February 1982. Through this statement a baccalaureate degree was recognized and accepted as an important credential for professional nursing.

The ANA has continued its efforts on behalf of individual nurses through its programs on economic and general welfare, its certification of practitioners, the development of standards for practice, and other significant activities in the areas of service, practice, education, and research. Although the organization's classic position paper issued in 1965 did much to aid the advancement of nursing, it also intensified controversy over the future direction of the hospital diploma program. This paper, prepared by the ANA Committee on Education, was adopted as a proposal for study by the ANA House of Delegates in 1964. It was released in 1965, proposed and approved by the ANA membership in 1966, and reaffirmed in 1978, when the ANA passed the Entry into Practice Resolution at the national convention. The statement and resolution, predicated on the need for improved nursing practice, concluded as follows:

> The education for all of those who are licensed to practice nursing should take place in institutions of higher education; minimum preparation for beginning professional nursing practice should be a baccalaureate degree; minimum preparation for beginning technical nursing practice should be an associate degree in nursing; education for assistants in the health service occupations should be short, intensive preservice programs in vocational education rather than on-the-job training.
>
> — AMERICAN NURSES ASSOCIATION, 1965

At the 1982 ANA convention the House of Delegates voted for a major bylaw change that mandated the restructuring of the ANA commencing in 1984. The essence of this change was that state nurses' associations would be the units of membership in the ANA; the individual member would belong to the ANA through state membership. Two objectives were to be achieved through this federation model: the strengthening of the ANA plus flexibility and autonomy for state nurses' associations.

All nursing organizations have served to effect some aspect of change and provide the necessary communication for collective action. Consolidation of the U.S. organizations was achieved in 1952 to increase efficacy and efficiency and to ensure collaboration. Since that time, additional associations have arisen, usually in response to a major issue facing a group or the entire profession. There is still concern that the current proliferation of nursing organizations may have diluted the power of a collective voice, diluted the profession, splintered nursing as a profession, and created disunity. The newer organizations are additional testament to the complexities and technologies that are being experienced in society and in the world as a whole. Most of the new groups are special-interest groups that arose to provide support for clinical practice. Space prohibits a discussion of all of these organizations, but the following are unique to an understanding of nursing's history.

NATIONAL BLACK NURSES ASSOCIATION

The National Association of Colored Graduate Nurses (NACGN) existed for almost 4 decades until the ANA House of Delegates voted in 1948 to remove all barriers that prevented full participation by racial minorities in the association. To bypass some state associations, the ANA offered individual membership to black nurses, and in 1949 ap-proximately 634 black nurses belonged to the organization. A special committee was also set up to explore comparable functions of the NACGN and the ANA. "Encouraged by the developments on the national level, the black nurses voted in 1949 to dissolve the NACGN, and formal dissolution occurred on January 31, 1951. The struggle for professional parity, they thought, was over. The dream of recognition and equality was finally to be realized" (Smith, 1975, p. 225).

The intent of black nurses was to become a part of the mainstream of organized nursing and of the ANA. This was apparently not the total answer for blacks and other minorities. "In many sections of the country, nurses are organizing in ethnically identifiable associations, because they have not felt they were integrated into the professional association" (Shaw, 1975, p. 8). The National Black Nurses Association, Inc., thus emerged in 1971 as a structure that would not duplicate the functions of the ANA but would complement them so as to meet the special needs of black nurses. This organization was begun through the efforts of Lauranne Sams as a vehicle to express the concerns of black nurses. Some of these concerns were the absence of black nurses in positions of leadership; limited opportunities for black nurses to share in shaping ANA policies and priorities; loss of identity of black nurses; and limited recognition of their contribution to nursing. Membership was open to all licensed nurses (registered nurses and licensed professional nurses) and nursing students. "Its future is uncertain, as would seem to be true of other emergent nursing organizations organized around race, sex, specialization, and division of labor" (Smith, 1975, p. 226).

Cultural diversity and cultural competency have become significant concepts in educational and practice settings in nursing. The creation of the National Black Nurses Association serves as a vivid reminder that great care must be taken to ensure the rights and privileges of all nurses, regardless of race, gender, ethnicity, or religion.

AMERICAN ASSOCIATION OF COLLEGES OF NURSING

Developments in professional nursing associations included the establishment in 1969 of the Conference of Deans of College and University Schools of Nursing. The name was changed in 1973 to the American Association of Colleges of Nursing (AACN) to indicate its separation from the NLN. The AACN, which is a national association of nursing deans of colleges and universities, was created to provide administrators of baccalaureate and graduate degree nursing programs with an outlet for review of developments in the health care field. Its numerous activities are executed to improve the practice of professional nursing by elevating the quality of degree programs. Schools of nursing are represented by their respective deans, who discuss common concerns. Through a concerted effort, the organization has continually influenced public policy related to nursing and nursing education. "In 1996, AACN launched a new alliance of multiple organizations to accredit nursing higher education programs in a more streamlined and uniform process. Alliance organizations include an autonomous arm of AACN, the Commission on Collegiate Nursing Education, which is the only national agency dedicated exclusively to the accreditation of bachelor- and graduate-degree nursing education programs" (www.aacn.nche.edu). AACN today represents more than 600 schools of nursing at public and private universities and senior colleges nationwide and has been a trendsetter in the area of nursing education.

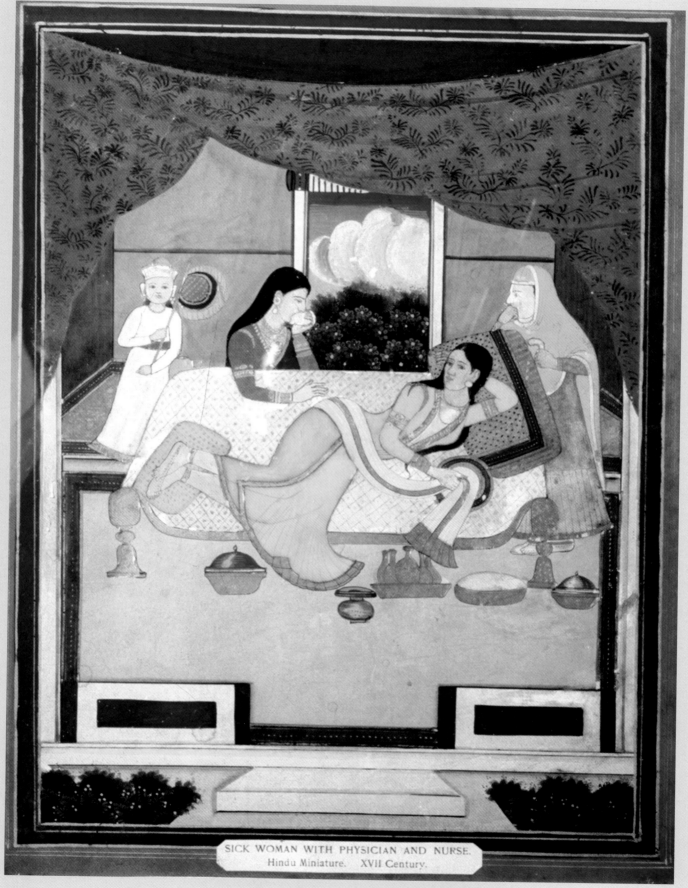

SICK WOMAN WITH PHYSICIAN AND NURSE.
Hindu Miniature.   XVII Century.

Sick woman attended by nurses, Indian.

Marc Charmet, *Sick Woman Attended by Nurses,* 17th century, painting, The Art Archive/Private Collection/Marc Charmet.

AMERICAN ACADEMY OF NURSING

The American Academy of Nursing was established in 1973 under the auspices of the ANA. Membership in this academy was originally limited to graduate nurses who were members of the ANA. Currently, applicants who are U.S. citizens must be current members of the ANA or an ANA constituent member association (state nurses' associations). International applicants must be members of one of the National Nurses Associations listed as member organizations of the International Council of Nurses.

A nurse who becomes a Fellow in the American Academy of Nursing has provided evidence of outstanding contributions to the improvement of nursing at the national or international level. Election to this group is considered an honor because members represent a selected group of leaders in the profession. The academy currently comprises more than 1500 top nursing leaders in the fields of education, management, research, and practice. Meetings are held annually, primarily to enter into dialogue about nursing issues and to work on reports, studies, and position papers related to major nursing and health care issues. The inclusion of members from around the world has enhanced the emphasis on nursing as an international discipline and as a profession working collaboratively to facilitate health care for all.

NURSES COALITION FOR ACTION IN POLITICS

Nurses for Political Action was started in 1972 as the first national organization of nurses to enter the political arena. It soon became affiliated with the ANA and has been regarded as its legislative and political action arm (Kalisch and Kalisch, 1978). The name was eventually changed to Nurses Coalition for Action in Politics in 1974. That group was organized as a nonpartisan and nonprofit association. Its expressed goal was the attainment of substantial political influence on national policy related to health care delivery. This group encouraged and assisted nurses in becoming social and political activists. It continues to strive for support for nursing from legislators and government officials. In 1986, to promote identification with the ANA, the name was changed to ANA/PAC.

AMERICAN ASSOCIATION FOR THE HISTORY OF NURSING

Early American nursing leaders supported and promoted the study of nursing history and advocated its incorporation into the curricula of schools of nursing. In particular, M. Adelaide Nutting, Lavinia L. Dock, and Isabel M. Stewart became known as authorities on nursing history through the publication of their classic works on the subject. Dedicated to fostering greater understanding of and respect for nursing's past, they were committed to the belief that to understand and deal with problems and trends in nursing education and nursing practice, nurses should be familiar with their histories. These leaders believed that no one can get a true picture of current situations without finding out how the issues developed and what their underlying causes were. This general philosophy was expressed by Stewart: "History can often help individuals to deal more effectively with persistent issues and conflicts by throwing light on their origins, and by indicating long-term trends that show the general direction in which things are moving. Educators who know something of the historical foundations of a system of education are also in a better position to evaluate the materials that have gone into it, to capitalize its assets and to eliminate what is no longer useful" (Stewart, 1943, p. viii).

There has been no consistent support for historical inquiry. In fact, emphasis on the historical foundations of nursing has decreased over time to the point where few nursing history courses are currently available in schools of nursing. Nor is there sufficient available nursing faculty prepared to teach them. In an effort to revive an interest in nursing history, a small number of interested nurses and historians began meeting as a historical methodology interest group in 1978 as part of a federally funded project for the development of nursing research in the Midwest. Originally called the International History of Nursing Society, the name of the group was changed in 1980 to the American Association for the History of Nursing. The membership comprises individuals, nurses and nonnurses, who are interested in achieving the purpose of the association—to educate the public about the history and heritage of the nursing profession. This movement, although slow, has begun to return nursing history to the curricula of schools of nursing; to foster historical research; and to collect, restore, and preserve historical materials relevant to nursing's rich heritage. In addition, historical nursing organizations, centers, and museums have been established with increasing frequency in countries all over the world.

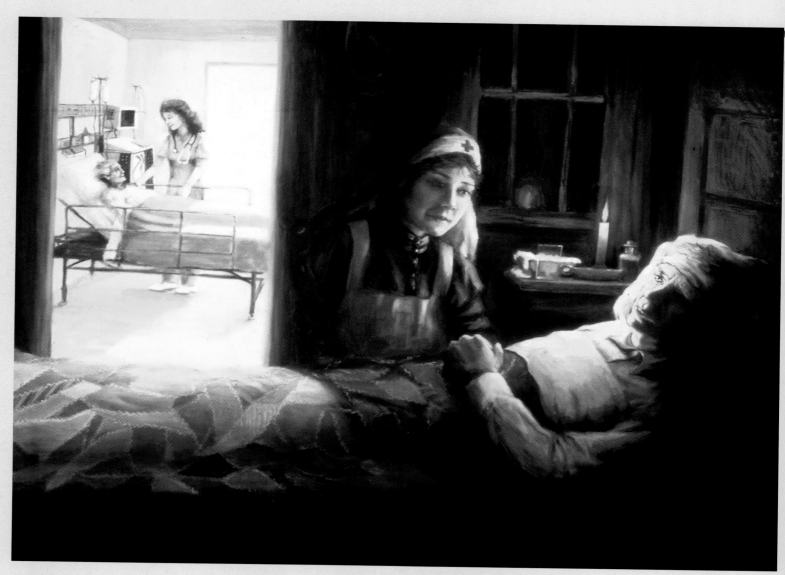

In the foreground, a turn-of-the-century nurse tends a patient at home in a quilt-covered bed. Light spills across the foot of the bed from the doorway where today's nurse tends a patient in the hospital. Beyond is another doorway opening to an intense light—the promise of an even brighter future for nursing. The original painting hangs in Pro-Nurse headquarters in Gaithersburg, Maryland.

Winona Chenevert, *Nursing: Yesterday, Today, Forever,* 1989, painting, 91.44 × 121.92, Pro-Nurse.

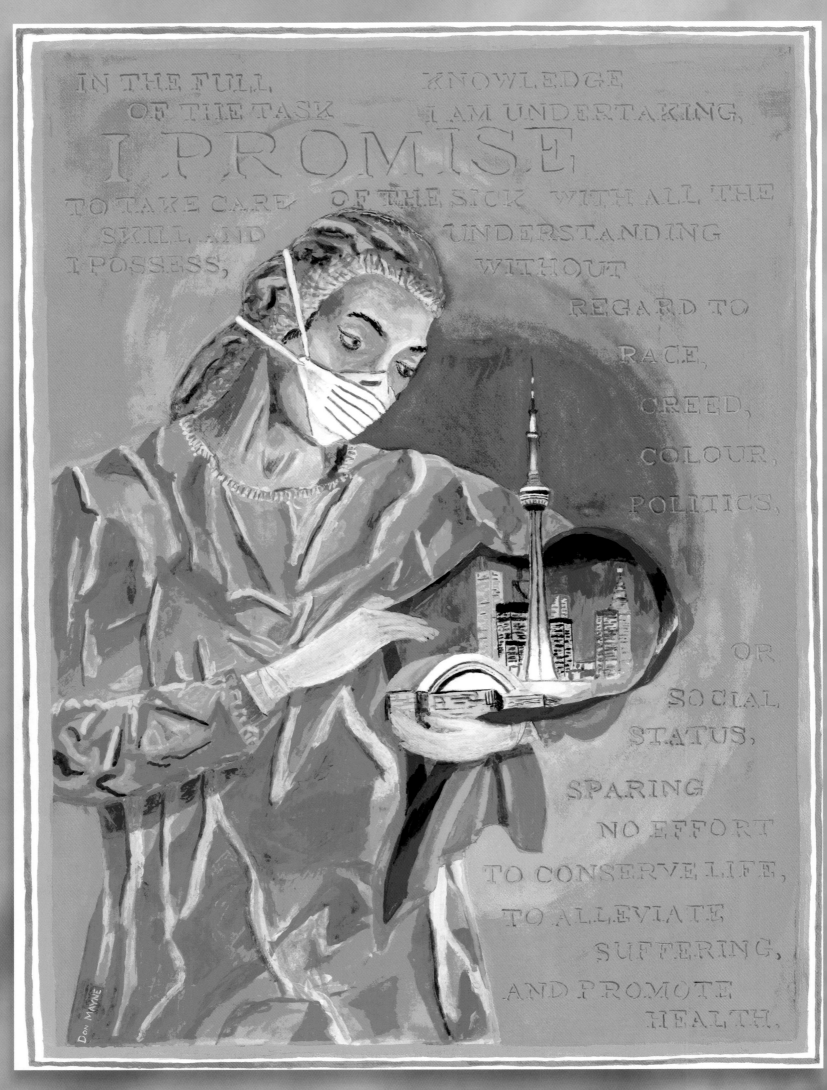

UNIT Seven

The Nursing Transformation

To accelerate the delivery of essential health services to the people of the world, particularly underserved populations, the transformation of the nursing profession is critical, and professional nurses must assume roles as leaders and active participants in change. Nurses must master the skills of visionary and strategic thinking to have an impact on institutional and political forces that control health development. The emergence of the phenomenon of transformation is providing a rare opportunity for nursing. Transformation provides a scenario for a new way of interacting, a new way of problem solving, and a means to developing a shared vision among health professionals in various settings.

— LILLIAN M. SIMMS

In 2003, the deadly SARS virus arrived in Toronto. The only defenses were quarantine and isolation orders. Nurses were called upon to care for suspected and confirmed cases of SARS. They donned double gowns, gloves, and masks. Hidden from photographers, they provided patient care, caring for a frightened city. Many nurses contracted the virus, and some died. Nurses wore masks at home to protect their families. Their spouses and children were shunned by friends, colleagues, and classmates. The entire city was shunned by the global community as world headlines published Toronto's daily death toll. The World Health Organization ordered a non-essential travel ban to and from Toronto. This is the story behind the *I Promise* portrait. It depicts the strength of the brave nurse at the start of her night shift. Concern in her eyes and compassion in her touch, she carefully adjusts the dark blanket separating her from the city life. The words carved into the sunset represent the goals of nurses worldwide and are taken from the pledge of the International Council of Nurses.

Don Mayne, *I Promise,* 2003, watercolor (gauche), 13.5″ × 15.5″, Toronto, Ontario, Canada.

	1996	1997
Nursing	**1996** Task Force on Doctoral Education formed **1996** John A. Hartford Foundation Institute for Geriatric Nursing established **1996** ABC Codes for billing systems recognized by ANA **1996** Arista 2: Nurses & Health: Healthy People—Leaders in Partnership held	**1997** National League for Nursing Accrediting Commission (NLNAC) established **1997** State funeral held in Calcutta India for Mother Teresa
Medicine and Health Care	**1996** European Commission bans exports of beef from U.K. due to outbreak of mad cow disease **1996** First live broadcast of laparoscopic surgery via Internet	**1997** Validation of I-beta-CIT in assessing dopamine transporters in the diagnosis of Parkinson's disease **1997** U.S. tobacco companies settle $368.5 billion claims by former smokers
Science and Technology	**1996** Web TV invented	**1997** 3D MR angiography developed **1997** DNA originally extracted from fossils in the Neander Valley in Germany in 1856 supports theory that modern humans diverged from Neanderthals about 600,000 years ago **1997** NASA spacecraft lands on Mars **1997** British scientists clone an adult sheep named Dolly **1997** Gas-powered fuel cell invented
The Visual Arts		
Daily Life	**1996** Bill Clinton reelected President of U.S. **1996** Yasser Arafat elected President in first Palestinian elections	**1997** Tiger Woods, 21, becomes the youngest person to win the Masters golf tournament **1997** President Bill Clinton apologizes to 399 African-American men in Alabama left untreated for syphilis as part of a government experiment from 1932 to 1972 **1997** Diana, Princess of Wales, dies in a car accident in Paris **1997** Madeleine Albright becomes first female U.S. Secretary of State

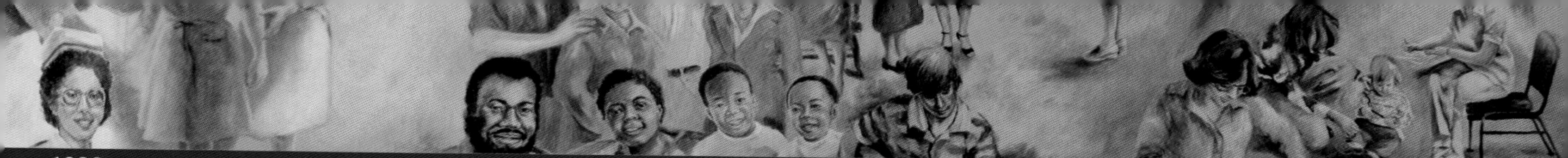

1998 Council on Accreditation of Nurse Anesthesia Educational Programs require all programs to be at the graduate level

1998 *Evidence-based Nursing* journal launched by colleagues in the U.K. and Canada

1999 Elnora D. Daniel becomes first black nurse elected president of a major university at Chicago State University

1999 First practice doctoral program opened at the University of Tennessee Health Science Center

1999 The International Centre for Nursing Ethics launched at the University of Surrey

---

1998 Viagra becomes the fastest-selling drug in U.S. history

1998 Dr. Nancy Dickey inaugurated as first female president of the AMA

1998 First vaccine for lyme disease developed

1999 Institute of Medicine released landmark report *To Err is Human: Building a Safer Health System*

1999 Doctors in Kentucky perform first human hand transplant in the U.S.

1999 National Center for Complementary and Alternative Medicine (NCCAM) established at NIH

1998 The Google Internet search engine goes online

1998 Vascular endothelial growth factor genes inserted into a human heart and form new blood vessels

1998 India and Pakistan begin testing nuclear weapons, sparking fears of an arms race in southern Asia

---

1998 Farnsworth Art Museum opens Center for the Wyeth Family in Maine

1999 Olga's Gallery becomes one of the largest and most comprehensive online collections

1999 Artcyclopedia presents museum-quality fine art on the Internet

1999 Stuckism, a radical art movement, founded in London to advance new figurative painting with ideas as the most vital artistic means of addressing contemporary issues

---

1998 President Bill Clinton impeached by the House for perjury and obstruction of justice

1998 El Niño blamed for scorching temperatures, drought, and tornadoes in the U.S.

1999 President Bill Clinton acquitted by the Senate

1999 Killing spree at Columbine High School

1999 Lt. Col. Eileen Collins is first woman astronaut to command a space shuttle mission

1999 NATO bombs Serbia

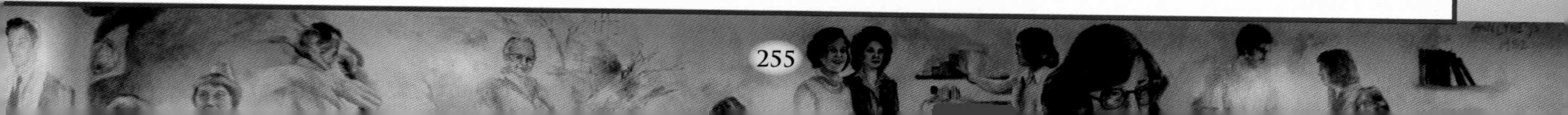

Even prior to the new millennium, transformation had been occurring everywhere—in organizations and corporations; in economic, political, social, educational, and religious institutions; and in health care delivery systems. Conflict, crisis, chaos, deterioration, and disintegration were some of the words being used to describe health care delivery systems, and they were consistent with the transformational phenomenon. These words provided a picture of massive change and turmoil that seemed to be out of control and to be promoting human degradation. Societies were seeking new information, new knowledge, new paradigms, and new ways of understanding and dealing with the forces that were driving important decision making. Even more critical, societies were searching for ways to improve the quality of life of present and future generations. Are societies also now in the process of *Creating a New Civilization* (1995), as suggested by the Tofflers? The Tofflers have been writing about the future since 1970, when their first best seller, *Future Shock*, was published. That work discussed the impact of accelerated change that was overwhelming and disorienting people and their societies. *The Third Wave* (1980) was even more startling because it contained a predictive framework. In it the information revolution was compared with the agricultural and industrial revolutions, two other great transformations in history. The Tofflers believed that the impact of this third historic wave of change was currently being felt and that a new civilization was being created.

There is no doubt that society is changing at a quickening pace, and experts predict that change will accelerate even more. The term *singularity* is now being used to describe this trend as "a watershed moment when accelerating technology becomes so advanced that it surpasses what the human brain can comprehend. And because it can improve its own programming, change happens instantly, almost without us being aware of it." (Youso, 2009, p. E1). According to Kurzweil

(2005, p. 7), who has written extensively on this concept, "Singularity in our future is increasingly transforming every institution and aspect of human life from sexuality to spirituality. [Singularity is] a future period during which the pace of technological change will be so rapid, its impact so deep, that human life will be irreversibly transformed." It is believed by some that singularity will be here by 2050, accompanied by enormous changes along the way. The impact will certainly affect health care and create increasingly sophisticated medical treatments and potentially "enhanced humans with better bodies." Nursing and its practice will also be affected by this rapid change but in ways yet unknown.

A new way of thinking about the future will be needed to meet the imminent challenges of change and transformation. An interesting book, *The Tyranny of Dead Ideas* by Miller (2009), although dealing with policy, politics, and economics, presents some salient ideas about ways of renovating thinking that will meet the challenges of the 21st century. Dead ideas are today's destructive conventional wisdom; people have grown comfortable with settled ideas about the way the world works and fail to adapt to new circumstances. But what is necessary, according to Miller, is a new way of thinking, which he calls "tomorrow's destined ideas," that will ultimately transform America in the years to come. Essentially, the key to future success in organizations, workplaces, and personal lives is the skill and speed with which people cope with new circumstances. Although this author is speaking primarily about the United States, his arguments apply to the whole world and to nursing in particular. The question for nursing becomes: What ideas in nursing are dead, are obsolete, yet remain entrenched in all facets of the profession, particularly in the areas of practice and education?

Nursing has not escaped this phenomenon and has been undergoing its own transformation in all areas. The numerous changes are representative of those occurring in society at large—patient and health care are being challenged by the emphasis on efficiency, effectiveness, and economy and by the plea for accessible and competent health care. As Simms stated in 1991, the transformation of nursing is critical, and nurses must assume responsibility as leaders and active participants in this massive process of change. They must be visionary, strategic, innovative, and creative in order to impact the numerous forces currently controlling health care and the development of healthy populations. In essence, nurses must be able to think critically and act independently in diverse settings and situations.

Historically, nursing has demonstrated great resiliency in the face of health care changes but has tended to be reactive rather than proactive. What must be emphasized and embraced is that nursing must capitalize on its unique position and focus on courageous and visionary directions in creative practices for health promotion and holistic care. Nursing is in a strategic position that allows it to promote and facilitate this paradigm shift in health care. Nursing can shape and provide primary health care. Nursing has been and still can be a strong social force and an advocate for

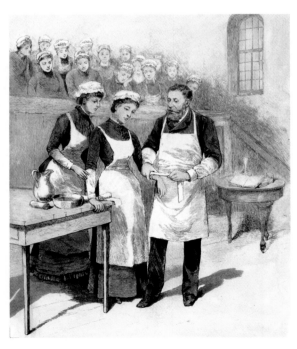

Nursing students are being taught how to apply bandages at the Blockley Training School for Nurses at Philadelphia General Hospital.

Nursing School, 1885. Image courtesy of the Granger Collection, NY.

Facing page, Ann Lyness, *Instruction,* 1998, mural, University of Pittsburgh, School of Nursing, Acute-Tertiary Care Department. The University of Pittsburgh Nursing School paintings are owned by the University of Pittsburgh, protected by copyright, and are reproduced with permission from the University of Pittsburgh.

change. Nurses have consistently risen to the task of overcoming barriers and meeting challenges. Their ultimate goal has always been concern and care for human beings, only some of whom were ill. If nurses are to continue this humanitarian tradition they will require a level of commitment and a degree of courage that will exceed those of previous circumstances, and a proactive stance on all issues involving health care will be mandated. Nursing has always had the power to accomplish such change, but it has continued to perpetuate the passivity of the past, to behave as an oppressed group, and to regard itself as a victim in the organizational structure of health care.

THE NURSING PERSPECTIVE: THE STATE OF THE ART IN THE NEW MILLENNIUM

During the last part of the 20th century and the beginning years of the 21st century, nursing has been intertwined with vast social problems, profound financial crises, and a health care system in a state of turmoil. Essentially, the issues of health care remain the same as they were when nursing was created, and they are related to accessibility, resources, division of labor, the caregiver pool, and reimbursement. Some of nursing's earlier issues have improved, been resolved, or are no longer problematic. The issue of entry-level education, for example, although not totally resolved, has improved, and more nurses are obtaining advanced degrees.

Hospital diploma programs are continuing to close or become affiliated with colleges and universities.

Educational programs are being examined around the world, and decisions are being made to move them into institutions of higher learning. However, the issue still involves controversy, and individuals who oppose educational change severely criticize the new generation of nurses who spend an "inadequate amount of time caring for patients" and spend "very few clinical hours" in their educational programs. These new nurses, it is said, are overeducated and have moved away from the bedside. This way of thinking also speaks to the issue of whether the number of clinical hours in the nursing program or the experiences received during clinical hours allows for more competent patient care; which is the primary factor that results in competency?

The primary difference between nursing today and that of the past is its maturity, which evolved over the course of the 20th century. Indeed, new concerns have periodically arisen that may cause nurses to pause and deliberate; for example, the increased use of unlicensed assistive personnel, the changed reimbursement systems, the presence of nursing information systems, and the return to alternative forms of health care and healing practices. What must be remembered constantly, however, is that change also brings opportunity, and that places nursing in a prime position to impact health care.

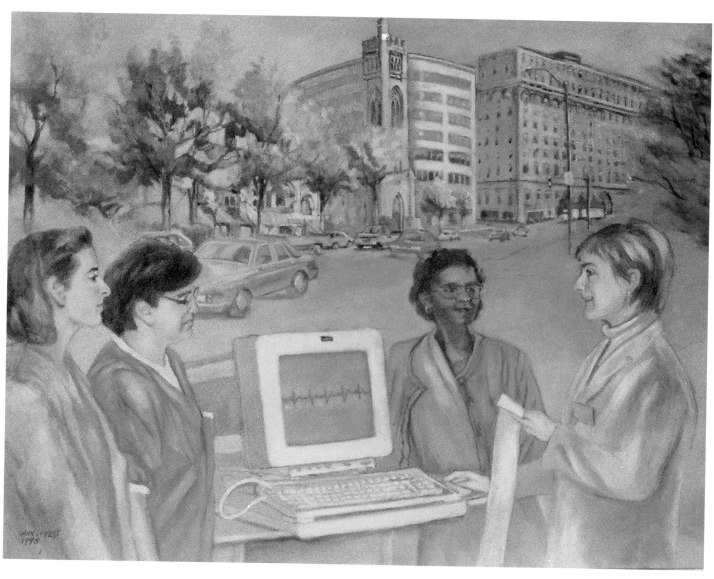

THE FORCES AT WORK

The nature of change must be understood and is paramount to the progression and survival of nursing. Both external and internal forces are involved in the process of change and directly or indirectly affect the nursing discipline. External forces are generally believed to be the strongest, although internal forces may have a positive or negative effect. Bullough and Bullough (1994) identified external and internal forces that were affecting the nursing profession and nursing roles and that are still applicable today.

External Forces

1. Developments in science and technology have made a wider array of health care procedures possible.
2. The continued restriction by medicine of its numbers has resulted in high incomes and in the almost exclusive deployment of physicians into specialty roles (Office of Technology Assessment, 1986).
3. Changing demographic patterns have created a range of unmet needs, with an aging population, a decreasing birth rate, and increasing immigration of refugees and peoples from developing nations.
4. Increased environmental hazards have appeared and there has been growth in the awareness of them.
5. A major pandemic of HIV/AIDS has developed along with epidemics of other sexually transmitted diseases.
6. The health care delivery system has failed to keep pace with needs, although there is now evidence that society may be ready to deal with some of the inequities in the system.
7. Expanded nurse practice acts were enacted, providing at least a limited increase in autonomy and responsibility for practice, although it is clear that further expansion of these acts would make better use of the talents of advanced practice nurses (Safriet, 1992).

Internal Forces

1. There have been expanding knowledge bases and growing sophistication on the part of nurses.
2. More functional and more cost-effective systems of nursing services have been established, including educational systems that prepare students to function on a variety of nursing levels.
3. A significant body of nursing research has been focused on developing theory and improving nursing practice (pp. 3-4).

Nursing's future will continue to be affected by the constant changes created by external and internal forces. Acknowledging this reinforces the fact that there is a close and indispensable alliance between nursing and society. In other words, nursing has and always will be linked to constantly occurring issues generated by changes in the medical and human sciences, in technology, in consumers' health care problems and needs, and in health care systems (Donahue, 2004).

When nursing hesitates to fill the needs created by change, other individuals or groups move in. Numerous examples throughout nursing's history attest to this phenomenon, and occurrences are cyclical. In the early 1970s, the American Medical Association (AMA) advocated the proposal that 100,000 nurses be upgraded to physician assistants. The American Nurses' Association (ANA)'s rebuttal was that nurses were already assisting physicians and did not need to be upgraded to do so. The confrontation ended when the AMA created the position of physician assistant; the ANA eventually created the position of nurse practitio-

ner. In the late 1980s, an attempt was made by the AMA to introduce a new type of caregiver, the registered care technologist (RCT). This occurred at the peak of the nurse shortage in the United States and was proposed as a method of providing a new type of bedside caregiver. According to some AMA members, the overemphasis on the education of nurses had moved them away from the bedside. The AMA, without input from or discourse with organized nursing, approved plans for four pilot projects, with the first class to begin in July 1989. High school graduates would be trained to give patient care. They would take tests and be registered in their states. Basic RCTs would receive 9 months of training; advanced RCTs would receive an additional 9 months. The basic RCTs would learn some higher-level skills such as oral medication administration; the advanced RCTs would also be taught to care for cardiac monitors and ventilators and to administer routine intravenous medications. Supervision of these activities was addressed, but the issue was not totally clarified. This was one occasion that prompted unity in the nursing community. Professional nursing associations exerted enormous pressure in opposition to the proposal. They were joined by the American Osteopathic Association and the Florida Medical Association. Although one pilot project was initiated at a Kentucky nursing home, the enrolled RCTs evidently never finished the program.

Nursing and nurses must direct attention to educational, legislative, and organizational changes that will have an impact on the profession. Nurses must increasingly recognize their responsibility to be active, participating members in mandates for health care, initiating actions as problems emerge. The time to react to changes is long past; the time to be proactive has arrived, and the transformation has begun.

THE PRACTICE ARENA

Nursing changes and grows in response to perceived social need, parallels the development of the social welfare system, and reflects society's attitudes toward sickness and health, lending credence to the fact that nursing is a reflection of social reality. Nursing is thus in a state of flux, which makes it extremely difficult to capture the essence of nursing—its true art and its caring spirit (Donahue, 2004). Its history documents the growth of an occupation in its quest for professionalization, an intimate view of the work experiences of women in a culture traditionally dominated by men, and the impact of nursing on patient care in hospitals. "Perhaps the most important single element in reshaping the day-to-day texture of hospital life was the professionalization of nursing. In 1800, as today, nurses were the most important single factor in determining ward and room environment. Nursing, like professional hospital administration changed modes of hospital financing, has played a key role in shaping the modern hospital" (Rosenberg, 1987, pp. 8-9). Historically, nurses have influenced patient care even in circumstances involving limited power, control, and resources.

During recent decades, nursing practice has been characterized by rapidly increasing responsibility, accountability, autonomy, and authority in patient care. It has been a time concerned with practice measurement and outcome research in health care. Potentially, further differentiation of roles will occur as relationships between nurses and physicians are transformed and new patterns of governance within the nursing hierarchy are established. Collaboration will, of necessity, be the byword because health professionals can no longer practice independently; boundaries are collapsing. Hospitals' need for nurses with strong technical skills will continue, but these nurses will, in all probability, be accountable for their practice to a nurse with advanced preparation who will serve as the case manager for a group of patients. Departmental governance and the participation of nurse representatives in institutional, agency, and practice policies will continue and must escalate. But will nurses' redefined roles be formally recognized and adequately compensated? Will advanced practice nurses be permitted to function with the full spectrum of their abilities and capabilities?

ADVANCED PRACTICE NURSING

The nurse practitioner movement has been one of the best illustrations of nursing's ingenuity in the face of societal upheaval and professional agitation. Created at a time of physician shortages in primary health care, it provided an opportunity for nurses to promote their professional agendas and embrace their service to society (Ford, 1992). One of the primary goals of the original pediatric nurse practitioner program that was begun in the United States in 1965 was to expand the nurse's scope of practice through increased depth of knowledge; clinical judgment and management would be emphasized. (The nurse practitioner role appeared in United Kingdom literature in the mid 1980s; in New Zealand and Australia in the 1990s.) It was, indeed, an

avenue to advanced clinical expertise. The success of the practitioner movement has been demonstrated by the dramatic growth in practitioner specialties. In addition, rapidly increasing numbers of different types of practitioner programs have been initiated in nursing educational programs for a variety of reasons. Perhaps the most significant reason is the paradigm shift in health care.

Nurse specialists are here to stay. How they will finally land in terms of hierarchy remains to be seen. In the past, nurses in administrative positions ranked above those with specialized clinical expertise. Now nurses with clinical expertise are usually ranked equal to or above those in administrative positions, and clinical nurse specialists may rank equal to or above traditional head nurses or supervisors. More and more attention is currently being paid to defining and describing advanced practice nursing because dramatic increases are occurring in the numbers of generalists, practitioners, and clinical specialists. Yet there is still a difference of opinion regarding what Bullough (1992) referred to as two models for specialization. The first is the nursing model, or clinical nurse specialist (CNS), which emphasizes advanced content in behavioral sciences, education, and nursing. The focus of this model is the caring role of the nurse. The second model, the collaborative model, builds on acquired nursing skills and includes advanced knowledge of medicine and the behavioral and biological sciences. Nurse practitioners, nurse-anesthetists, and nurse-midwives are included in this model, and some nurses believe that it is such

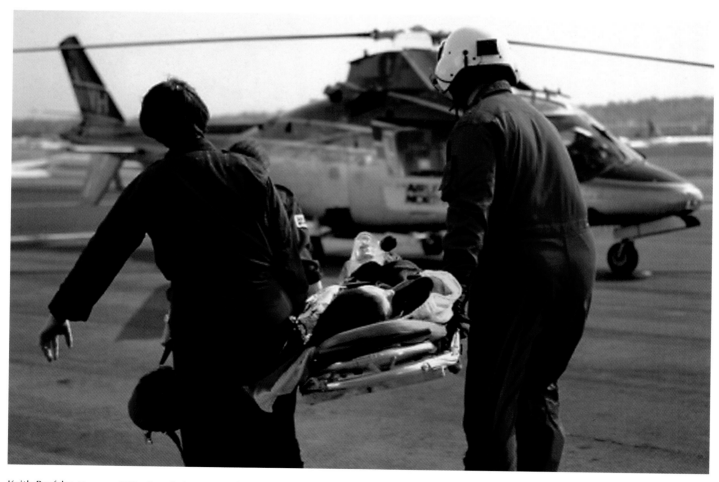

Keith Brofsky, *Nurses and Pilot Carry Patient on Stretcher to Helicopter,* photograph. Getty Images.

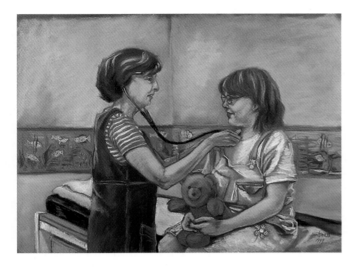

Pediatric nurse practitioner.

Ann Lyness, *Evolving a Nursing Program with a Vision,* 2001, mural (detail), University of South Carolina College of Nursing.

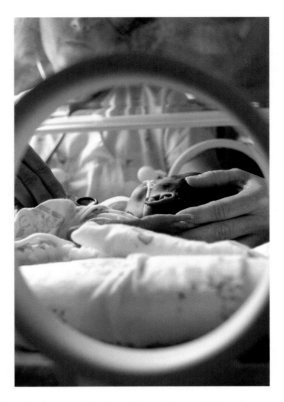

Theodore Anderson, *Infant Critical Care,* photograph. Getty Images.

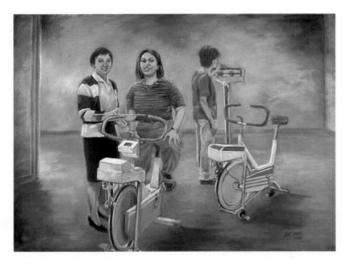

Adult nurse practitioner.

Ann Lyness, *Excellence in Nursing Is Timeless,* 2003, mural (detail), University of South Carolina College of Nursing.

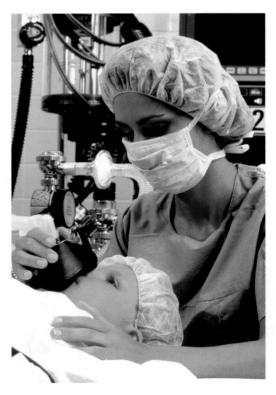

Nurse Anesthetist Prepares a Child for Surgery in the Operating Room.

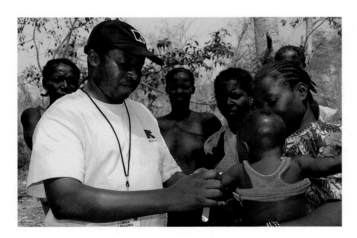

Central African Republic International Rescue Committee nurse practitioner Charles Muganda tests for malnutrition.

Central African Republic IRC Nurse Practitioner Charles Muganda Tests for Malnutrition, February 5, 2007, photograph, Central African Republic. Photo courtesy of International Rescue Committee, Inc., New York, NY.

Facing page, Thora Erichsen worked as a nurse anesthetist from 1914 until 1950. Nurse anesthetists were the only anesthetists in Norway and Scandinavia until 1950.

Roald Atle Furre, *Nurse Anesthetist Thora Erichsen,* 1924, painting, Haukeland University Hospital, Bergen, Norway, Roald A Furre/Christine Urquhart Furre/Pbase.com/alnsf.

inclusion that pushed nursing into a medical role. Styles (1992) critically commented on specialties, stating that "it can be seen that (1) professional, practice, and market forces are accelerating the development of specialties in nursing; (2) this proliferation is not occurring in an orderly manner overall; and (3) there are no universally recognized specialties, no accepted standards, and no common principle or authority" (p. 33). Rogers vehemently opposed the practitioner movement and abhorred nurses who surrendered to "blatant perfidy spawned by such terms as pediatric associate, nurse practitioner, family health practitioner, primary care practitioner, geriatric practitioner, physician extender, and other equally weird and wonderful cover-ups designed to provide succor and profit for the nation's shamans" (1975, p. 1834). Organized nursing was also not originally supportive of the advanced practice role, frequently referring to nurse practitioners as "physician substitutes." Adding to the turmoil was the fact that advanced practice nursing, for all practical purposes, had no common foundation; program admission criteria, educational preparation, credentialing standards, and regulatory mechanisms varied widely.

Advanced practice is actually a contemporary term for the traditional practice of nursing, that of simply caring for others. What has been extremely confusing, however, is the lack of consensus about which title really distinguishes advanced practice nursing. Numerous titles are used worldwide, including nurse-anesthetist, nurse-midwife, CNS, and nurse practitioner (NP). NPs are further designated by specialty, such as pediatric NP, adult NP, family NP, acute care NP, community health NP, and women's health NP, as well as by a host of other titles. Another debate that periodically arises concerns what an advanced practice nurse really is, especially when considering CNSs and NPs. Some literature suggests that these two roles should be merged under the umbrella term *advanced nurse practitioner* to eliminate the current confusion about titles. This, it is said, would provide consistency in titling, would decrease role ambiguity, and would pave the way for a better understanding of advanced nursing practice worldwide. What would be needed, however, if this were to occur, would be a careful review and evaluation of the various titles currently in use. Potentially, a new paradigm could be mandated.

Advanced practice roles are usually discussed from a historical perspective, using four categories: nurse-anesthetist, nurse-midwife, clinical nurse specialist, and nurse practitioner. One could argue that nurse-anesthetists and nurse-midwives are nurse practitioners, but because they are the earliest specialties on record, they are almost always discussed separately. Nursing's involvement with anesthesia administration has occurred in various time periods in different countries. For example, until 1950 nurse-anesthetists were the *only anesthetists* in Scandinavia. Nurses in the United States were not involved in anesthesia until the mid-1800s.

According to Bankert (1989), the nurse's role in anesthesia originated in 1877 with Sister Mary Barnard, who is recognized as the first official nurse-anesthetist to practice in the United States; she worked at St. Vincent's Hospital in

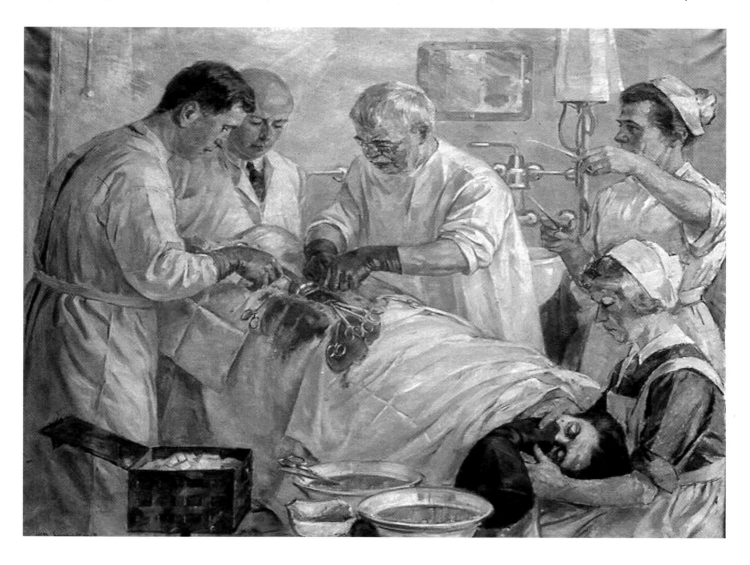

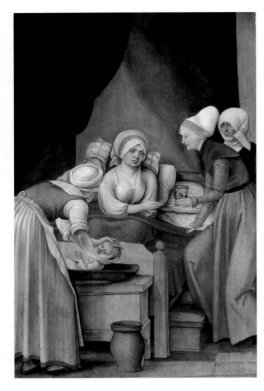

Nursing mother receives a drink from the midwife. An assistant attends to the child.

Hans Suss von Kulmbach, *Birth of the Virgin*, 1510-1511, oil on wood, 60.7 × 38 cm, Museum der Bildenden Kuenste, Leipzig, Germany. Photo courtesy of Bildarchiv Preussischer Kulturbesitz/Art Resource, NY.

Erie, PA. The first course for nurse-anesthetists was offered in 1909, and the American Association of Nurse Anesthetists was established in 1931. (There appears to be some controversy surrounding the accuracy of the Bankert publication, but this information is also provided on the association's website.) The nurse-anesthetist role developed at the request of surgeons who were searching for a solution to the high morbidity and morality rates attributed to anesthesia. Nurses were seen as professionals who could provide undivided attention to patient care during surgical procedures. Most significant, however, was the fact that no incentive existed for anyone with a medical degree to engage in such work because the surgeon collected the fees. So nurses became involved in the full range of surgical procedures, soon a standard practice in the operating room.

The history of midwifery is complex. Its original roots lie in European and African cultures. The lay practice of midwivery preceded the inception of nurse-midwives. Female relatives, neighbors, and friends as well as midwives, who functioned independently of doctors and hospitals, attended births, which were viewed as natural phenomena. Few individuals sought formal nursing education in order to provide assistance with childbirth, an event that was considered to be within the female province of innate skills. It was the establishment of male medicine in the 19th century that ultimately led to the demise of midwives.

Nurse-midwives were not introduced into the United States until 1925, through the efforts of Mary Breckenridge and the formation of the Frontier Nursing Service in Ken-

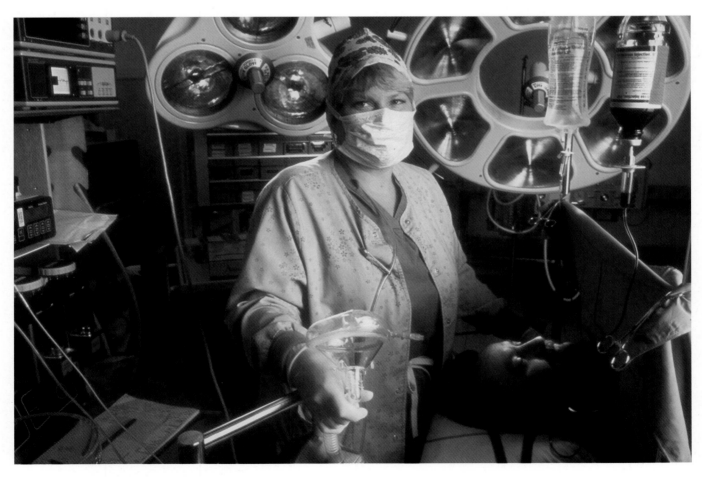

Nurse anesthetist Sharon Fassett in the operating room.

Alan Levenson, *Sharon Fassett,* photograph, Time and Life Pictures/Getty Images.

tucky. They are still somewhat of an anomaly in the 21st century, as is demonstrated by the fact that nurse-midwives attend a relatively small percentage of American births. It has been extremely difficult for nurse-midwives to obtain favorable legislation to practice because physicians in the United States have for decades been the sole legitimate providers of care during childbirth. Consequently, the majority of births occur in hospitals rather than in homes. On the other hand, nurse-midwives in other countries worldwide have been attending a significant percentage of births and

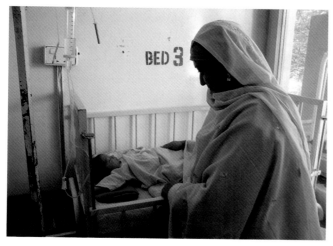

An angel of a nurse midwife who practices in a rural village in Afghanistan in 2008.

Ellyn Cavanagh, *Sonia—Midwife,* photograph, District Hospital, Jalabad, Afghanistan.

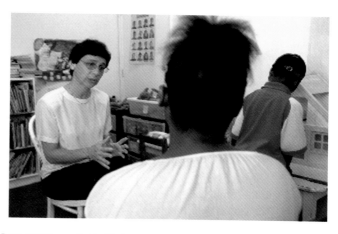

Barry Williams, *Robin Bledsoe Counseling a Client at the Community Advanced Practice Nurses Women's and Children's Clinic,* 2004, photograph.

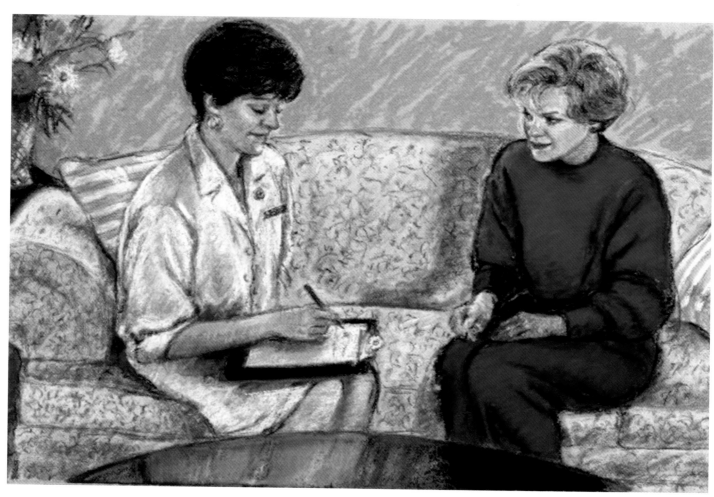

Counseling has been a vital component of the clinical nurse specialist's role since its inception.

Michele Warner, *Counseling.* Getty Images.

have been doing so for many years—prior to their initiation in the United States.

The Clinical Nurse Specialist program evolved as the result of technological advancements in psychiatry that emphasized interpersonal relationships with patients. New roles in mental health emerged, including the development of psychiatric nursing. Mental health issues in the 1930s and 1940s that resulted from war-related psychiatric problems also necessitated the need for specialized psychiatric nurses. The first master's-level degree CNS program was offered by Rutgers University in 1954 through the efforts of Hildegard Peplau, a strong nurse leader who envisioned a nurse prepared at the graduate level (CNS in psychiatric nursing) to provide direct care to psychiatric patients. Other CNS specialty programs followed. Training in a variety of specialty areas was offered; nurses would be trained to care for a patient population in a specific specialty.

These early CNSs functioned as consultants, educators, clinicians, and researchers and eventually served as role models and agents of change, once they had gained acceptance by health care organizations. They were experts in clinical care for a specific population of patients. Some CNSs would ultimately fulfill another role when health care providers instituted a case management role in the late 1980s to improve the quality of care and cut the costs and lengths of hospital stays. Although case managers could be registered nurses, advanced practice nurses, or social workers, in accordance with institutional policies and patient populations, the functions associated with this role were similar in a variety of aspects to those of the traditional CNS. This opened the door for CNSs to assume case management also.

As with other initiatives in nursing education, CNS programs experienced challenges that proved to be cyclical. During the 1990s, health care costs were escalating, hospital stays were becoming shorter, and acutely ill patients were being discharged earlier and in sicker conditions, resulting in the downsizing of the number of beds and personnel in

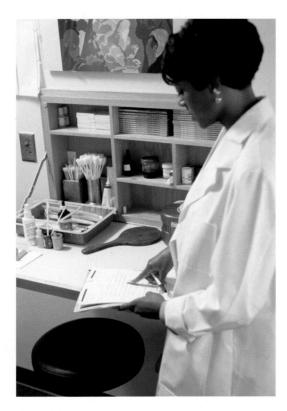

Keith Brofsky, *Clinical Nurse Specialist,* photograph. Getty Images.

hospitals. This shift to ambulatory care directly affected CNSs, who were thought to be unproven and too expensive. CNSs began losing positions nationwide. As NP programs increased in the mid 1990s, CNS programs dramatically declined. Many nursing education programs also began to combine the NP and CNS curricula. During the late 1990s, reports in the literature stressed the demand for and shortage of CNSs nationwide. A current concern of CNSs is the emerging role of the clinical nurse leader (CNL). Although there has been much discussion about the two roles, CNSs are concerned that the new CNL role duplicates the important nursing care provided by clinical specialists. To address questions raised by the nursing community about this issue, a group of individual CNSs, leaders in the field of nursing and CNS practice and education, were asked to work with the American Association of Colleges of Nursing (AACN) to develop a statement that would compare the roles of the CNL and the CNS—the similarities, differences, and complementarities (AACN, 2004). This document illustrates the distinct and complementary roles played by the CNS and the CNL. There is little reason to expect that these clinicians cannot work collaboratively to ensure that patients receive the best possible care.

The role of advanced practice nurse is not new but has changed greatly since its beginning. It predated modern professional nursing and focused on social injustices and on providing care for those in need. The role has evolved in response to numerous changes in the distribution of health care services. In general, these nurses have been ahead of their times in the areas of educational programming and legislative practices. In the 21st century, they continue to adhere to nursing's traditional values and commitments but still face challenges and struggles in their quest to shape the ongoing design of health care reform.

In the United States the first advanced practice nurses were involved in providing anesthesia, starting in the mid-1800s. Their education was controlled by and provided by physicians. Nurse-midwives appeared in the 1920s, CNSs in the 1950s, and NPs in the 1960s. In other countries, the dates vary as does the evolving presence of advanced practice nurses. Certainly, this evolution can be traced back to earlier eras in which practitioners such as lay midwives were not necessarily trained or educated in a formal sense and were not nurses, yet they served an important societal function. What does remain clear is that the role of advanced practice nurses is significant in the provision of health care alternatives to the populations of the world.

Advanced practice nurses are prepared to fulfill a variety of roles in which they provide expert clinical, educational, emotional, and supportive care. They provide safe and effective care within the scope of their practice, which is governed by protocols, and they seek consultation when necessary. Numerous functions performed by advanced practice nurses positively influence patient outcomes. These nurses:

- Serve as role models and agents of change.
- Manage high-risk patients and clinically complex cases.
- Are involved in the evaluation of costs and of the quality of outcomes.
- Are involved in promoting health and preventing disease.
- Communicate the effectiveness of expert nursing care.
- Devote extra time and attention to patients and families.
- Use a holistic approach to patient care.
- Perform high-quality primary care in the areas of their competence.

- Provide services where needs exist.
- Establish educational programs.
- Manage care in a variety of settings.
- Provide advice on the use of technological equipment.
- Provide and manage medication regimens.
- Act in their traditional advocacy role.
- Empower patients by providing the information they need so as to make informed choices.

Many other functions are also performed by APNs in accordance with their area of specialization that are equally valuable for quality health care.

In the United States, nursing is the only profession that offers certification both within and outside of the professional association. The ANA and approximately 25 other groups act as certifying bodies. The American Nurses Credentialing Center was an internal unit of the ANA from 1982 until 1991, when it was established as a separately incorporated subsidiary of the ANA. Nurses in other countries have been facing similar issues with regard to specialties and regulatory mechanisms, but for the most part their situations involve centralized authorities, such as ministries of health or professional associations. However, several events have prompted redefinitions of nursing's roles and functions. A 12-member European Community was established to oversee free movement by workers across national boundaries; international societies of nurse specialists were developed; new groups of technicians emerged; and nursing and postgraduate education programs moved into universities. In addition, the International Council of Nurses was addressing the definitions, titles, and credentialing of specialists worldwide (Styles, 1992).

The International Council of Nurses, through its International Nurse Practitioner/Advanced Practice Nursing Network (INPAPNN), has made strong efforts to facilitate worldwide understanding of advanced practice nursing, which it defines as follows: "A Nurse Practitioner/Advanced Practice Nurse is a registered nurse who has acquired the expert knowledge base, complex decision-making skills and clinical competencies for expanded practice, the characteristics of which are shaped by the context and/or country in which s/he is credentialed to practice. A master's degree is recommended for entry level" (ICN, 2002). The INPAPNN is an invaluable resource; it responds to current issues and trends, supports nurses and countries in the process of introducing the role of NP or APN, and makes readily available relevant and timely information about the roles. This is particularly important because the expertise, skills, and education associated with these roles vary widely and are specific to particular settings. For example, in certain countries the authority to write prescriptions is not customarily given to APNs.

Increased global interest in advanced practice nursing has occurred for a variety of reasons, including:

- The need for access to improved health care services;
- Primary health care initiatives that increasingly highlight nursing roles;
- Requests for cost-effective care;
- The view that nursing services improve the health care provided by a region or community;
- The expanding need for home care;
- Growing demands that rapidly escalating disease rates be addressed worldwide;
- Requests by well-informed health care consumers;
- The acceleration of specialization in nursing; and
- The expansion of nurses' roles, including writing prescriptions (Schober, 2004, pp. 73-74).

One of the most comprehensive global perspectives on advanced practice has been rendered by Schober (2004). She provides a summary of the International Council of Nurses INPAPNN international survey of nurse practitioner/advanced practice roles (ICN, 2001). The survey addressed the existence of the advanced practice role, the preparation for the role, the characteristics of the role, and the country's overseeing of and educational preparation for the implementation of the role. In addition, Schober describes advanced practice in Australia, Botswana, Canada, the Cayman Islands, the eastern Mediterranean region, Ireland, the Netherlands, New Zealand, the Republic of South Africa, South Korea, Taiwan, the United Kingdom (England, Northern Ireland, Scotland, Wales), West Africa, and the western Pacific region. The descriptions portray the unique and the common issues associated with advanced practice nursing in these countries and regions and further attest to the global diversity of the role (2004, pp. 76-92). Although this publication is 5 years old, it demonstrates the "evolving nature and growing presence of NP and [APN] roles globally."

The history of advanced practice nursing is commendable but is faced with continual challenges and barriers that threaten its existence at a time when nonphysician providers of care are in high demand. Licensure laws, regulations, and government policies have frequently limited the scope of practice of advanced practice nurses and restricted access to their services. This has created a situation in which consumers have far fewer choices of health care providers and pay higher prices for services. It happens in spite of the fact that advanced practice nurses can perform many health and medical services traditionally performed by physicians and can perform them in a variety of settings and with comparable health outcomes, lower costs, and high patient satisfaction. Havinghurst's statement, although made in 1986, still rings true: "Professional licensure laws have long made the provision of most personal health services the exclusive province of physicians. Obviously, such regulation limits consumers' options by forcing them to use highly trained, expensive personnel when other types might serve quite well" (p. 700).

Much still remains to be done regarding the policies, licensure procedures, and rules and regulations that govern advanced practice nurses. They must be expanded so that advanced practice nurses are able to fulfill the full spectrum of their scope of practice. This is especially true in terms of prescriptive privileges. This subject has created conflict, controversy, and some of the most heated debates about professional boundaries; the right to prescribe medications has fallen, historically, exclusively within the realm of the physician.

It must be noted, however, that there is little consistency regarding the role nurses should play in this field. In the United States, prescriptive authority was delegated by medical practice acts. (This is an example of giving one profession full veto power over the rules and regulations of its competitors.) Or it came from nurse practice acts. Some states have permitted nurses to prescribe medications independent of physicians; other states have not. In some countries, allowing nurses to prescribe medications is not always linked with their being advanced practice nurses or NPs. In these instances, nurses who are not advanced practice nurses may prescribe medications, particularly in underserved areas and in primary health care settings.

Other arguments concerning the advanced practice nurse have arisen and continue to escalate. Numerous physicians

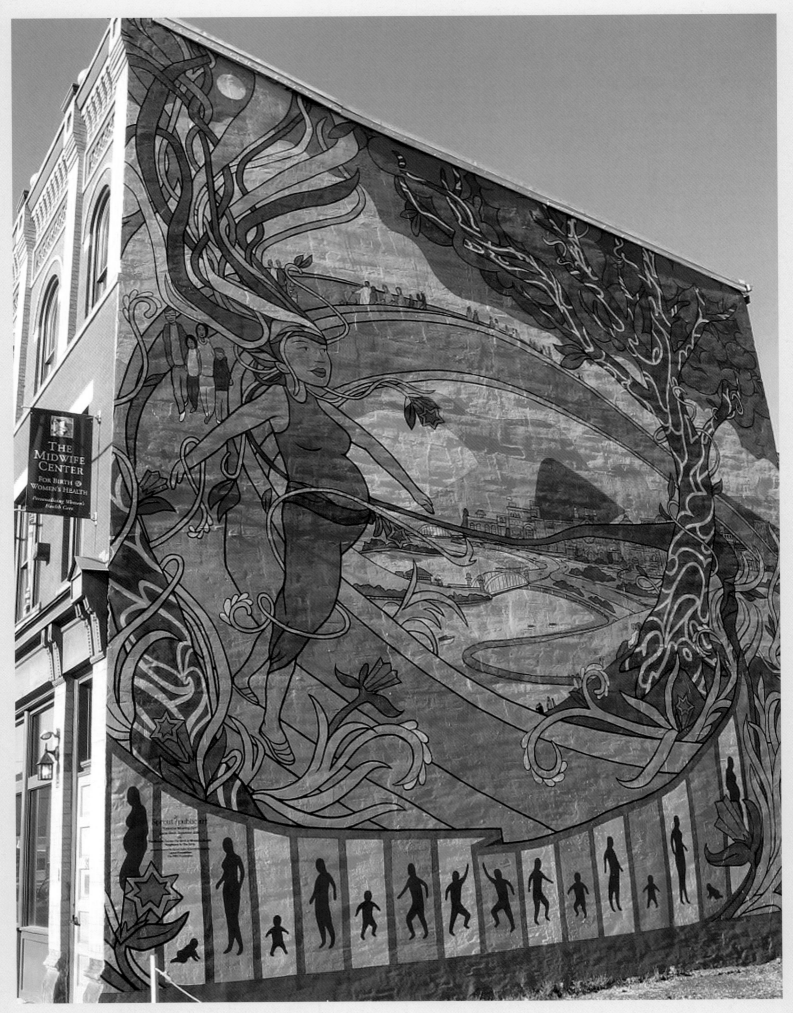

The Midwife Center for Birth and Women's Health mural *The Celestial Weaving Girl* displays themes of creativity, growth, phases of life, community, diversity, and families enjoying the local charm and architecture of the Strip in Pittsburgh. The Center is southwestern Pennsylvania's only licensed and accredited freestanding birth center offering well-woman gynecological care, prenatal care, and childbirth in a warm and supportive birth center. Care at the facility is provided by Certified Nurse-Midwives.

Lucas Stock, *Celestial Weaving Girl,* 2006, mural, 30' × 30', The Midwife Center, Pittsburgh, PA. A 2006 Sprout Public Art mural by Lucas Stock.

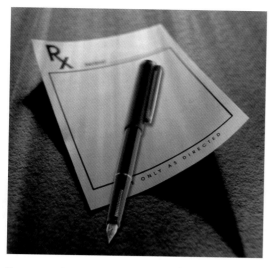

Nurse prescriptive privileges are still an ongoing issue.

Prescription Pad and Pen, photograph.

have expressed concern that these nurses are providing services beyond their abilities, that they are encroaching on medical practice, and that potentially, patients could be at risk. Yet no research studies have backed up these allegations. Instead, reports, research studies, and organizations' documents point out that the inclusion of advanced practice nurses is feasible, cost-effective, and safe and provides accessibility to those in need of health care. Indeed, the changes that have taken place since the advent of the advanced practice nurse have altered the way health care is perceived, practiced, and delivered.

The struggles to achieve legitimacy are not over for advanced practice nurses as they seek to obtain the independence and autonomy enjoyed by nurses prior to the rise of organized medicine. These struggles are reflected in Hayes' comments about nurse practitioners, which are still accurate and applicable to the whole of advanced practice nursing: "No role in nursing, or for that matter, in any field has been so debated in the literature, and possibly no other nursing function has ever been so obsessed about by those performing it as has been the NP role" (1985, p. 145). Nevertheless, these nurses have proved to be courageous, resilient, innovative, creative and, above all, committed to and compassionate about providing the most effective and highest quality of patient, family, and community health care services. They truly exemplify the attributes of the advanced nurse practitioner defined by Patterson and Haddad (1992):

> Those nurses who push beyond the known boundaries of their profession, who have the vision and flexibility necessary to consider new possibilities for improvement and/or expansion, who have the urge to ask questions and seek out the answers, who are willing to take the risks and face the challenges associated with breaking new ground, and who have the ability to articulate their thoughts clearly as they move ahead such that they contribute to the understanding and development of new knowledge and skills within nursing and thus lead their profession forward to meet the needs and demands of society.

MAGNET RECOGNITION PROGRAM

In the early years of the 21st century, one of the greatest shortages of nursing in U.S. history was predicted and ultimately, it would not be confined to the United States. A global shortage of health care workers would eventually occur, presenting a serious threat to the health of people around the globe and exacerbating the decline in the number of nurses in developing countries as a result of nurses' migration to more affluent nations. (*Brain-drain stress* is a term used to describe the impact on developing countries as their nurses are recruited to work in other countries.) Numerous factors contributed to this nursing shortage, including the continuous rise in the average age of nurses, the continuous drop in the rate of new nurses entering the profession, faculty retirement, dissatisfaction with working conditions, an increasingly elderly population, greater acuity on the part of hospitalized patients, and medical and technological advances in patient care. Even more startling was the practice of registered nurses themselves discouraging young people from considering nursing because of their own personal dissatisfaction with ongoing workplace problems.

In response to these issues, the American Academy of Nursing's Task Force on Nursing Practice in Hospitals conducted a study of 163 hospitals in 1983 to determine the variables that created an environment that attracted and retained well-qualified nurses. Of them, 41 were described as Magnet Hospitals because of their ability to attract and retain nurses. The 14 characteristics that differentiated these organizations became known as the Forces of Magnetism. These forces included quality of nursing leadership, organizational structure, management style, personnel policies and programs, professional models of care, quality of care, quality improvement, consultation and resources, autonomy, community and the health care organization, nurses as teachers, image of nursing, interdisciplinary relationships, and professional development that provided the conceptual framework for the Magnet appraisal process. They are thought of primarily as the outcomes that exemplify excellence in nursing. Each of the forces clearly defined the expectations for achievement in that specific area (ANCC, 2003).

The American Nurses Credentialing Center, through which credentialing programs and services would be offered, was established by the ANA in 1990. The ANA also approved an initial proposal for the Magnet Hospital Recognition Program for Excellence in Nursing during that same year, and a pilot project was launched. The outcome of that project was the designation, in 1994 by the American Nurses Credentialing Center, of the University of Washington Medical Center in Seattle as the first designated Magnet organization. The program's name was changed to the Magnet Nursing Services Recognition Program in 1997, and the name was officially changed to the Magnet Recognition Program in 2002. Eventually, the program was expanded to recognize nursing excellence in long-term care facilities and health care organizations abroad (ANCC, 2003).

Nurses, hospitals, and the nursing profession as a whole have benefited from this initiative. The success that followed from the designation of Magnet Hospitals was the result of key outcomes, such as increased retention of nurses, higher nurse-patient ratios, negative costs of operating a Magnet Hospital, lower recruitment costs, and nurses' reports of excellent or good patient care. But most important, health care organizations recognized that the nursing shortage was more of a quality and safety issue and not merely a workforce problem. Numerous studies particularly relevant to the nursing shortage were being conducted. One important study at the University of Pennsylvania found that in hospitals with high patient-to-nurse ratios, surgical patients experienced higher risk-adjusted 30-day mortality rates and failure-to-rescue rates, and nurses were more likely to experience burnout and job dissatisfaction (Aiken et al., 2002). An increasing amount of evidence also documented a significant association between the quality of health care that was provided and the educational level of the nursing staff. In a significant study by Aiken and associates (2003), surgical patients experienced lower mortality and failure-to-rescue rates in hospitals with higher proportions of nurses educated at the baccalaureate degree level or higher.

COMMUNITY NURSING CENTERS AND CLINICS

Nurses are making powerful contributions to health care through innovative community practices that promote health, accessibility, and lower costs and facilitate a high quality of care. Community nursing centers are key examples of these contributions to health care reform. The concept of nurse-managed care was conceived early in nursing's history by such visionary leaders as Lillian Wald at the Henry Street Settlement in New York City, Mary Breckenridge at the Frontier Nursing Service in Kentucky, and Margaret Sanger, who opened the first birth control clinic in the United States in Brooklyn, NY. These centers are classic examples of practice settings created and managed by nurses at the turn of the 20th century to provide care to under-served populations. They drew their inspiration from their observations of community needs and established the precedent of direct access by the consumer to professional nursing services.

The movement toward community nursing centers occurred in the middle to late 1970s in diverse locations, including Freeport, New York; Lehman College in Chicago; the University of Wisconsin-Milwaukee; Montana State University; and Arizona State University (Glass, 1989; Lundeen, 1994). It was influenced in part by changes in national health

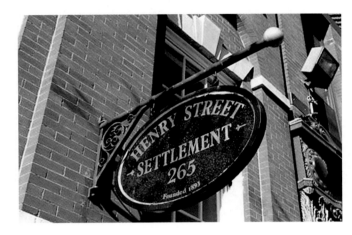

Julian Voloj, *Henry Street Settlement*, photograph.

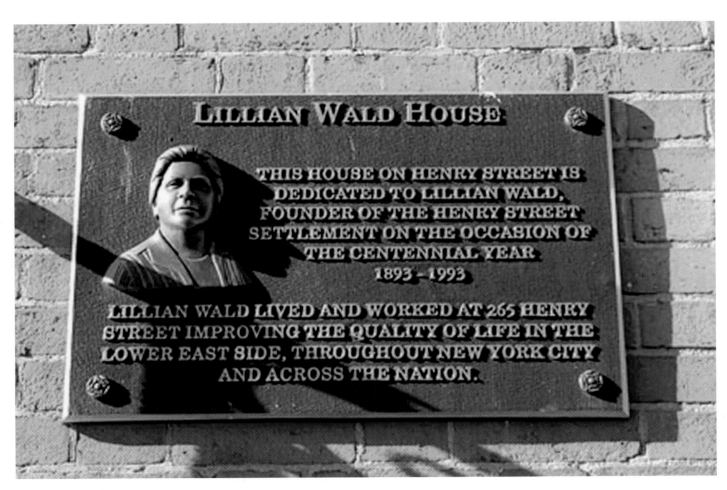

Julian Voloj, *Lillian Wald House*, photograph.

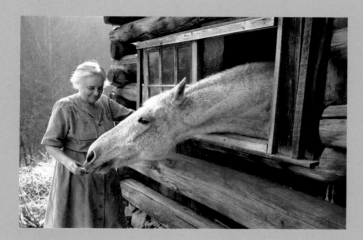

Mary Breckenridge, founder of the Frontier Nursing Service, petting her horse.

Eliot Elisofon, *Mary Breckenridge, who Runs the Frontier Nusing Service, Petting her Horse,* December 1, 1949, photograph, Time Life and QOOP.

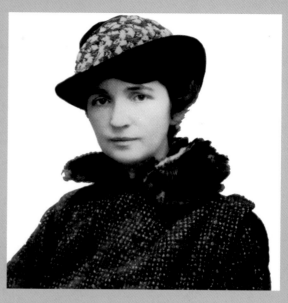

Margaret Sanger, photograph, Sophia Smith Collection, Smith Library.

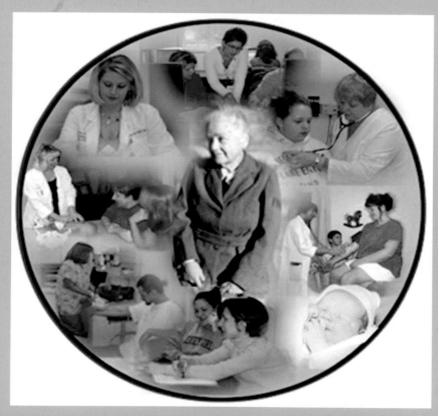

The Frontier Nursing Service celebrated 80 years of service to families in 2005.

Frontier Nursing Service, photo montage. With permission from the Frontier Nursing Service Inc.

care laws that began in the mid-1960s. As the number of centers steadily increased, two biennial conferences for nurse-managed centers were held in Milwaukee, one in 1982 and another in 1984. A variety of models of nursing centers were being developed, so an effort was made at the second conference to produce a consensus definition. The centers ranged from individual nurse-established clinics and disease-specific clinics to academically based nursing centers. In 1986, an ANA task force reviewed and modified the definition that had been developed with the assistance of a Delphi survey at the 1984 conference, with the following result:

> Nursing centers—sometimes referred to as community nursing organizations, nurse-managed centers, nursing clinics, and community nursing centers—are organizations that give the client direct access to professional nursing services. Using nursing models of health, professional nurses in these centers diagnose and treat human responses to actual and potential health problems, and promote health and optimal functioning among target populations and communities. The services provided in these centers are holistic and client centered and are reimbursable at a reasonable fee level. Accountability and responsibility for client care and professional practice remain with the professional nurse. Overall accountability and responsibility remain with the nurse executive.
>
> Nursing centers are not limited to any particular organizational configuration. Nursing centers may be freestanding businesses or may be affiliated with universities or other service institutions, such as home health agencies and hospitals. The primary characteristic of the organization is responsiveness to the health needs of the population.
>
> — ANA, 1987

Eventually the Council for Nursing Centers was formed within the NLN in 1989 as a more formalized structure within which nurses involved with centers could participate and function as an organized whole (Lundeen, 1994).

The potential for nursing clinics to assist effectively with community problems, both disease-related and social, is undeniable, and the advantages of community-based care are numerous: ease of accessibility; services and care that are sensitive to religious, racial, and cultural norms; community participation in the identification of needs; and increased comprehensive services through collaboration with social service agencies. Nurse-managed centers and clinics are run by nurses who have advanced practice degrees, including NPs, CNSs, nurse midwives, and public health/community health nurses. An additional element in centers affiliated with universities or schools of nursing is their use as sites for clinical experiences for both undergraduate and graduate students. Nursing educators may also use them as sites for faculty practice. As with the early settlement houses and nursing clinics, the philosophy that health issues are intricately and intimately connected with a variety of human issues is embraced. Family structure, social support systems, employment, education, environment, and choice of lifestyle are believed to contribute to the health and well-being of a community and its members. Thus the primary focus of nursing services is on the promotion of good health and on health education.

The varied opportunities associated with community nursing centers are far-reaching, and benefits to society and the nursing profession are numerous. An academic nursing center, the Silver Spring Community Nursing Center (University of Wisconsin-Milwaukee) and a community social service agency center, the Silver Spring Neighborhood Center, were established in 1986 and demonstrate a collaborative model of primary care. They provide a comprehensive program of primary health care to those who live in a federally subsidized residential development that houses approximately 2000 low-income persons and to those in the surrounding four census tracts of single- and multiple-unit dwellings. The original campus-based nursing center at the University of Wisconsin-Milwaukee is one of the earliest academic nursing centers, having been in operation since 1979 (Lundeen, 1993).

Another type of nursing clinic evolved from the Pine Street Inn, which was founded by Paul Sullivan in 1969 and was originally located on Pine Street in Boston to serve homeless male alcoholics. Nurses became involved because the majority of that population suffered from a variety of illnesses and wounds related to falling and fighting. The Pine Street Inn Nurses Clinic, a men's clinic, opened for a month-long trial run in Boston in 1972 as a volunteer operation. Services included basic nursing care as well as wound care, suture removal, and a variety of other types of medical and care options. As the inn expanded its services, women were seen in the men's clinic until 1987, when a shelter-based women's clinic, the Women's Inn, was opened to provide the same nursing services given in the men's clinic. Home health care, public health, and the addressing of emergent health issues were the major functions at this clinic, where an innovative nursing model promoted self-care. This model was different from those used in other community nursing clinics because originally it was not based on an advanced practice model. An additional aspect was an outreach van that traveled the city streets and alleys every night of the year to deliver food, clothing, and health care to the homeless people who would not come into the clinics.

The Pine Street Inn Nurses Clinic had an unfortunate ending; it was taken over by the Boston Health Care for the Homeless program. Discussions had begun between the two organizations in the beginning of 2001. It is interesting to note that an evaluation done by a consultant documented that the clinics generated approximately 120,000 reimbursable visits per year, thus establishing the fact that the clinics would be able to generate substantial monies. The clinic's nursing management had previously hired three nurse practitioners as a method of overcoming limited funding. Unfortunately, the future of the clinic was tied to economics, and its closure occurred in 2003 (Sered, 2003, 2004).

AID Atlanta, one of the largest AIDS service organizations, was founded in 1982. A number of its programs are in keeping with its mission of advocacy, education, and service. AID Atlanta is run by a nurse and based on nursing theory. A nurse practitioner functions in the early intervention clinic, which provides care for patients who have the human immunodeficiency virus but do not yet have AIDS. Issues of housing and other basic needs are addressed along with health care in this model. An interdisciplinary approach to case management provides for a continuum of care, including hospital- and community-based services. "This model seeks to fully integrate the nursing knowledge of the nurse practitioner into the overall case management model" (Sowell and Meadows, 1994).

It is apparent that the development of nursing centers puts nursing in a unique and important position in which it is possible to link hospital- and community-based services. Nursing centers also link educators, students, and schools of nursing with community practice settings where vital clinical experience can be obtained and joint-practice relationships can be understood. The centers offer holistic care of patients, a philosophy long emphasized in nursing's history. The growing movement to provide excellent health care to vulnerable populations and communities has allowed committed and compassionate nurses to join together to achieve that goal. One of several important organizations, the National Nursing Centers Consortium, an outgrowth of the Regional Nursing Centers Consortium formed in 1998, was established in 2002. Its mission is "to strengthen the capacity, growth and development of nurse-managed health centers, to provide access to quality care for vulnerable populations and to eliminate health disparities" (www.nncc.us, 2009). Another organization that has evolved is the Nursing Centers Research Network, founded in 2001 as a "practice-based research network composed of academic nursing centers in the Midwest United States." (www.uwm.edu/nursing).

Nursing centers have evolved worldwide; that attests to the importance of their services to vulnerable, at-risk populations and communities. Nurses are constantly on the front lines in a variety of settings and countries, providing care in clinics that deliver primary services in which all types of conditions are treated and providing specialized services, such as those dealing with diabetes, cardiology, and maternity. A remarkable and commendable program, the Wellness Center in Kampala, Uganda, was initiated in 2008. It was the result of a 3-year, public-private partnership among the U.S. President's Emergency Plan for AIDS Relief, BD (Becton, Dickinson and Company), and the International Council of Nurses. It will be managed by the Uganda National Association of Nurses and Midwives and will offer health and support services for health care workers and their families. The goals of this collaboration are to strengthen the health care system and address health worker shortages" (ICN, 2008). Doctors, nurses, and other health care workers are vulnerable to the impact of HIV/AIDS, tuberculosis, and malaria in this region. Many health care workers have become sick and have been unable to access health care easily. This wellness center will be an essential resource for them.

STANDARDIZED LANGUAGES AND CLASSIFICATION SYSTEMS

Now more than ever before it has become necessary to develop a standardized language that represents nursing. Concerns about the costs of health care and computerization will continue to force the nursing community to identify the structure and components of nursing practice and to clarify nursing's role for other health care professionals. The clinical, theoretical, and research dimensions of nursing must be brought together in a unified whole that recognizes the influence of and the need to shape the political, economic, and ethical domains. It is believed that professional advancement of the discipline can be achieved only when it is possible to use consistent language that represents the breadth and depth of nursing care and the management of that care in all settings and on all levels. Individuals, groups, and organizations have steadily moved toward that end and have developed systems of nursing language that have been appearing in the literature since the early 1970s.

Systems representing nursing languages have been described in a variety of terms, most commonly nomenclatures, vocabularies, classifications, and taxonomies that offer limited clarity about exactly which category best describes the language system. For the purposes of this discussion, the term *vocabulary* will be used to encompass these developments in nursing. Each vocabulary is developed with particular goals or purposes in mind. One of the early precursors to the development of nursing vocabularies was patient classifications for nurse staffing in the early 1950s. The usefulness of these vocabularies cannot be denied; enhanced communication, generation of research hypotheses, projections of trends, and other benefits can be realized by using them. Increasingly, they have been implemented in nursing education curricula, textbooks, research, administration and, most important, clinical practice. There has also been a significant movement to include these vocabularies in computer information systems used in health care agencies and hospitals to support the documentation of nursing care and the management of that care. Three types of vocabularies have been determined to be needed in health care: the point of care vocabulary, which occurs at the individual and practice level; the point of service vocabulary, which emphasizes the settings in which care is delivered; and the network, or reference, vocabulary, which links clinicians' documentation across integrated systems of care delivery (McCormick and Jones, 1998).

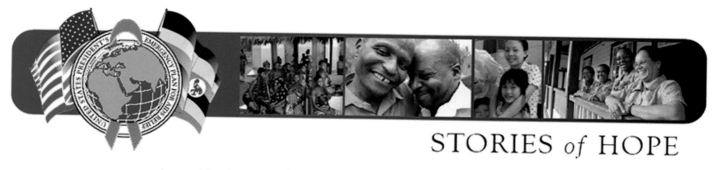

STORIES *of* HOPE

A new public-private partnership helps Ugandan health care professionals and their families.

Banner for U.S. President's Emergency Plan for AIDS Relief, electronic and photo, United States President's Emergency Plan for Aids Relief.

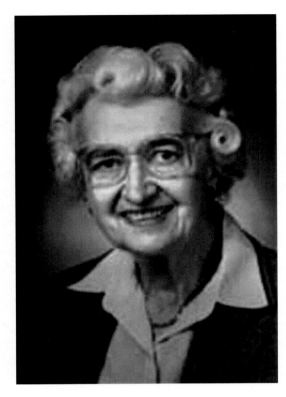

Harriet Werley, photograph.

Awareness of the need for nursing vocabularies and their focused development were strongly influenced by the identification of nursing's essential data needs. The initial work toward the development of the Nursing Minimum Data Set (NMDS) began in the 1970s. Based on the concept of the Uniform Minimum Health Data Sets, the NMDS was the initial attempt to establish uniform standards for the collection of comparable, minimally necessary, and essential nursing data. According to Werley and others (1994), it is "a standardized approach that facilitates the abstraction of essential, core minimum data to describe nursing practice. It is intended for use in any and all settings where nursing care is provided" (p. 113). Following earlier work, the NMDS was developed in the United States in 1985, and three broad categories of elements were identified: nursing care, patient or client demographics, and service. As the name itself implies, the NMDS consists of a minimum set of items that have uniform definitions and uniform categories concerning nursing practice (Werley and Lang, 1988). Through the use of this system, two primary goals potentially can be achieved: the description of the essence of nursing and the development of a database. Its importance is furthered highlighted by the establishment of national Nursing Minimum Data Sets in seven other countries—Australia, Canada, Belgium, Iceland, Switzerland, Thailand, and the Netherlands—as well as the development of an overarching international nursing minimum data set supported by the International Council for Nurses and the International Medical Informatics Association (http://www.icn.ch/matters_i-NMDS.htm). The emerging international nursing shortage and safety issues necessitate the systematic collection of nursing data that will present a clearer picture of nursing in all countries and allow for enhanced collaboration.

Although individual nurses were involved in diagnoses before the 1970s, the North American Nursing Diagnosis Association (NANDA) is considered the forerunner in this ac-

tivity. Since 1973, its members have endeavored to develop nursing diagnoses and classifications, thereby differentiating nursing from medicine. The NANDA Nursing Diagnosis Taxonomy has had great significance for the discipline of nursing and for the organization of its knowledge. Its development did become controversial for a variety of reasons, such as whether nurses' abilities to think critically about patients' problems would be decreased; whether *nursing diagnoses* is a static term incompatible with a dynamic system; and whether nurses will become lax in their observations because they will check diagnoses and indicators on a computerized list.

Since the First National Conference on Classification of Nursing Diagnosis in St. Louis (October 1973), a great number of nursing diagnoses have been approved for clinical testing. The North American Nursing Diagnosis Association's Taxonomy I was translated into the format used by the World Health Organization, the organization that revises and publishes the International Classification of Disease. This format provides for an organized international database for health care; the inclusion of nursing diagnoses assists the development of an international nursing database within the framework of the International Classification of Disease (Warren, 1994).

The Nursing Interventions Classification (NIC) was developed at the University of Iowa College of Nursing. The primary use of this classification of treatments performed by nurses is to plan and document nursing care, to communicate the nature of nursing, and to develop large databases for research related to the effectiveness of nursing care. In May 1992, the Nursing Interventions Classification was published. It listed 336 standardized direct-care nursing interventions. The classification applies to nurses in all specialty areas and in all settings and is meant to include the expertise of all nurses (Bulechek and McCloskey, 1994).

Evaluating the effectiveness of health care was one of the great challenges of the 1990s. Emphasis was placed on patients' outcomes, which have been studied primarily in relation to specific diagnoses, whether medical or nursing, and to specific interventions. The landmark research of Horn and Swain (1978) was a grand effort to organize nursing-sensitive patient outcomes. Their research was conducted to identify patient outcomes that had been influenced specifically by nursing care. Other research efforts have focused on the identification and categorization of the outcomes used to measure the effects of nursing care. In keeping with this emphasis on outcomes, the Nursing Outcomes Classification was developed at the University of Iowa College of Nursing. The overall purpose of this classification (NOC) was to identify, label, define, and classify patient outcomes and ultimately develop valid and reliable outcome measures (Johnson and Maas, 1994).

The driving force for coordination, standardization, and quality has been the ANA and its process of recognition through the Committee for Nursing Practice Information Infrastructure (CNPII). It recognized 13 systems, including 2 minimum data sets (NMDS and Nursing Management Minimum Data Set to capture the context of nursing care delivery) and 11 vocabularies, including those of the North American Nursing Diagnosis Association, the Nursing Interventions Classification, and the Nursing Outcomes Classification (Omaha System, 1992; Clinical Care Classification [formerly the Home Health Care Classification], 1992; Patient

Care Data Set, 1998; Perioperative Nursing Data Set, 1999; SNOMED-CT, 1999; International Classification for Nursing Practice, 2000; Alternative Link, 2000; Logical Observation Identifiers Names & Codes, 2002). This work has informed nursing at an international level (Thede, 2006).

Another significant development was occurring simultaneously at the international level. The International Classification for Nursing Practice (ICNP), a project of the International Council of Nurses, was initiated as a unified nursing language for worldwide use. The International Classification for Nursing Practice facilitates the development of and the cross-mapping of local terms and existing vocabularies and classifications, allowing comparisons, for example, of patient outcomes related to nursing interventions across various systems and health care delivery settings. The International Classification for Nursing Practice uses web ontology language, description logics, and associated software tools to support continuous development and maintenance of this growing terminology. At the point of care, the International Classification for Nursing Practice represents nursing diagnoses, interventions, and outcomes.

In October of 2008, the World Health Organization Family of International Classifications (WHO-FIC) approved the addition of the International Classification for Nursing Practice to the WHO-FIC as a related set of terminologies. The International Council of Nurses began development of the International Classification for Nursing Practice in 1989. Version 1.0 was released in 2005, and Version 2.0 was released in 2009. The purpose of the WHO-FIC is to promote the appropriate selection of classifications in the range of settings in the health field across the world. The International Council of Nurses will work with selected classification entities in an ongoing effort to harmonize the International Classification for Nursing Practice with other health care classifications. Its first project is to collaborate in mapping the International Classification for Nursing Practice and the International Classification of Functioning and Disabilities.

The description of nursing practice remains at the forefront of thought concerning nursing. Standardized language is believed to be the answer to facilitating that description and to making it operational and measurable. The preceding examples of vocabulary systems and the others that exist may provide the mechanism for achieving this goal as linkages among diagnoses, interventions, and outcomes are identified in the developmental processes. Perhaps most beneficial, standardized vocabularies can be computerized. This is particularly significant because information system activities and the drive toward computer-based patient records are influencing, and will continue to influence, the day-to-day practice of nurses. The Institute of Medicine had set the year 2000 as the date for the achievement of a computer-based patient record in the United States and defined it in the following manner:

> ... an electronic patient record that resides in a system specifically designed to support users through availability of complete and accurate data, practitioner reminders and alerts, clinical decision support systems, links to bodies of medical knowledge, and other aids. This definition encompasses a broader view of the patient record than is current today, moving from the notion of a location or device for keeping track of patient care events to a resource with much enhanced utility in patient care (including the ability to provide an accurate longitudinal account of care), in management of the health care system, and in extension of knowledge.
>
> — DICK AND STEIN, 1991

Nurses must continue to focus their energy on synthesizing the multiple standardized vocabularies into comprehensive yet flexible uses. The emphasis is now on the use and integration into reference terminology systems (SNOMED CT) to support the use of one, some, or all of these vocabularies as needed. As yet, there are no computer systems available in the world with the ability to integrate vocabulary, classifications, and language from the point of service to network to universal levels.

NURSING RESEARCH

Research is not a new phenomenon in nursing. Its evolution, however, has gone through numerous shifts and stages that have contributed to its overall development. At various periods in history the emphasis in nursing research was on the development of nursing education and administration, on the goals and the mission of nursing and, more recently, on clinical practice. At certain periods the idea of replication of studies was viewed in a negative light. Current thought about replication is that it is necessary so as to build on the results of other studies and to confirm achieved results. Programs of research were either virtually unheard of or did not exist. Collaborative research with nursing colleagues or researchers from other disciplines was a rarity. Often the so-called research was not of a high caliber; nurse researchers were few or were not adequately prepared to conduct research. In retrospect, nursing has come a long way in its research endeavors. Nursing now has a sound research tradition. Funding agencies give much more than lip service to nurse researchers, and federal funding has increased. Centers for nursing research have developed in various loca-

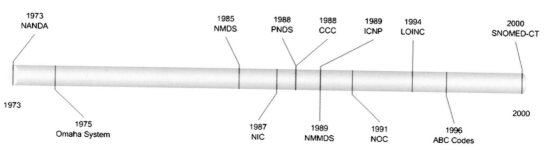

Bonnie Westra, Connie White Delaney, Debra Konicek, and Gail Keenan, *Nursing Terminology Development Timeline,* from *Nursing Outlook,* September/October 2008, p. 259.

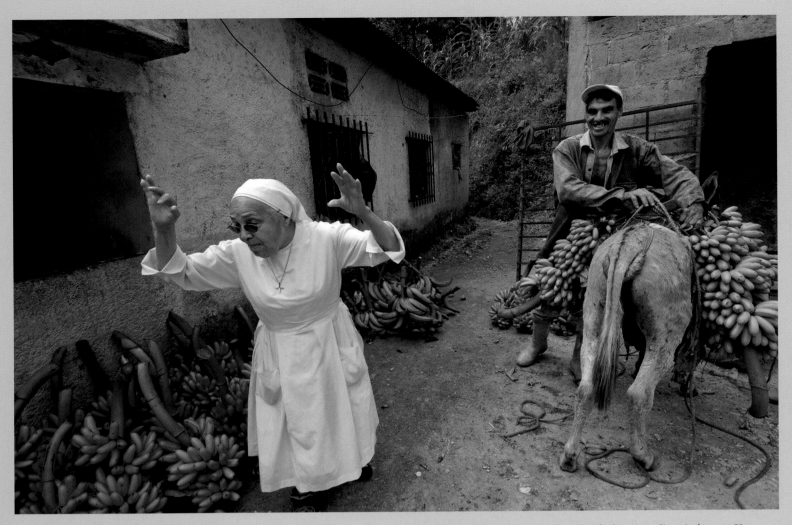

Throwing up her hands, Sister Isolena gives in to a local banana seller, who, out of respect, refuses to accept payment from her for his wares. Sister Isolena, an 80-year-old nurse, serves a wide community scattered across northeastern Venezuela.

Karen Kasmauski, *Sr. Isolena (Venezuela), Researcher,* photograph, from *Nurse: A World of Care,* 2008, p. 96.

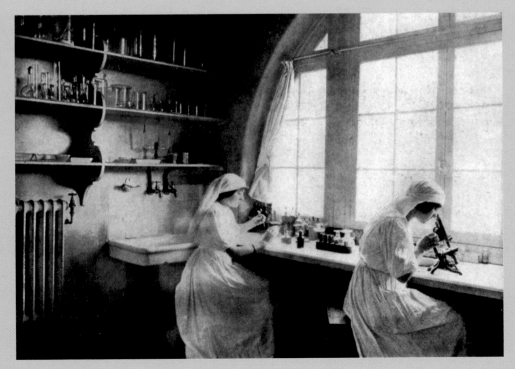

Nurses were engaged in research work for the benefit of French soldiers during WWI.

Paul Thompson, *Women Engaged in Research Work for the Benefit of French Soldiers,* 1917, photograph, National Geographic Magazine, p. 327.

tions and the number of doctorally prepared nurses has gone up significantly. Research is now accepted as being legitimate in the eyes of the nursing community. But one thing remains clear: "There is no longer any question that the priorities and goals for nursing research must be based on predictions about future consumers of nursing services, evolving systems for health care delivery, and the context within which nurse's practice" (Felton, 1989, p. 276).

A milestone was reached in the United States with the advent of the National Center for Nursing Research in 1986. The center became a reality through an intensive effort by nurses across the country and organized national, state, and specialty nursing associations. A Congressional override of a presidential veto was necessary to enact legislation that established the center at the National Institutes of Health in Washington, D.C. The purpose of the center was threefold: to provide a focal point for promoting the growth and quality of research related to nursing and patient care; to provide leadership that would expand the pool of experienced nurse researchers; and to promote closer interaction with other bases of health care research (NLN, 1985; Congress overrides veto, nursing gets center for research, 1986). The center was elevated to the status of an institute in June 1993 by the National Institutes of Health Revitalization Act of 1993. The National Institute of Nursing Research conducts and supports research and research training in universities and research centers across the country and at the National Institutes of Health. Its budget, however, has remained modest by the standards of the National Institutes of Health.

Nursing must not be satisfied with its efforts to establish research and its accomplishments in research. Commentary can still be heard that there continues to be little evidence of the use of research in practice and little evidence of demand for research by practicing nurses. The acceptance and the valuing of nursing research cannot be mandated for the majority of nurses or the general public. It will be valued only when people see that it makes a difference. And what of the future for nursing research? Lindeman (1989) depicted the hypothetical challenges of nursing research for the late 1990s or early 2000s as they are reflected in the literature about the future:

1. Knowledge derived from health care research will double every 2 to 3 years. Researchers taking longer than 2 to 3 years to complete a study will produce knowledge that is obsolete.
2. Performance records on all health professionals will be maintained in a national data base. Those data will be used to determine research access to human subjects.
3. Telematics will link epidemiological and environmental data, enabling new understanding of the causes of illness and reducing infectious diseases by the very early detection of outbreaks.
4. Computer-applied quality-assurance standards will determine whom to treat and by what means.
5. A small number of super-experts will update intelligent machines; other health professionals will use them.
6. People will become their own primary care practitioners and their own primary care systems.
7. Automation and robotics will bring hospital staffing to less than two [full-time equivalents] per occupied bed.
8. Research will be conducted through computer simulations and data banks controlled by the federal government.
9. Books, journals, and face-to-face conferences will become obsolete; people will network through computer systems or teleconferencing (p. 3).

It is perhaps time to reexamine these hypotheses. Although this list was generated just 20 short years ago, the majority of these hypothetical challenges are current realities; the rest appear to be perfectly feasible and are in the process of happening. Nursing research must not ever become an elitist endeavor. Researchers must not conduct research in isolation from practitioners but must continue to develop and increase partnerships in scholarly and scientific inquiry. It is the practitioners who are faced with the social realities involved in health care and who must deal with them daily. Research, too, does not exist in a vacuum. Its focus must change as the economic, political, and ethical influences impinge on societal needs and the delivery of health care. Consequently, the type of research that nurses must be focused on now concerns primary health care issues and health care policy.

To be effective, research must be communicated, disseminated, tested, and adopted. Nurse researchers have a responsibility and an obligation to provide opportunities for practicing nurses to be involved in research as participants in the discussion, the testing, and the use of findings. A cautionary note: adoption of research findings can be time consuming. A number of years ago, Barnard (1982) commented that nursing was in the early phase of the discipline of nursing. She said that we have a good beginning and that

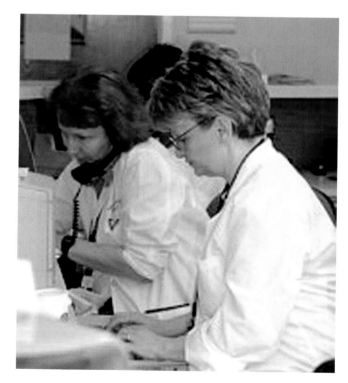

Patricia Swanson and Rose Goodwin, stem cell transplant research nurses at the National Heart, Lung, and Blood Institute and the Clinical Center.

Patricia Swanson and Rose Goodwin, Stem Cell Transplant Research Nurses, photograph, National Heart, Lung, and Blood Institute, Bethesda, MD.

increasingly, research is focusing on issues of practice. She continued:

> We must guard against impatience, expecting the answers from research to be instantly translated. History of other disciplines is instructive; it reveals the many years it takes for a science to build explanatory theories and have empirical evidence. Nurse researchers must continue with their creative work, which deals with the most complex of all phenomena, the human being, and at the same time be encouraged to search for proof and the empirical evidence that will eventually lead to scientific bases for nursing practice (p. 11).

EVIDENCE-BASED PRACTICE

The movement of evidence-based health care has evolved over time. Its birth can probably be traced to Thomas Beddoes (1760-1808), an English physician who called for a comprehensive system for the management of medical information. He was followed by Pierre Charles Alexandre Louis (1787-1872) who apparently performed a type of chart review that produced evidence to undermine beliefs about blood-letting. His publications and methods provided a cornerstone for clinical evaluation. It was not until the middle of the 20th century, however, that medical science developed the randomized clinical trial for generating information that could be turned into evidence. A turning point occurred in 1979 when Archie Cochrane, a British epidemiologist, criticized health professionals for the many years of interruption in translating evidence into practice, stating that evidence should be linked to clinicians (Goodman, 2003). His criticism resulted in a significant initiative, the Cochrane Collaborative, an international and virtual organization. This collaborative has practice-specialty groups evaluate studies and communicate findings in abstracts easily accessible on the Cochrane website.

During the past 50 years, efforts to generate evidence-based practice have intensified and expanded greatly around the world. They involve the movement from the use of evidence from a single study to the use of evidence from a body of studies from which conclusions about an intervention can be drawn. Sackett and colleagues (1996) are usually credited with defining the term *evidence-based medicine* in an editorial in the *British Medical Journal*. Evidence-based practice is clinical decision making in which the clinician critically appraises the available pertinent research. So evidence-based practice is a method of translating effectively and efficiently the best existing evidence and research into clinical practice. This method is distinguished from opinion-based decision making that is based on values and reserves. Consequently, the essentials of efficiency, quality improvement, cost containment, and increasing effectiveness in health care are addressed. Its overall goal is the improvement of patient outcomes. Yet the translation from research into practice may take as long as 17 years (Balas and Boren, 2000).

Two leaders in nursing's history are usually associated with the movement toward evidence-based nursing practice— Florence Nightingale and Virginia Henderson. Nightingale used statistics to demonstrate the evidence of nursing's effectiveness. She recognized that logical reflection combined with empirical research would lead to the development of scientific knowledge about nursing. Henderson's thinking concurred with that of Nightingale; logical reflection and empirical research are instrumental in the development of a

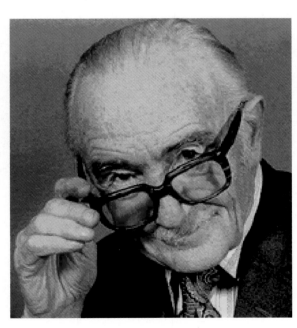

A.L. Cochrane was the first to clearly set out the vital importance of randomized controlled trials (RCTs) in assessing the effectiveness of treatments. His work led to the establishment of the Cochrane Collaboration, a worldwide endeavor dedicated to tracking down, evaluating, and synthesizing RCTs in all areas of medicine.

Professor Archibald Leman Cochrane CBE, FRCP FFCM (1909-1988), photograph, The Cochrane Collaboration.

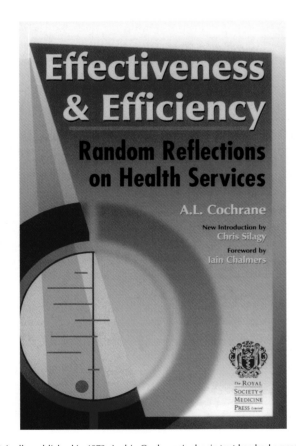

Originally published in 1972, Archie Cochrane's classic text has had a profound influence on the practice of medicine and the evaluation of medical interventions. Few doctors and other health care professionals were familiar with the term "evidence-based practice" prior to its publication.

Effectiveness and Efficiency: Random Reflections on Health Services, 1972, book cover, Royal Society of Medicine Press.

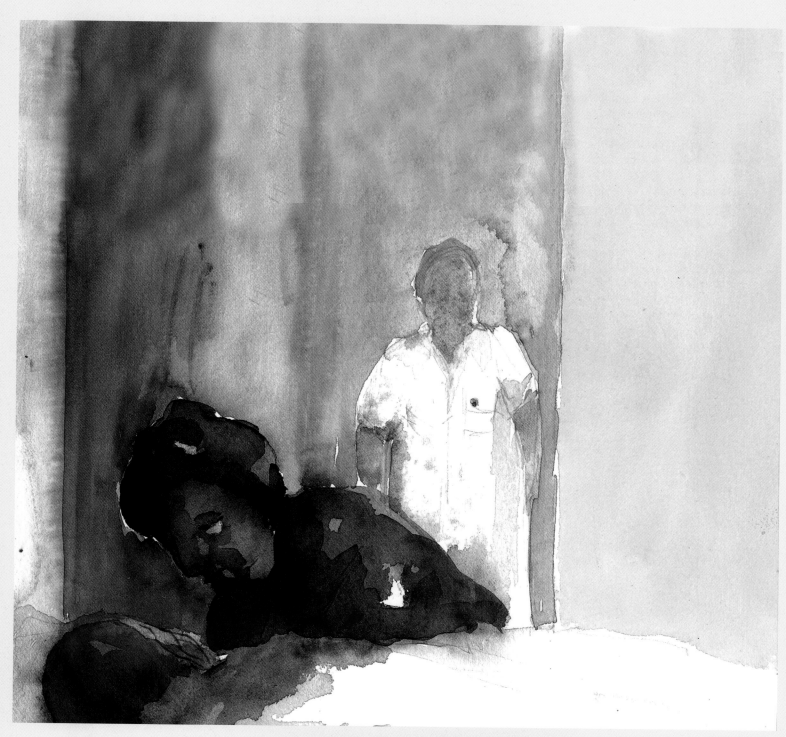

Jorit Tellervo, *Hospice,* painting, Denmark.

scientific nursing knowledge base (Evers, 2001). Her description of nursing "to assist individuals (sick or well) with those activities contributing to health, or its recovery or to peaceful death, that they perform unaided, when they have the necessary strength, will, or knowledge; to help individuals carry out prescribed therapy and to be independent of assistance as soon as possible" (Henderson, 1960) was accepted by the International Council of Nurses.

The development of evidence-based nursing is closely related to the evolution of evidence-based health practice and evidence-based medicine. Although evidence-based practice currently resonates in the field of nursing, it is not a new concept. The implementation of research findings into clinical nursing practice was being discussed as far back as 1976 and has continued for several decades among researchers and practitioners alike. The discussion, however, has not been without controversy, criticism, and issues concerning the applicability of evidence-based practice to nursing. MiJa Kim (2000) identified some of the major criticisms, with references and corresponding responses:

- Evidence-based health care overemphasizes randomized controlled trials and systematic reviews.
- Emphasis on routinization of evidence-based nursing may work against strategies of professional authority and autonomy embedded in the new nursing.
- Third-party payers may ask, Should we pay for care that has not been validated as the best way to improve the patient's health status?
- Evidence-based nursing isn't new.
- Evidence-based nursing leads to "cookbook" nursing and a disregard for individualized patient care.
- The emphasis is on current best-care practice. This is because today's golden truth may easily be tomorrow's inaccurate, or even inappropriate, information.

- Is evidence-based nursing the same as research utilization?

Other challenges involve ensuring that existing practitioners are knowledgeable about and use evidence-based practice when educating the next generation of nurses.

As evidence-based nursing practice has almost become the norm, several models for translating knowledge into practice have been used to assist in the transition. They include the Promoting Action on Research Implementation in Health Services model developed by the United Kingdom's Royal College of Nursing Institute; the Iowa Model of Evidence-Based Practice to Promote Quality Care, which was initially used at the University of Iowa Hospitals and Clinics; the Ottawa Model of Research Use; and the ACE Star Model, which was developed at the Academic Center of Evidence-Based Practice of the University of Texas Health Science Center at San Antonio, Texas. Bliss-Holtz (2007) provides a synopsis of each of the models in her comprehensive article on evidence-based practice. New models continue to be developed worldwide.

It is believed that evidence-based nursing will continue to be a significant part of nurses' everyday practice. This will occur with the ongoing development of clinical guidelines.

REDESIGNING NURSING EDUCATION

Throughout nursing's history, one element has been identified consistently as a freeing force and a powerful agent. That element is education, which the nursing discipline constantly redesigns in response to the changing needs of society, the increasingly complex mechanism of the modern hospital, the issues generated by changes and trends in the medical and human sciences, technological advances, consumers' health care problems and needs, and the paradigm shifts in health care delivery. Nursing is truly a reflection of

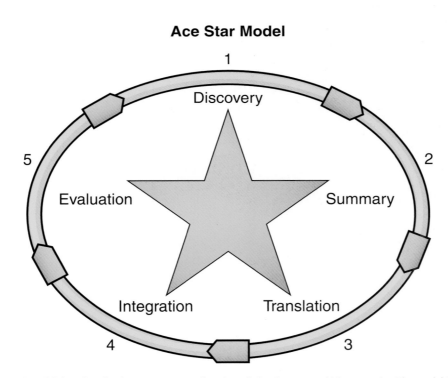

Ace Star Model

1 Discovery
2 Summary
3 Translation
4 Integration
5 Evaluation

The Ace Star Model is a conceptual model that identifies key stages to transform knowledge (i.e., research) into practice. The model illustrates five major stages of knowledge transformation: (1) knowledge discovery, (2) evidence summary, (3) translation into practice recommendations, (4) integration into practice, and (5) evaluation. Evidence-based processes and methods vary from one point of the Star Model to the next.

K.R. Stevens, *Ace Star Model*, 2004, digital image. Used with express permission.

social reality in that it is involved in a cyclical process of responding to social changes of all types. Nursing and society will continue to engage in this close and indispensable relationship, which demands a reconceptualization of both nursing education and nursing practice so as to generate the type of leadership that is mandated by the dramatic changes in health care.

It is interesting to note that Isabel Maitland Stewart expressed serious concerns about nursing leadership in the petition for educational reform she wrote more than 50 years ago:

> It is evident . . . that leadership in nursing . . . is of supreme importance at this time. Nursing has faced many critical situations in its long history, but probably none more critical than the situation it is now in, and none in which the possibilities, both of serious loss and of substantial advance, are greater. What the outcome will be depends in large measure on the kind of leadership the nursing profession can give in planning for the future and in solving stubborn and perplexing problems. . . . if past experience is any criterion, little constructive action will be taken without intelligent and courageous leadership.
>
> — STEWART, 1943, P. 326

Stewart also referred to leaders as crusaders and fighters and pondered the fate of future nursing pioneers:

> As I remember some of the older leaders, it seems to me they were a little more ready to stand up for unpopular causes and fight for what they believed in even if they were considered queer or radical by their associates. I realize that times have changed and that causes and crusades are no longer the fashion even among the young. Perhaps they will come in again, and we shall develop more crusaders like Isabel Hampton and Lavinia Dock, Adelaide Nutting, and Annie Goodrich.
>
> — STEWART, 1943, PP. 144-145

Traditionally, nursing curricula have focused on the development of leadership skills at the end of the educational program. The renewed recognition of the importance of these skills now mandates a focus on leadership development throughout the entire program of study.

Nurse educators are currently being forced to break away from established educational patterns and to envision and create new, innovative approaches to nursing education. A variety of factors have contributed to this trend, primarily the need for nurses to have more knowledge, education, and skills as well as preparation for enhanced clinical leadership, as distinct from management and advanced practice roles, and for outcomes-based practice.

CLINICAL NURSE LEADER

Two events in the United States in 1999 fostered a study by the AACN: (1) nurse educators were faced with years of declining enrollments in baccalaureate programs in nursing; (2) the Institute of Medicine released its landmark report, *To Err is Human: Building a Safer Health System*. This report called on health care systems to reduce medical errors and improve patient safety. The Board of Directors of the AACN was concerned that nursing had not succeeded in differen-

The Iowa Model of
Evidence-Based Practice to Promote Quality Care

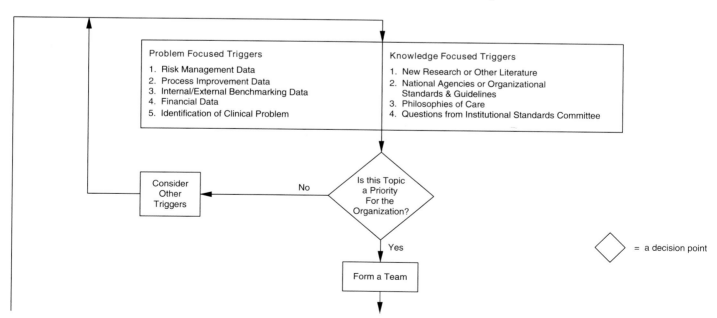

The Iowa Model has several distinct advantages; it provides a guide for clinical decision making, it provides details regarding implementation of evidence-based practice, and it includes both practitioner and organizational perspectives.

The Iowa Model of Evidence-Based Practice to Promote Quality Care (partial view) 1998, digital line drawing, book by Titler, Kleiber, Steelman, Rakel et al., 2001. Copyright of the Iowa Model of Evidence-Based Practice to Promote Quality Care will be retained by Marita G. Titler, PhD, RN, FAAN and the University of Iowa Hospitals and Clinics.

tiating the practices of registered nurses who had had various education preparations; that numerous reports had shown that the care provided to patients was not of high quality; that the knowledge base for nurses had increased dramatically; and that the health delivery system had become much more complex. The first Task Force on Education and Regulation for Professional Nursing Practice (TFER #1) was thus established (www.aacn.nche.edu/). The task force studied nursing education and issues concerning regulation and practice and sought input from and consultation with AACN members, regulators, nursing practice leaders, and other health professionals. Based on the results, TFER #1 determined that a new nursing role was needed, a role that would include nurses educated beyond the 4-year baccalaureate program. In July 2002, the AACN Board created the TFER #2 task force to continue the work begun by TFER #1. This task force's work on the examination of what the new nurse would look like resulted in the publication of the draft white paper, the Role of the Clinical Leader, in May 2003. Representatives from nursing education and practice were then invited to participate in a discussion of the proposed role at AACN's fall semiannual meeting in October 2003 and at other stakeholder meetings.

The clinical nurse leader (CNL) would be able to coordinate, manage, and evaluate effectively the care of groups of patients in complex health systems. The CNL would be a leader in the health care delivery system across all settings in which health care is delivered, not just the acute care setting. A master's degree education was proposed as the

preparation for this role. What had to be understood, however, was that the CNL would not be an advanced practice nurse; the CNL would be an advanced generalist. This fact was and has been an important point of confusion, because a master's degree in nursing is generally associated with advanced practice nurses who are specialists and have extensive education and clinical practice experience with specific patient populations. The generalist, on the other hand, would provide direct patient care and care management in health care settings and, as part of an interdisciplinary team, would implement evidence-based practice to ensure high-quality patient care. The role of the CNL is defined by AACN as follows:

> The CNL is a leader in the health care delivery system, not just the acute care setting but in all settings in which health care is delivered. The implementation of the CNL role, however, will vary across settings. The CNL role is not one of administration or management. The CNL assumes accountability for client care outcomes through the assimilation and application of research-based information to design, implement, and evaluate client plans of care. The CNL is a provider and manager of care at the point of care to individuals and cohorts of clients within a unit or healthcare setting. The CNL designs, implements, and evaluates client care by coordinating, delegating and supervising the care provided by the health care team, including licensed nurses, technicians, and other health professionals.

> — *AACN, 2007, p. 10*

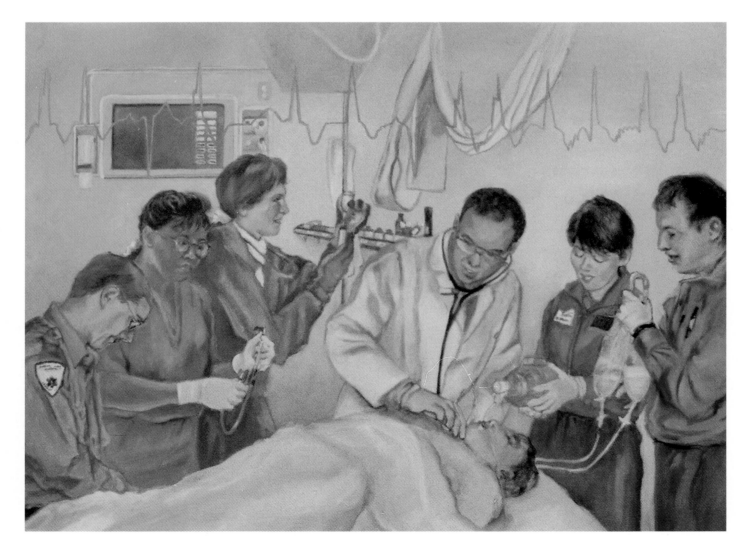

Numerous pathways to becoming a CNL were designed, and models were developed for baccalaureate graduates, associate degree graduates, graduates with baccalaureate degrees in other disciplines (second-degree students), and others involving post-BSN and post-MSN certificates. A comprehensive curriculum was developed; it stipulated all aspects of the educational program, including assumptions, core competencies, core knowledge, professional values, liberal education, and role development. After successful completion of the formal CNL education program, including a 10- to 15-week immersion experience, the CNL graduate will be eligible to sit for the CNL certification examination developed under the auspices of the AACN. As of March 2009, more than 75 CNL master's degree programs were in existence in the United States, and some were partially or completely online.

Although the CNL role has been accepted by many in the nursing community, some nurses are not convinced that the creation of this role has been an advantage to the nursing profession but has been a disadvantage. The primary issue is additional role confusion for the general public as well as for nurses. Instead of simplifying entry-into-practice standards, greater misunderstanding about nursing roles, practice, and educational degrees will occur. Certainly, confusion already exists because the CNL prepares at the master's degree level, as have CNSs and NPs. Other issues will in all probability involve salaries, the lack of understanding by hiring agencies as to what these graduates are prepared to do, the transition of the graduates into practice, whether nurses and health care agencies are ready for this "new nurse," and the answer to the question "Is the CNL the answer to clinical leadership?" Only time will tell!

DOCTOR OF NURSING PRACTICE

The emergence of the Doctor of Nursing Practice (DNP) is described in a variety of ways. Hathaway, Stegbauer, and Graff (2006) state that the DNP is being described as "a disruptive innovation that is altering the landscape of nursing and health care and creating a great deal of controversy within and beyond the profession of nursing." But they propose that the DNP "is actually the natural evolution of a larger disruptive innovation begun in the late 1960s with the advent of the nurse practitioner programs" (p. 487). The current debate about DNPs is therefore likened to the controversy surrounding the introduction of NP programs in the 1960s. Moreover, those who perceive the introduction of the DNP as a threat to the status quo and perceive themselves as being displaced adamantly oppose its establishment. Comments in the professional literature refer to the role as one that will open up new opportunities and say that it is important for nurses to have nurse practice doctorates, that the driving force of the DNP is the increasing emphasis on evidence-based practice, and that the practice doctorate will provide for the translation of evidence into clinical practice. The ever constant issue is that of the creation of role confusion between the PhD and the DNP and role confusion about nursing in general. The degrees, however, are different in that the PhD prepares nurses to generate the evidence and the DNP educates nurses to be the expert users of evidence to improve patient outcomes.

The first nurse practice doctorate, originally conceived of as a professional degree, was established at Case Western Reserve University in 1979 with the degree of Nursing Doctorate. This program was developed to prepare college graduates as nurses who would rank on levels similar to those of other health professionals who held doctoral programs, such as doctors, dentists, and others. Early programs that followed included those at Purdue University, Columbia University, the University of Kentucky, and the University of Tennessee—Memphis. Rush University, the University of South Carolina, and the University of Colorado developed additional programs to prepare expert leaders in evidence-based practice, health policy, management, or education. After an examination in 2002 of the issues surrounding these emerging programs, the AACN recommended phasing out Nursing Doctorate as a title and accepting Doctor of Nursing Practice as the title for the practice doctorate. It was to be a graduate degree in preparation for advanced nursing practice, including but not limited to the four current roles of the advanced practice nurse: clinical nurse specialist, nurse-anesthetist, nurse-midwife, and nurse practitioner.

The organization's *Position Statement on the Practice Doctorate in Nursing* was endorsed by the membership in October 2004. It distinguished practice as:

> The term *practice*, specifically nursing practice, as conceptualized in this document refers to any form of nursing intervention that influences health care outcomes for individuals or populations, including the direct care of individual patients, management of care for individuals and populations, administration of nursing and health care organizations, and the development and implementation of health policy. Preparation at the practice doctorate level includes advanced preparation in nursing, based on nursing science, and is at the highest level of nursing practice.
>
> — *AANC POSITION PAPER, 2004, P. 3*

This decision called for changing the level of preparation necessary for advanced nursing practice from master's degree to doctorate degree by the year 2015. The change was made in response to the complex nature of the current health care system, which entangles informatics, technology, health policies, business practices, and a general environment that necessitates the highest level of scientific knowledge and practice expertise to ensure high-quality patient outcomes. The DNP curriculum was built on the traditional master's degree programs; it provides education in evidence-based practice, quality improvement, systems leadership, interdisciplinary collaboration for improving the health care outcomes of patients and populations as well as other key areas. The degree was designed as a terminal degree in nursing practice and serves as an alternative to research-focused doctoral programs. Consequently, the DNP may serve to increase the number of nurses with doctoral degrees and may even generate more interest in the PhD. Finally, DNP graduates who possess exceptional clinical knowledge and skills may ease the faculty shortage by making up the majority of nursing faculty in the future.

A proliferation of DNP programs has begun, and more than 100 programs are currently in place in the United States (AACN, 2009). The AACN *Essentials of Doctoral Education for Advanced Nursing Practice* was endorsed by member institu-

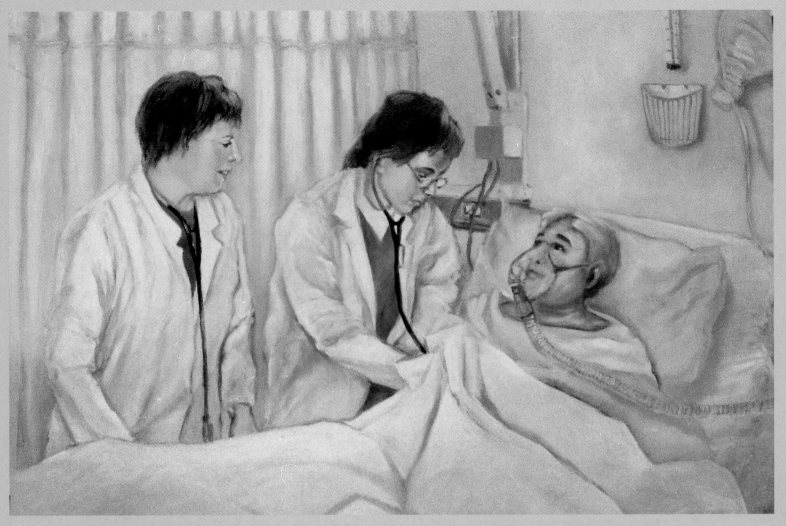

Ann Lyness, *Recovery*, 1997, mural, University of Pittsburgh, School of Nursing, Acute-Tertiary Care Department. The University of Pittsburgh Nursing School paintings are owned by the University of Pittsburgh, protected by copyright, and are reproduced with permission from the University of Pittsburgh.

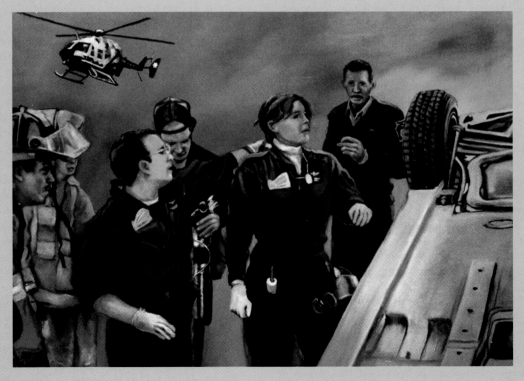

Ann Lyness, *Arrival*, 1982, mural, University of Pittsburgh, School of Nursing, Acute-Tertiary Care Department. The University of Pittsburgh Nursing School paintings are owned by the University of Pittsburgh, protected by copyright, and are reproduced with permission from the University of Pittsburgh.

tions in October 2006. The process of accreditation of DNP programs by the Commission on Collegiate Nursing Education, an arm of the AACN, was initiated in the fall of 2008. What will be the future of this movement? It is innovative, exciting, and ambitious but certainly not without challenges. One such challenge concerns whether DNP graduates should or should not use the title *doctor*. Certainly, physicians have loudly expressed their concern about the DNP role. Doctors at the AMA House of Delegates annual meeting in 2008 left little room for doubt about their views on the appropriate role of nurses in patients' medical care: "Although nurses—including those with a terminal degree in nursing—are welcomed as part of the medical team, physicians still need to take the lead." The point was also made that the use of the term *doctor* in a clinical care setting would mislead patients if it is not reserved solely for physicians. The full impact of the DNP role will not be known immediately, and its global status has yet to be determined. What is known is that it is opening up great opportunities for graduates to respond effectively to new demands in clinical practice, to deliver the highest level of care in all situations and environments, and to influence the future of the health care system.

NURSING IN THE SHADOWS

The issue of an inaccurate image has long been among nursing's struggles. Few nurses would disagree that nursing is frequently misrepresented in the media, as they remember Nurse Ratchet, Hot Lips Houlihan, and nurses in soap operas and television exposés, including "The Nightingales" in 1989. The focus of this TV series was five pretty nursing students with active libidos and their boss, Leonore, all living together in a villa called Nightingale House, located in Los Angeles. Each seems to have a troubled past, and they all spend an inordinate amount of time getting into and out of their uniforms. Needless to say, they had the types of problems that do not portray nurses in a positive light. What is positive is that nurses now are more frequently uniting in common cause to eliminate some of these negative stereotypes. "The Nightingales" was pulled from the air (after 4 months) as the result of protests by individual nurses and by nursing organizations; they believed that the negative portrayal of the nurses diminished public respect and discouraged talented people from seeking careers in nursing. Nurses and other "women in white" were featured in the November 1983 issue of *Playboy* magazine. This display

brought angry reactions from nurses in the form of letters to the editor. In addition, the nurses who were featured in the centerfold were criticized for betraying nursing and further contributing to the perpetuation of nurses as sex objects. Yet some people contend that nurses create their own images. In other words, information about nurses is acquired from their interactions with patients and visitors.

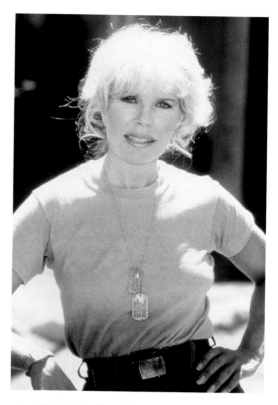

The character of "Hotlips Houlihan," played by Loretta Swit, was inspired by the real-life Korean War MASH head nurse "Hotlips Hammerly," a very attractive blonde from El Paso, Texas. She was not shy about using her romantic contacts with superior officers in efforts to get her way. Over time, Margaret softens from a completely "by-the-book" head nurse to a more laid-back member of the cast who softens her authority with humanity.

MASH, photograph. Photo courtesy of The Picture Desk.

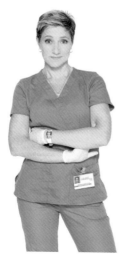

Nurse Jackie, 2009, photograph. With permission from Showtime, The Kodal Collection, and Christian Weder.

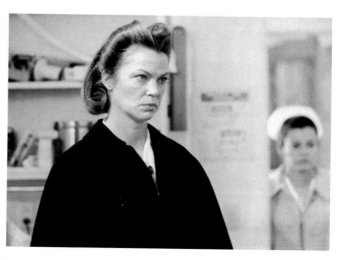

Upon arrival at a mental institution, a brash rebel rallies the patients together to take on the oppressive Nurse Ratched, a woman more a dictator than a nurse. She is a cold, sadistic tyrant who has become a popular stereotype of the nurse as battle axe. She has also become a popular symbol for the corrupting influence of power and authority in establishments such as the mental institution where the movie takes place.

One Flew over the Cuckoo's Nest, photograph. Photo courtesy of The Picture Desk.

Various strategies can be used to inform the public of the true image of the nurse, but nurses must take the initiative. Although many individual nurses and nursing organizations have been creative in attempts to educate the public about nursing, Sigma Theta Tau's *Nursing Approach* (1993) was unique. *Nursing Approach* was the first national television news series created for and about nurses. Coproduced by Sigma Theta Tau International and Samuel Merritt College's Studio Three Productions of San Francisco, the weekly half-hour show was billed as "the single most important national forum for nurses." It was televised on CNBC's American Medical Television. More than 110 news stories were aired during the 14-month life of the show. Segments focused on the work of nurses and included updates of recent research findings. This was an exceptional example of nursing's being proactive rather than reactive.

Historically, the image of nursing has been closely associated with the image of women because at its inception nursing was a job held almost exclusively by females. Women typically cared for the sick, the helpless, the weak, the elderly, and anyone else in need. Society viewed nursing as "women's work," which dissuaded men from entering the discipline, devalued nurses' work, and served as a repressive force against women with higher aspirations. Cultural conditioning, stereotypes, and the continual depiction of the female image of nurses in literature and in the media continued to contribute significantly to society's identification of nurses as females. These ideas and beliefs were consistently perpetuated and severely hindered the progress of nursing. An additional factor that had a detrimental effect on nursing was the misconception that the female mind was inherently inferior to the male mind and that intellectual growth would be harmful to women. After all, women were born to be wives and mothers, and intellectual thought would severely harm their reproductive organs, leaving them barren and psychologically impaired. It was not until their caring function was recognized as being crucial to the workings of hospitals and other health care organizations that nursing began to be recognized as an honorable profession that women could pursue. Ultimately, nursing heroines such as Florence Nightingale, Lillian Wald, Clara Barton, Dorothea

Dix, and others emerged to become excellent role models for the establishment of nursing as an honorable and respected service to humankind. "No other occupation open to women could match [nursing's] glamour, its image of dedication, its service, even its freedom" (Bullough and Bullough, 1984, p. 23).

Images of nurses abound in the media, movies, books, and the news. In the majority of instances these images are ill conceived and misrepresentative of the realities of nursing. The most common images portray nurses as ministering angels, physicians' handmaidens, bimbos, naughty nurses, or stereotypical sex objects who have no boundaries. A controversial event, an exhibition of Richard Prince's *Nurse Paintings*, was held in a variety of galleries and museums in 2008. It created a great deal of fervor among nurses, some of whom regarded it as being akin to a horror movie. The paintings were actually figures from mid-20th century covers of pulp-fiction paperback novels about nurses that had been published in the 1950s and 1960s. Prince painted the original white-uniformed nurses in an especially gory manner, with white surgical masks on their faces, with layers of magenta, wine red, and deep purple paint bleeding off parts of their bodies, and with some suggestive titles, such as "Nympho Nurse," "Surfing Nurse," and "Man-Crazy Nurse." The meaning of these paintings is open to speculation because they can be viewed in a number of ways, including that of a game of irony. Nurses may also perceive them in a positive light, portraying the state nursing is in today and depicting nurses as gagged, oppressed, silent, and stereotypical victims.

Around the world, nurses have struggled with their generally poor image, which is considered to be a significant problem that is tied to professional identity. Negative images of nursing also impact recruitment efforts, the quality of persons who choose nursing, decisions of policymakers who enact legislation that affects nursing, and the allocation of resources for nursing practice. More important, the images fail to inform consumers of the variety of vital services nurses perform. Unfortunately, nurses also continue to be more invisible in the media than other cultural and professional groups. The 1997 Woodhull Study conducted by Sigma Theta Tau International found that of 1153 health care stories in 16 major newspapers, only 11 included references to nurses. Pesut (Quoted in Sussman, 2000) commented that the Woodhull Study showed nursing in the shadows; nurses, caring, and the role of nursing were in the background. Typically, the media images place physicians, patients, and organs in the foreground, rather than nurses.

More current nursing research studies are revealing that nurses are now beginning to be portrayed in a more positive light. A study titled Celluloid Angels: A Research Study of Nurses in Feature Films 1900-2007 by Stanley (2008) found that recent films are more likely to portray nurses as strong, passionate, assertive, and self-confident professionals rather than as early films' portrayal of nurses as "self-sacrificial heroines, sex objects and romantics." This research was a massive undertaking in which Stanley reviewed more than 36,000 feature film synopses; 280 relevant feature films were identified. Most of the films were made in the United States and the United Kingdom. The Image of the Nurse on the Internet, a study by Kalisch, Begeny, and Neuman (2007), had a twofold purpose: "to examine the image of nursing on the Internet and to compare the image of nursing on the Internet in 2001 and 2004" (p. 183). Overall, the study revealed a

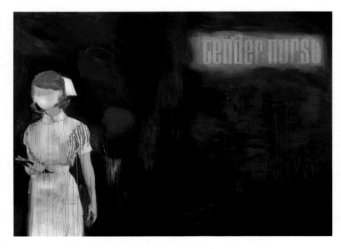

This work is part of Richard Prince's 19-painting series known as "The Nurse Paintings" that he completed between 2002 and 2003. It sold for $2,256,000 on Nov. 16, 2006, reportedly by Adam Sender.

Richard Prince, *Tender Nurse*, 2002, inkjet print and acryllic on canvas, 75" × 103". Copyright Richard Prince. Courtesy Gladstone Gallery, NY.

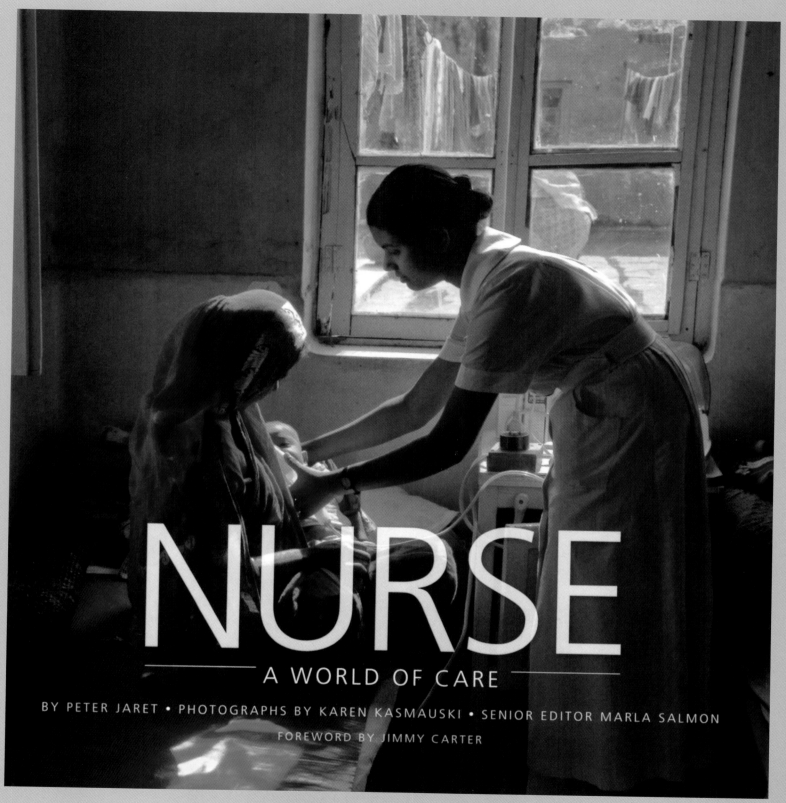

Karen Kasmauski, *Nurse: A World of Care*, book cover, 2008.

relatively positive image of nursing. "Approximately 70% of the Internet sites showed nurses as intelligent and educated, and 60% as respected, accountable, committed, competent, and trustworthy. Nurses were also shown as having specialized knowledge and skills in the majority of the websites in both years of the study" (p. 186). Of particular significance is the finding that the portrayal of nurses on the Internet is much more positive than it is in entertainment media. Numerous factors may have accounted for the rise in the status of the nursing profession in entertainment media and on the Internet but perhaps the most compelling is the fact that nurses are now more likely to have advanced degrees and to provide more of the care physicians have traditionally given.

A stunning and powerful work published in 2008 vividly portrays nurses globally in a more than positive light. *Nurse: A World of Care* documents and celebrates the vital and frequently invisible work of nurses worldwide. The faces and voices of nurses are captured in gripping detail by photographer Karen Kasmauski and writer Peter Jaret. Marla Salmon, Dean at Emory University School of Nursing, envisioned this exquisite work during her 30-year nursing career, citing the book as a wake-up call for the world so that it may understand the dangers of the nursing shortage and the critical role nurses play in community health and stability. The book truly demonstrates a team effort, not only with regard to the photographs and text but also in its publication. Emory University, with generous assistance from the Johnson & Johnson Campaign for Nursing's Future, published *NURSE: A World of Care*; Sigma Theta Tau International is the distributor. Proceeds from the sale of the book benefit the education of nurses worldwide. This book cannot help but inspire individuals to raise their voices in support of nursing, which is critical to the delivery of health care in all corners of the globe. In addition, it cannot help but inspire individuals to learn more about the real world of nursing.

The impact of the current and projected nursing shortage along with the drop in enrollment in and graduation from nursing education programs in the latter half of the 1990s created the impetus for an innovative approach to the problems. The Johnson & Johnson Company launched its Campaign for Nursing's Future in February 2002 with the stated goals being to: "enhance the image of the nursing profession, recruit new nurses and nurse educators, and to retain nurses currently in the system" (Johnson & Johnson, 2002). Campaign actions included a wide variety of initiatives, including:

- The development and distribution of recruitment materials, such as brochures, pins, posters, and videos that were free of charge;

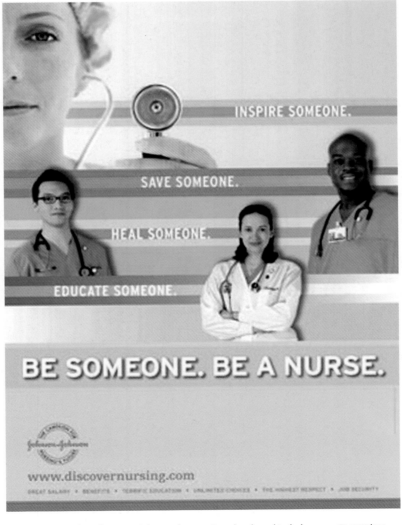

Inspire is one of the Johnson & Johnson free posters developed to help promote nursing.

Inspire, poster, 18" × 24", Johnson and Johnson.

- National television, print, and interactive advertising campaign in English and Spanish, celebrating nursing professionals and their contributions to health care;
- A website about the benefits of a nursing career, featuring links to hundreds of nursing scholarships and accredited nursing educational programs;
- Research project sponsorships;
- Broadcasts during the 2002 Winter Olympics and prime-time national television shows; and
- Fundraising for student scholarships and faculty fellowships.

The campaign was relaunched in 2007 with all new commercials, videos, and materials and a new website highlighting nurse and nurse faculty retention. Johnson & Johnson remains committed to its corporate credo: "We believe our first responsibility is to the doctors, nurses and patients, to mothers and fathers and all others who use our products and services . . . and [we are] committed to a continuing relationship with the nursing profession." This initiative has been a prime example of private sector involvement in addressing not only the image of nursing but also the current and projected nursing shortage.

LOOKING AHEAD

Although we cannot predict with certainty all of the tough issues nurses will face in the remaining years of the 21st century, trends that will have a direct bearing on nursing and health care can be observed. Emphasis on cost containment will continue, and the allocation of scarce resources will prompt an even greater increase in ethical concerns. New types of managed care will continue to develop, along with a shift to outpatient services. Environmental concerns will escalate, as will consumer focus on personal physical and mental fitness. Consumers will be even more involved in decision making about their own care and treatment and will strongly consider the use of alternative health care methods. Some hospitals have previously designed care units that combine traditional medicine with alternative techniques. On such units, complementary modalities grounded in research and posing little risk to the patient are being used.

Relationships among hospitals, health care providers, businesses, and industries will continue to be sought. In all this change, a vital place exists for nurses. Opportunities for nurses are limitless if they but grasp them or create them. Nurses can be, are prepared to be, and should be the front-runners in the primary health care movement.

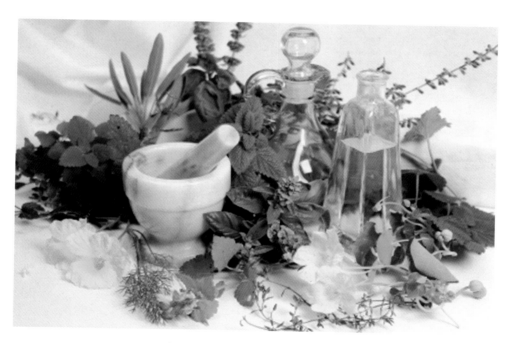

Alternative Medicine Therapies, photograph.

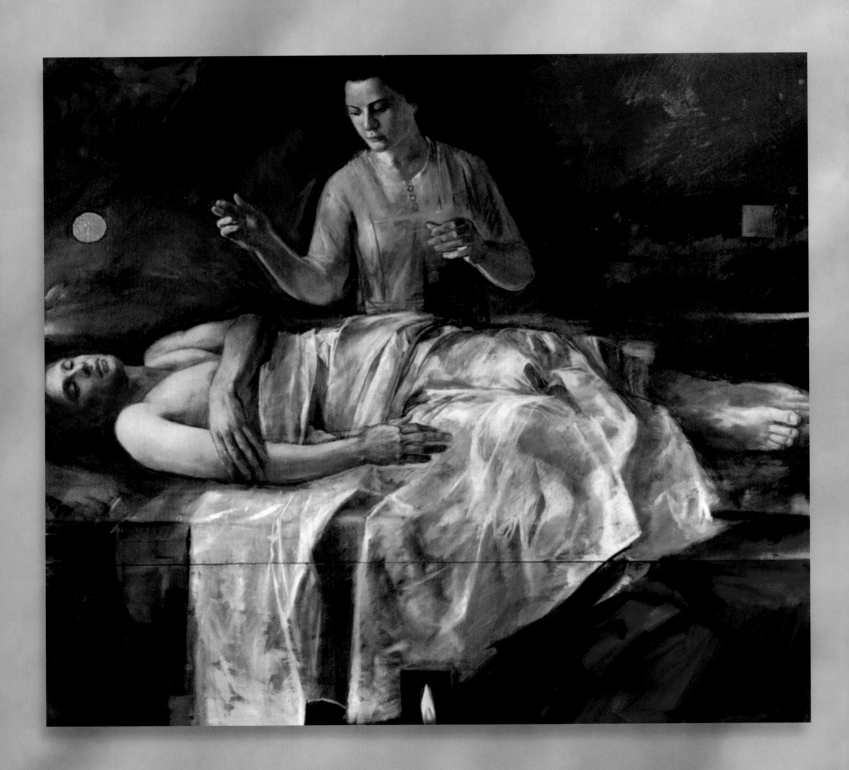

UNIT Eight

The Healing Spirit of Nursing

Nurses, now more than ever, will need to be risk takers to take up the challenge of nursing's future—to be leaders in the movement to balance the humanistic and traditional values of nursing with the highly technological, specialized care delivery system in which they practice. They will need to be visionaries, dreamers, innovators, and creators of new patterns in order to have a pivotal role in determining the health care system of the future. Nurses will need to be politically involved to steer health policy toward greater social harmony, to alleviate those social dilemmas created by competing or changing sets of values. Nurses can have an impact on institutional and political forces that control health care and its development.

– M. Patricia Donahue

Trevor Southey, *The Healer's Art,* mural, Brigham Young University.

	2000	**2001**	**2002**
Nursing	**2000** NSNA House of Delegates reaffirms BTN Project's efforts to recruit younger populations into nursing **2000** Systemized Nomenclature of Medicine—Clinical Terminology (SNOWMED—CT) reference terminology recognized by ANA **2000** Task Force on Education and Regulation for Professional Nursing Practice #1 (TFER #1) established by AACN	**2001** Arista3: Nurses and Health: A Global Future begun as a 3-year initiative **2001** University of Kentucky starts DNP program	**2002** Nursing and Midwifery Council takes over from UKCC as the U.K.'s regulatory body **2002** Johnson & Johnson Campaign for Nursing's Future launched **2002** Nursing Knowledge International established as a subsidiary of STTI
Medicine and Health Care	**2000** AIDS becomes epidemic in Africa	**2001** Artificial liver invented by Dr. Kenneth Matsumura and Alin Foundation	
Science and Technology	**2000** Pasko Rakic discovers astrocytes are brain cells that arose from stem cells and differentiated into neurons **2000** Announcement made that genome map is completed	**2001** Roger Cayrel reports age of the universe to be at least 12.5 billion years, give or take 3 billion **2001** Apple Computers announce their portable music digital player, the iPod **2001** Nuvaring birth control invented by Organon **2001** Segway Human Transporter invented **2001** Stem-cell research becomes political issue in the U.S.	**2002** Edward Teller, "Father of the H-bomb," dies
The Visual Arts		**2001** Superflat, a postmodern art movement, founded by the artist Takashi Murakami and influenced by manga and anime	**2002** Relational Art, an emerging movement, identified by Nicolas Bourriaud, a French philosopher
Daily Life	**2000** Hillary Clinton wins U.S. Senate seat in New York **2000** Dot-com businesses bust **2000** World population increases to 6.2 billion	**2001** New York's World Trade Center attacked on 9/11 **2001** George W. Bush elected President of U.S. **2001** U.S. bombs Afghanistan and topples the Taliban government after linking the World Trade Center attacks to Osama bin Laden	**2002** "Reality television" format dominates network television **2002** Catholic Church scandalized by revelations of child molestation by priests and cover-ups by the Church **2002** Enron declares bankruptcy, the largest in U.S. history **2002** President Bush labels Iran, Iraq, and North Korea an "axis of evil" and declares U.S. will wage war against states that develop weapons of mass destruction **2002** U.S. and allied forces invade Iraq in Operation Iraqi Freedom **2002** Euros, the currency of the new European Union, begin circulation

2003 Clinical Nurse Leader (CNL) proposed by AACN

2003 Nightingale Initiative for Global Health formed

2003 Institute of Medicine (IOM) report "Keeping Patients Safe: Transforming the Work Environment of Nurses" released

2004 Alliance for Nursing Informatics (ANI) established

2004 AACN member institutions vote to change preparation for advanced nursing practice from master's degree to Doctor of Nursing Practice (DNP) by 2015

2005 TIGER (Technology Informatics Guiding Education Reform) initiative created

2005 Essential nursing competencies and curricula guidelines for genetics and genomics established by consensus panel

2005 Columbia University starts DNP program

2003 SARS virus (severe acute respiratory syndrome) starts in China and spreads to Europe and North America

2003 Canadian researchers announce first successful sequencing of the genome of the coronavirus believed to cause SARS

2004 Researchers may have discovered what causes psoriasis, a common and irritating skin ailment

2004 Acupuncture proven effective as osteoarthritis treatment

2005 Cancer replaces heart disease as top cause of death for people ages 85 and under

2005 U.S. Food and Drug Administration (FDA) approve Entecavir for the treatment of hepatitis B

2005 Numbers of hospitals start to use remote surveillance with video cameras on patients

---

2003 U.S. Human Genome Project completed

2003 *Columbia* space shuttle explodes over north-central Texas as it returns from a mission

2003 Toyota's Hybrid Car developed

2004 Scientists create two new chemical elements named ununtrium (element 113) and ununpentium (element 115).

2005 Researchers construct a hydromechanical device the size of and emulating the basic function of the cochlea structure of the mammalian ear

---

2004 *Garçon à la Pipe* (1905) by Pablo Picasso sells at Sotheby's New York for $104.2 million, the highest priced painting ever sold at auction

2005 Flickr becomes the best online photo management and sharing application in the world

---

2003 U.S. invades Iraq, supposedly based on intelligence that Saddam Hussein is concealing weapons of mass destruction.

2003 Saddam Hussein captured, but weapons of mass destruction are never found

2003 Six million people across West Africa's semiarid Sahel region face famine due to invasion of locusts followed by severe drought

2004 Tsunami devastates Indonesia

2004 Tom Brokaw signs off as anchor of NBC News after 21 years

2005 Condoleezza Rice becomes first African-American female Secretary of State

2005 Iraqi people hold first free elections in more than 50 years

2005 Hurricane Katrina strikes U.S. gulf coast in one of the worst natural disasters in the nation's history

2005 Cyclist Lance Armstrong wins seventh consecutive Tour de France

2005 YouTube, the online video sharing and viewing community, established

2005 Pope John Paul II dies

2005 Benedict XVI becomes the next pope

2005 Saddam Hussein goes on trial for the killing of 143 people in the town of Dujail, Iraq, in 1982

ursing has long been involved in social activism. Its history is full of examples of nurses fighting against social injustices and agitating for positive social change. Many of these nurses are identified throughout this book, but their stories provide only a small sample of the many accomplishments that have been achieved, sometimes against overwhelming odds. The current events in health care around the world can, indeed, leave us with a feeling of dread—so many changes, all of them happening too fast, and chaos seemingly everywhere. Yet nursing has always struggled with the challenges of change. Without question, nurses have become strong, and with their strength and resiliency, they have continued their long legacy of humanitarian service. Yes, things could always be better, but it is time that we herald nursing's glories.

Nursing currently presents a complex and impressive picture in its quest not only to care for the sick but also to protect health. Its healing spirit has always provided the impetus to overcome the numerous trials and tribulations experienced throughout its history and to promote a discipline in which innovation, creativity, inventiveness, and visionary leadership have been promoted and recognized. The work of nursing is extremely intimate, bodily and spiritually, and therein lies its beauty. It embodies the traditional values of caring, compassion, commitment, advocacy, and quality of care. These values provide the foundation for the humanistic aspects of care, the aspects that impart awareness of the patient as a human being. This humanitarianism, a philosophy that asserts the worth and dignity of the individual, has consistently guided nursing in its caring functions and has long been a motive for rendering nursing care.

Care and caring are considered to be the most valuable aspects of nursing. Caring is the essence of nursing—caring for, caring with, and caring about. Caring in nursing encompasses the totality of the human being: the body, the mind, and the spirit. Nursing care thus involves attention to all facets of the human being, including the physical, biological, cultural, social, psychological, spiritual, and economic aspects. It mandates consideration of and provision of a holistic approach to patients. It mandates attention to individuals during times of sickness, during times of health, during times of need. Whatever the circumstances, nurses always can care, whether or not the patient can be cured.

The heritage of nursing is a rich one. Its history is a record of pioneering that reflects new advancements in all areas of nursing practice with each generation. From its beginning, the nursing profession has continuously endeavored to excel in patient care but has also grown and developed into a discipline that studies, researches, and creates new knowledge. In the early years of the 21st century, nursing stands poised between the past and the future. What lies ahead is open to speculation, but it is clear that this century has already been marked by many changes in the healing arts, some of which embody striking contrasts with earlier epochs. Yet many of the extraordinary innovations that have occurred are continuations of contributions from the past. These changes have resulted from the interplay of numerous factors that have arisen in an increasingly technological age. There is little doubt that nursing has been and will be forced to make severe accommodations to the larger societal context, with its increased knowledge and shifting attitudes and values.

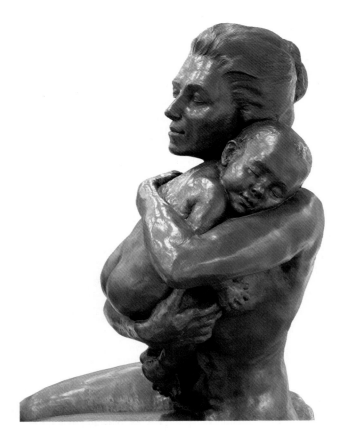

Judi Charlson, *Caring Sculpture* (side view), sculpture, lobby of Victoria Hall. Reproduced with permission from the University of Pittsburgh.

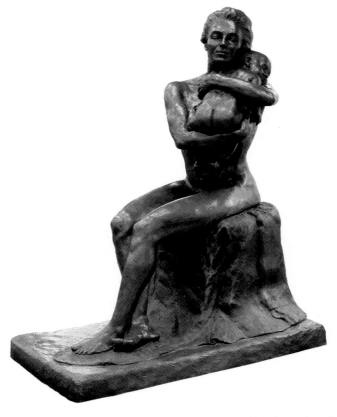

Judi Charlson, *Caring Sculpture* (full view), sculpture, lobby of Victoria Hall. Reproduced with permission from the University of Pittsburgh.

Nurses of today are expected to be many things to many people and to function in a variety of settings. They are to be excellent caregivers, adequate researchers, seekers of knowledge, and thinkers grounded in scientific and logical thought. Nurses are involved with scientific and technological advances and with all types of new roles that have broadened their opportunities but increased the scope of their responsibilities. This electronic age of the 21st century offers nurses and nursing the potential of a foundation for health care delivery unlike any previously known. Technology is transforming health care, and the nurses who understand it can guide its power to impact health care reform. Nurses are currently humanizing technology and ensuring that technology complements nursing care without replacing it. Nursing informatics plays a crucial role in defining the relationship between nursing and information technology and in accessing the knowledge that can be gained when these domains work together to create a truly healing environment. Nursing informatics is a vital facet of every part of nursing; nurses are at the heart of information flow in health care. There is no doubt that the healing spirit of nurses will continue to guide them as they create innovative ways to ensure the holistic care of patients.

THE INFORMATION REVOLUTION

It is almost an impossible task to determine the total impact of information technology on society, let alone on health care and nursing. At first, many people did not know what to make of the "new technology." Some were confused; others realized that it would help people communicate in ways they had never dreamed possible. Currently, not a day goes by without the appearance of a publication concerning the

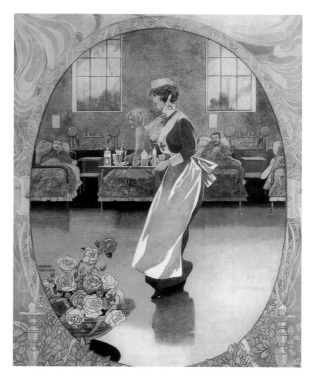

In this 1915 drawing, a nurse makes the rounds with an angel on her medicine tray.

Charles Robinson, *The Great Elixir*, 1915, drawing. Image courtesy of Pronurse.

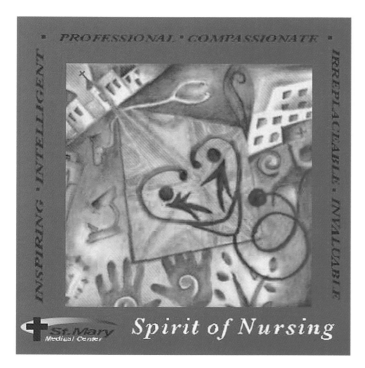

The fourth annual Spirit of Nursing Distinction in Excellence Awards ceremony was held in May of 2008 at St. Mary Medical Center in Langhorne, Pennsylvania. Nurses were nominated by their peers for promoting excellence in nursing practice and nursing research and enhancing the image of nursing.

Spirit of Nursing, 2008, logo, St. Mary's Medical Center.

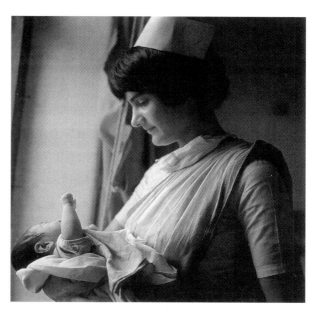

An International Health Organization nurse caring for a newborn child. The IHO is a non-government, non-profit, tax-exempt organization for the health and development of the Indian Subcontinent (India, Nepal, and Bangladesh).

Avinash Pasricha, *IHO Nurse Caring for a Newborn Child*. Photograph courtesy of the American Center, New Delhi.

wonders of the new information age and the development of new hardware, software, and electronic devices of all types. It is even difficult to keep up with the evolution of terminology that is coming forth so rapidly. For example, the term *cyberspace* has now caught on to describe not a science-fiction fantasy but today's increasingly interconnected computer systems, particularly those plugged into the Internet. *Cyberspace* has come to be synonymous with other terms—such as the *net,* the *web,* the *cloud,* the *matrix,* the *electronic frontier,* and the *information superhighway*—that have been bestowed on that nebulous space where all computer data reside. Some individuals go so far as to embrace cyberspace as the "land of knowledge."

Cyberspace encompasses millions of personal computers connected by modems to local area networks, e-mail systems, commercial online services, cell phones, and the Internet. Contrary to what some think, cyberspace is not the wires and the cables. It is about people using the new technology to communicate with one another. So advanced is the transformation that several of the most recent innovations are already being taken for granted. The most prominent, the Internet, exemplifies the paradigm shift into this information society, a world based on electronics. Physical presence is no longer necessary for communication.

The Internet was initiated more than 30 years ago in the United States as a Department of Defense experiment. On its release in 1984, it spread rapidly, nearly doubling every year. "Today, the Internet is certainly the most valuable information resource there is, with over 800 million people using it everyday. When the Internet originally was developed 30 years ago, it was mainly used by governments, scientists, researchers and university teachers. Today, the Internet is used by people in all walks of life" (Internet Trends, 2009). Remarkably, the Internet has made possible entirely new forms of social interaction with websites such as Myspace and Facebook. E-mail has long been the most widely used Internet application and for some people, their most common form of communication. More than a decade ago, approximately 30 to 40 million people in more than 160 countries had, as a minimum, e-mail access to the Internet. Since

then, there has been more than a 1000% increase in the number of users in New Zealand, Japan, and parts of Europe. One of the reasons for the success of the Internet is that it is open, or nonproprietary. It is owned by no one, and no single organization controls it. It crosses national and international boundaries.

Information technology has, in a sense, also revolutionized health care delivery. It comprises hardware and software that are used to manage and process information. The information systems in the field of health care are labeled to specify the disciplines and purposes they serve. Hospital information systems support hospital functions such as financial and other operational aims of the institutions. Nursing and medical information systems manage information that is necessary for clinical practice. They store data that are relevant and necessary to bolstering practices and informing decision making. It has become increasingly common for computerized information systems to replace patients' paper charts and various other types of paper and telephone communications, such as requisitions and memos. Computerization has entered health care and will continue to expand. In addition to hospitals, insurance companies, payers, regulators, and health care personnel have seen benefits in using computerized data for medical and patient information. Correspondingly, the specialized field of nursing informatics has become a reality; courses and entire programs of study in informatics have been developed in nursing education. Nursing informatics combines computer science, information science, and nursing science to support the practice of nursing and the delivery of nursing care.

By using advanced computer technology, a significant contribution to nursing was made through the joint efforts of Sigma Theta Tau International and the Online Computer Library Center Electronic Journals Online Service with the publication in 1994 of *The Online Journal of Knowledge Synthesis for Nursing.* This was the first peer-reviewed electronic journal to be published in the field of nursing; it was

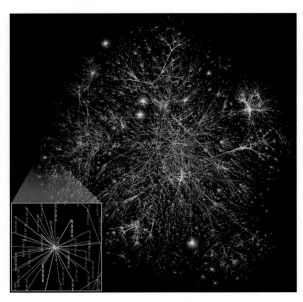

A visualization of the various routes through a portion of the Internet.

Matt Britt, *Partial Map of the Internet,* 2006, digital rendering, Wikipedia.

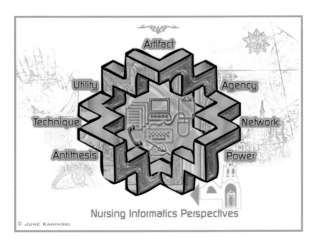

Nursing Informatics Perspectives

The Nursing Informatics Perspectives Conceptual Model. Themes derived from a literature review were fashioned into a conceptual framework that focuses on seven significant perspectives of informatics: antithesis, artifact, utility, technique, agency, networks, and power. All seven of these views present a unique yet interwoven body of analysis that helps to shape the experience and adoption of nursing informatics when applied to the context of nursing practice, education, research, and administration. (June Kaminski)

June Kaminski, *Nursing Informatics Perspectives Conceptual Model,* 2006-2007, digital image. Used with permission from June Kaminski.

the second in the field of health care. The journal, which transmits via computer linkages, provides critical reviews of research literature that are pertinent to the problems of clinical practice. Its primary importance is that knowledge is disseminated rapidly, and new knowledge is continuously available. The potential for additional innovations in nursing exists and is limitless. Conferences, list-serves, bulletin boards, and courses for credit have already found their way into the information revolution in nursing worldwide.

Consumers of health care have also entered the age of information. Individuals, families, and communities are turning to computers for advice about everyday illnesses. The practice of thumbing through clumsy, heavy reference books is becoming obsolete. With computer technology the search for medical, health, and fitness information is not only possible but rapid, and the information is generally more extensive and easier to read. The question being raised, however, pertains to the reliability of the programs, which should be regarded as another educational tool. Programs include *Mayo Clinic Medical Information and Tools for Healthy Living, The Doctor's Book of Home Remedies, Healthy Place, Medical House Call,* and *The Family Doctor.* The difficulty with the increase in this type of program lies in the fact that laypeople are providing some of the information. Their advice may or may not be accurate and may or may not contain a cautionary statement that directs users to consult their physicians for more information, rather than substituting software information for professional treatment.

The use of computer technology is, indeed, reordering the health care system, as was discussed by Lesse (1981) in *The Future of the Health Sciences.* He envisioned a system in which consumers will monitor their own care, technology will be the primary care modality, and vast storage banks of scientific data will be available to ensure that each person's good health will become a near certainty. The impact of such a system on health care professionals would be profound. Intense competition for employment would potentially occur as the number of people needed to provide care would greatly decrease, and only the most competent would be retained and advanced. There have already been significant effects on nursing since computer-assisted nursing practice has mandated changes in knowledge acquisition. Nurses now need additional knowledge in mathematics and statistics and in the biophysical and behavioral sciences. In addition, they must learn to use computers effectively and to understand their relationship to practice and research.

Major problems exist with the use of computer information systems of any type: confidentiality, security, liability, data loss, and ethical considerations. Currently, these issues are particularly sensitive in health care because the identification and resolution of ethical issues and the legislation of laws related to the use of such information are still somewhat in their infancy. As time passes, the criticism that this technology is potentially dangerous because of the loss of the human element may also be laid to rest in one way or another. Be that as it may, nurses will have to be constantly vigilant for possible misuse or misinterpretation of information that is retained in various types of databases. In addition, they will have to help ensure that technology does not become an end in itself that results in the dehumanization of patients in the health care system.

The inevitability of remarkable changes in health care

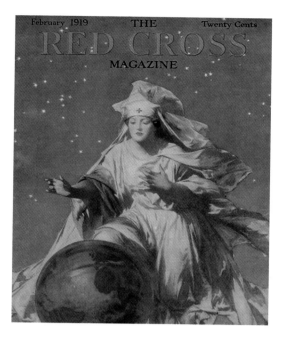

Nursing Is Universal, February 1, 1919. Image courtesy of Pronurse.

systems will continue to confront the nursing profession worldwide, particularly in relation to the impact of information and technology. This is a reality that must be understood by nurses, as must awareness that through contact with one another, through unity, and through diversity, they can be advocates and a primary force in making changes that are consistent with nursing's traditional values and will lead to good health care for all.

THE FIELD OF INFORMATICS

Information is a word and a concept that has been used from the earliest of times with immeasurable frequency. According to the *Oxford English Dictionary*, its first known historical meaning in English was the act of informing or giving form to the mind as with education or instruction. Yet no clear and precise definition of *information* currently exists because it has a diversity of meanings, depending on context, and is closely related to such concepts as communication, knowledge, meaning, and representation. In terms of data, it can be defined as a collection of facts from which conclusions may be drawn. Often the word is used without careful consideration of these various meanings. In spite of this, the information age is forcing health professionals to understand information and its relationship to health and other aspects of the human experience. In a sense, the proliferation of information today is reinforcing the need for a commitment to life-long learning. In all probability, the word *information* will continue to be redefined and processed as the use of technology expands, and it may be viewed differently in the future.

Current literature is now focusing on *informatics*, a word that also has various definitions. Europeans have long used the term *informatics* (or *informatika*) to define the study of science and the application of information technology to various disciplines. This term, in the form *informatik*, was created by a German scientist in 1957. It is said to have been originated to describe the science of automating information interactions. Makhhailov and colleagues (1967) argued for a broader meaning that would include study of the use of information technology in various communities and of the interactions between technology and human organizations: "Informatics is the discipline of science which investigates the structure and properties (not specific content) of scientific information, as well as the regularities of scientific information activity, its theory, history, methodology and organization." The usage of the term *informatics* eventually led to the modification of this definition by removing the restriction to scientific information. In addition, computation is now central to informatics because currently most information is digitally stored as well as created, transformed, and managed. Finally, the representation, processing, and communication of information have been added as objects of investigation.

The concept of informatics continues to evolve along with additional and newer definitions as the science is explored, developed, and applied. The term is most commonly used with the name of a discipline, as in medical informatics, nursing informatics, and health care informatics, where it symbolizes the relationship of informatics to that discipline. A significant point is that the term *informatics* applies not just to computers themselves but also to their optimal structure, function, and use and to the data, information, and knowledge managed and processed by computers. Informatics is the unique and required involvement of both information science and computing.

NURSING INFORMATICS

Nursing informatics began to evolve in the second half of the 20th century as information technology became integrated into health care. The actual term *nursing informatics* was originated by Scholes and Barber in 1980 (Scholes et al., 1983); Graves and Corcoran formally defined the term in 1989 as "a combination of computer science, information science, and nursing science designed to assist in the management and processing of nursing data, information, and knowledge to support the practice of nursing and the delivery of nursing care" (p. 227).

As with most events in nursing's history, the processing of information is not a new phenomenon. Frequent references in nursing informatics literature refer to Florence Nightingale as having compiled and compressed data for reports and military statistics as early as 1857. Her words echo her frustration about the lack of obtainable information related to health care that prevented evaluation of the influence of the hospital on patient-care outcomes:

There is a growing conviction that in all hospitals, even in those which are best conducted, there is a great and unnecessary waste of life. . . . in attempting to arrive at the truth, I have applied everywhere for information, but in scarcely an instance have I been able to find hospital records fit for any purpose of comparison. If they could be obtained, they would enable us to decide many other questions besides the one alluded to. . . . [I]f wisely used, these improved statistics would tell us more of the relative value of particular operations and modes of treatment than we have any means of obtaining at present. They would enable us, besides, to ascertain the influence of the hospital . . . upon the general course of operations and diseases passing through its wards; and the truth thus ascertained would enable us to save life and suffering, and to improve the treatment and management of the sick.

— *FLORENCE NIGHTINGALE, 1863, PP. 175-176*

Ozbolt and Saba (2008, p. 199) claim that these words of Nightingale "planted the seeds of 3 intertwined health sciences: health services research, evidence-based practice, and nursing informatics." They also point out the fact that this occurred 137 years before the Institute of Medicine's (2000) report estimated that as many as 98,000 hospitalized Americans were being killed annually by medical errors.

Since Graves and Cocoran's initial formal definition of nursing informatics, various additional definitions have been proposed. A widely accepted definition arose from the International Medical Informatics Association-Nursing Informatics Special Interest Group, which was adopted in 1998: "Nursing Informatics is the integration of nursing, its information and information management with information processing and communication technology to support the health of people worldwide." A more recent definition is that of the *American Nurses Association's Scope and Standards for Nursing Informatics Practice*, published in 2008: "Nursing Informatics is a specialty that integrates nursing science, computer science and information science to manage and communicate data, information, knowledge and wisdom in nursing practice." This is consistent with the American Nurses' Association (ANA)'s approval of nursing informatics as an official nursing specialty in 1992 as well as the establishment of basic certification in nursing informatics by the American Nurses Credentialing Center in 1998. This specialty designation clearly demonstrates that nursing informatics is a critical component of health care and of effective decision making and high-quality nursing practice. The research results of this area of expertise will be particularly significant in the improvement of patient care, good health, and well-being.

The field of nursing informatics began in the early 1970s and has grown exponentially. It is integrated into all aspects of nursing care and across all nursing specialties and has forced the creation of courses and programs in nursing informatics (NI). The first official NI program was established as a master of science degree at the University of Maryland School of Nursing in 1989 to develop nursing expertise in the application of computer-based information systems in hospitals, industry, and other health care organizations (Heller, Romano, and Moray, 1989). Numerous programs

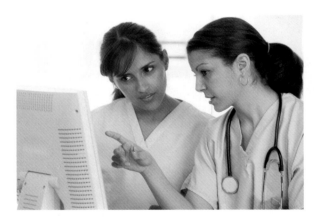

A nurse using the Online Journal of Nursing Informatics.

Nursing Informatics, photograph, Online Journal of Nursing Informatics. Image courtesy of Fotosearch

have developed since this first initiative. The expansion has resulted in various nursing education program options: individual NI courses at the undergraduate and graduate levels; undergraduate and graduate programs with concentrations in NI; graduate programs with a specialty in NI; and NI certificate programs. In addition, the importance of NI has received global recognition and NI organizations have been established in countries around the world, including Brazil, Australia, Europe, Hong Kong, the United Kingdom, and Switzerland.

Nurses with expertise in informatics are referred to as nurse informaticians or nurse informaticists. They play a key role as interpreters between the worlds of health care and computer science and ensure that information systems in health care work to support patient care. Their role also includes ensuring the representation of nursing practice in computerized systems and ensuring that these systems support the information needs of nurses. Saba presents a most compelling argument for informatics' advancing the field of nursing by "bridging the gap from nursing as an art to nursing as a science" (2001, p. 177) and believes that a future challenge for nursing professionals will be to "utilize virtual reality technology to provide real world models for teaching the 'art and science of nursing' " (p. 185). Nursing informaticists are truly in the forefront of this endeavor. They define the relationship between nurses and information technology. Their value to health care organizations lies in their understanding of technology and its power to transform the health care workplace.

Nursing informatics has escalated in all areas of nursing practice, education, administration, and research to the point where it is extremely difficult to relate its story adequately and accurately. A comprehensive description is certainly beyond a small section in this unit, so a selected list of significant events, not previously identified, highlights the centrality of informatics in the transformation of nursing in the information age.

1950s

- Implementation of the first hospital information system (HIS) occurred.
- Harriet Werley, the first designated nurse researcher at Walter Reed Army Research Institute, was asked by IBM to provide consultation about possible uses of computers in health care.

1960s

- Computer-assisted instruction (CAI) to teach obstetrical nursing by means of a simulation exercise was developed.
- *American Journal of Nursing* published "Automating Nursing's Paperwork" (1965) and "Automating Nurses' Notes" (1966), the first articles written by nurses.

1970s

- Five nursing papers were presented at the first Medical Informatics Conference in Sweden, 1974.
- The first undergraduate nursing informatics elective was established at the University of Buffalo, New York, in 1977.
- *Eclypsis*, formerly *Technicon HIS*, one of the first HISs that documented patient care and included nursing care protocols, was adopted and implemented in the Clinical Center of the National Institutes of Health in 1978.

1980s

- The ANA formed the Council on Computer Applications in Nursing in 1986.
- The journal *Computers in Nursing* was created in 1984.
- A course titled Computer Technology in Nursing was introduced on undergraduate and graduate levels at Georgetown University School of Nursing.
- The International Medical Informatics (IMIA) Association sponsored the first triennial conference on nursing informatics in 1982.
- Judy Ozobolt was the first nurse elected to the board of directors of the Symposium on Computer Applications in Medical Care (SCAMC).
- One of the first conferences in the United States concerning the subject, Computers in Nursing Care, was held at the National Institutes of Health.
- The personal computer was introduced in 1980.
- Rita Zielstorff compiled one of first textbooks about computer applications in 1980.
- Susan Grobe, the first nurse to write about incorporating NI competencies into education, published an article, "Nursing Informatics Competencies," in 1989.
- Virginia Saba organized a track for nursing papers at the Symposium on Computer Applications in Medical Care in 1981.
- Judith R. Graves, the first formally educated nursing informaticist, completed the National Library of Medicine postdoctoral study at the University of Minnesota in 1988.

1990s

- The ANA published *Scope of Practice for Nursing Informatics* in 1994.
- The ANA Congress on Nursing Practice formed the Database Steering Committee to Support Nursing Practice in 1990.
- The Nursing Informatics Special Interest Group became a formal special-interest group in the American Medical Informatics Association (AMIA), replacing the Symposium on Computer Applications in Medical Care.
- Charlotte Weaver was hired as the first chief nursing officer in the health care information technology industry in 1999.

2000s

- Technology Informatics Guiding Educational Reform (TIGER) was created, and the first invitational conference was held in 2005.
- Judith Warren was appointed to the National Committee on Vital and Health Statistics.
- Delaney and associates exemplified knowledge building through data mining using standardized nursing classifications embedded in a hospital nursing information system.
- Alliance for Nursing informatics (ANI) was established in 2004.
- The American Association of Colleges of Nursing required literacy in informatic systems in bachelor of science in nursing and doctor of nursing practice programs.
- Great growth occurred internationally in graduate nursing programs in informatics. (Osbolt and Saba, 2008; Saba, 2001; Weaver et al., 2006; Zytkowski, 2003).

It is apparent that nurse informaticians are leaders in nursing and have embraced both the art and the science of nursing with their use of technology along with the human interface. Across the globe they are dedicated to enabling the nursing profession to facilitate the transformation of health care, to support the health of people worldwide, and to function as one with their healing spirit. The recognition of their value in the design, implementation, and evaluation of information systems argues for rapidly increasing the numbers of these nursing specialists.

ELECTRONIC HEALTH RECORD

"Around the world, there is a major movement under way to make this the 'Decade of Health Information Technology.' Various governments are making billion-dollar investments to establish electronic health networks" (McBride, 2006, p. 5). The impetus for this global trend in developing electronic health records (EHRs) has arisen from accelerating costs associated with health care delivery, record management, growing demands for health care data, and the unprecedented evolution of information technology to support these trends. This drive for the implementation of computerized records is also prompted by an increased emphasis on quality, effectiveness, and efficiency in the provision of care and the mandate for safe care. Health care organizations and governments worldwide are adopting EHRs and thereby moving toward the elimination of paper-based patient clinical records. Historically, these paper-based records have had serious drawbacks, including access issues, a single copy for use by many people for various purposes, legibility, security and confidentiality breaches, and the episodic nature of the record. These factors and others increase the risk of serious errors and potential harm to patients. Computerized records, on the other hand, can and do reduce the problems associated with paper records and increase the quality of patient care.

Hippocrates developed the first known medical record in the fifth century BCE. He prescribed two goals: a medical record should accurately reflect the course of disease; a medical record should indicate the probable cause of disease (Green, Saunders, and Wilson, 2005). This, of course, was a paper record that preceded the advent of electronic records and also preceded the demand for the shared decision making of an interprofessional health care team. Although these goals are still appropriate, it is important to understand that electronic health records systems serve additional purposes for data use that were previously unattainable.

Multiple terms have been used to define electronic patient care records, which began to appear in the 1960s and continued to be developed in the early 1970s. These terms include the EHR, electronic medical record, computer-based patient record, and computer-based health record. They refer essentially to the same thing, although some individuals designate the term *EHR* a global concept and the term *electronic medical record* a localized record, the electronic version of the paper patient record. The EHR is defined by the Health Information Management Systems Society as:

> The Electronic Health Record (EHR) is a longitudinal electronic record of patient health information generated by one or more encounters in any care delivery setting. Included in this information are patient demographics, progress notes, problems, medications, vital signs, past medical history, immunizations, laboratory data and radiology reports. The EHR automates and streamlines the clinician's workflow. The EHR has the ability to generate a complete record of a clinical patient encounter, as well as supporting other care-related activities directly or indirectly via interface—including evidence-based decision support, quality management, and outcomes reporting.
> — NATIONAL INSTITUTES OF HEALTH NATIONAL CENTER FOR RESEARCH RESOURCES, 2006, P. 1

This is a standard, widely accepted definition in the field of informatics.

The emergence of standardized nursing terminology and EHR systems has provided the nursing profession with a marvelous opportunity never before imaginable. "These two forces, the EHR and the availability of a standard nursing terminology, will enable nursing to make its practice visible, to show its contribution to patient outcomes, and to demonstrate what is uniquely nursing" (Weaver et al., 2006, p. xxv). Nursing's role in patient, family, and community health as well as in health care can finally become visible and enable nursing's contribution to be considered in health care policy. The time when only a few people understood what good nursing care is about will be replaced by an understanding that nurses are the eyes and ears of ongoing patient assessment, that they generate new knowledge through research, and that they use data and research findings for support of clinical decisions. The involvement of nurses, particularly those immersed in the field of informatics, in the selection and design of information systems has indeed paved the way for the nursing discipline to be recognized as the true innovator of patient- and family-centered care within the vision of health care for all.

TECHNOLOGY AND NURSING

Numerous influences have shaped nursing's history and continue to impact nursing practice and nursing education. Foremost among these influences are nursing's identification with religion and religious orders, the effects of militarism on nursing, and the impact of technology that has shaped the work of nurses. Currently, advancements in technology are moving at an unprecedented pace and forc-

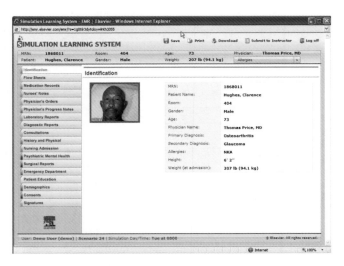

A sample patient record view from an image-based electronic health record.

Sample Electronic Medical Record. Image taken from Elsevier's Simulation Learning System.

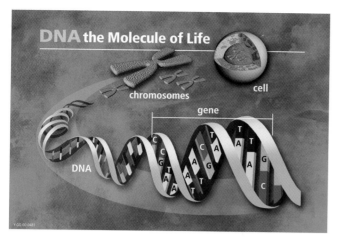

DNA: The Molecule of Life, U.S. Department of Energy Genome Program's Genome Management Information System (GMIS), http://genomics.energy.gov.

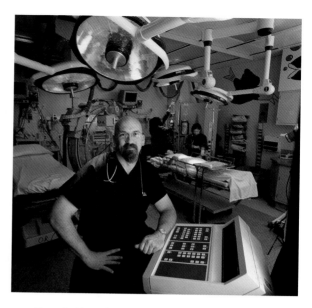

Nurse Amidst Technology, photograph. Copyright Corbis.

ing nurses to become highly skilled in and knowledgeable about increasingly sophisticated technology, including computer and information technology and genetic engineering.

Essentially, technology and information technology are revolutionizing nursing and mandating that nurses learn to care in new and different ways. This presents a shift from nursing's past relationship to technology, with its emphasis on tools, instruments, appliances, and machines, to a new type of relationship that encompasses a broader meaning of *technology* and provides the opportunity of creating new and more sophisticated dimensions of nursing. This inexorable link between nursing and technology is vividly described in the comprehensive work of Margaret Sandelowski (2000), *Devices and Desires: Gender, Technology, and American Nursing* Sandelowski asserts that nursing has been shaped by technology and that historically, nursing has been defined by others and by nurses themselves:

> Nursing has been identified—in deed, word, and image, by others and by nurses themselves—both with and against technology and thus, in an ironic way, with and against itself. Early in their history, American nurses identified nursing with technology in order to align themselves with an entity associated with science and progress and thus highly valued in Western culture. Physicians identified nursing with technology and thereby appropriated the nurse's body and mind as instruments of medicine. Yet nurses have also positioned nursing against technology to disassociate nursing from an entity that, especially after World War II, was increasingly viewed as dehumanizing patient care. But, in order to separate themselves from technology, nurses realigned their practice with an entity traditionally denigrated in Western culture: feminine caring (p. 178).

These statements are consistent with the increasing amount of literature that stresses the impact of technology on professional roles, responsibilities, and relationships.

The increasingly fast pace of technology is challenging nurses to retain the humanistic aspects of nursing care. What remains to be seen is whether nurses can continue to maintain their ability to care for patients in a humane manner while using technology. This question is particularly significant because a majority of nursing work involves interpersonal relationships in which communication with pa-

tients, families, and communities is essential. Currently, there are two prominent schools of thought: technology viewed as being an extension of and readily incorporated into humanistic nursing practice; and technology viewed as being incompatible with the nursing discipline. These concerns about the impact of technology on the nurse have been evident for quite some time. In 1977, Gadow voiced a note of caution:

> The perspective of history is essential in helping clarify the extent to which the traditional role of the nurse as steadfastly caring and minimally technical has been a function of the level of technology involved in health care. Without question, the role of the modern nurse encompasses far more knowledge and skill concerning equipment and apparatus than has ever before been the case. Does the advancement of technology in nursing signify a necessary nonconcomitant; a decline in the customary caring which has characterized nursing? Is nursing faced with a decision between preserving its commitment to *caring*, on the one hand, and following the progress of medical science with more technically intricate *curing*? (p. 8)

What is being addressed here is the fact that the intricacies of technology intimately influence aspects of nursing in every setting and directly challenge caring as the essence of nursing.

Numerous factors are involved in any discussion of technology, including a consideration of whether it is a liberating or an oppressing force. Certainly, its promise to conserve time and energy has not always been fulfilled. In fact, in some cases, technology has actually increased the time expended and produced unexpected labor. In addition, technological advancements are useless if nurses cannot access them or don't know how to use them. With the technological explosion in the health care workplace during the 20th century, nurses were forced to acquire a variety of high-tech skills as advanced tools, such as the digital thermometer, IV pumps, and life-saving machinery, were developed. Technology also changed diagnostic procedures and introduced alternative and noninvasive surgical techniques such as laser surgery. Nurses in the 21st century, however, are

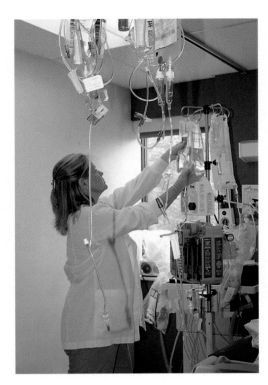

ICU. Photograph courtesy of Hunterdon Healthcare.

forced not only to quickly adapt to the rapid changes in technology but also to be Internet savvy, computer literate, and technologically fluent and competent.

TECHNOLOGY IN NURSING EDUCATION

The technological advances in health care and in nursing practice have had profound effects on nursing education. Nurse educators are faced with new challenges because they must be informed about new technologies and their usefulness in enhancing student education. They must know the best ways of implementing and using new types of technologies and must identify outcomes that are best achieved through the use of technology. A crucial element that has been unfolding is the need to bridge the gap between faculty members who did not grow up in the computer age and learners who are computer literate and electronically connected. This is particularly problematic now, when a faculty shortage exists. Faculty already burdened by a variety of issues in nursing education, along with pressure to become proficient in newer and more advanced technology, are voicing increased dissatisfaction with the educator role, and that could potentially hasten their departure from schools of nursing.

Nursing education began incorporating computer and electronic technologies into teaching strategies in the early 1990s. PowerPoint presentations, for example, were initiated and e-mail became an almost universal standard for communication. Students entering nursing programs were already using computers for both personal and academic applications and expected to continue to do so. In addition, avoiding the use of technology in health care was no longer an option, and that forced those in nursing education to evaluate their approach to the preparation of students for work in a highly technological environment. The challenge for nursing and nursing education rapidly became the issue of how to balance "high touch with high tech" and thus ensure that nurses would retain their abilities to communicate and maintain relationships. Nasbitt, Nasbitt, and Philips

(1999) expressed concern about the impact of technology on lives in the 21st century in their book *HighTech/High Touch: Technology and Our Search for Meaning.* Their view is that technology at its best "supports and improves human life, and warning that, at its worst, it alienates, isolates distorts, and destroys" (pp. 2-3).

DISTANCE EDUCATION

Distance education (sometimes referred to as e-learning) is not a new phenomenon but its history demonstrates that its evolution has been difficult, complex, and beset with challenges. It has also been faced with problems related to the implementation and acceptance of new types of educational innovations. The history of distance education has followed more than one path; a wide range of approaches have been used. The earliest form occurred in the early 1700s as correspondence courses. They were delivered by the postal service and provided a way of offering instruction to students geographically separated from campus. Later, instruction by radio, two-way audio, and television was added to a growing list of distance-education technologies. In more recent years, videoconferencing, webconferencing, interactive computer networking, handheld wireless devices, the Internet, the web, and e-mail have emerged. They provide an increasing number of options for meeting a wide variety of educational and communication needs effectively and conveniently. In 2006 the Sloan Consortium reported that more than 96% of the largest colleges and universities in the United States offered online courses; almost 3.2 million U.S. students were taking at least one online course during the fall 2005 term. In addition, online universities were beginning to appear on the scene.

Distance education courses and programs for the delivery of nursing education have increased and will continue to increase in the years to come. These initiatives have been influenced by a variety of factors, including the changing demographics of nursing students, the need for off-campus accessibility by students, issues concerning the constraints involved in combining study and parenting, and the shortages of practicing nurses and teachers. There is speculation that distance education will decrease and eventually eliminate the nursing shortage by educating more nurses for practice and by preparing future nurse educators and researchers. An added benefit is the opportunity for collaboration by nursing faculty in all areas of the nursing discipline through the use of technological advances. Of primary importance, however, is finding ways of keeping faculty members up to date in their knowledge of the changing technologies in both education and health care.

Historically, nurses have never been hesitant in seeking the most recent methods of obtaining the education needed to remain current. Distance education presents a vehicle that facilitates this goal so the challenges of health care can be met. It provides a mechanism whereby nursing students can use Internet resources to support clinical decisions, access information, support evidence-based practice, and plan care.

Facing page, Instructor Eva A. Crowdis, RN, teaching at Hartford Hospital Training School for Nurses, shows student nurses the Chase doll, 1921.

Instructor Eva A. Crowdis, RN, Teaching at Hartford Hospital Training School for Nurses, 1921, photo, Connecticut Nurses Association. Photo courtesy of The Hamilton Archives at Hartford Hospital.

CLINICAL SIMULATION

Clinical simulation is a teaching/learning strategy that has been used in nursing education since its inception. It is defined by Gaba (2004) as "an educational technique that presents a simulated patient or part of a patient and interacts appropriately with the actions taken by the simulation practitioner." Elements of the real world are integrated to achieve specific goals related to learning or evaluation. It is thus important to note that "the spectrum of simulation typology varies in complexity and fidelity, ranging from the use of static human models to human patient simulators. This spectrum can include task trainers, computer-based programs, virtual reality, high-fidelity human patient simulators, and standardized patients" (Decker et al., 2008, p. 75). The current focus in nursing education is on high-fidelity simulation that incorporates a computerized full-body mannequin that can be programmed to provide extremely realistic, physiological responses to a practitioner's actions.

Early in nursing's history, the infamous Mrs. Chase, the proxy patient, was a type of simulation in which beginning students learned and practiced their basic psychomotor nursing skills, such as bathing and bed making. The use of this mannequin was indeed an educational strategy, albeit not one that incorporated computer technology. Mrs. Chase is vividly remembered by nurses who were enrolled in schools of nursing between the early 1900s and the 1970s, during which time the mannequins were modified as new

materials came into existence and as nursing procedures became more varied and intricate. The real Mrs. Chase (née Martha Jenks Wheaton) was born in Pawtucket, Rhode Island. Her talent for making dolls evolved into the production of mannequins manufactured by the Chase Factory. The first "Chase Hospital Doll was sent to the Hartford Hospital Training School for Nurses in 1911" (Hermann, 1981).

The use of clinical simulation is rapidly gaining momentum in nursing education worldwide. Advances in this technology have been continual and have escalated during the past 40 to 45 years. The first simulators were computer based and were used by industry and the military. In the United Kingdom, Mrs. Chase was the first simulator to teach student nurses the skill of physical assessment (Peteani, 2004). Harvey, a cardiology mannequin, was first demonstrated in 1968 at the American Heart Association Scientific Sessions. It simulates 27 cardiac conditions and is the earliest part-task trainer for medical skills (Cooper and Taqueti, 2004). Resusci-Anne was created in the early 1960s for training in mouth-to-mouth ventilation. It has been widely used to train nurses and other medical personnel and ultimately became the vehicle for training in cardiopulmonary resuscitation. The first truly computer-controlled simulator did not achieve acceptance; only one was manufactured. The Sim-One was a remarkably lifelike mannequin invented in 1969 primarily to allow practice of endotracheal intubation for

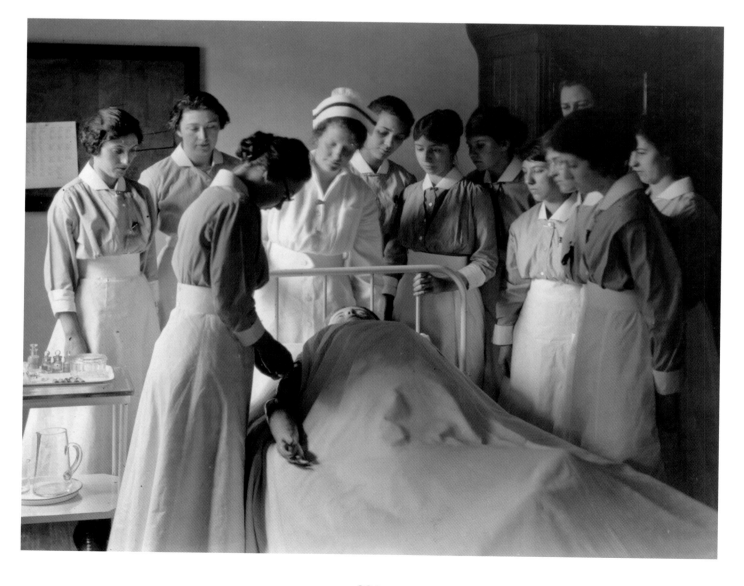

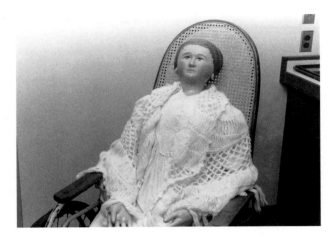

The Chase doll in retirement at Hartford Hospital, 1976.

The Chase Doll in "Retirement" at Hartford Hospital, 1976. Photo courtesy of The Hamilton Archives at Hartford Hospital.

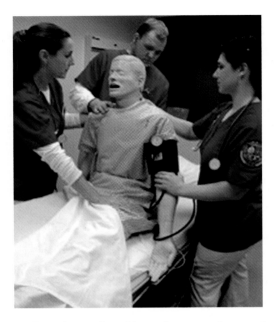

SimMan provides students and practitioners the opportunity to practice a wide variety of scenario-based training/learning needs.

Laerdal SimMan, photograph. Photo courtesy of the University of New England.

anesthesia (Cooper and Taqueti, 2004; Peteani, 2004). Since that time, advances have continued to be made in simulation technology; now there are high-fidelity human-patient simulators.

Human-patient simulators such as SimMan and SimBaby have been used in nursing schools since the mid-1990s. They are fully computerized mannequins that can be programmed to teach pathophysiology, pharmacology, and comprehensive scenario testing for one or more critical health incidents. The full scope of their use is as yet unknown, but future mannequins will be more sophisticated and possess even more realistic features and practical applications. What is known is that clinical simulation offers students rich and authentic clinical experiences in a safe, nonthreatening environment. The future of clinical simulation and the use of human-patient simulators in nursing is promising but not without challenges. Of primary concern is the percentage of real clinical time that can be accounted for through the use of simulation. Will a critical point be reached that will mandate the use of simulation for the majority of clinical time spent in nursing education programs? This issue has been fueled by the decrease in available clinical sites; the rules and regulations required by health care agencies and regulatory bodies; and patient safety. Finally, a determination must be made about how simulation fits in as a core component of, rather than an add-on to, teaching, learning, and assessment strategies.

NURSE INVENTORS, INNOVATORS, AND ENTREPRENEURS

Labels are normally used to identify leaders and to describe their superior qualities. This has been true throughout nursing's history; leaders were defined by their contributions to the growth and development of nursing in a variety of ways. They were commonly visionaries possessed with unusual discernment or foresight. They were faced with innumerable challenges that have been documented in articles, texts, biographies, reports, and studies. They were unified in their efforts to develop and shape a viable and respected nursing art. They found a congenial cause and ample scope in nursing and nursing education. These leaders believed that knowledge, not service, should be the driving force of education. Knowledge would prepare the nurse to care for patients but would also prepare the nurse for life in a diverse and complex society. In addition, the educational structure would be founded on a sound economic base that balanced the art, the science, and the spirit of nursing. The labels that describe these leaders are evident in nursing literature:

> Numerous individuals have been identified as leaders throughout nursing's history. They have been referred to as nurse leaders, nurse influentials and innovators (Fitzpatrick, 1983), nurse heroines (Christy, 1969), and the developers of nursing's legacy. In addition, Hamilton (1994) refers to a large group of eminent leaders as nurse inventors as she conceptualizes nurses' "thinking," the thoughts and the thinking patterns of the leaders who designed nursing as a vocation for women" (p. 240). These nurse inventors formed a certain set of core ideas consistent with their social context. These ideas were deliberately chosen, as they were deemed appropriate for nursing practice, for society, and for themselves.
>
> — Donahue, 2004, p. 22

These leaders in nursing shared thoughts, ideas, and resources and were committed to the future development of nursing as a profession. Although the word *inventor* is normally associated with an individual who conceptualizes and creates devices, it is particularly appropriate for these leaders, who frequently addressed the interrelationship of thought and action. They were, in truth, the inventors of ideas and thoughts that would serve as a solid foundation for nursing practice. Annie Goodrich (1932) was most profound in her comments on this topic:

To the nurse, working in the different levels of the social structure, in touch with the fundamentals of human experience, is given a unique opportunity to relate the adventure of thought to the adventure of action—this to the end that the new social order to which we are committed by our forefathers may be realized. To effectively interpret the truly great role that has been assigned her, neither a liberal education nor a high degree of technical skill will suffice. She must also be master of two tongues, the tongue of science and that of the people (p. 14).

The element of social justice was clearly an aspect of thought and deed, and it was illustrated through their work in effecting changes in public health, education, and school

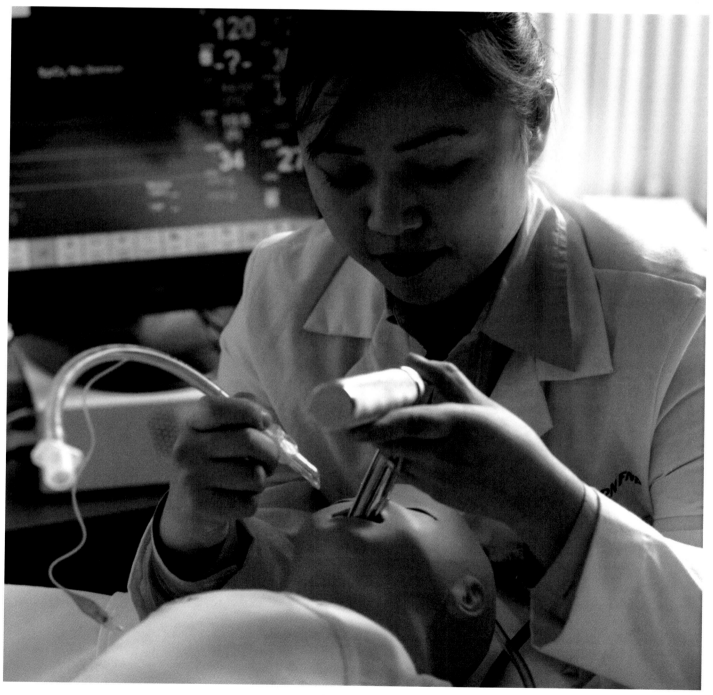

Technological advancements in educational tools such as SimBaby enable students to experience "real-life" scenarios without the risk, providing them with confidence when responding to living patients.

Nanette Bedway, *Advancement,* photograph, Nannette Bedway Studio, Cleveland, OH.

and industrial health and in the founding of settlement houses. "The social and ethical significance of nursing" thus became firmly implanted in nursing practice and nursing education.

NURSE INVENTIONS

It is somewhat difficult to differentiate among the terms *inventor*, *innovator*, and *entrepreneur* because they are commonly used interchangeably. In addition, an inventor can also be an innovator and entrepreneur; an innovator, an inventor and entrepreneur; and an entrepreneur, an inventor and innovator. This section focuses on inventions by nurses that involve primarily devices and equipment.

First of all, invention is not a new phenomenon in nursing. A rich tradition of nurse inventors pervades nursing's history as far back as Florence Nightingale's development of the polar-area diagram, which was used to illustrate causes of death that had occurred in the British Army. It is, however, difficult to determine the exact number of patents that have been granted to nurses because the United States Patent and Trademark Office does not maintain records according to occupation, nor can its official data base be directly searched for nurse inventors. There are also numerous inventions by nurses that have never been patented or advertised, an indication that the information about nursing interventions is potentially inaccurate. According to Metier (2005), more than 130 U.S. patents, ranging from food items to surgical instruments, have been issued to nurses. This number would certainly swell if information from countries around the world were readily available.

It is important to note that the majority of inventions by nurses have been created to improve patient care and to ensure patient privacy and dignity. Financial gain has not been the driving force behind their development. In fact, in many instances, a large sum of money is needed to get the patenting process under way. For example, provisional filing costs can range from $2000 to $4000 or more; utility filing fees for U.S. patents can range from $10,000 to $25,000 or more. These sums do not include the capital needed to produce and market the invention. Yet nurse-inventors have consistently been creative in their efforts to improve what wasn't or isn't working in health care. Their inventions enhance and improve clinical practice by increasing patient comfort, enhancing treatment, and facilitating care. Nurses' continual observations of and close relationships with patients and their families have been the impetus for this creativity.

The spectrum of nurse inventions is extensive and has had profound effects on health care. It is, however, beyond the scope of this book to detail all of these important and significant inventions. However, they include such items as the following:

- Med Search Hand Guard (hemoshield), a protective device for use when injecting blood into the rubber tops of vacutainers; developed by Alice Dicks in 1993.
- Bili Bonnett (photo therapy eye mask), a device to protect infants' eyes from exposure to the ultraviolet light used for premature babies undergoing treatment for jaundice; developed by Sharon Rogone in 1997.
- Puddle Guppy, a device used to aspirate fluid from floors; developed by Dan Tribastone in 1999.
- IVease, a stabling device; developed by Renée Duplessie-Miller.

- Embo-Optics Fluid Illuminator, a multihook device that illuminates the fluid chambers of IV solutions; developed by Joanie O'Donnell.
- SwaddleKeeper, a wrap to keep babies snuggled in a swaddle that won't come undone; developed by Kim Stolte.
- Snugli, a soft baby carrier; developed by Ann Moore in 1969.
- The Vollman Prone Positioner, a lightweight frame that can easily turn patients and enhance proning; developed by Kathleen Vollman (Farella, 2001; Johnson and Walsh, 2005).

Perhaps one of the most serendipitous ideas that translated into a product for women was the development of Kotex sanitary pads. This product was the result of a new use for the Cellucotton being used to bandage wounds by Army nurses serving in France during World War I. These nurses observed the wonderful absorbency of the cellulose material and began making sanitary pads from it for their own uses. Following the war, the Cellucotton Products Company experimented for 2 years and ultimately marketed the new sanitary pads known as Kotex, according to an ad that appeared in a 1921 issue of *Cosmopolitan*. There is no doubt that the future holds many inventions that will have been developed by nurses to facilitate and improve patient care.

NURSE ENTREPRENEURS

Entrepreneurship is a relatively new and developing area in nursing. A growing number of nurses are searching for more satisfying and fulfilling ways to contribute to health care, and they view entrepreneurship as the vehicle for accomplishing this goal. They are establishing businesses and are contributing to the effectiveness of health care delivery. Although numerous definitions of the concept exist in professional literature, the primary emphasis by nurse entrepreneurs is that of nurse control of practice and patient care (Riesch, 1912). In addition, both entrepreneurship and intrapreneurship nursing ventures exist. Entrepreneurship ventures include such entities as independent nurse practices and nurse-owned nursing homes and consultancy agencies.

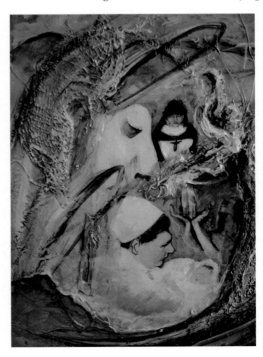

Hazel Mary Cope, *The Skilled Midwife*, 2009, mixed media.

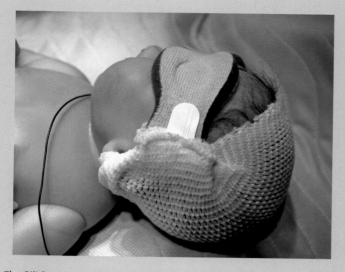

The Bili-Bonnet, created by Small Beginnings, is a photo-therapy mask that molds to the preemie/newborn's face to prevent light from coming in around the sides. It is currently the only mask with zero light penetration, while it also removes pressure from the occular space. These masks are being used in NICUs worldwide for premature infants suffering from bilirubin excess.

Bili-Bonnet, photograph. Image courtesy of Small Beginnings

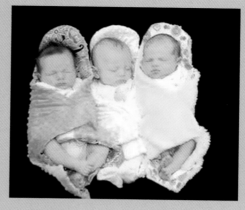

The SwaddleKeeper was designed to make swaddling easier and benefits the baby by supporting a "back to sleep" position with head support.

Karen Holt, *Swaddlekeeper,* June 2007, invention, SwaddleKeeper, Hood River, OR.

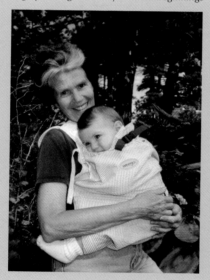

The original soft baby carrier—the Snugli—was created by Ann Moore, who was intrigued by the way African mothers carried their babies in fabric slings tied to their backs.

Ann Moore, *Ann Moore with a Baby in a Weego (Snugli),* invention, Smithsonian Institution/National Museum of American History/Archives Center, Washington, DC.

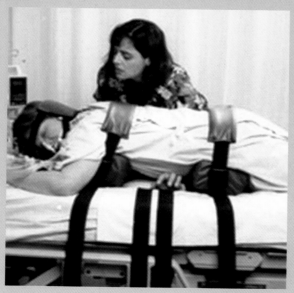

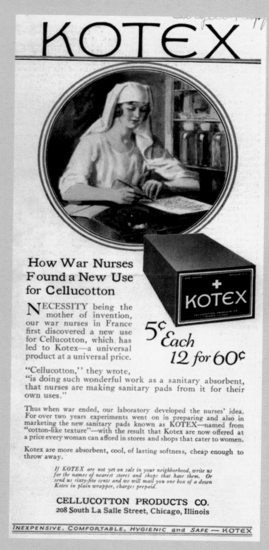

Cellucotton Products Co., *How War Nurses Found a New Use for Cellucotton,* 1921, advertisement. With permission from Duke University.

At left, The Vollman Prone Positioner was developed to help facilitate the turning and prone positioning of critically ill patients. The prone position has been shown to improve pulmonary oxygenation of patients with acute respiratory distress syndrome (ARDS).

Kathleen Vollman, *The Vollman Prone Positioner,* 1997, photograph, Henry Ford Hospital, Detroit, MI.

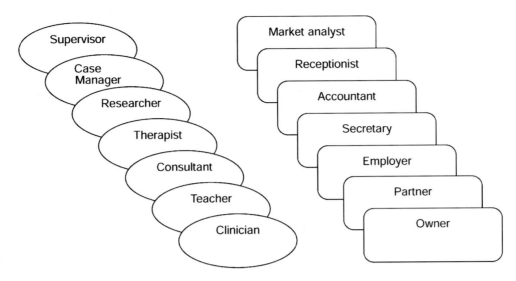

The nurse entrepreneur assumes a multitude of roles directly linked with the professional and business aspects of the practice and provides a wide range of services. Taken from the Internal Council of Nurses *Guidelines on the Nurse Entre/Intrapreneur Providing Nursing Service,* 2003.

International Council of Nurses, *Nurses' Roles in Entrepreneurship,* digital line drawing, International Council of Nurses, Geneva, Switzerland.

Intrapreneurship ventures, on the other hand, include entities such as nurse-led rehabilitation units, emergency services, clinics, and telephone consultation services (Kingma, 1998). Entrepreneurship and intrapreneurship are essentially the same; context is the differing factor between the two.

Nurse entrepreneurship is not a new phenomenon; it dates back to the turn of the 20th century. Prior to World War II, many nurses in a number of countries were in independent practice, particularly in the role of private-duty nurses. They practiced in public health and in home nursing and were highly valued by society. Social and economic changes following the war forced nursing practice to be, for the most part, institutionalized. Nurses became employed by hospitals and community health agencies, the standard that still predominates in health care delivery today. The role and education of nursing students, of necessity, also changed (ICN, 2004). But now the ranks of nurse entrepreneurs are growing as a result of the increased autonomy and job satisfaction that are realized. Particularly significant is the resultant outcome of providing needed services and high-quality, cost-effective care.

Another type of entrepreneurial undertaking involves the establishment of schools, especially for girls, in the forbidding terrain that gave birth to the Taliban, the remote regions of Pakistan and Afghanistan. Greg Mortenson, a trauma nurse from San Francisco and a mountaineer, failed in his attempt in 1993 to climb the world's second highest mountain, Pakistan's K2 in the Karakoram range. As a result, his life changed forever. As he was being embraced by the kindness of the inhabitants of the area, he saw a group of children sitting in the dirt, writing in the sand with sticks. Mortenson made a promise to help them build a school. Since then, he has dedicated his life to that promise and has initiated a remarkable humanitarian campaign that has led to the establishment, as of 2008, of 78 schools in rural and often volatile regions of Pakistan and Afghanistan. His remarkable story is told in *Three Cups of Tea: One Man's Mission to Promote Peace . . . One School at a Time* (2006).

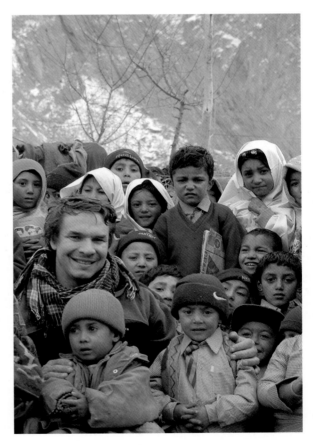

Greg Mortenson with Khanday community school students, Hushe Valley, Karakoram Mountains, Pakistan.

Greg Mortenson with Khanday Community School Students, December 2006, photograph, Hushe Valley, Karakoram Mountains, Pakistan. Image courtesy Greg Mortenson, Central Asia Institute.

Facing page, *Three Cups of Tea,* 2007, book cover. Image courtesy Greg Mortenson, Central Asia Institute.

The International Council of Nurses stated that "it appears that 0.5% to 1% of working nurses are nurse entrepreneurs" (2004, p. 9), but statistical data concerning nurse entrepreneurs are difficult to acquire and compare. A number of factors account for this difficulty. Various countries use different definitions; private-duty nurses may or may not be incorporated into the data; nurses owning businesses may no longer be considered nurses and so may be excluded. Furthermore, data concerning nurse entrepreneurs are available only in countries that have in place a system for recording the nursing workforce in a consistent manner.

The social, cultural, economic, ethical, and legal perspectives of each country also determine the relevance and prevalence of the nurse entrepreneur.

Although the original focus of nurse entrepreneurs was basic nursing skills delivered in the home or in a hospital setting, relatively few of today's independent practitioners in industrialized countries focus exclusively on the treatment of medical ailments (Robson, 1993). These nurses offer a wide variety of services anchored in creativity, initiative, self-reliance, and assertiveness. They assume a multitude of roles that are directly linked to the business and professional

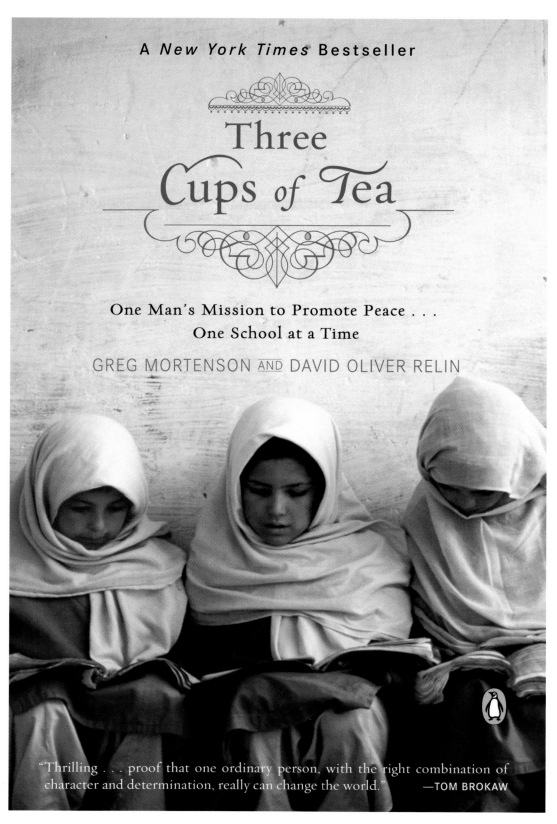

aspects of the practice (ICN, 2004). Their role is not without risk, but the opportunities for their services in health care are unparalleled because of the massive changes occurring in the field, and this will continue to facilitate growth in the numbers of nurse entrepreneurs. Overall, they have established a positive public image as advocates for patients, families, and communities and as counselors, educators, and expert clinicians. Future advancements in health care cannot help being facilitated by nurse entrepreneurs.

NURSING AND POLITICS

There seem to be two schools of thought regarding nursing's involvement in the political arena. One focuses on the whole of nursing which, historically, has presumably failed to be a consistent and viable political force. Numerous factors have contributed to this particular idea but the primary reason is the reality that women have continued to dominate the profession. Women, including nurses, have typically been viewed by society as being nonpolitical, and efforts to change that image have been slow to have effects. In addition, women's involvement in politics was considered inappropriate and unfeminine. In some instances, nurses themselves have had contempt for politics and have regarded politics as dirty and unprofessional (Lewenson, 2002; Mason, 1990). What has been recognized is the undeniable fact that involvement in politics can be a vital positive influence on nursing and its health care agenda and that the overall challenge for nurses and all women has always been to increase their representation in political offices and emerge from the fringes to fill powerful political positions. During the past several decades this process has begun to occur, and it will continue as nurses embrace the concept of politics as power, understanding that it can effect major changes in health care delivery.

The second thought regarding nursing involvement in the political arena is that nursing has a long and rich heritage of political achievement attained by nursing leaders in the early part of the 20th century. These achievements are documented by specific nursing heroines, the work of nursing organizations, nurses' involvement in legislative issues,

the interface of nursing with the feminist movement, and the growing number of publications on the subject of power and politics (Kalisch and Kalisch, 1982; Lasseter, 1999; Lewenson, 1998; Mason, 1990). An examination of nursing's past shows that there have been nursing role models who were involved in politics. Prominent among them was Florence Nightingale, an accomplished politician who initiated considerable reforms and used statistics as a political strategy to persuade government officials. She used her network of influential friends to help her achieve her goal of relieving the common people of suffering and neglect.

Lillian D. Wald regarded legislation as a way of resolving social and health problems and as a mechanism whereby some measure of justice could be ensured for so-called unfortunates. "Throughout her life she had opposed political and social corruption and supported those measures that would improve the health, wealth, and happiness of humanity" (Donahue, 1996, p. 307). She also developed important relationships with government officials, friends, and philanthropists who helped to facilitate her work. She was regarded as one of the most influential health workers of her time.

Lavinia Lloyd Dock completed a study of laws under which professional organizations could operate, contributed powerful articles to professional journals on a variety of social issues, and fought as a zealous suffragist for women to achieve the vote. She was convinced that nursing could never reach its full potential if women did not have the right to vote. She as well as other nursing leaders recognized that without the vote, nursing's future would be dictated by others. She urged that nurses and nursing associations become involved in the effort because, in her eyes, the nursing profession had become "an intelligent army of workers, capable of continuous progress and fitted to comprehend the idea of social responsibility . . . it would be a great pity for them to allow one of the most remarkable movements of the day to go on under their eyes without comprehending it" (Lewenson, 1998, p. 49). There is no doubt that Dock was a risk taker and that she engaged in unpopular causes and frequently used her pen as a political force.

Although many nurses have made outstanding contributions to the health of society through their political skills, Sojourner Truth was regarded as an orator who could use her voice to effect change. She unceasingly traveled across the country to influence thought about human rights. Relying on her experience as an abolitionist and suffragist, she strove to demonstrate the interrelationship between freedom and health. Her skill as an orator was indeed used to change discriminatory practices toward women and people of color (Carnegie, 1986). The power of her words proved to be an effective vehicle for the shaping of public opinion and policy.

It is true that nursing's organizational efforts also played a major role in emphasizing the importance and strength of collective action. This was particularly evident during "the fateful decade," that 10-year time period (1890-1900) that was marked by numerous important events and fateful decisions in nursing's history. The societal context presented the industrial revolution, exceedingly high illness and death rates, epidemics of cholera, diphtheria, typhoid and other illnesses that had to be addressed. As Hamilton (1994) remarked, ". . . the society of the 'fateful decade' resonated to an anxious but hopeful rhythm in which ideas of reform, progress, democracy, idealism, good women, and justice

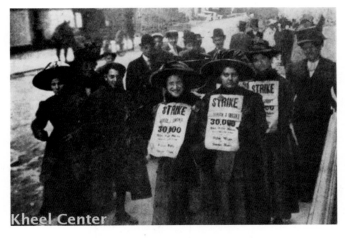

Lavinia Dock and Lillian Wald protest child labor and unsafe conditions in New York.

Lavinia Dock, RN and Lillian Wald, RN, Founder of Public Health Nursing, Protesting Child Labor and Unsafe Conditions in New York, photograph, International Ladies Garment Workers Union Archive, Kheel Center, Cornell University.

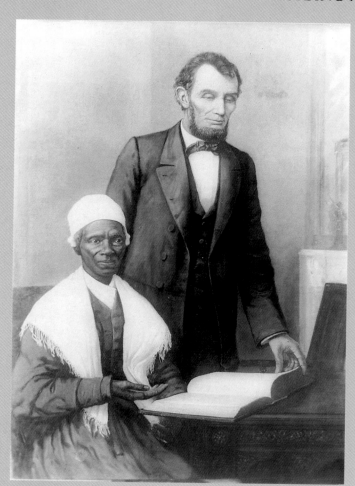

Abraham Lincoln showing Sojourner Truth the Bible presented by colored people of Baltimore, Executive Mansion, Washington, DC, October 29, 1864.

A. Lincoln Showing Sojourner Truth the Bible, October 29, 1864, photograph. Photo courtesy of the Library of Congress.

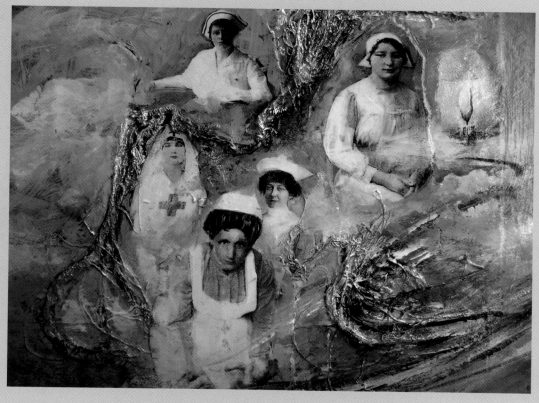

Hazel Mary Cope, *In Birth and in Death—the Nurse,* 2009, mixed media, 10 × 13 cm.

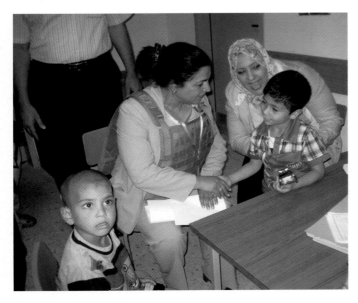

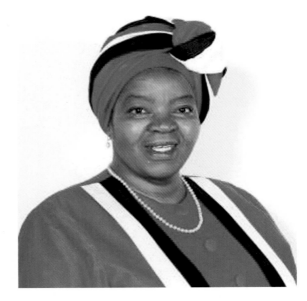

Dr. Al-Gasseer is a Bahraini national who has served as the World Health Organization (WHO) representative in Iraq since 2003.

WHO Iraq Representative Dr Naeema Al-Gasseer Talking with Patients at a Baghdad Hospital, 2008. Photograph courtesy of the World Health Organiztion.

Dr. Sheila Dinotshe Tlou serves as a member of Parliament in Botswana. She served as Botswana's Minister of Health from 2004 to 2008.

Sheila Dinotshe Tlou, PhD, RN, photograph, American Academy of Nursing.

harmonized" (p. 12). The time was ripe for the initiation of marked interventions to resolve these issues.

The impact of nursing's achievements during this time is almost immeasurable. It was as though a cataclysmic occurrence had taken place. Great leaders emerged, organized nursing was born, the *American Journal of Nursing* was initiated, and nurse-training schools proliferated. Early leaders quickly realized that nursing's power and potential would be realized through an organized effort of united individuals. Through a concerted effort, the American Society of Superintendents of Training Schools for Nurses was formed in 1893; the Nurses Associated Alumnae of the United States and Canada was formed in 1896. These two organizations paved the way for extensive changes in both nursing practice and education and demonstrated the influence of professional organizations as a political force.

Although numerous events that included nurses' political involvement occurred, one of the most significant was the successful campaign for legislation and registration. This was an initiative directed toward achieving control of the practice of nursing in order to protect the public and standardize the preparation of nurses. The first licensing laws were enacted in the United State in 1903 in four states. Campaigns for registration and licensure had also begun or were taking place during this time in other countries, such as Great Britain and South Africa.

Currently, nurses are becoming politically sophisticated and recognizing that politics is a professional and social responsibility. They understand that politics involves more than issues concerned with government and elections; politics is a part of everyday life and is intimately associated with power. It is also useful to remember that this is the first time in the history of health care that a nursing crisis and a call for major transformation in the health care delivery system have coincided. This presents a time of immense opportunity because the nursing shortage has served to increase nursing's power in the workplace. Lasseter (1999) encapsulated these thoughts: "True today as it was then, both the external and internal systems in which the practice of nursing exists

are complex, and it is important for nurses to understand and participate in the processes that affect their practice. Early nurses possessed courage, tenacity, and vision that resulted in an inspiring legacy for today's nurses to continue political efforts to advocate for their patients and their profession" (p. 905).

NURSING: A CARING AND HEALING PROFESSION

Nursing's legacy is that of a caring and healing profession that involves taking care of individuals in a holistic manner. Nurses are healers principally through the caring relationships they form with patients. Their healing presence encompasses being conscious and compassionate when in the present moment with others and believing in their potential for wholeness in life. Historically, nurses have committed their lives to caring, treating, and preserving others in mind, body, and spirit. This is consistent with the traditional values of nursing in which care and healing have more to do with the person than with the disease. This perspective emphasizes the nurse-patient relationship as being of a healing nature and the nursing practice as being healing work. Numerous forces have mandated a return to the examination of what it means to be human, what it means to be healthy, what it means to be healed, and nursing's role in the healing process.

The concept of healing is viewed in a number of different ways. It is, however, necessary to understand its definition in relation to the practice of nursing. The words of Dossey, Keegan, Guzzetta, and Kolkmeir (1995) capture the beauty of this relationship:

> Healing is not just the curing of symptoms. It is the exquisite blending of technology with caring, loving, compassion and creativity. Healing is a lifelong journey into understanding the wholeness of human existence. . . . Healing is learning to open what has been closed so that we can expand our inner potential. . . . A nurse healer is one who facilitates another person's growth toward wholeness (body-mind-spirit)

or who assists another in the recovery from illness or in the transition to peaceful death. (p. xxvi)

Although these authors were actually differentiating between curing and healing, their words resonate with the attributes of the healing spirit of nursing. They speak to the belief that a person may have been judged to be healed but still has an illness. Also essential to capturing this caring-healing relationship is what Koerner (2007) refers to as the healing presence of the nurse: "The unifying, underlying essence of our work is the timeless and profound healing presence we offer that enhances the exploration and creation of meaning in the inevitable health challenges faced by individuals, families, and groups whose lives we are privileged to touch" (p. xviii).

COMPLEMENTARY AND ALTERNATIVE MEDICINE

The growth of interest in complementary and alternative medicine (CAM) is currently progressing at a rapid pace, although its roots reach deep into the history of many cultures; its use spans almost the entire history of humankind. Complementary and alternative therapies flow from primitive medicine, mythology, and folklore and are based on the medical systems of ancient peoples, including the Egyptians, Chinese, Asian Indians, Greeks, and Native Americans. They have been used worldwide for many years, although they are a more recent addition to Western medicine. Ayurvedic medicine, for example, is more than 5000 years old and combines lifestyle and dietary modifications in the search of balance. It originated in India and has been a major influence on Chinese and Greek medicine. Acupuncture, too, is more than 5000 years old and originated in Asia. The practice involves the use of fine needles to stimulate points along the energy meridians of the body. Other practices, such as naturopathy, the use of plants, herbs, and natural substances; homeopathy; osteopathy; and chiropractic medicine, are not as ancient but reach back into the 18th century. All such practices rely on natural remedies and on the body's own ability to help itself heal. CAM practices are typically grouped into five major categories:

- Alternative medical approaches involving complete medical systems that include theory and practice, such as ayurveda and naturopathy
- Biologically based therapies involving the use of substances found in nature, such as herbs, aromatherapy, diet, vitamins, and so forth
- Mind-body interventions that enhance the mind's capacity to affect bodily functions, such as meditation, imagery, and music and art therapy
- Manipulative and body-based methods involving manipulation or movement of one or more parts of the body, such as acupressure, massage, chiropractic, and osteopathy
- Energy therapies involving the use of electromagnetic fields, or energy fields, around the body, such as therapeutic touch, reiki, and qigong.

At right, The Hukpiri, a traditional Korean ocarina, is among instruments used to help reduce patient suffering. The power of music can alleviate anxiety and ward away pain.

Nanette Bedway, *Healing*, photograph, Nannette Bedway Studio, Cleveland, OH.

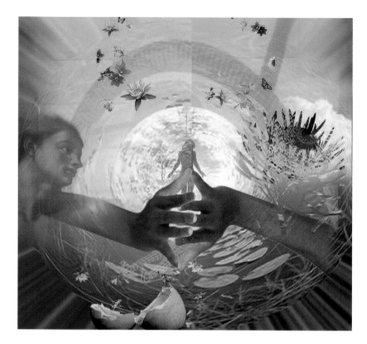

David Stirts, *Healing Presence*, book cover, 2007.

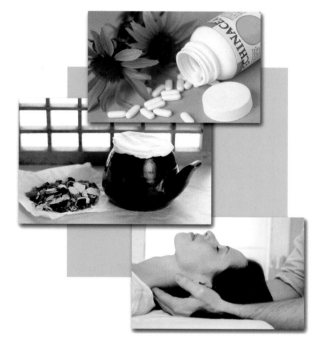

Alternative Medicine. Photographs courtesy of photos.com.

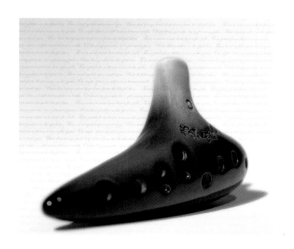

The terminology used in complementary and alternative therapies can be confusing, particularly for the general public. It must be understood that complementary therapies are used together with conventional therapies to complement them, and alternative modes of medical treatment are *usually* meant to replace traditional Western medicine. The primary goal, however, is to provide for patients a host of benefits that are achieved by combining the best of both worlds. This is why patients and the general public are asking to try these techniques. Most commonly, patients turn to CAM when they have chronic problems that conventional medicine hasn't completely cured; when they have side effects that are caused by conventional medicine and have not decreased; when they are looking for less invasive therapies; and when they desire more control over their treatment regimes and their lives. Healthy individuals are also turning to CAM, believing that the CAM techniques can improve overall well-being and potentially can prevent illness or ensure a more healthful lifestyle. This trend will affect health care delivery and nursing practice for the foreseeable future, and there is an increasing demand for holistic health professionals.

NURSES AND HOLISM

Historically, nurses have embraced a holistic approach to nursing practice that encompasses the whole person, including the mind, emotions, body, and spirit. With the explosive interest in and demand for CAM, nurses are in a unique position to bridge the gap between them and conventional therapies. Although all nurses can be viewed as holistic practitioners because of the nature of the profession, the specialty of holistic nursing has emerged. It promotes the education of nurses in all aspects of holistic caring and healing, including the use of ancient healing arts.

Holistic nursing is defined as "all nursing practice that has healing the whole persons as its goal" (American Holistic Nurses' Association, 1998). Holistic nurses are considered to be instruments of healing and facilitators in the healing process. These nurses may integrate CAM into clinical practice along with conventional therapies, thus providing the greatest healing potential for those under their care. Or they may venture into entrepreneur opportunities such as establishing their own holistic practices. According to the American Holistic Nurses Association, holistic nursing can be practiced in any setting. Demographics in the United States

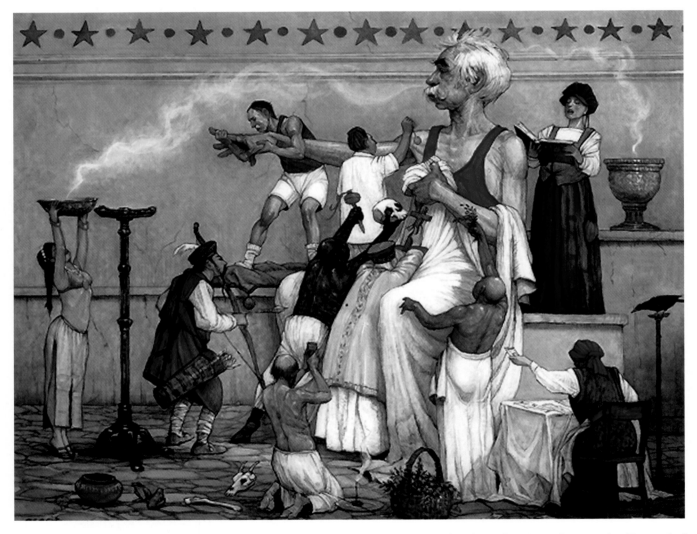

Alternative medicine refers to all those methods of treatment that fall outside the sanction of conventional medicine. This painting shows a senior citizen perfectly at ease as the numerous alternative practitioners minister to his needs.

Jose Perez, *The Alternative Practitioner,* painting, 24" × 30", WRS Group Ltd., Waco, TX.

show that 39% of holistic nurses work in hospitals; 23% in private practice; 15% in academia, education, or research; and 11% in hospice, palliative, or long-term care facilities; 9% are students. Opportunities for their services are limitless and even extend to practice in beauty and health settings, such as spas, cruise ships, and wellness centers.

Holistic nurses are usually required to have additional education that is focused on techniques that promote psychological, spiritual, and mental health. Courses in CAM are being offered with increasing frequency in both undergraduate and graduate programs in nursing, and holistic certification now exists. At the graduate level, nursing schools are offering academic degrees or certificate programs in holistic nursing or complementary therapies. In December of 2006,

Holistic nursing was officially recognized by the ANA as a nursing specialty with a defined scope and standards of practice, acknowledging holistic nursing's unique contribution to the health and healing of people and society. This was achieved through the efforts of the American Holistic Nurses Association, which was established in 1981. Efforts to establish holistic nursing associations have now begun in other countries such as New Zealand. Holistic nursing has become a reality worldwide, and it illustrates the blending of the Eastern and Western healing traditions.

At the forefront in the advancement of important initiatives relative to health and healing is the Center for Spirituality and Healing located at the University of Minnesota and established in 1995 as part of the Academic Health Center. It

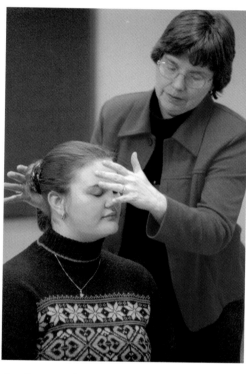

A nurse performing a complementary therapy.

Generating New Knowledge Through Research, photograph, Center for Spirituality and Healing University of Minnesota.

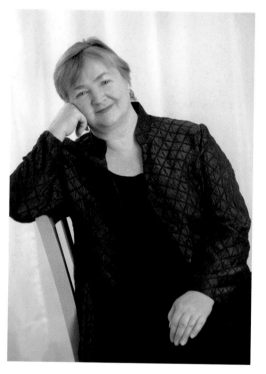

Dr. Mary Jo Kreitzer, founder and director of the Center for Spirituality and Healing.

Mary Jo Kreitzler, 2008, photograph, Center for Spirituality and Healing University of Minnesota.

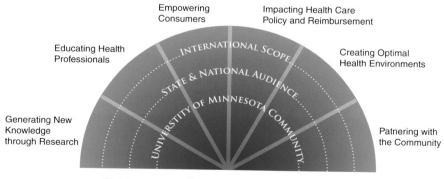

Empowering Consumers

Impacting Health Care Policy and Reimbursement

Educating Health Professionals

Creating Optimal Health Environments

INTERNATIONAL SCOPE

STATE & NATIONAL AUDIENCE

UNIVERSITY OF MINNESOTA COMMUNITY

Generating New Knowledge through Research

Patnering with the Community

CENTER FOR SPIRITUALITY & HEALING

The Center for Spirituality and Healing has been designated by the NIH as a Developmental Center for Research on Complementary and Alternative Medicine, a distinction attained by only five institutions in the United States.

Center for Spirituality and Healing Model, University of Minnesota Center for Spirituality and Healing.

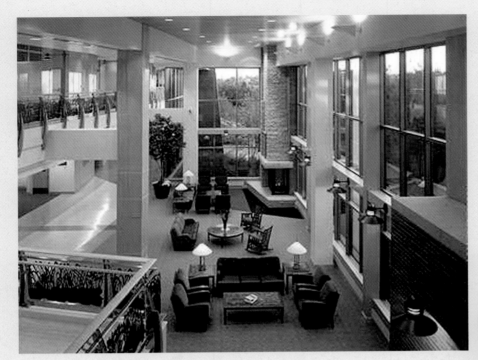

Town Center, photograph, Woodwinds Health Campus, Woodbury, MN.

Inside Fireplace, photograph, Woodwinds Health Campus, Woodbury, MN.

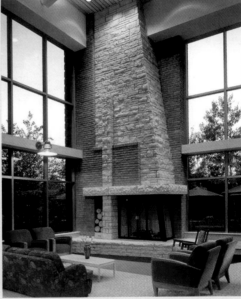

The fireplace area and multi-denominational chapel at Woodwinds Health Campus in Woodbury, Minnesota. Woodwinds opened in August 2000, the only hospital in the southeast metro area. At Woodwinds Health Campus, an unprecedented healing environment revolves around the needs of patients and their families. Its philosophy of holistic care recognizes and respects the role of the individual and family in the health care experience. Its purpose is to promote health and healing of body, mind and spirit for all through relationships, choices and learning. Woodwinds is a primary example of the integration of high-tech medicine with whole person healing. It offers a variety of healing art therapies, including: essential oils, healing touch/energy-based therapies, guided imagery, healing music, acupuncture, acupressure, and massage. Woodwinds Health Campus was named the 2009 Best Minnesota Hospital Workplace by the Minnesota Hospital Association.

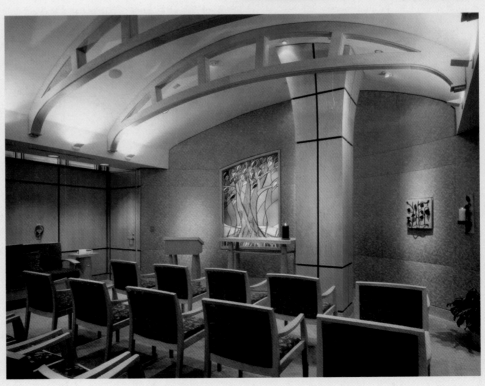

Chapel, photograph, Woodwinds Health Campus, Woodbury, MN.

includes 50 faculty members drawn from more than 12 academic units of the university. They have appointments at the center, which holds the goal of enhancing "health and well-being by educating health professionals, empowering consumers, and fundamentally transforming the delivery of health care through the creation of interdisciplinary academic, research, clinical care, and outreach programs that advance integrative health and healing" (Center for Spirituality and Healing, 2009). It has been designated by the National Institutes of Health as a Developmental Center for Research on Complementary and Alternative Medicine, a distinction attained by only five institutions in the United States. The center has received worldwide recognition, and its resources are used by individuals in countries around the world. Dr. Mary Jo Kreitzer, a tenured professor in the School of Nursing is its founder and director. This initiative is a wonderful statement about nursing's participation in the holistic movement that is circling the globe.

Lest we forget—hospitals are also reexamining their approaches to health care, and some are involved in creating the best patient experience possible. Healing environments are the priority in these hospitals, and they revolve around patients and their families. A holistic health care model and philosophy are incorporated into the delivery of services in which patients and families participate. Traditional medicine and state-of-the-art technology work in tandem with natural approaches to wellness and health. Healing art therapies or CAMs that are consistent with an individual patient's healing process are readily available. Nurses practicing in these hospitals use a holistic model of care and truly embrace a patient-centered approach to health care.

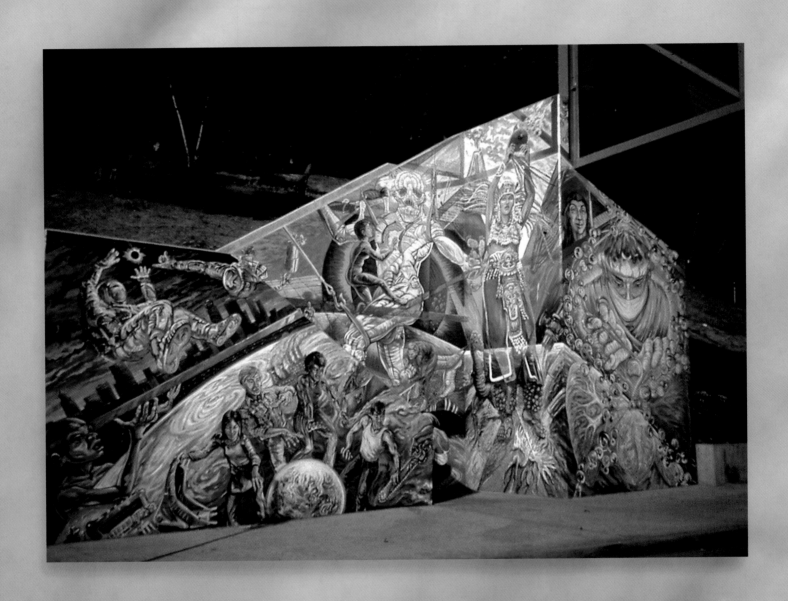

A Global View of Nursing and Health Care

What the world needs now is connectedness. There is a need for a global network that is multicultural, multidimensional. It is centered in individual and local partnerships and is always shifting, changing, and open to new perspectives. Nursing is in a position to facilitate such a network. Our tradition of caring, nurturance and understanding of love as the highest level of consciousness makes it possible for nursing to be the connecting link in the needed reformulization of health-care systems as one of cooperation, collaboration, and partnership.

The underlying implicate order of nursing's mission—caring in the human health experience—is the transforming pattern. In the unfolding of it, we are its transforming presence.

— **MARGARET E. NEWMANN**

The *Stairway to Global Health* mural was created in 1991 by the East Los Streetscrapers based in East Los Angeles, California. The mural is located on four walls surrounding a stairway across the street from the entrance to the Francisco Bravo Medical Magnet Senior High School. In it, an Aztec shaman uses traditional healing.

East Los Streetscapers (Healy, Wayne, Botello, David, Raya, and Rich), *Stairway to Global Health,* 1991, acrylic on concrete, 21' × 30', East Los Streetscapers, Los Angeles, CA.

	2006	2007
Nursing	**2006** TIGER Summit convenes **2006** Essentials of Doctoral Education for Advanced Nursing Practice is endorsed by AACN **2006** International Centre for Human Resources in Nursing (ICHRN) is established	**2007** Johnson & Johnson Campaign for Nursing's Future relaunches
Medicine and Health Care	**2006** Avian flu in humans poses public health threat to parts of Asia, the Middle East, and Oceania; Western countries prepare for possible outbreaks **2006** U.S. approves drug Gardasil as first vaccine against cervical cancer **2006** Merck abandons HIV vaccine trials **2006** Ex-Marine Claudia Mitchell becomes first woman fitted with a truly bionic arm	
Science and Technology	**2006** Pluto loses status as a planet and is reclassified as a dwarf planet **2006** CeBIT consumer products showcase the "mental typewriter," a brain-to-computer interface that translates thoughts into cursor movements on a computer screen **2006** U.S. researchers calculate the speed of data transfer from eyes to brain and clock it at 8.75 megabits per second	**2007** Scientists announce five planets found circling a star 41 light-years away from Earth in the constellation Cancer **2007** Scientists confirm global warming **2007** House passes bill on stem cell research in favor of legislation that eases restrictions on federal funding of embryonic stem cell research
The Visual Arts	**2006** *No 5* (1948) by Jackson Pollock sells privately for $140 million, making it the most expensive painting ever sold. **2006** Tate attracts more than seven million visitors across its four galleries in 2006/2007, making it the most visited modern art museum in the world	
Daily Life	**2006** Saddam Hussein is convicted of crimes against humanity by an Iraqi court and hanged in Baghdad	**2007** Minimum wage increases to $5.85, up from $5.15 **2007** Minneapolis, MN bridge collapses into the Mississippi River **2007** Cristina Fernández de Kirchner becomes first woman president in Argentina **2007** Former vice president Al Gore shares Nobel Peace Prize for work on human-caused climate change and for outlining ways to reverse global warming

2008 The Essentials of Baccalaureate Education for Professional Nursing Practice revised and approved by AACN

2008 The World Health Organization Family of International Classifications (WHO-FICP) approves the addition of the International Classification for Nursing Practice (ICNP®) to the WHO-FIC as a related terminology

2009 International Nurses Day focus is Delivering Quality, Serving Communities: Nurses Leading Care Innovations

2008 Doctors in England give woman a new windpipe with tissue grown from her own stem cells, eliminating the need for an anti-rejection drug

2008 Researchers decode the genome of a cancer patient

2008 *Triptych* (1976) by Francis Bacon sells at Sotheby's New York for $86.3 million, becoming the most expensive post-war work of art sold at auction and the highest priced work by an Irish artist

2008 Democratic candidate Barack Obama becomes first African-American to be elected President of U.S.

2008 Economic recession

2008 Hundreds die in tribal violence in Kenya

2008 Castro resigns as President of Cuba

2008 Unemployment rate reaches highest level in 5 years in U.S.

2008 U.S. Senate passes bailout plan

2008 Police break up a global organ trafficking scheme and hunt for alleged mastermind Dr. Amit Kumar

Transformation is occurring across the planet. The world becomes smaller and smaller each day. Individual countries can no longer remain isolated and concerned only with issues that arise within their own boundaries. Now that international travel has become commonplace, there is deep knowledge of cultural similarities and differences and at the same time keen awareness of the need for greater understanding and communication. Global interaction is indeed progressing at a rapid pace, a pace that has been spurred on by technological developments, particularly in the area of information systems. It will become even more important to understand and clarify language systems that are essentially developed not only to describe the world but also to define it. Languages represent unique ways of perceiving reality.

People everywhere are searching for new directions and for alternatives to their current states of being, as numerous titles in various types of literature attest. New paradigms are being created that seem to be leaning more toward greater emphasis on human respect and human caring. Authors are proposing that an era of true spiritual awareness or a spiritual renaissance is occurring as people are attempting to find meaning in their lives. Redfield's *The Celestine Prophecy* (1993) provided one such view of the changing world. Its popularity was directly linked to predictions associated with relationships, international affairs, and insights that, if grasped, could provide a new image of human life and a vision for protecting and preserving the environment. All this current spiraling activity is also exhibited in the search for health-promotion therapies and a shift away from disease-oriented care. Health care reform is but one aspect of change; holistic and alternative approaches to care and cure are being investigated and accepted. In a number of instances people are returning to health care practices and systems that were used thousands of years ago. An increasing emphasis on preventive medicine and health promotion is taking place.

It is essential to create international links among nursing communities because all nurses around the globe are facing common issues and experiencing increasing social pressures. The environments in which nurses work worldwide have changed drastically and now present even greater challenges. Nursing's vision for the future must embrace the building of a healthy international society in which adequate care is available to and provided for everyone. Nursing's choice for the 21st century remains clear: we can participate in health care for a few or health for all (Maglacas, 1988, 1989). Nurses are strategically placed to support health care for all and to support one another in creating conditions for change.

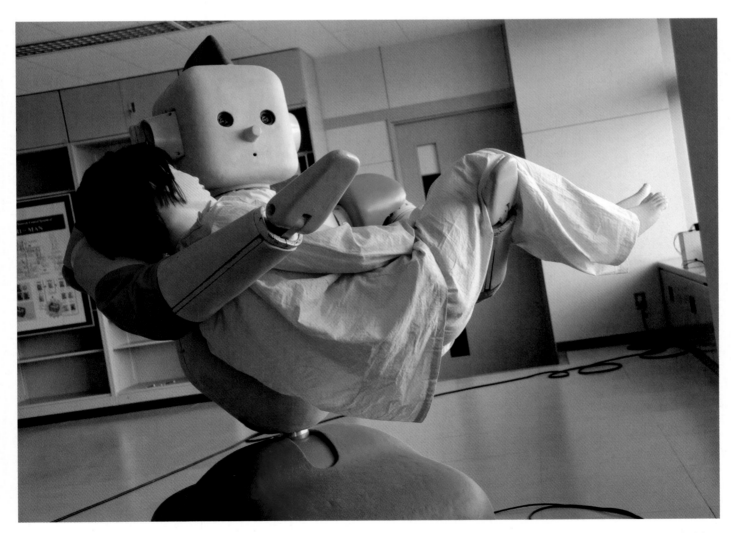

Health care of the future may well include the use of robots. Japan has been in the forefront of engineering a variety of robotic caretakers that may be used for lifting patients, bathing patients, or performing other caregiving skills. As with all technology, will their use save nurses time and energy and will patients accept nonhuman caregivers?

Karen Kasmauski, *Japanese Robotics,* photograph, from *Nurse: A World of Care,* pp. 216-217.

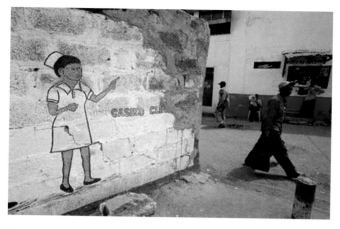

The Casino Clinic is a public treatment centre for sexually transmitted infections in Nairobi, Kenya.

Jonathan Torgovnik, *Nairobi, Kenya (Casino Clinic)*, 2006, photograph, 40 × 60 cm, UNAIDS Secretariat, permanent collection, Geneva, Switzerland.

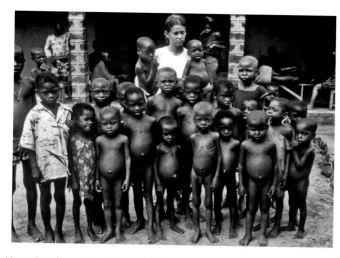

Nurse Standing with a Group of African Children Showing Symptoms of the Protein-Deficiency Disease Kwashiorkor, late 1960s, photograph, Nigeria. With permission from Image Envision.

WORLD HEALTH ISSUES

At the 30th World Health Assembly in 1977, member states of the World Health Organization (WHO) established a broad common goal: "Health for all by the year 2000." Primary health care was declared the mechanism for achieving this goal as it was articulated in the Declaration of Alma-Ata in 1978. A global strategy was formulated at the 34th World Health Assembly in 1981. Inherent in the strategy was the continuous, progressive improvement of the health status of populations through national health care systems that provide health promotion, disease prevention, and curative and rehabilitative services to all. The following themes were targeted:

1. All people in every country will have ready access at least to essential health care and first-level referral facilities.
2. All people will be actively involved in caring for themselves and their families as far as they can and in community action for health.
3. Communities throughout the world will share with governments responsibility for the health care of their members.
4. All governments will assume overall responsibility for the health of their people.
5. Safe drinking water and sanitation will be available for all people.
6. All people will be adequately nourished.
7. All children will be immunized against the major infectious diseases of childhood.
8. Communicable diseases in the developing countries will be of no greater public health significance in the year 2000 than they were in developed countries in the year 1980.
9. All possible ways will be applied to prevent and control noncommunicable diseases and promote mental health through influencing lifestyles and controlling the physical and psychosocial environment.
10. Essential drugs will be available to all.

— *U.N. Chronicle*, 1992, p. 45

Since the Alma-Ata Declaration on Primary Health Care was promulgated, 31 years have passed. Although progress toward the goal has been made, barriers to its accomplishment still exist. Two reports regarding the implementation of the strategy were written; the first was completed in 1984; the second covered 1985 through the middle of 1988. A substantial improvement was noted in the status of health worldwide, as demonstrated by decreasing infant mortality rates and increased life expectancy at birth. The WHO Expanded Programme on Immunization had been successful in protecting the lives of children by administering vaccines against poliomyelitis, measles, tuberculosis, diphtheria, whooping cough, and tetanus. Of all infants worldwide, 80% had been vaccinated against the six diseases. Malaria remained one of the major and most serious of the world health problems, and other tropical diseases (cholera, yellow fever, and dengue) continued to wreak havoc on human populations. Noncommunicable diseases such as cardiovascular disease, stroke, cancer, and chronic respiratory infection were decreasing in developed countries but increasing in developing countries. The common denominator of risk for these diseases is lifestyle, so more healthful lifestyles continued to be promoted. Campaigns and programs for the provision of safe water and uncontaminated food continued, along with emphasis on better sanitation. Improvements had been made in these areas, particularly in the availability of safe water and in rural water supplies. Unfortunately, achievements in access to health care were extremely uneven, and the health gap between the least developed countries and other developing countries was increasing. Downward economic trends grossly affected economic welfare and health status in the developing countries (Maglacas, 1989; U.N. Chronicle, 1992).

Unfortunately, those who were visionary thinkers in 1978 could not have foreseen the numerous world events that would transpire: an oil crisis, a global recession, and the shifting of national budgets away from social services, including health care. As resources for health diminished, the intended aim of reshaping health care moved to selective interventions. In addition, the emergence of HIV/AIDS and the resurgence of diseases such as tuberculosis moved the focus from broad-based programs to the management of emergencies that involved high mortality rates. A review by the WHO in 1994 of changes in health care developments determined that the goal of health for all by 2000 would not be met. Yet the concept of primary health care became known as an extremely relevant strategy in the struggle to provide health care for all.

In October 2008, the WHO issued its World Health Report on primary health care to coincide with the 30th anniversary of the Alma-Ata Declaration. The report stressed that health systems are not performing as well as they could or as well as they should. It requested that political leaders pay close attention to the rising social expectations of fair and efficient health care and that they reinforce the values articulated in the Declaration of Alma-Ata. It clearly articulated the message that health systems must respond faster and more efficiently to a changing world by means of primary health care. Nursing and nurses have critical roles to play in the provision of primary health care, and they are well prepared to fill those roles.

ADVOCACY REVISITED

Societal trends, the complexities of life, technological innovations, and health care issues and dilemmas make the need for advocates as important as ever. Nurses must be staunch advocates for clients, families, and communities, just as they have been in the past. Early nurse leaders were patients' advocates "concerned about and committed to human rights, dignity, humanitarianism, and accountability" (Donahue, 1978, p. 146). Their definition of nursing included autonomy, advocacy, and independent practice that focused on the prevention of illness as well as the maintenance of health. Although the word *advocacy* might not have been used, nursing's history is rich with examples of the advocacy role.

> One need only read about such individuals as Lavinia Dock and Lillian Wald to realize that nursing not only was concerned about patient advocacy but also practiced it. Delving even further into the roots of nursing, one cannot help but be impressed with the endeavors of Florence Nightingale, the founder of modern nursing. She was truly an independent practitioner who viewed herself as the patient's advocate. She thoroughly understood the importance of economics and the stratagems of power, and sought to establish a system whereby nurses themselves controlled nursing practice and nursing education. In her book, *Notes on Nursing: What It Is and What It Is Not* (1860), she set forth a clear, concise charge to nurses for a broad definition of nursing; caring for and caring about, encompassing the care of the whole individual. It has taken the focus on consumer protection and human rights, however, for the emphasis on patient advocacy to resurface within nursing.
>
> — DONAHUE, 1985, P. 341

Nurse advocates exist today and must exist to help society face challenges and battles against enemies such as AIDS. Barbara Fassbinder, RN, was infected with HIV in 1986 while assisting with the treatment of a patient in the emergency department of Memorial Hospital in Prairie du Chien, Wisconsin. Her personal courage and her sense of professional responsibility were the driving forces behind her decision to make her story public. With the support of her family, she spent her remaining time as an outspoken advocate in the fight against AIDS. She traveled extensively, educating health care workers about HIV and its consequences for the U.S. health care system. In 1991, she spoke out against mandatory HIV testing of health care workers in her testimony before Congress. In 1992 she received national recognition from the U.S. Surgeon General and the Department of Health and Human Services for her efforts in AIDS education. Her death in 1994 was a great loss to the nursing profession and to humankind.

Advocacy is an important concept in nursing practice. Commonly, it describes the nurse-client relationship. It is an ethic of practice stemming from the philosophy of nursing that emphasizes supporting an individual to promote his or her own well-being as understood by that individual. Nurses have consistently advocated for health care improvements related to infection control, practice environments, patient care environments, access to care, and high-quality health care. They have always been advocates for patients' health, safety, and rights. Some nurses may also be involved in advocacy that is aimed at influencing social and governmental institutions; they work in political arenas to establish health policies. What must be remembered is that the concept of advocacy is complex; it is subject to ambiguity of interpretation, there are difficulties in its operationalization, and it may create challenges for the practicing nurse.

Nurses are continually rising to the challenge to combat pressing problems in health care. The time is ripe for the nursing profession to make a major difference. In the face of inadequate and dwindling resources, however, different and more creative strategies must be developed if primary health care for all is to be achieved. New ideas, approaches, and knowledge in nursing must be shared with colleagues around the world even as adaptations are made to conform with the variations in health systems in each country. Because of the humanistic approach and educational preparation of nurses in areas of both care and cure, they are the best-qualified group to take the leadership role in developing and providing health care services. Nurses can no longer be bound by local, regional, or national borders but must join together as one united, global community. Health care issues are not unique to specific countries, and nurses cannot afford to isolate themselves from the world. They must work in unity to be agents of change, health care policy makers, and key participants in health care reform. They must be staunch advocates for all peoples and all countries of the world in the quest for fair and efficient health care.

ETHICAL CONCERNS

Political, social, and economic realities are important elements that underlie both the determinants of health and ethical decision making. They can inhibit or enhance the achievement of good health and sound ethical practices. Scientific advancement, technological innovations, and crises such as conflicts and wars are having profound effects internationally on health care and on nursing in this time of rapid change. Ethical issues are thus arising from a variety of sources and are being created by a variety of circumstances. Progress itself has been one of the key factors.

Nurses must make ethical decisions every day. They are now being forced to examine ethics even more deeply and from a worldwide point of view. It is one thing to understand and appreciate the ethical ramifications of decisions made in one's own setting; it is another to think about them from a global perspective. This becomes particularly difficult because the ways in which societies view and think about ethical issues are affected by political and economic circumstances and how they change. What's more, the definitions of ethical conduct vary widely in accordance with culturally accepted practices. Is keeping someone alive with machines and drugs better or worse than assisting someone to die when he or she is terminally ill and in severe pain? Is scarification better or worse than breast augmentation? In some countries, abortion and prostitution are legal; in others they are not. In some countries, age limits and ability to pay determine whether treatments or procedures such as dialysis and organ transplantation will be carried out.

What is becoming obvious is that for thousands of years adherence to standards of ethical behavior applied to very small groups, possibly only to individual acts. Then it encompassed families and with time, tribes, regions, and finally entire nations. Currently, the world is in the throes of making a giant leap in the definition of *ethical behavior*, and it is essentially embracing all of humankind. With new and improved methods of communication, people become aware of ethical crises no matter where they are occurring. No longer are regions and nations isolated. News reports of atrocities, violations of human rights, and wars such as the one waged in Bosnia-Herzegovina in 1992 are constantly being broadcast and received all around the globe. In a sense the world is now a community of which everyone is a member. What happens in that world is a concern to all cultures in all geographical locations. Global ethics has all but become a reality. Again, however, it must be remembered that humans develop their ethics by the method of public discussion, which leads to public acceptance of what appears to be right and good and rejection of what is judged to be wrong and bad. Consequently, differences of opinion exist regarding ethical concerns. In addition, the concept of what is ethical, right, and good changes in the light of new knowledge, new technology, and continuing debate. Problems also arise because of differences in interpretation.

Ethical issues of international concern occur at an even more fundamental level, and nurses everywhere have a responsibility to consider them. Holleran (1994), in her provocative discussion of the difficulties that arise when dealing with international ethical issues, provided insights on a few subjects that she believed to be of concern to nurses worldwide:

- The usefulness of and need for drugs, in particular, the export of outdated drugs, the export of drugs not yet certified as being safe and effective for distribution, and the promotion and aggressive sale of nonessential drugs
- The promotion of infant formula and weaning foods in poor countries
- The sources of organs used in transplants
- Awareness of cultural differences
- The safety of nurses working in prisons
- The safety of nurses working in situations that put them at risk

She effectively used specific examples to illustrate that nurses must consider all aspects of situations " . . in which they might be asked to withhold their services . . . in times of war . . . or in caring for or refusing to care for people with certain diagnoses, such as AIDS" (p. 766). In addition to presenting a strong argument in favor of all nurses' developing political savvy, Aroskar (1987) effectively summarized these points: "Dealing with ethical concerns in the world of nursing practice and service requires dealing with the political dimension as well. Ethics and politics interface and overlap.

. . . Isn't ethics about right or good action and politics about power and manipulation?" (p. 268).

As part of a global discipline, nurses are vitally interested in reducing and ultimately eliminating disparities in health care so better health is achieved for all peoples. It is thus necessary to consider the need for a global ethic that encompasses social justice, human rights, and freedom and emphasizes both the individual good and the common good. Crigger (2008) identified five qualities or characteristics in the literature that may facilitate a viable and just statement of global nursing ethics:

- **Inclusion and Balance:** This involves a balanced methodology of inclusive decision making. Global ethics discussions should include people from multiple countries and multiple disciplines.
- **Balance of Community and Individual:** This involves the establishment of a balance between community and individual interests and rights. A consideration of the social context and cultural variety must be present so that views and beliefs in differing countries are valued.
- **Use of Reflexivity:** Reflexivity is an important characteristic that can be used to see our world and ourselves realistically. It is the ability to see from another's point of view. It is also the ability to reflect critically on everything, including one's self or one's own perspective.
- **Openness to New Approaches to Human Rights:** This involves a lack of consensus on what rights are due to all human beings and the shift to a more inclusive theory of human rights. This discussion identifies how Sen and Nussbauma differ in how they present the "capacity approach" to human rights.
- **Business and Technology:** Business and technology must not be allowed to stand as barriers to social justice and the common good. Although advancements in business and technology have benefits, the problems they give rise to have been identified in nursing and other disciplines. They should be positioned to benefit all people rather than to exploit marginalized and poor people.

— (CRIGGER, 2008, PP. 21-25)

According to Crigger, there is no doubt that these characteristics of a global ethic can guide nurses and society to respond more adequately to the inequities of today's world and to adjust their responses to human rights abuses and poverty. They will also be more responsive to differences in health resources and resource distribution.

The current nursing shortage (termed a global crisis since 2002) has presented another ethical concern that has been particularly devastating in developing countries. Although the international mobility of nurses is not a new phenomenon, the increasing recruitment of nurses by developed countries, such as the United States, the United Kingdom, Ireland, and Australia, to counteract domestic shortages is a current development. Countries that have been devastated by natural disasters and pandemics have been more acutely impacted because they can ill afford to lose nurses. Nurses involved in this situation have been forced into involuntary migration as refugees because they fear persecution at home or have been aggressively wooed by promises of a better life in another country. The latter situation concerns ethical recruitment. All nurses must understand this concept and work together to facilitate ways of ethically and legally supporting the nursing workforce in every country. The underlying point in this entire discussion is that high-quality health care is directly dependent on an adequate supply of qualified and committed nursing personnel!

The ethical recruitment of nurses internationally is a major concern and is without precedent. If the best and the brightest nurses are recruited for international work, the quality of care in their own countries will be profoundly affected. The WHO, the International Council of Nurses (ICN), and other organizations are studying this brain drain of critically needed nursing personnel in countries struggling to provide health care services. One study completed in 2003, *International Nurses Mobility: Trends and Policy Implications*, was funded by the WHO, the ICN, and the Royal College of Nursing. Inadequate working conditions (poor pay, excessive workloads, and violence in the workplace) and aggressive recruiting efforts (better salaries, career opportunities, professional development, and improved conditions of employment) were specified as the push-pull forces that have stimulated damaging international nurse migration patterns (ICN, 2003).

The nursing shortage is not a new occurrence; it has been documented throughout nursing's history. In past shortages, however, either an increasing demand or a decreasing supply was the primary factor. Currently, a number of factors—varying definitions of *shortage*, the small number of other health professionals, and the fact that both supply and demand are involved equally—pose a complex and far-reaching problem that must be resolved. Compounding the problem is that nurses are leaving the profession because of poor practice environments and because the nursing population is aging and retiring; what's more, they sense a lack of support, have little autonomy, and feel devalued. All these factors affect the entire scope of the nursing discipline. To achieve resolution of this dilemma, a unified nursing voice and concentrated action at all levels—locally, regionally, and nationally—are required. Equally important is retaining nurses in active practice and in nursing education in both developed and developing countries.

The position statement and guidelines for ethical nurse recruitment issued by the ICN in 2001 (revised and reaffirmed in 2007) acknowledges "the adverse effect that international migration may have on health care quality in countries seriously depleted of their nursing workforce" yet recognizes "the right of individual nurses to migrate, and confirms the potential beneficial outcomes of multicultural practice and learning opportunities supported by migration" (paragraph 2). These statements serve as standards that facilitate the protection not only of nurses but also of the health care systems in which they practice worldwide. They are consistent with the ICN Code for Nurses, which provides the foundation of ethical nursing practice throughout the world.

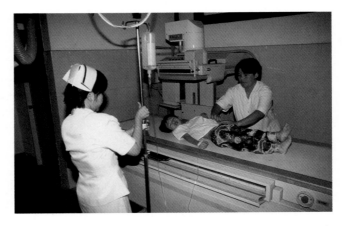

Two nurses at Sawanpracharuk Hospital, Nakorn Sawan, prepare a young boy with dengue for an x-ray in order to observe the degree of internal plasma leakage.

Andy Crump, *Sawanpracharuk Hospital, Nakorn Sawan: Two Nurses Prepare a Boy with Dengue for an X-Ray,* 2000, photograph, TDR Document Centre, World Health Organization, Geneva, Switzerland.

DISEASES AND EPIDEMICS

Throughout the history of humankind, bacteria, parasites, and viruses have swept through cities, devastated populations, and ultimately transformed politics, public health, and economies. The threat of disease outbreaks caused by these agents is always present. When the threat becomes a reality, history may be altered and a tremendous burden placed on societies. Currently, the emergence of diseases has been accentuated by the movement of people, the result of increased globalized trade, the ease of world travel, and the fluctuations of waves of refugees and immigrants. In addition, resistant strains of bacteria and viruses have arisen, and previously preferred treatments have become ineffective for a variety of reasons.

Many of the diseases that exist in the world today have varying degrees of virulence. The diseases that used to be contained in specific areas and countries are now being transported to foreign locations because of the increasing mobility of people. Today a healthy or sick individual can travel from one country to another in a matter of hours. Diseases can be spread in ways that were unimaginable in the past. It is difficult to predict what lies ahead as far as world-changing diseases are concerned, but the hope is that we will be better prepared for them than we were in the past. The WHO continues to be a significant resource because it is the directing and coordinating authority for health within the United Nations system. As such, the organization provides the most up-to-date health and disease information readily available and it monitors outbreaks. Access to this current information facilitates earlier preventive measures.

Nurses are faced with more infectious diseases, epidemics, and pandemics and are at the forefront in caring for those afflicted. Their dedication, even under the most difficult of circumstances and often at great risk to their own health, is constant and unwavering. There are relatively few examples in nursing's history of situations in which nurses have refused to care for or have walked away from contagious patients. They have cared for patients with infectious diseases prior to the development of vaccines, cared for patients with newly emergent diseases about which little was known, and too frequently contracted those diseases and died. They have always been engaged in disease investigations in which they performed surveillance, collected specimens, administered immunizations, wrote reports, and educated individuals, families, and communities. Nurses have contracted syphilis, smallpox, polio, and any number of other diseases. They were not immune just because they were caregivers. What is extremely important in today's world is that nurses and all other health care workers must be vigilant and stay informed about global occurrences of diseases.

New challenges related to world health arise constantly, such as the emergence in April 2009 of a novel influenza A virus (H1N1 strain) not previously observed in humans. Initially referred to as the swine flu, the WHO declared a global pandemic on June 12, 2009. The virus is contagious, and as of the publication date, 30,000 cases have been confirmed in 74 countries. The virus preferentially infects youths; the majority of cases have occurred in people younger than 25 years of age. Worldwide, the number of deaths has been low; the severe and fatal infections have occurred in adults between the ages of 30 and 50 years (WHO, 2009). Other flu pandemics have occurred in the past:

- Spanish flu, 1918: considered to be one of the deadliest outbreaks, with deaths estimated between 20 million and 50 million people
- Asian flu, 1957: 2 waves of illness, the first hitting primarily children and the second affecting mostly the elderly, killing about 2 million people
- Hong Kong flu, 1968: affecting mainly the elderly, killing about 1 million people
- Swine flu, 2009: about 150 people have died so far

Cholera pandemics have sent waves of the disease across the planet since the 1800s. The world is currently in the midst of the seventh pandemic of cholera, which began in Indonesia in 1961. Death is caused by dehydration that results from severe diarrhea. Poor sanitation, lack of sewage systems, and lack of clean water are the mechanisms for the

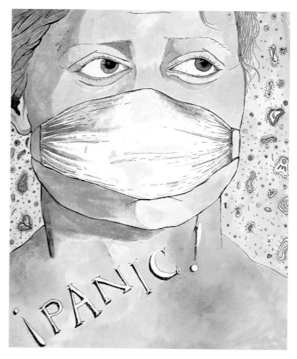

This painting represents one person's thoughts about H1N1 in Mexico.

Genevieve Roudane, *Panic,* watercolor on paper, San Cristobal de Las Casas, Chiapas, Mexico.

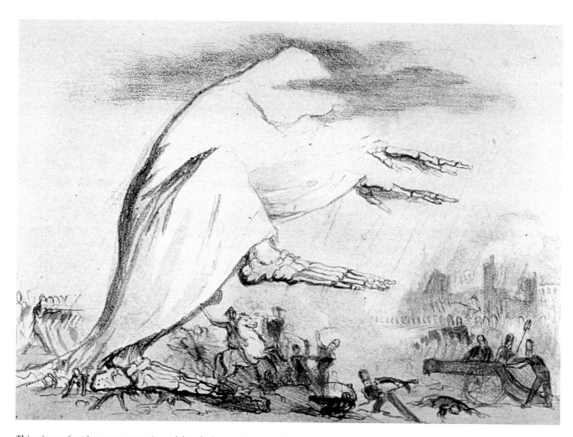

This piece of art is a representation of the cholera epidemic of the nineteenth century. Before 1830, cholera was unknown in the western hemisphere, but it became one of the most feared epidemic diseases of the nineteenth century.

Robert Seymour, *Cholera: Tramples the Victors and the Vanquished Both,* 1831, lithograph, 10 × 12 cm, originally in *McLean's Monthly Sheet of Caricatures,* October 1, 1831, p. 2, no. 22. Image courtesy of the National Library of Medicine.

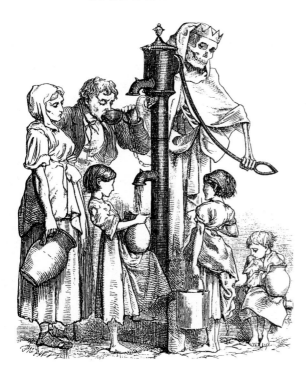

This powerful drawing was a preparatory sketch for an illustration published in the English magazine *Fun* during the outbreak of cholera in London in 1866. By 1866, most physicians and public health officials were convinced that cholera was communicated through the water supply.

Death Dispensary, 1830, engraving, private collection. Photo courtesy of Bridgeman Art Library.

spread of the disease. Unfortunately, more than 1 billion people in the world do not have access to safe drinking water, and 2.5 billion lack adequate sanitation (WHO, 2009). Cholera is considered an old enemy because it has been described in the ancient Chinese, Greek, and Sanskrit literatures. One of the worst cholera epidemics, which occurred in London in 1854, killed more than 10% of the city's inhabitants in less than 2 weeks. This devastating historical event is vividly described in Steven Johnson's (2006) book *The Ghost Map: The Story of London's Most Terrifying Epidemic—and How It Changed Science, Cities, and the Modern World.* Along with being well researched, the book reads like a medical thriller and epidemiological detective story that not only details the outbreak but also outlines its implications for today. Historical research such as this informs the global society and particularly health care professionals about the impacts of diseases and the scientific miracles that have counteracted their effects. In this instance, the story traces the efforts of John Snow, a scientist and anesthetist, who was determined to find out how cholera was transmitted.

Malaria continues to be one of the major causes of morbidity and mortality in the world today. It is one of the most lethal infectious diseases in history and causes as many as 3 million deaths a year. Today approximately 40% of the world's population, mostly those living in the world's poorest countries, is at risk for malaria. Of the deaths caused by

Field-research nurse Sister Isolena and a local "malaria hunter" track signs of malaria that lurks in the swampy tidal flats of Venezuela. Sister Isolena's research focuses on health problems in the homes of the poor and in the laboratory.

Karen Kasmauski, *Sr. Isolena (Venezuela) in Malaria Swampy Tidal Flats,* photograph, from *Nurse: A World of Care,* pp. 26-27.

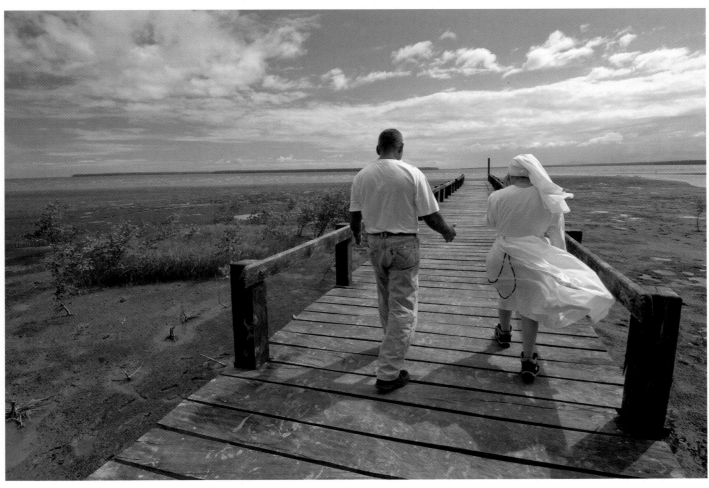

malaria, 90% occur in Africa south of the Sahara, and most deaths occur in young children. Usually, people get malaria by being bitten by the *Anopheles* mosquito, the only mosquito that can transmit the disease. The first effective treatment was quinine, an antimalarial drug derived from the bark of the cinchona tree. In 1955, the World Health Assembly submitted a proposal to eradicate malaria worldwide; it focused on spraying houses with insecticides, on providing antimalarial drug treatment, and on surveillance. The long-term maintenance of the effort was eventually abandoned for a variety of reasons, including difficulties in obtaining sustained funding from donor countries.

"Half of the world's population is at risk of malaria, and an estimated 247 million cases led to nearly 881,000 deaths in 2006. . . . The combination of tools and methods to combat malaria now includes long-lasting insecticidal nets (LLIN) and artemisinin-based combination therapy, supported by indoor residual spraying of insecticide (IRS) and intermittent preventive treatment in pregnancy (IPT)" (WHO, 2008,

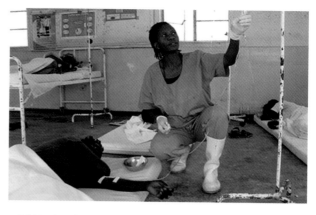

Nurse Diki Dudzai checks the intravenous fluid infusion for a cholera patient at the Katanaga Utano Cholera Treatment Centre in the district of Norton, about 40 kilometers from Harare, Zimbabwe.

Nurse Diki Dudzai Checks the Intravenous Fluid Infusion for a Cholera Patient at the Katanga Utano Cholera Treatment Centre in the District of Norton, photograph, World Health Organization.

At right, A nurse gives tuberculosis medicines to patients at the Beijing Chest Hospital.

Nick Otto, *A Nurse Gives Tuberculosis Medicines to Patients at the Beijing Chest Hospital in China,* photograph, World Health Organization.

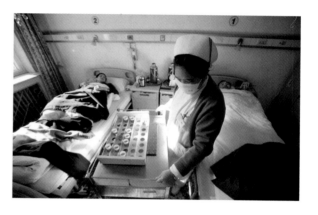

Below, The basic tenets of compassion and love are put into practice at a hospice adjacent to the temple at the Wat Pra Bahpnampu Buddhist Monastery outside of Lop Buri City, Thailand. Nurse Wiliawan Khantiwongse lovingly cares for a patient, although she also supervises a staff of practical nurses.

Karen Kasmauski, *Thailand Hospice/AIDS,* photograph, from *Nurse: A World of Care,* p. 145.

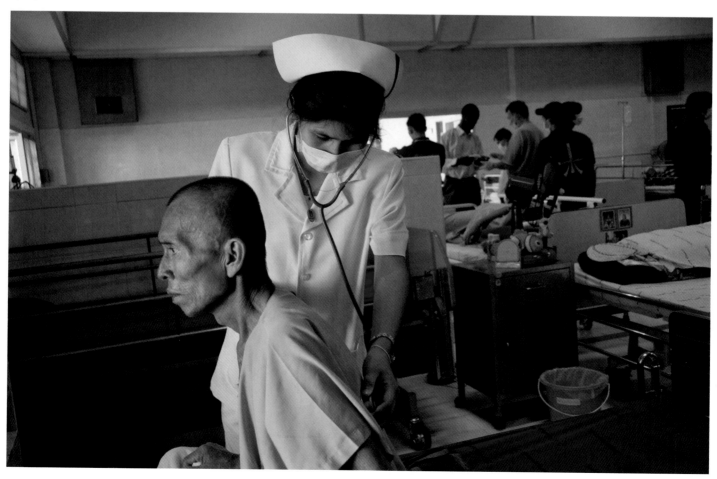

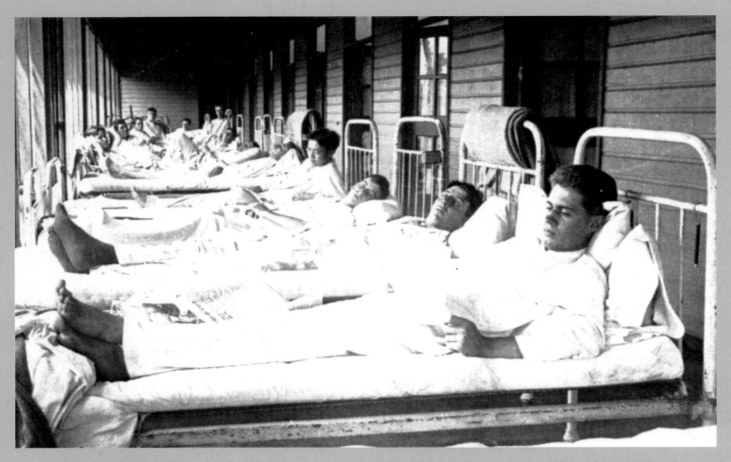

Treatment for tuberculosis in the early 1900s was primitive. With antibiotics unobtainable, the only available protections were natural cures. Since health care providers believed that fresh air, sunshine, and rest provided the best treatment, patients spent the majority of their time in solarium-like porches.

Oakdale Sanitarium, West Porch, Oakdale Sanitarium, Oakdale, IA. With permission from the Iowa City Lion's Club.

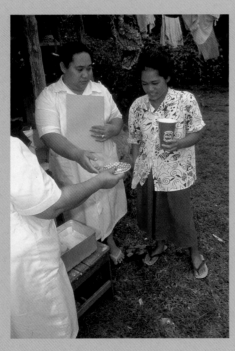

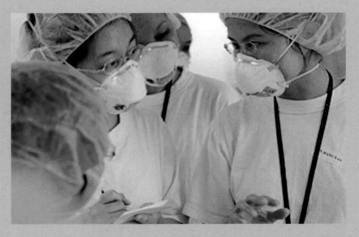

Nurses at Beijing Ditan Hospital in Beijing, the center for dealing with the SARS virus.

Nurses Discuss the Care and Treatment for People with SARS in the Tan Tock Seng Hospital, 2006, photograph, Tan Tock Sang Hospital. Image courtesy of the World Health Organization.

Samoan district health nurses hand DOTS tablets to a young tuberculosis patient.

Andy Crump, *District Health Nurses Hand DOTS Tablets to a Young Tuberculosis Patient in her Garden during a Home Visit to Dispense Anti-Tuberculosis Treatment,* 1999, photograph, TDR Document Centre, World Health Organization, Geneva, Switzerland.

p. vii). Unfortunately, the number of available insecticidal nets is far below the number needed, especially in Africa; and access to treatment, especially artemisinin-based combination therapy, was inadequate in all countries surveyed in 2006.

An old enemy, tuberculosis (TB), is once again spiraling out of control. It has spread dramatically as a result of overcrowding and poverty, the spread of AIDS, and the resurgence of TB strains resistant to drugs. TB and HIV are a lethal combination, each speeding the other's progress. HIV weakens the immune system, thereby creating a situation in which a person who is HIV-positive and infected with TB bacilli is many times more likely to become sick with TB than is a person infected with TB bacilli who is HIV-negative. It was estimated that by the end of the 1990s, TB would speed the occurrence of death in one third of people who have AIDS; approximately 14% of cases of TB would be caused by AIDS. The vast majority of the projected HIV infections and AIDS cases would occur in developing countries by the year 2000. It is unfortunate that these estimates have become reality. One thing remains clear: the world pandemic can be contained only through strong commitment by all communities, national and international. Disease and ill health recognize no borders.

TB is one of the most dangerous diseases on the planet and is again spreading rapidly. Historically, the struggle against TB stimulated some of the first quests for antibiotics, promoted pasteurization to heat and thereby kill TB and other pathogens that contaminate milk, and prompted the building of sanatoriums where people could be isolated and treated. In the 1950s, TB was no longer a major public health threat, so most sanatoriums had reached the end of their useful lives and were demolished.

This is an example of benefits that can be achieved by efforts to control or eliminate diseases. Nurses played a unique role in the era of the TB sanatorium. Not only did they take primary responsibility for the care of patients, they also risked their lives. Globally, one person is newly infected with TB bacilli every second; one third of the world's population is currently infected with the TB bacillus (WHO, 2009). Tuberculosis has also become drug-resistant and is a public health issue in many developing countries because of the necessity of longer treatment and the need for more expensive drugs. The WHO declared TB a global health emergency in 1993.

The epidemic of severe acute respiratory syndrome, known as SARS, was a global threat that occurred in 2002. Caused by a virus, the epidemic appears to have started in Gguangdong Province, China; the first reported case originated in Shunde, Foshsan, Guangdong in November of 2002. China's lack of openness about the epidemic and its failure to inform the WHO of the outbreak until February of 2003 caused delays in attempting to control the epidemic. Within a matter of weeks in early 2003, SARS had spread from Guangdong Province and had rapidly infected individuals in some 37 countries around the world, including North America, South America, Europe, and Asia. Between November 2002 and July 2003 there were 8096 known cases and 774 deaths (WHO, 2003).

Smallpox, believed to have originated more than 3000 years ago in India or Egypt, is one of the most devastating diseases known to humanity. For centuries, repeated epidemics swept across continents, decimating populations and changing the course of history. No effective treatment

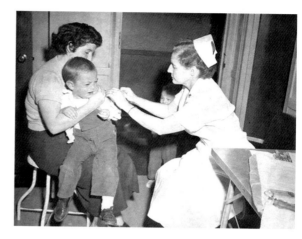

A child receives a smallpox vaccination at a local health department.

Child Receiving a Smallpox Vaccine, 1960s, photograph, Centers for Disease Control and Prevention.

was ever developed for smallpox and as many as 30% of those infected died. Between 65% and 80% of survivors were marked with deep scars (pockmarks), most prominently on the face. In 1798, Edward Jenner demonstrated that inoculation with cowpox could protect against smallpox. As a result, a vaccine was developed that ultimately facilitated the elimination of the disease. It was officially declared eradicated in 1979. This was achieved by a collaborative global vaccination program led by the WHO. The last known natural case was diagnosed in the small coastal town of Merka in southern Somalia in 1977. Since that time, the only known cases were caused by a laboratory accident in 1978 in Birmingham, England, which killed one person and caused a limited outbreak.

What the future holds for the world regarding diseases and epidemics is difficult to predict. The world, however, will continually be faced with the reemergence of "old" diseases and the emergence of "new" diseases. Total eradication of diseases such as cholera, AIDS, and TB may never occur because numerous factors, such as a lack of resources, insufficient numbers of health care professionals, and funding limitations, continue to prevent their elimination. Nurses worldwide will, however, continue to be at the forefront in the fight to overcome diseases and will be advocates for the vulnerable populations most at risk for contracting them.

DISASTERS AND CATASTROPHES

Disasters can be caused by humans (resulting from armed conflicts, industrial accidents, terrorism, or plane crashes) or by natural circumstances (resulting from floods, earthquakes, volcanoes, or droughts). Regardless of the source, essential services, such as electricity, water, sewage removal, transportation, and so forth can seriously affect the health, social, and economic networks of communities and whole countries for an extended time; the outcomes are devastating. In some instances, disasters may be considered chronic in that they have been ongoing for a long period. The African nation of Kenya is an example of this kind of situation, and food shortages and subsequent malnutrition are the result. Disasters cause excessive morbidity and mortality rates and seem to be occurring with greater frequency than ever before. In the United States and its territories alone, there have been 1841 declared disasters since 1953 and 583 declared disasters since 1990 (FEMA, 2009). No individuals and no countries are immune from natural catastrophes or other forms of disaster. In 2001, it was estimated that 3 million people had died in natural disasters since 1990, and many more were affected (ICN, 2001).

Recent world events have created a new perspective with which to view nursing's role in emergency management. Disaster-response teams have usually developed locally and regionally but have also expanded to incorporate an international concept. These teams involve civilian volunteers, including health care professionals. Nurses are in a unique position to participate in all aspects of disaster response because of the skills they have that are related to patient triage, stabilization, state-of-the-art care, and evacuation. Their education, experience, and practice qualify them to be first responders, care givers, and leaders in any large-scale public health emergency. However, the roles of nurses in disasters vary with the specific situations and may present some difficult challenges because disaster responses occur in diverse settings and under the starkest physical conditions and include intense psychological responses. Nurses must prepare themselves to be there for the victims during all stages of a disaster.

The frequency of disasters continues to increase globally. Situations have included anthrax mailings, bioterrorism, earthquakes, tsunamis, hurricanes, and those fueled by world political events that have led to wars. Although nurses have historically been a vital part of emergency responses, it is essential that the nursing profession take leadership roles in treatment decisions and care for victims during times of disasters. Weiner's article (2006), "Preparing Nurses Internationally for Emergency Planning and Response," highlights

the numerous challenges nurses currently face in responding to disasters. So it is imperative that content relating to disasters be included in nursing program curricula; currently, such content is limited. Nursing literature emphasizes that undergraduate and graduate programs in nursing should include content and courses on the subject and that continuing education programs should be available for all nurses. A number of schools now offer programs in disaster preparedness, and one of them is the University of Glamorgan in Wales, U.K. This university collaborated with other schools in the United Kingdom to offer a comprehensive curriculum delivered in an online format. A master of science degree in disaster health care relief and a postgraduate certificate or postgraduate diploma are offered (Weiner, 2006). In 1999 the University of Ulster (U.K.) offered the first academic program in disaster nursing available to nurses. The first postgraduate nurses trained in disaster relief graduated in 2002 (University of Ulster, 1997, 2002). Hyogo University in Japan was designated as a 21st Century Center of Excellence for the training it offers in disaster relief.

Nurses will continue to be the key players in disaster response throughout the 21st century. Their most important attribute is the fact that they intuitively know how to care for people and know who needs their care. They are not, however, immune from the psychological stress that accompanies disasters and may suffer posttraumatic stress disorder.

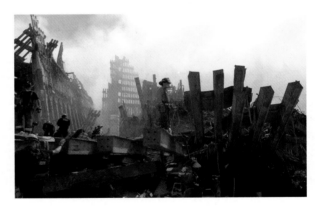

Andrea Booher, *Fire Fighters and Urban Search and Rescue Workers Continue to Battle Smouldering Fires and Search for Survivors at the World Trade Center,* September 14, 2001, photograph, FEMA, byAndrea Booher/FEMA News Photo.

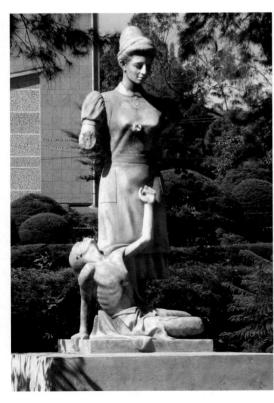

This beautiful sculpture is at the Ethiopian Addis Ababa National Museum. Ethiopia has suffered from famines brought on by periodic droughts.

Nurse with Starving Child, 1930-1970, sculpture, Addis Ababa Ethiopia National Museum, photograph taken by Kathleen Cohen.

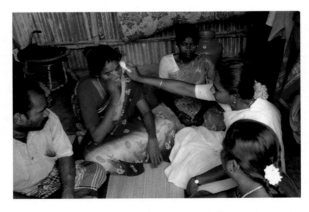

Village health nurse Mrs. R. Rani (in white) visiting shelters to give psychosocial counseling to women who have been affected by the tsunami in Akirapettal shelter, Nagapattinam. Here she tries to console a woman who lost her 16-year-old son.

Pallava Bagla, *Village Health Nurse Visiting Shelters After Tsunami,* photograph, World Health Organization.

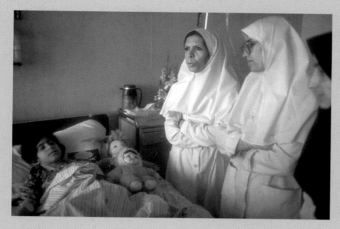

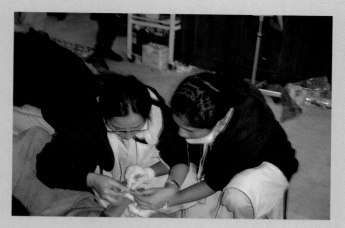

Nurses at the bedside of a young earthquake victim at Al Shahati Hospital.

William Foley, *Nurses at the Stuffed-Animal-and-Doll-Adorned Bedside of a Young Earthquake Victim at Al Shahati Hospital in Tehran, Iran,* photograph, Time and Life Pictures/Getty Images.

Aga Khan University nurses responded under less-than-ideal conditions to the physical needs of Kashmir earthquake victims.

Rafat Jan Rukanuddin, *Pain Management,* 2006, photograph, Reflections (STT). Photo courtesy of Rafat Jan Rukanuddin.

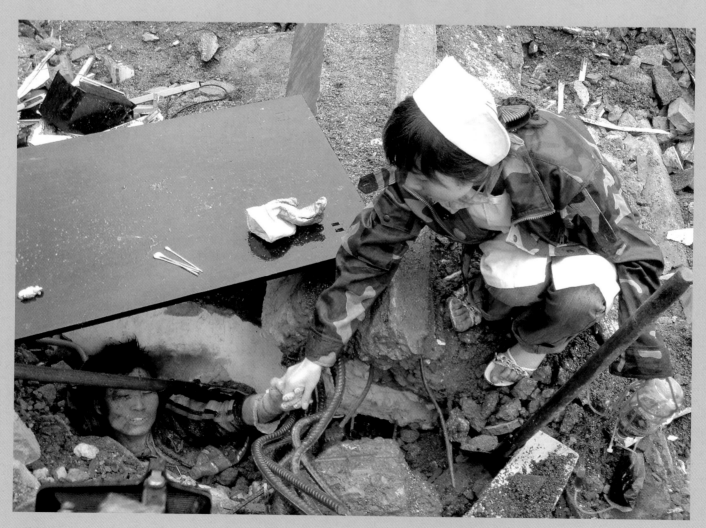

A Chinese nurse helps a trapped youth in the earthquake-hit region of Beichuan, southwest China's Sichuan province on May 13, 2008. Rescue workers sifted through tangled debris of toppled schools and homes for thousands of victims as the death toll from China's worst earthquake in over 3 decades climbed to over 12,000.

Xinhua, *A Chinese Nurse Helps a Trapped Youth,* photograph, photographed in China's Sichuan province. Getty Images.

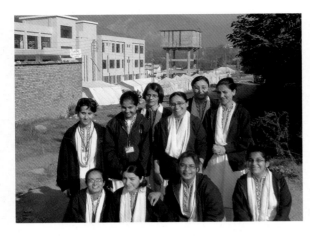

The team of Aga Khan University who responded to the earthquake disaster in Kashmir: Sitting (l-r) Ambreen Noorani, Zahida Haji, Nadia Mulji and Hamida Ismail; middle row (l-r), Sobia Perveen, Methtab Qutubddin, Rafat Jan Rukanuddin, Gul Sharif; and back row (l-r), Shadia Nazar and Rozina Ddulat.

Rafat Jan Rukanuddin, *The Team of AKU Nurses who Responded to the Earthquake Disaster in Kashmir,* 2006, photograph, Reflections (STT). Photo courtesy of Rafat Jan Rukanuddin.

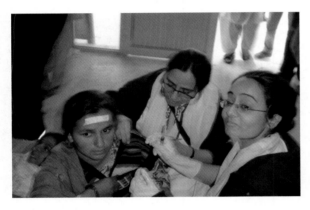

Aga Khan University nurses caring for Kashmir earthquake victims.

Rafat Jan Rukanuddin, *Nurses in Action,* photograph, Reflections (STT).

Overall, nurses provide the foundation for humanistic caring in times of great distress and devastation.

THE AGING POPULATION

One of the most significant demographic events of the 20th century was the aging of the population. Older individuals became a larger percentage of the total population because of a worldwide decline in fertility; major reductions in the prevalence of infectious and parasitic diseases; a decline in mortality rates; the increasing costs of raising children; later marriages; and the longer lives of older people. Consequently, the older population has been growing faster than the total population in virtually all of the developed and developing countries of the world.

The expression *demographic winter* is used to denote the worldwide decline in birthrates, which is also referred to as birth-dearth. Philip Longman, in his book *The Empty Cradle: How Falling Birthrates Threaten World Prosperity and What to Do About It* (2004), comments, "The ongoing global decline in human birthrates is the single most powerful force affecting the fate of nations and the future of society in the 21st century. . . . Worldwide, birthrates have been halved in the past 50 years. There are now 59 nations, with 44% of the world's population, with below-replacement fertility" (Feder, 2008). The elderly, on the other hand, are living longer; life

expectancy has risen around the world. It is projected that by the midpoint of the 21st century, 16% of the world's population will be older than 65, and there will be 400 million Chinese by 2040 (Feder, 2008). This demographic decline will change the face of civilization as numerous challenges arise. The major challenge is to make certain that all peoples will be able to age with security and dignity and receive appropriate health care as needed. But the primary question is Who will care for the graying population?

As life expectancy increases, the growing number of aging people will challenge the capacities of health care providers, policy makers, governments, and society as a whole. What's more, it is logical to assume that as the population of the world ages, the cost of health care in most countries will escalate. Future long-term care for the aging will be the primary challenge for all nations because older populations generally experience higher instances of chronic illness and disability. The quality of those lives then becomes extremely important to consider. Will they be healthy longer lives or longer lives filled with disabilities? It will certainly be a challenge for health care professionals, including nurses, who will be the key players in the response to this global issue.

Historically, nurses have always had an investment in the care of the elderly, who have unique needs. In the 1980s, it was recognized that this population required health care providers who had specific expertise in geriatrics. A movement was begun, and it eventually led to the development of the role of gerontological nurse practitioner (GNP). But originally, these practitioners had been registered nurses, and they had been recruited from nursing facilities for gerontological education and training through continuing education. One initiative that occurred in the United States was sponsored by the W.K. Kellogg Foundation and administered by the Mountain States Health Corporation in Boise, Idaho. The project was conceived by Barbara Lee, a Kellogg Company officer, in collaboration with John Gerdes. Recruitment was the responsibility of Dr. Priscilla Ebersole, the only nurse involved in this phase of the project. The recruited nurses received a certificate of completion upon graduation and were eligible to take the GNP exam offered by the American Nurses Credentialing Center. They were to return to their respective facilities as full-time GNPs (Ebersole, 2006; Rapp, 2006). A marked difference in the care of elderly people occurred. Attention was immediate, GNPs were available, and clinics were established in apartment buildings, senior centers, and so forth. Eventually, GNP certification became available only through graduate nursing programs.

Currently, nursing programs are providing content, courses, and degrees that focus on care of older persons. Nursing students at all educational levels and in all countries are being provided with strong clinical experience in geriatric settings. Student exchange programs with other countries are being developed and implemented so as to facilitate students' understanding of cultural differences among the aged of various nationalities. New models of care are being researched with the goal of providing alternatives to the typical nursing home and permit the aged to live in home-like environments or to remain in their own homes, where they can continue to have control over their lives. The Aging in Place model is one such innovation; it allows the elderly to access health and personal care services, which are delivered to them while they reside at home (Karek and Rantz, 2000). These are prime settings for GNPs and other registered nurses to assess, organize, and implement high-quality care. The future may hold a world in which GNP clinics exist everywhere and are managed and served by nurses, even in some cases owned by nurses.

Organizations and corporations are also involved in facilitating the development of innovative strategies for elder care. The John A Hartford Foundation, established in 1929, has been at the forefront of innovations in training, research, and service systems that promote the health and independence of America's older adults. This foundation has funded the five original Hartford Centers of Geriatric Nursing Excellence since 2000. The aim of these centers is to ad-

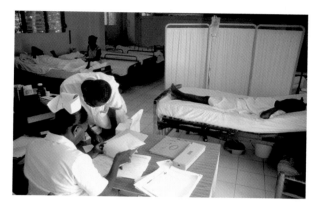

Patients and nurses inside the ward at the sociomedical complex in Cange, Haiti.

Andy Crump, *Cange: Patients and Nurses Inside the Ward at the Sociomedical Complex,* 2001, photograph, TDR Document Centre, World Health Organization, Geneva, Switzerland.

vance geriatric nursing through education, research, practice, and policy making. Four new centers were funded in 2007. Sigma Theta Tau International received a $1.6 million dollar grant from the foundation to launch the Geriatric Nursing Leadership Academy. Many national nursing associations (NNAs) have also been instrumental in promoting initiatives for access to and delivery of services to the aged.

During the past 25 years, immense advances have occurred in elder care worldwide. Many of these initiatives have resulted from the vision, leadership, innovation, collaboration, research, and specialized skills of GNPs and other registered nurses who are devoted to ensuring safe, dignified, and expert care.

THE GENETICS REVOLUTION

The major advances in the field of genetics present great opportunities for the improvement of health care. Nearly all health problems have a basis in genetics; trauma is the exception. The tremendous amount of knowledge that has been gained in this field is beginning to shift health care from diagnosis and treatment to prediction and prevention. The Human Genome Project, which was completed in the spring of 2003, identified the estimated 30,000 genes in human DNA and determined the sequence of the more than 3 billion chemical base pairs (known as A, C, G, and T) that combine in DNA strands. The project had been launched through a joint effort of the National Institutes of Health and the U.S. Department of Energy. "During the early years of the HGP, the Wellcome Trust (U.K.) became a major

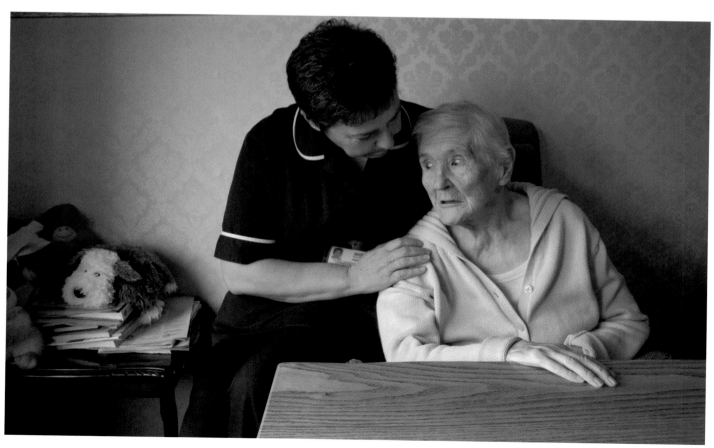

An elderly Scottish woman receives care in her home from a community health nurse.

Karen Kasmauski, *Scottish Community Health Nurse,* photograph, from *Nurse: A World of Care,* pp. 220-221.

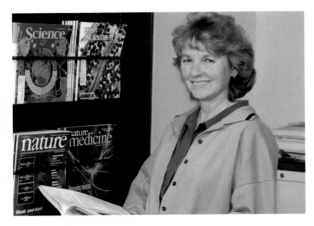

Jean Jenkins, PhD, RN, FAAN, Senior Clinical Advisor to the Director, National Health Genome Research Institute.

Maggie Bartlett, *Dr. Jean Jenkins,* photograph.

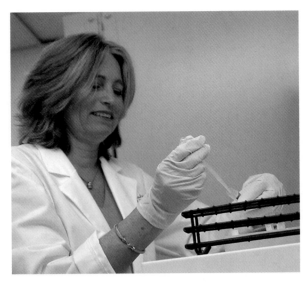

Ann Cashion, PhD, RN is discovering that genetics has a far greater reach than she had imagined as she works in the lab at the University of Tennessee Health Science Center.

Ann Cashion, PhD, RN, photograph, University of Tennessee Health Science Center.

partner; additional contributions came from Japan, France, Germany, China, and others" (Human Genome Information, 2008).

Several years of debate about ethical and social issues and whether the project had any real scientific value preceded its start. A companion ethics program was initiated in conjunction with the project to investigate the consequences of scientific knowledge of genetics. This program would ultimately provide the basis for the development of policies related to potential harm that could result from complex ethical, legal, and social implications. The major concerns include stigma, discrimination, stereotyping, and misuse of genetic data to promote racism; lack of access for research purposes to discoveries because of the patenting of genes; a simplistic view of humans as assemblages of genes; attribution of behavioral and social ills to genes; and lack of respect for individuals, families, and populations (ICN, n.d.). The primary concerns for nurses and health care professionals are privacy, confidentiality, access to health care, and informed decisions concerning health.

The Human Genome Project is responsible for some of the most significant discoveries of applications of genetic information, such as "a new and better understanding of the genetic contribution to disease, the development of targeted drug therapy (pharmacogenetics) and the development of genetic tests that identify those who may have or be at risk for genetic diseases" (Greco and Mahon, 2003, p. 4). Genetic approaches are being used to diagnose diseases and manage disease risk. Commercial testing for susceptibility genes, such as the predisposition genes for breast and colon cancer, is being conducted. The project that was once considered absurd, dangerous, and impossible is now being proclaimed the crown jewel of 20th century biology.

Historically, nurses have always provided care to individuals and families who had or were at risk for genetic conditions. It must remembered, however, that for many years genetics was associated primarily with childbearing decision making and with caring for children who had genetic disorders; medical genetics involved hereditary disorders that affected a small segment of the population. Genetic advances and knowledge are impacting practicing nurses in very different ways now that genetics is understood to play a greater role in common and complex disorders. Consequently, nurses must understand that concerns relating to genetics are present in all clinical settings; favor no age groups; pose

ethical, legal, and social considerations, and are an important component of nursing education and practice.

The genetic revolution has opened the door to new opportunities for nurses as the science is being incorporated into patient care and research. Since the 1960s, nurses have participated in the management of genetic information when providing care for children with genetic disorders and for their families. The surge in nursing literature related to this field began in the 1960s when genetics was conceptualized as being an important component of nursing practice, especially for community health and pediatric nurses. These publications also discussed the nurse's role in the field of genetics and the subject of conducting genetics research. The 1980s revealed a great deal of activity in this area of nursing. The role of clinical nurse specialist in genetics originated in the 1980s. The Genetics Nursing Network was incorporated in 1984 and became the International Society of Nurses in Genetics in 1988. In 1997, genetics was designated an official nursing specialty by the American Nurses Association. In 1998, the international society published *Scope and Standards of Genetics Clinical Nursing Practice* and approved the formation of the Genetic Nursing Credentialing Commission. Soon—in 2001—the first Advanced Practice Nurse in Genetics was credentialed (Greco and Mahon, 2003).

It is no longer acceptable merely to mention genetics in nursing education programs. All patients, families, and communities are impacted by genetics, so nurses must be exposed to content concerning genetics. Currently, nursing programs are offering courses, continuing education classes, certificate programs, and degrees in nursing genetics. More and more nurses have achieved credentials in genetics and are collaborating with nurses worldwide to integrate genetics into education, practice, and research. They are articulating the significance of the work done by genetics nurses and its relationship to nursing practice in general: "Genetic nursing is a holistic practice that includes assessing, planning, implementing, and evaluating the physical, spiritual, ethical,

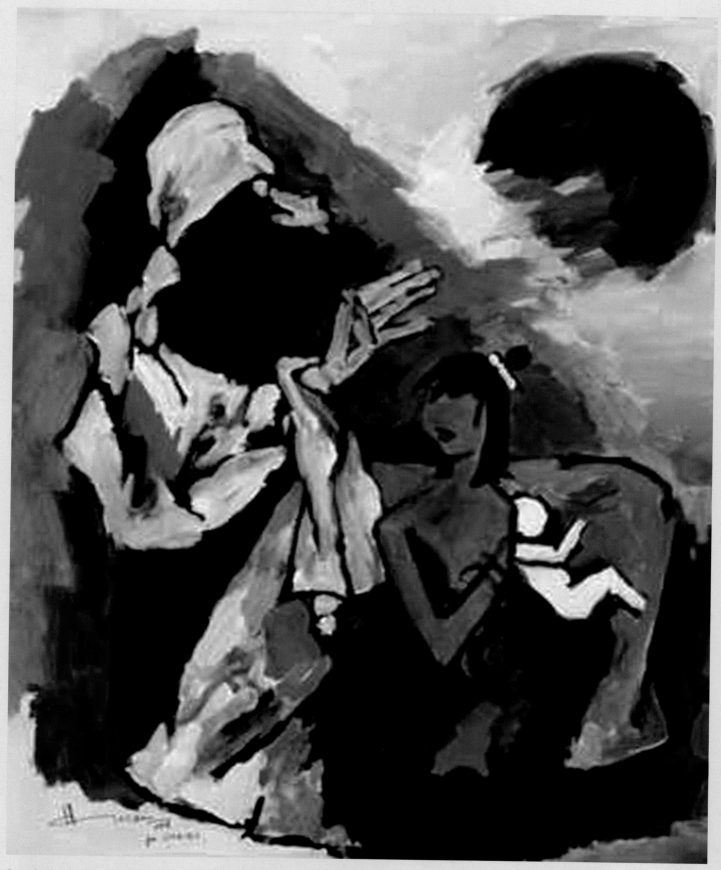

One of India's best known artists, Maqbool Fida Husain, does not shy away from controversy as he creates art in many formats from oil on canvas to documentaries and performance art installation. In this piece Mother Teresa, a mother, and a child are shown together, symbolizing the hope that exists in the response to AIDS

Maqbool Fida Husain, *Mother Teresa,* 2006, oil on canvas, 104 × 92 cm, UNAIDS Secretariat, permanent collection, Geneva, Switzerland.

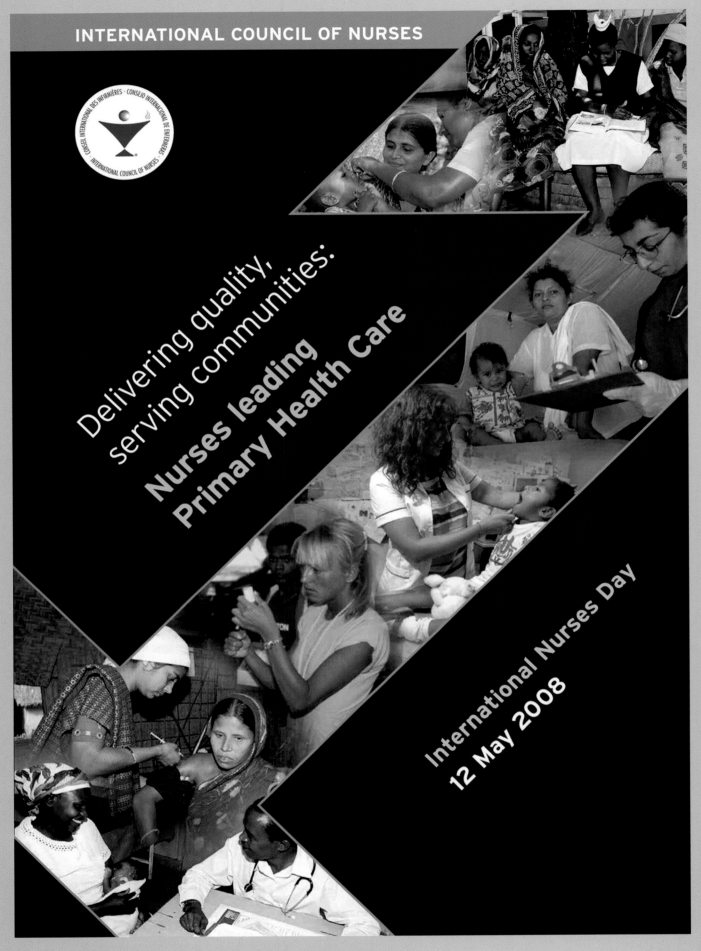

ICN International Nurses Day poster.

International Council of Nurses, *Delivering Quality, Serving Communities,* 2008, International Council of Nurses, Geneva, Switzerland.

and psychosocial aspects of patients and families who have genetic concerns"(Anderson, Read, and Monsen, 2000). Genetics nurses may function in a variety of roles in which they provide genetic counseling, genetic testing, and education; take detailed family histories and construct pedigrees; become involved with clinical trials; and do genetic research. They must stay well informed because the field of genetics is ever changing, and analysis of the data from the genome project will continue for many years. Above all else, however, these nurses care for vulnerable patients and their families with care and compassion.

WORLDWIDE NURSING

Nursing was one of the first groups to understand the significance of primary health care and to progress toward its implementation. This is true even though, in some instances, nurses were not enthusiastic about the movement. Yet as gaps in primary health care have occurred, nurses have been willing and able to fill them and provide a highly cost-effective and high-quality service. The numbers of advanced practice nurses and their areas of clinical expertise have been steadily increasing since the 1960s. The number of nursing specialty areas is remarkable. Much to their credit, nurses have for some time emphasized preventive and primary health care rather than high-tech medical interventions. They have also been more prone to practice in disadvantaged areas with disadvantaged socioeconomic groups. Thus, nursing is well positioned to lead the way toward the resolution of issues concerning accessibility, quality of care, and cost. The question is whether nurses are willing to intellectually view the future from a position of strength, for the

time is ripe for creating a major impact on patient care. Are nurses willing to rise to the challenges of change and chaos and seize the opportunities available in the current situation? Although things may at times appear bleak, Ferguson's words are significant: "At first the idea of creating a new order by perturbation seems outrageous. . . . Yet our traditional wisdom contains parallel ideas. We know that stress often forces new solutions, that crisis often alerts us to opportunity; that the creative process requires chaos before form emerges; that individuals are often strengthened by suffering and conflict, and that societies need a healthy airing of dissent" (Ferguson, 1980, p. 313). Current developments in nursing establish that nurses are rising to the challenges and obstacles in health care that are being presented globally. Nurses are coming from a position of strength as they unite nationally and internationally to impact health care delivery in ways that allow the most efficient and effective care to be given.

HEALTH FOR ALL: PRIMARY HEALTH CARE

A high priority was given to nursing in the early years of the WHO, which was established in Geneva, Switzerland, in 1948 as a specialized agency of the United Nations. A nursing unit headed by a chief nursing officer was set up in 1949; nursing officer positions were later set up in six regional offices. Nurses from numerous specialty areas and countries provided consultation, conducted studies and research, and even engaged in nursing practice in several demonstration projects. However, in 1972, both the nursing unit and the position of chief nursing officer were abolished. The nurses were transferred to functional units within the organization. For years thereafter, the role of nursing was barely recognized. The reemergence of nursing's influence was greatly assisted by Amelia Mangay Maglacas, a nurse from the Philippines, who for 14 years held the position eventually designated Chief Scientist for Nursing. Maglacas was experienced in the fields of teaching, administration, research, and international nursing. By the time of her retirement, nursing's

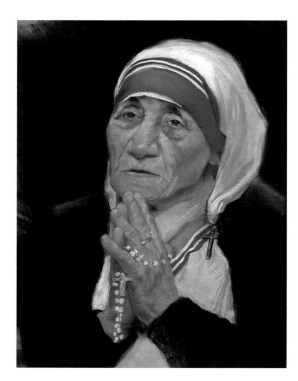

Mother Teresa Bojaxhiu was born in the Yugoslavian region of Skopje and joined the Sisters of Loreto order of the Roman Catholic Church in 1928. After teaching in Calcutta for 17 years, she left the Sisters and went to live and work among the poor in the slum district of Matizhi. There she founded The Missionaries of Charity organization; its first hospice opened in 1952.

Mark Sanislo, *Blessed Mother Teresa of Calcuta,* 2001, pastel drawing, 22″ × 28″. Image courtesy of Mark Sanislo.

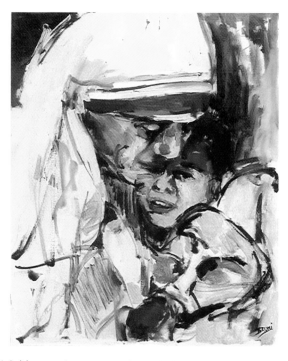

Bruni Sablan, *Mother Teresa: Mother and Child IV,* oil on canvas, 22″ × 28″, Bruni Gallery, Campbell, CA.

status and influence within the organization had grown and flourished. By 1985, nursing's value to the Health for All objective and to the strategy of primary health care to achieve it had been recognized. According to Halfdan Mahler, then Director General:

> If the millions of nurses in a thousand different places artic-ulate the same ideas and convictions about primary health care, and come together as one force, then they could act as a powerhouse for change. I believe that such a change is coming, and that nurses around the globe, whose work touches each of us intimately, will greatly help to bring it about. WHO will certainly support nurses in their efforts to become agents of change in the move towards Health for All. But if the full potential of nursing's contributions to pri-mary health care is to be realized, it is paramount that gov-ernments accept and encourage the placement of nurse leaders where they can have a voice at the policy and decision-making levels.
>
> — WHO, 1985

INTERNATIONAL NURSING EDUCATIONAL PROGRAMS

The Health for All objective called for an international view of nursing that had educational ramifications. A course or an elective concerning international nursing in the curricula of nursing education would no longer suffice. It became neces-sary for an international dimension of health and nursing to be a vital component of all types of nursing education in all parts of the world. Much can be gained by understanding the merits of a variety of nursing education programs and health care systems, including those that are nationalized, such as the Western European welfare type, and those in which priva-tization is operating. More countries are actually examining privatization as a possible way of providing greater efficiency and offering services to immigrant workers from developing countries. The nursing literature has frequently reflected a growing commitment to such an endeavor. Models for iden-tifying the conceptual components of both graduate and un-dergraduate international nursing programs and for integrat-ing international and transcultural content into nursing curricula are now available (Andrews, 1988; Lindquist, 1990; May and Meleis, 1987; Salmon, Talashek, and Tichy, 1988). They greatly facilitate the work of faculty members who are involved in the revision or development of nursing curricula.

Equally important will be further development in the area of international exchange, which has occurred among schools of nursing for many years. Numerous models of in-ternational exchange in schools of nursing currently exist, with wide structural variations. They include formal and in-formal contacts; the sharing of courses, materials, and re-sources; faculty exchanges; and activities such as consulta-tion and joint research and publication (Fenton, 1994; Lindquist, 1984, 1990). The numbers of students receiving degrees in other than their home countries has risen and should continue to increase. However, innovative strategies for student and faculty exchanges must be developed, and additional avenues for funding international nursing activi-ties should be investigated and obtained. This is particularly important considering the current economic situation fac-ing all countries. International exchange contributes to the development of nursing curricula and research consistent with contemporary issues and facilitates collaborative ef-forts to enhance worldwide health care. Its importance can-not be denied.

Additional creative ventures involving the international-ization of nursing continue and will ultimately become stan-dard components of educational programs. For example, Central Finland College of Health in Jyväskylä became in-creasingly international: a joint International Nurse Program between the College and Lancashire College of Nursing and Health Studies in Preston, England, was designed, with im-plementation beginning in August 1994. The 4-year program conformed to the educational standards of both Finland and the United Kingdom; exchange visits were intended to occur in the fourth year. The Central Finland College of Health had international partners in Sweden, Norway, Denmark, Hol-land, Belgium, Great Britain, Estonia, and Hungary (Central Finland College of Health, 1994). This joint curriculum and collaborative effort was a step forward for the development of other explorations and developments in the field.

In 2003, a joint European project was launched by Jyväs-kylä Polytechnic, located in central Finland, and Lucian Blaga University of Sibiu in Romania. The project was coordinated by the University of Central Lancashire and focused on the development of a Romanian community nursing program. This project involved the planning of the community nurs-ing curriculum in accordance with European Union direc-tives concerning European nursing education and the train-ing of Romanian teaching personnel. Faculty members of both institutions shared responsibilities related to course development and information exchange (ESTIA-Net, 2003).

Another type of international nursing education initiative involves the University of Alabama's Pan American Health Organization (PAHO)/WHO Collaborating Center for Inter-national Nursing. The school was initially designated as a WHO collaborating center in 1993 and was redesignated in 1997 and most recently in 2007. Graduate nursing education and collaborative research are the primary focuses of the program. The school's collaborative relationships with Bra-zil, Chile, Colombia, Guatemala, Honduras, Korea, Taiwan, Thailand, Zambia, and many other countries have included visiting scholars, visiting professors, student exchanges, and international research programs. The terms of reference for 2007 to 2011 include the following:

> 1. Design and facilitate implementation of educational pro-grams for nurses and health care workers to strengthen nursing capacity in meeting priority health needs of children and families, with special emphasis in the PAHO region.
> 2. Strengthen leadership in nursing education and practice to meet priority health needs of children and families.
> 3. Build capacity for generation, utilization, and dissemina-tion of nursing knowledge to promote best nursing practice in meeting the health needs of children and families.
> 4. Enhance leadership development among faculty and stu-dents in the UAB School of Nursing in mentoring the terms of reference work of the PAHO/WHO Collaborating Center.
>
> — UNIVERSITY OF ALABAMA SCHOOL OF NURSING, 2009

Numerous other international initiatives are taking place at the University of Alabama School of Nursing, including pro-gram that offers a PhD degree in nursing in collaboration with Chiang Mai University in Thailand. Such programs are also oc-curring among countries all over the world, and they demon-strate the establishment of a truly global nursing community.

ORGANIZATIONAL EFFORTS

The ICN celebrated its 100 years of existence in 1999. The organization is the international voice of nursing and stands strong beside other intergovernmental organizations like the WHO and the International Labor Organization. The ICN was organized in 1899 as an independent, nongovernmental federation of NNAs. In the early years emphasis was placed on education, as attempts were made to develop definitions of *nursing* and of *nurse*. Although nursing education is still an important facet of the work of the ICN, other programs have contributed to its emergence as a primary societal force in many countries of the world. The ICN functions to promote the development of nursing as a profession and to serve the health needs and promote the health status of humankind. International nursing leadership has been demonstrated throughout the years by the organization's 10 executive directors and 22 presidents.

EXECUTIVE DIRECTORS OF THE INTERNATIONAL COUNCIL OF NURSES

Name	Country	Years
Lavinia L. Dock	United States	1900-1922
Christianne Reimann	Denmark	1922-1934
Anna Schwarzenberg	Austria	1934-1947
Daisy Bridges	United Kingdom	1948-1961
Helen Nussbaum	Switzerland	1961-1967
Sheila Quinn	United Kingdom	1967-1970
Adele Herwitz	United States	1970-1976
Barbara Fawkes	United Kingdom	1977-1978
Winnifred Logan	United Kingdom	1979-1981
Constance Holleran	United States	1981-1986
Judith Oulton	United Kingdom	1986-2008
David Benton	Scotland	2008-current

Source: *Annual Reports,* ICN.

PRESIDENTS OF THE INTERNATIONAL COUNCIL OF NURSES

Name	Country	Years
Ethel Gordon Bedford Fenwick	United Kingdom	1900-1904
Susan McGahey	Australia	1904-1909
Agnes Karll	Germany	1909-1912
Annie Goodrich	United States	1912-1915
Henny Tscherning	Denmark	1915-1922
Sophie Mannerheim	Finland	1922-1925
Nina Gage	China	1925-1929
Leonie Chaptal	France	1929-1933
Alicia Lloyd Still	United Kingdom	1933-1937
Effie Taylor	United States	1937-1947
Gerda Hojer	Sweden	1947-1953
Marie Bihet	Belgium	1953-1957
Agnes Ohlson	United States	1957-1961
Alice Clamageran	France	1961-1965
Alice Girard	Canada	1965-1969
Margarethe Kruse	Denmark	1969-1973
Dorothy Cornelius	United States	1973-1977
Olive Anstey	Australia	1977-1981
E. Muringo Kiereini	Kenya	1981-1985
Nelly Garzon	Colombia	1985-1989
Mo-Im-Kim	Korea	1989-1993
Margretta Madsen Styles	United States	1993-1997
Kirsten Stallknecht	Denmark	1997-2001
Christine Hancock	United Kingdom	2001-2005
Hiroko Minami	Japan	2005-2009
Rosemary Bryant	Australia	2009-current

Source: *Annual Reports,* ICN.

The ICN is a federation of NNAs currently representing nurses in more than 128 countries (ICN, 2009). When the organization was initiated, it was comprised of three countries. Only one NNA per country could belong. The ICN introduced a different membership structure for this new millennium. Three membership models presented by the Board of Directors were approved by the Council of National Representatives (CNR) in June 2001. Each NNA and future NNAs are offered the opportunity to choose the model that best meets their needs:

Model 1: Alliance

Under the alliance model, national nursing organizations in the country decide to form a new national nursing organization for international purposes. Banded together in an international alliance, the alliance becomes the ICN member. It determines its makeup and may include national generalist and specialist organizations. The new national nursing organization sets its own internal operating rules while complying with all of ICN's requirements.

Model 2: Collaboration

Under the collaboration model, the current NNA remains the ICN member and continues to carry the CNR vote. However, it speaks from the informed perspective of selected national nursing collaborating organizations. The current NNA selects national generalist and specialist organizations with whom it wishes to collaborate on international issues and establishes national operating rules for doing so. The NNA seeks input from the collaborating organizations prior to forming its national position on international issues.

Model 3: Traditional

Under the traditional model, only one NNA per country may be part of ICN and it must be the most representative generalist nursing organization in the country (ICN, 2009).

Under all membership models, ICN maintains the system of one vote per country.

The original purpose of the ICN remains the same: "to provide a medium through which the interests, needs, and concerns of member national nurses' associations can be addressed to the advantage of the public and nurses" (Ohlson and Styles, 1994, p. 408). Its mission is to represent nursing worldwide, advancing the profession and influencing health policy. It has the distinction of being the first international professional organization in the health care field. The ICN has served nursing well over the past century, particularly through its consultative status with the WHO. Close working relationships have been developed with other United Nations agencies, other nongovernmental organizations, and international foundations.

The ICN quickly accepted nursing's responsibility for primary health care in response to the Health for All global agenda. A number of activities were carried out to assist with nurse preparation and successful implementation. Between 1983 and 1985, seven regional workshops were organized to prepare nursing leadership. Another outcome of these workshops was the development of a resource book for primary health care nursing, which included guidelines for policy making, education, and practice. The response of the ICN to societal trends, health care crises, and varied challenges has been phenomenal. Its strength and timing have proven to be particularly significant to the progression of nursing's role in health care.

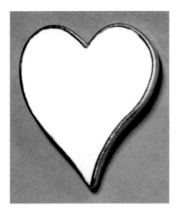

The white heart is the universal symbol for nursing. It is meant to characterize the caring, knowledge and humanity that infuse the work and spirit of nursing. The white heart is also a unifying symbol for nurses globally. White was selected because it brings together all colors, demonstrating nursing's acceptance of all people. White also has a worldwide association with nursing, caring, hygiene, and comfort. The heart shape communicates humanity and the central place that nursing has in quality health care.

The White Heart Pin, International Council of Nurses.

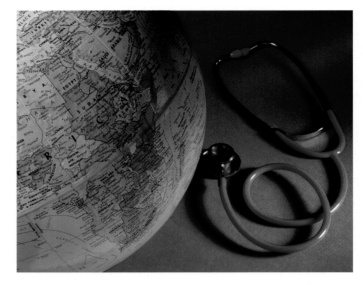

Regions around the world are flooding the Institute for Johns Hopkins Nursing with requests for international collaboration and assistance.

George Peters, *Global Positioning,* photograph.

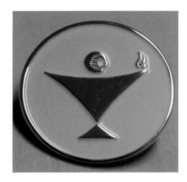

The ICN logo brings together the person (both the nurse and the people nurses serve) and the lamp, a symbol of nursing in many countries, representing the nurse working with people. Taken together, the four elements (base, lamp, flame, and globe) also represent unity, strength, wholeness, and equilibrium. This modern logo reflects the dynamism and flexibility of ICN as an organization.

The ICN Logo Pin, International Council of Nurses.

The ICN continues to be involved in a far-reaching project, the International Classification for Nursing Practice (ICNP). In a 1989 CNR meeting in Seoul, Korea, the American Nurses Association (ANA) and the Canadian Nurses Association proposed the resolution to the ICN that led to the project's development. Essentially, the resolution expressed "nurses' concerns about the effects of nursing's inability to define the problems to which it addresses its activities and the distinctive contribution it makes to solving them. The resolution asked that ICN encourage member NNAs to become involved in developing classification systems for nursing care, nursing information management systems, and nursing data sets to provide tools that nurses in all countries could use to describe nursing and its contributions to health" (Clark, 1994, p. 146). Considerable activity was involved in developing a common language that can be used across borders to describe and organize nursing data. Major contributors to the work of the ICNP are the North American Nursing Diagnosis Association; Nursing Interventions Classification; Saba's Home Health Classification (1992); and

The Omaha System (Martin and Scheet, 1992). Additional information about the ICNP can be found in Unit 8.

Other types of professional nursing groups and organizations have also been extensively involved in numerous enterprises that include international conferences, participation in the development of public policy, development of strategies to improve nursing's image, and the protection of the economic and general welfare of nurses. National nursing organizations are collaborating and are coordinating efforts to ensure the future of the nursing profession; they continually emphasize high-quality and cost-efficient care. The ANA established an International Nursing Center in 1991 in its Washington, DC, office. Two significant developments led to its institution: ". . . increasing trends throughout the world toward regionalism and globalism in political, economic, and labor sectors, and a realization among ANA leadership of ANA's need to respond to these trends with renewed focus on its international activities" (American Nurses Association, 1991). Sigma Theta Tau International Honor Society of Nursing became an international organization in 1988.

THE GLOBAL SCENE

Nursing and nurses around the world are the same, yet different. Nursing personnel in most countries represent a potentially powerful force capable of initiating changes in health care delivery and arousing public opinion. Most important, they are in constant contact with the people they care for in every type of environment imaginable. Nurses in various countries are not alone in facing challenges that have occurred as the result of organizational changes and economic constraints. The majority of local, regional, and national issues are also global issues. It may well be that the emphasis on primary health care will be the motivating force that will unify nurses nationally and internationally.

The nursing profession will continue to be bombarded by giant forces that are political, sociological, technological, epidemiological, and ethical in nature. Some of these forces will escalate, but others will change direction. Nurses must be flexible; they must be prepared to change course as the situation warrants. Nurses must be visionary and anticipate the waves of the future. Styles (1993) projected the following macrotrends—a combination of forecasts by professional futurists and impressions gathered through personal observations: health care reform; motivation of the workforce; gender issues; quality care and the empowerment of the consumer; and organizational transformation. These are consistent with other projections that appear in the literature. They are also compatible with the major implications for nurses in the face of health care reform, as identified by Buchan (1993): ". . . employment opportunities will grow more slowly; shift of care from the acute sector to outpatient and community care; more appropriate use of nursing staff; greater potential for autonomous health practice; and increasing emphasis on management skills" (p. 21). Although speaking of Canadian and United Kingdom nurses, the implications are applicable to nurses everywhere and are discussed frequently. Other trends have taken their toll on the nursing workforce—the increasing use of unlicensed assistive personnel, the cross-training of personnel, and the regulation and licensure of new types of technical workers. The rationale for these trends may not be universal; nonetheless, they have ramifications for nursing. In addition, as the macrotrends and their major implications are examined, along with workplace trends, it becomes apparent that nurses worldwide share common concerns about their workplaces and practices.

Because of continually changing statistics, it is often difficult to ascertain adequately and accurately at any given moment the global picture of nursing. A report about the global nursing workplace from *The Global Shortage of Registered Nurses: An Overview of Issues and Actions* by Bachan and Calman (2005) notes the following:

A Global Overview

- There is huge variation in the nurse-to-population ratios throughout the world.
- At country level, the reported nurse-to-population ratio varies in different countries from fewer than 10 nurses per 100,000 people to more than 1000 nurses per 100,000 people, a variation of more than 100-fold.
- The average ratio in Europe, the region with the highest ratios, is 10 times that of the regions with the lowest ratios, Africa and Southeast Asia.
- The average ratio in North America is 10 times that in South America.
- The average nurse-to-population ratio in high-income countries is almost 8 times greater than in low-income countries.
- The minimal availability of nurses in many developing countries is exacerbated by geographical maldistribution; even fewer nurses are available in rural and remote areas.

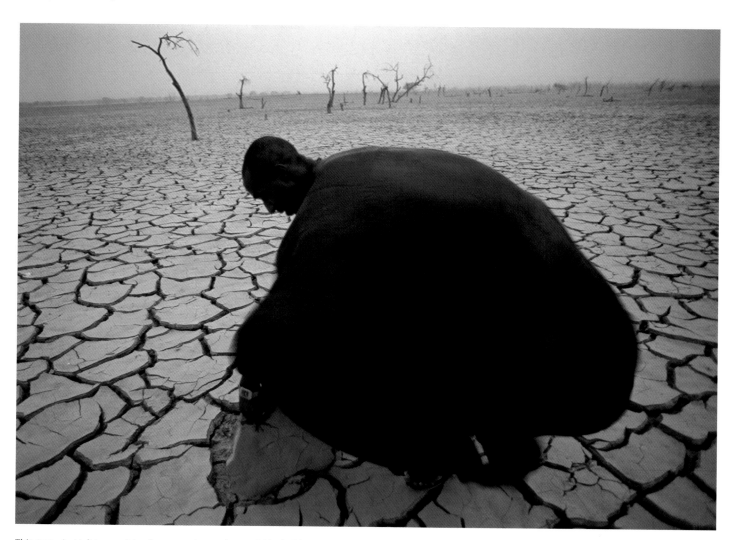

This nurse in Mali is searching for any moisture that could be hidden in a dry lakebed. Waiting for the dry season to end is an annual ordeal in much of Africa. The lack of water results in dehydration, poor hygiene, and the spread of disease.

Karen Kasmauski, *Searching for Water in Mali,* photograph, from *Nurse: A World of Care,* pp. 30-31.

342

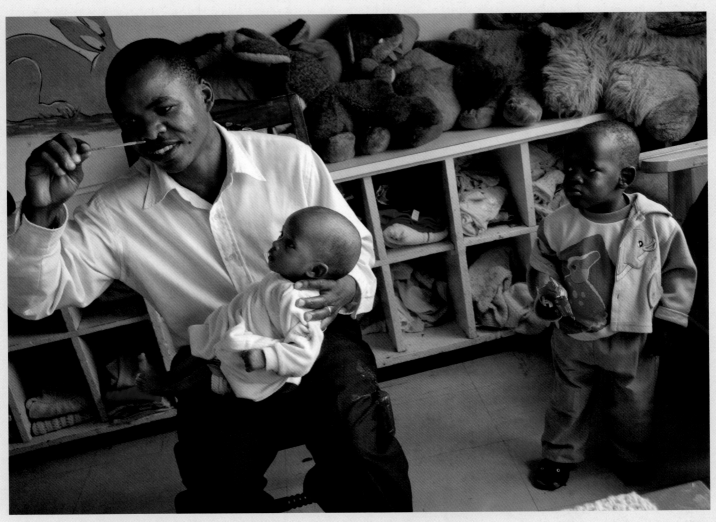

Boaz Sikobe works in a private children's clinic in Nairobi but volunteers at the Mama Ngina Kenyatta Children's Home. He originally expected to assist with a CDC-sponsored safe-water project. Observing, however, that many babies coming to the orphanage received no medical evaluation, he began giving the children check-ups.

Karen Kasmauski, *Nairobi Children's Home,* photograph, from *Nurse: A World of Care,* p. 171.

"The report [itself] presents a global picture of the distribution of nurses, based on an analysis and interpretation of data on nurse:population ratios, collated by the World Health Organization (WHO). The data collated by WHO from some countries includes midwives under the broad category of nurses, whilst in other countries only registered nurses are included. For some, it is also likely that the data may include auxiliary and unlicensed personnel. The nurse:population ratio gives a very broad indication of the level of availability of professional nursing skills in each country" (p. 2). Since this report was published in 2005, the data will have undoubtedly changed but to what extent is unknown.

Nursing shortages are being experienced in many of the African nations, consistent with the overall picture of limited numbers of all types of health workers. Most nurses are employed in urban areas because environmental, educational, and family and working conditions in rural areas are less than desirable. The majority of nurses are women, although nursing used to be a predominantly male profession there. Salaries are extremely low. The supply of nurses varies considerably within the Americas. Countries in North America are well supplied with nurses, whereas Latin American countries are not, although the situation various among these countries. A number of areas have resorted to the use of unlicensed assistive personnel to perform nursing tasks. A gross imbalance of nurses exists between oil-producing countries and the other countries in the eastern Mediterranean region. The immigration of nurses from India, Egypt, and the Far East accounts for the highest density of nurses in the oil-producing countries. The heavy migration of nurses out of Egypt is the result of low financial and moral rewards and poor working conditions. The European region has the highest density of nurses. The highest ratios occur in the Nordic countries. Differences in health care coverage are the least noticeable in this region. Human resources in Southeast Asia are generally poor. There is an extremely low ratio of nurses to population, although Thailand is an exception. There are well-developed nursing programs in Thailand, and nurses are leaders in primary health care. A number of countries in the western Pacific enjoy a high nurse-to-population ratio as compared with other regions of the world. The highest ratios occur in Australia, Japan, and New Zealand. Australian nurses have improved their conditions through the united voices of strong nursing unions that have made them effective in lobbying. Nurses' wages are low in Japan, where they work long hours, but efforts are being made to improve their economic and general welfare. The Philippines continue to lose nurses to countries that are willing to pay higher salaries. Filipino nurses receive no health benefits, have no job security, and work under extremely stressful conditions. Since the 1980s, Chinese nurses have been rebounding from the effects of communism, which cut off their contact with the West. Nurses are currently controlled by the medical profession.

Societies have witnessed a number of conflicts and crises as well as the information revolution. Health care delivery systems worldwide have been caught in a web of social problems, financial crises, and scarce resources that is forcing a major transformation in the rendering of care. Nursing must adapt to these shifting realities as it has in the past, while taking into account the need for internal change to meet new opportunities created by such upheaval. Challenges and visions once again have become important components in the fostering of nursing's evolution. Although much about nursing will continue to change, much will remain constant. But the changes will be a result of the unified effort of a global nursing community that is strong and resilient in its devotion to health care for all.

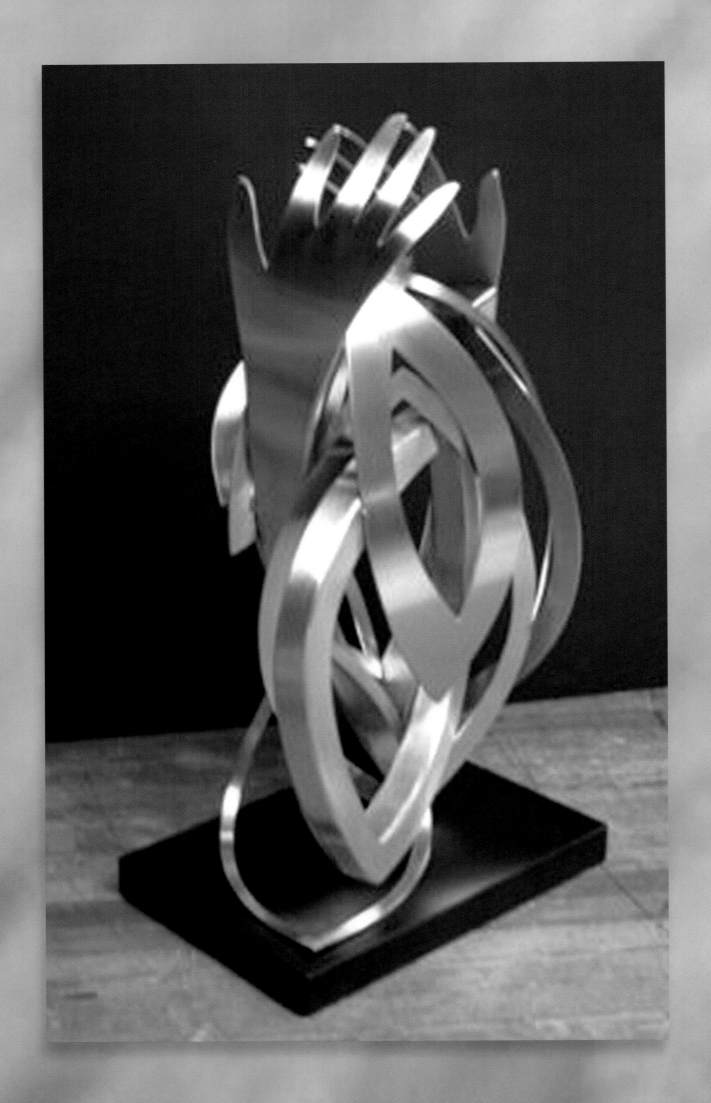

ℰPILOGUE

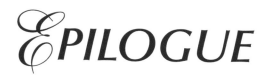 t is important to remember that nursing is a social mandate and has been part of the communal fabric since the dawning of civilization. Birth, death, and health-illness are part of the legacy of humankind, which requires the assistance of others. Exciting developments in science and technology have made the role of the nurse richer and more complex. We now have an array of tools and services to offer those we care for that were not possible for our predecessors. But the unifying, underlying essence of our work is the timeless and profound healing presence we offer that enhances the exploration and creation of meaning in the inevitable health challenges faced by individuals, families, and groups whose lives we are privileged to touch.

– JO ELLEN GOERTZ KOERNER

Gloria Tew, *The Enlightened Touch*, stainless steel sculpture, University of Minnesota School of Nursing.

This journey through nursing's history is a humbling epic in which the care of strangers and the protection of health are paramount. Central to the story are the women and men who chose the calling of nursing and paved the way for nursing to transition from an apprentice-type occupation to a recognized, respected, and accepted health care profession. What is reflected in this history is nursing's devotion to and responsibility to society, no matter what the circumstances—two qualities that often seem to be nearly extinct in today's world. The history also clearly reveals the close and indispensable alliance that has continuously existed between nursing and society. Although nursing emerged with altruism as its motivation, it is now a profession that mandates the acquisition of sophisticated knowledge and the skills necessary for the provision of high-quality care. This is no easy task as knowledge development continues at an amazingly rapid rate and technology emerges as a force with as yet unimaginable consequences.

Nursing's historical legacy is that of a caring-healing profession that embraces healing environments as well as attention to the wholeness of human beings. Its caring is defined by significant concepts that exemplify the attributes that are consistently exhibited by nurses in their practice. The concepts include compassion, commitment, competence, trust, tenderness, science, and touch—and these concepts represent a mere fraction of the words and concepts that portray the inherent qualities of nurses. All of these concepts are embedded within nursing's commitment to the health and well-being of humanity and are deep-seated in the philosophy that each and every human being is entitled to safe, efficient, and competent care. This care strongly emphasizes lack of bias, that each individual will receive care without regard for race, creed, sex, social or economic status, personal attributes, or the nature of the health problems. Consequently, throughout history, nurses have been involved in both popular and unpopular causes that have concerned health and social welfare and have consistently risen to challenges so as to bring about social reform.

A significant event in the history of nursing occurred in 2009—the University of Minnesota School of Nursing's Centennial Celebration. In 1909, through the influence of Dr. Richard Olding Beard, the School of Nursing became the first nursing school organized as an integral part of a university. Nursing students were admitted and registered as regular students of the university, with all university requirements and privileges. This event set the trend toward the housing of nursing education in institutions of higher learning, and the acquisition of college degrees by student nurses eventually occurred. The sculpture *Enlightened Touch* was commissioned to commemorate this occurrence, and it contributes to an understanding of the essence of nursing. It is true that the perception of artwork does remain with the eye of the beholder, but in this instance, no one can deny the impact of these uplifting and beautiful hands that personify the spirit of nursing. The hands are all-encompassing and are a protective force that brings healing to the global community of human beings, which are represented by the strong circular strands of steel. The hands touch so tenderly, representing the caring and healing relationship between the nurse and the patient. This wonderful personification of human touch defines the holistic and humanistic aspects that are vital to understanding nursing. My interpretation of the sculpture in no way denies the importance of science and technology to nursing because they too are components of the steel strands that blend and provide the strength to create the skill, the science, and the spirit of nursing. But the primary emphasis of the sculpture is on the healing touch so crucial to the practice of nursing in a renewed and enlightened period of history.

Touch has always been an integral and significant part of nursing and its history, but the meaning of the word can sometimes be difficult to articulate. In general, *touch* is used in a variety of ways: to indicate comforting, soothing, feeling, appreciating, understanding, respecting, and healing. The use of touch as a vehicle of communication, however, remains unsurpassed, particularly in the discipline of

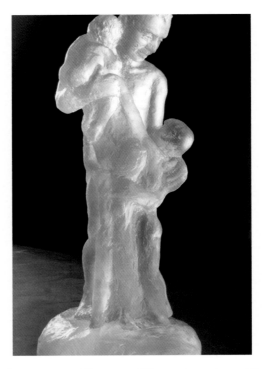

Judi Charlson, *Devotion* (side view), 2009, kiln cast glass sculpture, 14" × 6" × 6".

Judi Charlson, *Devotion* (full view), 2009, kiln cast glass sculpture, 14" × 6" × 6".

nursing. No matter whether a patient is conscious or unconscious, young or old, ambulatory or immobile, literate or illiterate, deaf or blind, nurses are able to communicate through touch. Nurses know that with a simple and gentle touch, more love and understanding can be conveyed than could have been communicated with any number of words. This has become extremely important as society and patients increasingly confront a world of high technology. The challenge for nurses has thus become the creation of a viable approach to balancing technology with touch and, first and foremost, to facilitating patient-centered care.

Nursing practice has always been strengthened by the use of touch as an act of understanding that provides energy, love, respect, and dignity to those who are vulnerable and whose lives are entrusted to nurses. Touch is also an intimate act that permits nurses to rise above social taboos. Nurses touch the private parts of their patients' bodies, and that signifies a formation of trust and closeness that can be almost spiritual. Physical touch not only provides a mechanism for the assessment of patient status and the provision of nursing acts such as bathing but also conveys the emotional element of caring so crucial to the well-being of patients. Intimacy is confined not only to the physical realm of patient care in nursing practice. Nurses also are privileged to hear the most private, intimate, and confidential aspects of patients' and families' personal lives. Nurses are trusted to provide care in such a manner as to protect human dignity under the most dire of circumstances.

Throughout nursing's history, change has been continuous, inevitable, and inescapable. Yet nursing has consistently recognized that forces occur over which there is little control and that these events must be turned into windows of opportunity. In essence, it is far better to embrace change than to waste energy resisting it; far better to embrace change as an opportunity rather than reject it as a threat. It has not always been easy, however, for nursing to embrace change, as is evidenced by periods of caution and hesitancy that sometimes impeded its progress. There have been instances in which new initiatives were opposed or rejected by members of the nursing profession. There have been instances in which compromises had to be made. Campaigns for better nursing education, for example, have been long and not without struggle. But overall, the primary factor in nursing's history of resolving issues of change has been concern for patient welfare and social justice.

It is almost impossible to reiterate totally the progress and positive changes that have occurred in nursing since its inception and the numerous changes in health care that have impacted both nursing practice and education. The identification of a selected few, however, renders some understanding of the complex issues that have been addressed:

- Patients became consumers of health care.
- Hospitals became big businesses.
- Nursing education moved into institutions of higher learning.
- Advanced degrees in nursing became a reality.
- The Doctor of Nursing Practice and the Clinical Nurse Leader became the newest educational initiatives in nursing.
- Continuing education requirements for health professional licensure renewal occurred.
- Intensive care and specialized care units were created.

- Advanced practice nursing came into its own.
- Nurses moved into many sectors of society and held positions of power.
- Complementary therapies once again became popular as individuals looked for other avenues to attain and maintain health.
- The fields of ethics, computer science, informatics, and genetics arrived on the scene.
- E-learning was created, changing the face of educational institutions and the way students learn and are taught.
- Technology continued to explode, impacting every area of life and living.
- Globalization occurred, and it mandated that nursing and health care be viewed in an entirely different manner.

The future of nursing is difficult to predict because of the almost certain demands of a reformed health care and public health system that will be emerging worldwide. Nurses will have to be risk takers, visionaries, dreamers, innovators, and creators of new practice models. They will have to be increasingly involved in the development of health care policy and more readily acknowledge the power that lies in politics. They must respond to challenges in ways that will maintain nursing as a caring-healing profession in which the humanistic and traditional values of nursing are balanced with the highly technological and specialized care-delivery systems. The key to nursing's future lies in recognizing the critical role nurses must play in solving many of the complex issues involved in health care and in reconceptualizing the role of nurses as being necessary in providing the holistic care that is vitally needed by patients, families, and communities. Task forces are currently being constructed in countries throughout the world to address the future of nursing, an issue that is considered to be of extreme importance.

Newly emerging leaders in nursing have a formidable task—to continue the work initiated years ago by the early nursing leaders. They must become the role models, the innovators, the nurses who provide inspiration and motivation and use their collaborative efforts to shape, develop, and implement viable nursing for the future. They must provide the structure whereby nurses will be united, will face uncharted territory, and will be engaged in practice that truly represents the spirit of nursing of the past, the present, and the future. They will be benefitted by knowledge of nursing's history, for as Tarnas (2002) states, "For us to participate fully and creatively in shaping our future, we need to better understand the underlying patterns and influences of our collective past."

Early and contemporary leaders in nursing consistently refer to nursing as an art as well as a science. Art in this context, however, is more than a static, linear concept. It involves a type of perception that is active, dynamic, and developing. An emotional quality guides the transformation of the material in art, but the role of intelligence and thinking is stressed. Isabel M. Stewart frequently wrote about nursing as an art. She stressed that the nurse as a true artist was essential to the progression of nursing into something other than a highly skilled trade. Stewart realized that numerous individuals thought of art and technique as a single entity, but she emphasized that a piece of work could be technically perfect, yet fall short of being a work of art. Technique, soul, mind, and imagination were all essential in the formation of a true artist.

The real essence of nursing, as of any fine art, lies not in the mechanical details of execution, nor yet in the dexterity of the performer, but in the creative imagination, the sensitive spirit, and the intelligent understanding lying back of these techniques and skills. Without these, nursing may become a highly skilled trade, but it cannot be a profession or a fine art. All the rituals and ceremonials which our modern worship of efficiency may devise, and all our elaborate scientific equipment will not save us if the intellectual and spiritual elements in our art are subordinated to the mechanical, and if the means come to be regarded as more important than ends.

— *Stewart, 1929, p. 1*

The heritage of nursing is rich. Although the entire story of the development of nursing has not been told in these pages, it is hoped that the reader will be able to envision the beauty and essence of its art as captured by some of the greatest masters in the world, whether they be painters, sculptors, or photographers. This wide range of artwork adds significantly to an understanding of nursing itself because the history of nursing portrayed by art demonstrates the most valuable aspect of nursing: care and caring. Caring is an essential component of nursing—caring for, caring with, and caring about. The pages of this book, through discussion and artwork, reflect the history of that caring as it has varied according to societal events and needs throughout the ages. No one, however, by pen or canvas, will ever be able to capture entirely the true art and the caring spirit of nursing. Both defy expression.

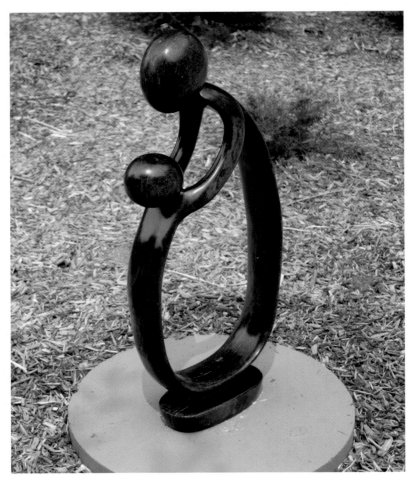

The Daisy Award for Extraordinary Nurses was created by the Daisy Foundation to recognize the superhuman work nurses do every day. Each month, in numerous hospitals and medical facilities around the United States, award recipients are chosen by their nurse administrators, peers, physicians, patients, and families. These nurses receive a unique, hand-carved Shona stone sculpture, entitled *A Healer's Touch*. As of July 2009, over 4500 nurses have received The DAISY Award. The Daisy Foundation purchases the sculptures from Zimbabwe where they are produced. They represent the nganga, or village healer believed to have the power to heal those who are physically ill, suffering misfortune, or spiritually weak. The flowing, connectedness of the sculpture reminds people of the bond of care and trust that exists between healer and patient, unbroken, one flowing into the other in the unique, caring reliance.

A Healer's Touch, sculpture. Photo courtesy of the DAISY Foundation.

Nursing is an art; and if it is to be made an art,
it requires as exclusive a devotion, as hard a preparation,
as any painter's or sculptor's work;
for what is the having to do with dead canvas or cold
marble, compared with having to do with the living
body—the temple of God's spirit?
It is one of the Finest Arts;
I had almost said, the finest of the Fine Arts.

—FLORENCE NIGHTINGALE

List of Plates

LIST OF PLATES

UNIT TEN

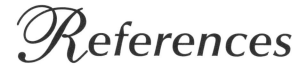

References

UNIT ONE

Alexander, W. (1782). *The history of women from earliest antiquity to the present time.* London: C Dilly.

Berdoe, E. (1893). *The origin and growth of the healing art.* London: Swan, Sonnenschein & Co.

Bhishagratna, K.K.L. (1907). *The sushruta samhita* [The father of surgery]. Calcutta: J.N. Bose.

Davison, W.C. (1943, April). Nursing as the foundation of medicine. *North Carolina Medical Journal,* 4, 141-143.

Dock, L.L. & Stewart, I.M. (1925). *A short history of nursing* (2nd ed.). New York: G.P. Putnam's Sons.

Dolan, J.A., Fitzpatrick, M.L., & Hermann, E.K. (1983). *Nursing in society: A historical perspective* (15th ed.). Philadelphia: W.B. Saunders Co.

Edwards, A.B. (1892). *Pharaohs, fellahs, and explorers.* New York: Harper & Brothers.

Frank, Sister C.M. (1953). *The historical development of nursing.* Philadelphia: W.B. Saunders Co.

Goodnow, M. (1942). *Nursing history.* Philadelphia: W.B. Saunders Co.

Hermann, P. (1954). *Conquest by man.* New York: Harper & Brothers.

Jamieson, E.M. & Sewall, M.F. (1950). *Trends in nursing history.* Philadelphia: W.B. Saunders Co.

Jones, W.H.S. (1909). *Malaria and Greek history.* Manchester: Manchester University Press.

Kaviratna, A.C. (n.d.). *Charaka-Samhita.* [trans.]. Calcutta: J.N. Bose.

Lyons, A.S. (1978). Medicine in Roman times. In A.S. Lyons & R.J. Petrucelli, *Medicine: An illustrated history.* New York: Harry N. Abrams, Inc.

Mason, O.T. (1894). *Woman's share in primitive culture.* New York: D. Appleton & Co.

Nutting, M.A. & Dock, L.L. (1937). *A history of nursing* (vol. 1). New York: G.P. Putnam's Sons.

Reinach, S. (1930). *Orpheus: A history of religions.* New York: Liveright, Inc.

Robinson, V. (1946). *White caps: The story of nursing.* Philadelphia: J.B. Lippincott Co.

Rosen, G. (1958). *A history of public health.* New York: MD Publications, Inc.

Seymer, L.R. (1932). *A general history of nursing.* London: Faber & Faber Ltd.

Stewart, I.M. & Austin, A.L. (1962). *A history of nursing* (5th ed.). New York: G.P. Putnam's Sons.

Shryock, R.H. (1959). *The history of nursing: An interpretation of the social and medical factors involved.* Philadelphia: W.B. Saunders Co.

Stewart, I.M. (1918). How can we help to improve our teaching in nursing schools? *Canadian Nurse,* 22, 1593.

Taylor, H.O. (1922). *Greek biology and medicine.* Boston: Marshall Jones Co.

UNIT TWO

Austin, A.L. (1957). *History of nursing source book.* New York: GP Putnam's Sons.

Butler, A. (1934). *The lives of the saints.* (12 vols.). H. Thurston & A. Attwater (rev. ed.). London: Burns, Oates & Wasbourne, Ltd.

Chesterton, G.K. (1924). *St. Francis of Assisi.* New York: George H Doran Co.

Christy, T.E. (1976). Historical perspectives on accountability. In J.A. Williamson (Ed.), *Current perspectives in nursing education.* St Louis: The CV Mosby Co.

Dock, L.L. & Stewart, I.M. (1925). *A short history of nursing* (2nd ed.). New York: G.P. Putnam's Sons.

Dolan, J.A., Fitzpatrick, M.L., & Hermann, E.K. (1983). *Nursing in society: A historical perspective* (15th ed.). Philadelphia: W.B. Saunders Co.

Donahue, M.P. (2004). Turning points in nursing history. In L. Haynes, T. Boese, & H. Butcher, *Nursing in contemporary society* (pp. 2-34). Upper Saddle River, NJ: Pearson Prentice Hall.

Eckenstein, L. (1896). *Women under monasticism.* Cambridge: Cambridge University Press.

Frank, Sister C.M. (1953). *The historical development of nursing.* Philadelphia: W.B. Saunders Co.

Fuller, J. (1968). *The days of St. Anthony's fire.* New York: Macmillan Publishing Co., Inc.

Garrison, F.H. (1913). *An introduction to the history of medicine.* Philadelphia: W.B. Saunders Co.

Haeser, H. (1857). *Geschichte christlicher krankenpflege und pflegerschaften.* Berlin: Anmerkungen.

Jamieson, E.M. & Sewall, M.F. (1950). *Trends in nursing history.* Philadelphia: W.B. Saunders Co.

Lord, J. (1885). *Beacon lights of history* (vol. 5, *Great women*). New York: Fords, Howard & Hulbert.

Nutting, M.A. & Dock, L.L. (1937). *A history of nursing* (vol. 1). New York: G.P. Putnam's Sons.

Petrucelli, R.J. (1978). Art and science. In A.S. Lyons & R.J. Petrucelli, *Medicine: An illustrated history.* New York: Harry N. Abrams, Inc.

Putnam, E.J. (1921). *The lady.* New York: G.P. Putnam's Sons.

Robinson, V. (1946). *White caps: The story of nursing.* Philadelphia: J.B. Lippincott Co.

Sellew, G. & Nuesse, C. J. (1946). *The history of nursing.* St. Louis: The C.V. Mosby Co.

Shryock, R.H. (1959). *The history of nursing: An interpretation of the social and medical factors involved.* Philadelphia: W.B. Saunders Co.

Stewart, I.M. & Austin, A.L. (1962). *A history of nursing* (5th ed.). New York: G.P. Putnam's Sons.

Tuker, M.A. & Malleson, H. (1900). *Handbook to Christian and Ecclesiastical Rome.* New York: The Macmillan Co.

Walsh, J.J. (1929). *The history of nursing.* New York: P.J. Kennedy & Sons.

UNIT THREE

Cohen, I.B. (1984). Florence Nightingale. *Scientific American,* 250, 128-137.

Cook, E. (1913). *The life of Florence Nightingale* (vols.1-2). London: The Macmillan Co.

Devane, R.S. (1948). *The failure of individualism.* Dublin: Browne & Nolan, Ltd.

Dickens, C. (1910). *Martin Chuzzlewit.* New York: The Macmillan Co.

Dock, L.L. & Stewart, I.M. (1920). *A short history of nursing* (2nd ed.). New York: G.P. Putnam's Sons.

Dolan, J.A., Fitzpatrick, M.L., & Hermann, E.K. (1983). *Nursing in society: A historical perspective* (15th ed.). Philadelphia: W.B. Saunders Co.

Evans, A.D. & Howard, L.G.R. (1930). *The romance of the British voluntary hospital movement.* London: Hutchinson & Co. Ltd.

Frank, Sister C.M. (1953). *The historical development of nursing.* Philadelphia: W.B. Saunders Co.

Goldsmith, M. (1937). *Florence Nightingale: The woman and the legend.* London: Hodder & Stoughton.

Howard, J. (1791). *An account of the principal lazarettos in Europe.* London: Johnson, Dilly & Cadel.

Hunt, L. (1889). *Essays—the monthly nurse.* London: Frederick Warne & Co.

Jamieson, E.M. & Sewall, M.F. (1950). *Trends in nursing history.* Philadelphia: W.B. Saunders Co.

Petrucelli, R.J. (1978). Art and science. In A.S. Lyons & R.J. Petrucelli, *Medicine: An illustrated history.* New York: Harry N. Abrams, Inc.

Martineau, H. (1859). *England and her soldiers.* London: Smith Elder.

Nightingale, F. (1859). *Notes on hospitals.* London: John W. Parker and Sons

Nightingale, F. (1860). *Notes on nursing.* New York: D. Appleton & Co.

Nutting, M.A. & Dock, L.L. (1907). *A history of nursing* (vol. 2). New York: G.P. Putnam's Sons.

Nutting, M.A. & Dock, L.L. (1937). *A history of nursing* (vol. 1). New York: G.P. Putnam's Sons.

On the genius and character of Hogarth, (1818). In *The works of Charles Lamb.* London: Printed for C. and J. Ollier.

Quoted in Dalton, R. (1900, January). Hospitals: Their origin and history. *Dublin Journal of Medical Science,* 109, 17-27.

Robinson, V. (1946). *White caps: The story of nursing.* Philadelphia: J.B. Lippincott Co.

Seacole, M. (1857). *The wonderful adventures of Mrs. Seacole in many lands.* London: James Blackwood Paternoster Row.

Seymer, L.R. (1932). A general history of nursing. London: Faber & Faber Ltd.

Shryock, R.H. (1959). The history of nursing: An interpretation of the social and medical factors involved. Philadelphia: W.B. Saunders Co.

Smith, F.B. (1982). *Florence Nightingale: Reputation and power.* London: Croom Helm.

Strachey, G.L. (1918). Florence Nightingale. In *Eminent Victorians.* London: G.P. Putnam's Sons.

Stewart, I.M. (1939). Florence Nightingale—educator. *Teachers College Record,* 41(3), 208-223.

Whitney, J. (1936). *Elizabeth Fry.* Boston: Brown & Co.

Woodham-Smith, C. (1951). *Florence Nightingale.* New York: McGrawHill Book Co.

UNIT FOUR

American Medical Association, House of Delegates. (1930). *Proceedings of the eighty-first annual session of the House of Delegates* (pp. 35-41). Chicago: American Medical Association.

American Nurses Association. (1941). *The A.N.A. and you.* New York: American Nurses Association.

Andrews, C. (1919). *The fathers of New England: The chronicles of America* (vol. 6). New Haven, CT: Yale University Press.

Ashley, J. (1975). Nursing and early feminism. *American Journal of Nursing,* 75, 1465-1467.

Ashley, J. (1976). *Hospitals, paternalism, and the role of the nurse,* New York: Teachers College Press.

Association of Collegiate Schools of Nursing. (1943). Proceedings of the tenth annual meeting: Association of Collegiate Schools of Nursing.

Brown, E.L. (1948). *Nursing for the future.* New York: Russell Sage Foundation.

Bush, L.P. (1890). Reminiscences of the Philadelphia Hospital and remarks on old time doctors and medicine. *Philadelphia General Hospitals Reports,* 1, 68-77.

Carlisle, R. (1893). *An account of Bellevue Hospital.* New York: Society of Alumni of Bellevue Hospital.

Christy, T.E. (1969a). *Cornerstone for nursing education.* New York: Teachers College Press.

Christy, T.E. (1969b, January). Portrait of a leader: M. Adelaide Nutting. *Nursing Outlook,* 17, 20-24.

Christy, T.E. (1969c, October) Portrait of a leader: Isabel Maitland Stewart, *Nursing Outlook,* 17, 44-48.

Committee on Nursing and Nursing Education in the United States. (1923). *Nursing and nursing education in the United States.* New York: The Macmillan Co.

Committee on the Grading of Nursing Schools. (1928). *Nurses, patients, and pocketbooks.* New York: Committee on the Grading of Nursing Schools.

Dock, L.L. (1901). History of the reform in nursing in Bellevue Hospital. *American Journal of Nursing,* 2(2), 89-98.

Dolan, J.A., Fitzpatrick, M.L., & Hermann, E.K. (1983). Nursing in society: A historical perspective. Philadelphia: W.B. Saunders Co.

Donahue, M.P (1981). Isabel Maitland Stewart's philosophy of education. (Doctoral dissertation, The University of Iowa). *Dissertation Abstracts International,* 42:5, p. 2018A. (University Microfilms No. 8123310).

Donahue, M.P. (2004). Turning points in nursing history. In L. Haynes, T. Boese, & H. Butcher. *Nursing in contemporary society* (pp. 2-34). Upper Saddle River, NJ: Pearson Prentice Hall.

Eason, F. (2004). Licensure. In L. Haynes, T. Boese, & H. Butcher. *Nursing in contemporary society* (pp. 417-434). Upper Saddle River, NJ: Pearson Prentice Hall.

Fitzpatrick, M.L. (1983). *Prologue to professionalism.* Bowie, MD: Robert J Brady Co.

Frank, Sister C.M. (1953). *The historical development of nursing.* Philadelphia: W.B. Saunders Co.

Gibbon, J.M. & Mathewson, M.S. (1947). *Three centuries of Canadian nursing.* Toronto: The Macmillian Co. of Canada Ltd.

Grippando, G.M. (1977). *Nursing perspectives and issues.* Albany: Delmar Publishers, Inc.

Hale, S. (1871). Lady nurses. *Godey's Lady's Book and Magazine,* 82, 188.

Henrietta, Sister (1939). A famous New Orleans hospital. *American Journal of Nursing,* 39(3), 249-256.

Jamieson, E.M. & Sewall, M.F. (1950). *Trends in nursing history.* Philadelphia: W.B. Saunders Co.

John, E. & Pfefferkorn, B. (1934). *An activity analysis of nursing.* New York: New York Committee on the Grading of Nursing Schools.

Kalisch, P.A. & Kalisch B.J. (1995). *The advance of American nursing* (3rd ed.). Philadelphia: J.B. Lippincott Co.

Kansas State Nurses' Association. (1942). *Lamps on the prairie: A history of nursing in Kansas.* Emporia, KS: Emporia Gazette Press.

Kenton, E. (Ed.). (1925). *The Jesuit relations and allied documents (1610-1791).* New York: A & C Boni.

Lyons A.S. (1978). The nineteenth century (the beginnings of modern medicine). In A.S. Lyons & R.J. Petrucelli, *Medicine: An illustrated history,* New York: Harry N Abrams, Inc.

Mollett, W. (1888). On the necessity of legal registration for nurses. *Nursing Record.* London.

Munson, H.W. (1948). Linda Richards. *American Journal of Nursing,* 48(9), 551-555.

Nightingale, F. (1883). Nurses, training of. In R. Quain (Ed), *A dictionary of medicine.* New York: Appleton and Co.

Nutting, M.A. (1905, June). Some results of preparatory courses for nurses. *American Journal of Nursing,* 5, 654.

Nutting, M.A. (1925, October 27-29). In Souvenir programme of the annual convention of the New York State Nurses' Association. Greeting at the New York State League for Nursing. The New York Organization for Public Health Nursing, Albany, NY.

Nutting, M.A. (1926). *A sound economic basis for schools of nursing.* New York: G.P. Putnam's Sons.

Nutting, M.A. & Dock, L.L. (1907). *A history of nursing* (vol. 2). New York: G.P. Putnam's Sons.

Petrucelli, R.J.: *Medicine: An illustrated history.* New York: Harry N. Abrams, Inc.

Proceedings of the American Medical Association. (1869, May). New Orleans. (Reprinted from *Medical News,* 20, 339, 351.)

Rathbone, W. (1890). *History and progress of district nursing.* New York: The Macmillam Co.

Roberts, M.M. (1954). *American nursing: History and interpretation.* New York: The Macmillan Co.

Roberts, M.M. (1956). Lavinia Lloyd Dock: Nurse, feminist, internationalist. *American Journal of Nursing,* 56(2), 176-179.

Robinson, V. (1946). White caps: The story of nursing. Philadelphia: J.B. Lippincott Co.

Shryock, R.H. (1959). The history of nursing: An interpretation of the social and medical factors involved. Philadelphia: W.B. Saunders Co.

Sigerist, H.E. (1934). *American medicine*. New York: W.W. Norton & Co., Inc.

Stewart, I.M. (1921, November). Popular fallacies about nursing education. *The Modern Hospital*, 18, 1-2.

Stewart, I.M. (1943). *The education of nurses*. New York: The Macmillan Co.

Stewart, I.M. (1961). *Reminiscences of Isabel M. Stewart*. New York: Oral History Research Office, Columbia University.

Stewart, I.M. (Undated). Letter from Stewart to Lillian A. Hudson.

Stewart, I.M. & Austin, A.L. (1962) *A history of nursing* (5th ed). New York: GP Putnam's Sons.

Wald, L.D. (1915). *The house on Henry Street*. New York: Henry Holt & Co.

Walsh, J.J. (1929). *The history of nursing*. New York: P.J. Kennedy & Sons.

Woolf, S.J. (1937, March 7). Miss Wald at 70 sees her dreams realized. *The New York Times*, 22.

UNIT FIVE

Alcott, L.M. (1863). *Hospital sketches, camp and fireside stories*, Boston: James Redpath.

Austin, A.L. (1957). *History of nursing source book*. New York: GP Putnam's Sons.

Aynes, E.A. (1973). *From Nightingale to eagle*. Englewood Cliffs, NJ: Prentice-Hall, Inc.

Baker, N.B. (1952). *Cyclone in calico: The story of Mary Ann Bickerdyke*. Boston: Little, Brown & Co.

Bamford, J. (1983). *Puzzle palace: AA report on America's most secret agency*. New York, New York: Penguin Group (USA) Incorporated.

Bamford, J. (2005). Pretext for war: 9/11, Iraq, and the abuse of America's intelligence agencies. New York, New York: Random House.

Beeber, L.S. (1990). To be one of the boys: Aftershocks of the World War I nursing experience. *Advances in Nursing Science*, 12(4), 32-43.

Blair, A.H. (1992). *At war in the gulf*. College Station, TX: Texas A&M University Press.

Boardman, M.T. (1915). *Under the Red Cross flag at home and abroad*. Philadelphia: JB Lippincott Co.

Bodansky, Y. (2004). *The secret history of the Iraq War*. New York, New York: Harper Collins Publishers.

Bradford, S. (1961). *Harriet Tubman: The Moses of her people*. New York: Corinth Books.

Christy, T.E. (1970). Portrait of a leader: Annie Warburton Goodrich. *Nursing Outlook*, 18(8), 46-50.

Chow, R.K., Hope, G.S., Nelson, E.A., Sokoloski, J.L, & Wilson, R.A. (1978). Historical perspectives of the U.S. Air Force, Army, Navy, Public Health Service, and Veterans Administration Nursing Services, *Military Medicine*, 143(7), 457-463.

David, P. (1991). *Triumph in the desert: The challenge, the fight, the legacy*. NewYork: Random House.

Davis, M.B. (1886). *The woman who battled for the boys in blue—Mother Bickerdyke*. San Francisco: Pacific Press Publishing House.

Donahue, M.P. (1995, Spring). An introduction: Faintly heard and little noted. *Caduceus*, 11(1), 3-10.

Dreves, K.D. (1975). Nurses in American history: Vassar Training Camp for nurses. *American Journal of Nursing*, 75(11), 2000-2002.

Fischer, J. & Stone, R. (1986). *Images of war*. Boston, 1990, Boston: Boston Publishing Company.

Flikke, J.O. (1943). *Nurses in action: The story of the Army Nurse Corps*. Philadelphia: J.B. Lippincott.

Frank, Sister C.M. (1953). *The historical development of nursing*. Philadelphia: W.B. Saunders Co.

Freedman, D. & Rhoads, J. (Eds.). (1987). *Nurses in Vietnam: The forgotten veterans*. Austin, TX: Texas Monthly Press.

Goodnow, M. (1942). *Nursing history*, Philadelphia: W.B. Saunders Co.

Goodrich, A.W. (1932). The school of nursing and the future, Proceedings of the thirty-eighth annual convention of the National League of Nursing Education. New York: National Headquarters.

Goostray, S. (1954). Isabel Maitland Stewart, *American Journal of Nursing*, 54(3), 302-306.

Hardaway, R.M.(1988). *Care of the wounded in Vietnam*. Manhattan, KS: Sunflower University Press.

Hine, D.C. (Ed.). (1985). *Black women in the nursing profession: A documentary history*, New York: Garland Publishers.

Hiro, D. (1992). *Desert shield to desert storm*. New York: Routledge.

Holm, J.M. & Wells, S.P. (1993, November). Air Force women in the Vietnam War. In *Celebration of patriotism and courage: Dedication of the Vietnam Women's Memorial*. Washington, DC: Vietnam Women's Memorial Project.

Joint Committee on Nursing in National Security. (1951). Mobilization of nurses for national security. *American Journal of Nursing*, 51(2), 78-79.

Judson, H. (1941). *Edith Cavell*. New York: The Macmillan Co.

Kalisch, P.A. & Kalisch, B.J. (1978). *The advance of American nursing* (3rd ed.). Philadelphia: J.B. Lippincott Company.

Kalisch, P.A. & Kalisch, B.J. (1987). *The changing image of the nurse*. Menlo Park, CA: Addison-Wesley Publishing Company.

Kalisch, P.A. & Kalisch, B.J. (1995). *The advance of American nursing* (3rd ed.). Philadelphia: J.B. Lippincott Company.

Kalisch, P.A. & Scobey, M. (1983, Winter). Female Nurses in American wars: Helplessness suspended for the duration. *Armed Forces and Society*, 215-255.

Lippard, L.R. (1990). *A different war*. Seattle, WA: The Real Comet Press.

Lippmann, W. (1944, December, 19). American women and our wounded men, *Washington Post*. Reprinted in the *Congressional Record* as an extension of the remarks of Hon. Edith Nourse Rogers.

Murray, W. & Scales, R.H. (2005). *The Iraq war: An elusive victory*. Cambridge, Massachusetts: Harvard University Press.

Norman, E.M. (1990). *Women at war: The story of fifty military nurses who served in Vietnam*. Philadelphia: University of Pennsylvania Press.

Pilcher, J.E. (1907). The Red Cross. *Military Surgery*, 20, 230.

Proceedings of the eighteenth annual convention of the American Society of Superintendents of Training Schools for Nursing (1912), New York: The Society.

Roberts, M.M. (1954). *American nursing: History and interpretation*. New York: The Macmillan Co.

Robinson, V. (1946). *White caps: The story of nursing*. Philadelphia: J.B. Lippincott Co.

Shields, E.A. (Ed.). (1981). *Highlights in the history of the Army Nurse Corps*. Washington, DC: U.S. Army Center of Military History.

Spelts, D. (1986). Nurses who served—and who did not return. *American Journal of Nursing*, 86(9), 1037-1039.

Stewart, I.M. (1943). *The education of nurses*. New York: The Macmillan Co.

Taft, W.H. (1917, September). A distinct call to women. *Ladies Home Journal*, 34, 5.

U.S. Council of National Defense: First annual report of the Council of National Defense [fiscal year 1917]. Washington, DC: U.S. Government Printing Office.

Vietnam Veterans' Association (1984, October). Women vets profiled in new VA study, *Veteran*, 5.

Vreeland, E.M. (1950). Fifty years of nursing in the federal government nursing services. *American Journal of Nursing* (anniversary issue), 50(10), 626-631.

Walsh, J. & Aulich, J. (Eds.) (1989). *Vietnam images: War and representation*. Houndmills, Basingstoke, Hampshire, England: Macmillam Press Ltd.

Whitman, W. (1961). *Leaves of grass* [selections]. New York: Crown Publishers.

UNIT SIX

American Nurses Association. (1965). First position paper on education for nurses, *American Journal of Nursing*, 65(12), 106-107.

American Nurses Association. (1980). *Nursing: A social policy statement*. Kansas City, MO: American Nurses Association.

American Nurses Association. (1988). *Nursing case management*. Kansas City, MO: American Nurses Association.

Bower, K. (1988). Managed care: Controlling costs, guaranteeing outcomes, *Definition*, 3, 14.

Buchan, J. (1993). The same but different. *Nursing Standard*, 7, 21.

Bulger, R.J. (1988). *Technology, bureaucracy, and healing in America: A postmodern paradigm*. Iowa City: The University of Iowa Press.

Bullough,V.L. & Bullough, B. (1984). *History, trends, and politics of nursing*, Norwalk, CT: Appleton-Century-Crofts.

Dennison, C. (1942). Nursing service in the emergency room. *American Journal of Nursing*, 42(7), 774-784.

Dock, L.L. (1901). Letters to the editor. *American Journal of Nursing*, 2(3), 231-232.

Duffield. C. (1988). Nursing in the 1980s and 1990s: A challenge for managers. *International Journal of Nursing Studies*, 25(2), 125-134.

Fitzpatrick, M.L. (1983). *Prologue to professionalism*. Bowie, MD: Robert J Brady Co.

Grace, H.K. (1978). The development of doctoral education in nursing: A historical perspective. In N.L. Chaska (Ed.), *The nursing profession: Views through the mist*, New York: McGraw-Hill Book Co.

Haldeman, J.C. & Abdellah, F.G. (1959, May). Concepts of progressive patient care. *Hospitals*, 33(10), 38-42.

Hall, L. (1963). A center for nursing. *Nursing Outlook*, 11, 805-806.

Harris, N. (2006). *Alice Magaw: The mother of anesthesia*. Unpublished doctoral dissertation, The University of Iowa, Iowa City, IA.

Henderson, V. (1966). *The nature of nursing*. New York: Macmillan Publishing Co., Inc.

Himali, U. (1995). More than 25,000 RNs march on Washington, issuing a wake-up call to consumers and lawmakers. *The American Nurse*, 27(1), 20-21.

Kalisch, P.A. & Kalisch, B.J. (1978). *The advance of American nursing*. Boston: Little, Brown & Co.

Kalisch, P.A. & Kalisch, B.J. (2004). *American Nursing. A history* (4th ed.). Philadelphia: Lippincott Williams & Wilkins, A Wolters Kluwer Company.

Krampitz, S.D. (1981). Clinical specialization: Historical antecedents of today's issues. In J.C. McCloskey & H.K. Grace, *Current issues in nursing*. Boston: Blackwell Scientific Publications, Inc.

Lambertsen, E.C. (1953). *Nursing team organization and functioning*. New York: Teachers College, Columbia University.

Magaw, A. (1899, May 15). Observations in anesthesia. *Northwestern Lancet*. 19, 207-210.

Magaw, A. (1900). Observations on 1092 cases of anesthesia from Jan.1, 1899 to Jan. 1, 1900. *The St. Paul Medical Journal* 2, 306-311.

Magaw, A. (1901). A report of 245 cases of anesthesia by nitrous oxide gas and ether. *The St. Paul Medical Journal*. 3(4), 231-233.

Magaw, A. (1904). Observations drawn from an experience of eleven thousand anesthesias. *Transactions of the Minnesota State Medical Association, (36th annual meeting)*, 91-102.

Magaw, A. (1906, December). A review of over fourteen thousand surgical anaesthesias. *Surgery, Gynecology and Obstetrics*, 3(6), 795-799.

Manthey, M., Ciske, K., Robertson, P., & Harris, I. (1970). Primary nursing: A return to the concept of "my nurse" and "my patient." *Nursing Forum*, 9(1), 65-84.

Marram, G., Barrett, M. & Bevis, E. (1979). *Primary nursing: A model for individualized care* (2nd ed.). St. Louis: The C.V. Mosby Co.

McCrary, L. (1995, March 31). Nurses to protest in D.C., saying job cuts erode care. *The Philadelphia Inquirer*, pp. A1, A20.

McManus, R.L. (1962). Isabel M. Stewart—Foremost researcher. *Nursing Research*, 11(4), 6.

Metarazzo, J.D. & Abdellah, F.G. (1971). Doctoral education for nurses in the United States. *Nursing Research*, 20, 404-414.

Newton, M.E. (1949). *Florence Nightingale's philosophy of life and education*. Unpublished dissertation, Leland Stanford Junior University.

Nightingale, F. (1860). *Notes on nursing*, New York: D Appleton & Co.

Reeder, S.J. (1978). The social context of nursing. In N.L. Chaska (Ed.), *The nursing profession: Views through the mist*. New York: McGraw-Hill Book Co.

Rogers, M.E. (1970). *An introduction to the theoretical basis of nursing*. Philadelphia: F.A. Davis Co.

Rosenberg, C.E. (1987). *The care of strangers*. New York: Basic Books, Inc.

Smith, G.R. (1975). From invisibility to blackness: The story of the National Black Nurses' Association. *Nursing Outlook*, 23, 225-229.

Stewart, I.M. (1929): The science and art of nursing [editorial]. *Nursing Education Bulletin*, 2, 1.

Stewart, I.M. (1943). *The education of nurses*. New York: The Macmillan Co.

Stevens, R. (1989). *In sickness and in wealth: American hospitals in the twentieth century*. New York: Basic Books.

Streef, M.B. (1994). Third-party reimbursement issues for advanced practice nurses in the '90s. In J. McCloskey & H.K. Grace (Eds.), *Current issues in nursing* (4th ed., pp. 437-449). St. Louis: Mosby.

Styles, M.M. (1977). Doctoral education in nursing: The current situation in historical perspective. In *National Conference on Doctoral Education in Nursing*. Philadelphia: University of Pennsylvania.

Styles, M.M. (1993). Macrotrends in nursing practice: What's in the pipeline? *Journal of Continuing Education in Nursing*, 24(1), 7-12.

Whitehead, A.N. (1929). *The aims of education and other essays*. New York: The Macmillan Co.

Zander, K. (1994). Nurses and case management. To control or to collaborate? In J. McCloskey & H.K. Grace (Eds.), *Current issues in nursing* (4th ed., pp. 254-260). St Louis: Mosby.

UNIT SEVEN

Aiken, L.H., Clarke, S.P., Cheung, R.B., Sloane, D.M., & Silber, J.H. (2003). Education levels of hospital nurses and patient mortality. *Journal of the American Medical Association*, 290, 1617-1623.

Aiken, L.H., Clarke, S.P., Sloane, D.M., Sochalski, J., & Silber, J.H. (2002). Hospital nurse staffing and patient mortality, nurse burnout, and job dissatisfaction. *Journal of the American Medical Association*, 288(16), 1987-1993.

American Association of Colleges of Nursing. (2004, October). AACN position statement on the practice doctorate in nursing. Available at www.aacn.nche.edu/DNP/pdf/DNP.pdf.

American Association of Colleges of Nursing. (2007, February). White Paper on the Education and Role of the Clinical Nurse Leader. Available at www.aacn.nche.edu/Publications/WhitePapers/CNL2-07.pdf.

American Association of Colleges of Nursing. (2009, April). The doctor of nursing practice. *Fact Sheet*. Available at www.aacn.nche.edu/Media/FactSheets/dnp.htm.

American Nurses Association. (1987). *The nursing center: Concept and design*. Kansas City, MO: American Nurses Association.

American Nurses Credentialing Center. (2003). *Magnet Nursing Recognition Program for Excellence in Nursing Service—Acute Care*. Washington, DC: American Nurses Credentialing Center.

Balas, E.A. & Boren, S.A. (2000). Managing clinical knowledge for healthcare improvements. In International Medical Informatics Association. *Yearbook of medical informatics* (pp. 65-70). Stuttgart, Germany: Schattauer Publishing Company.

Barnard, K. (1982). The research cycle: Nursing, the profession, the discipline. In *Communicating nursing research* (vol. 15, *Nursing science in perspective*). Boulder, CO: Western Interstate Commission for Higher Education.

Bliss-Holtz, J. (2007). Evidence-based practice: A primer for action. *Issues in Comprehensive Pediatric Nursing*, 30, 165-182.

Bulechek, G.M. & McCloskey, J. (1994). Nursing interventions classification (NIC). Defining nursing care. In J. McCloskey & H.K. Grace (Eds.), *Current issues in nursing* (4th ed., pp. 129-135). St. Louis: Mosby.

Bullough, B. (1992). Alternative models for specialty nursing practice, *Nursing and Health Care*, 13, 254-259.

Bullough, B. & Bullough, V.L. (Eds.). (1994). *Nursing issues for the nineties and beyond*. New York: Springer Publishing Company.

Bullough, V.L. & Bullough, B. (1984). *History, trends, and politics of nursing*, Norwalk, CT: Appleton-Century-Crofts.

Congress overrides veto, nursing gets center for research. (January, 1986). *The American Nurse*, 1, 24.

Dick, R.S. & Stein, E.B. (Eds.) (1991). *The computer-based patient record: An essential technology for health care*. Washington, DC: National Academy Press.

Donahue, M.P. (2004). Turning points in nursing history. In L. Haynes, T. Boese, & H. Butcher, *Nursing in contemporary society* (pp. 2-34). Upper Saddle River, NJ: Pearson Prentice Hall.

Evers, G.C.M. (2001). Naming nursing: Evidence-based nursing. *Nursing Diagnoses* 12(4), 137-142.

Felton, G. (1989). Nursing: A profession to celebrate. *Journal of Professional Nursing*, 5(5), 273-278.

Ford, L.C. (1992). Advanced nursing practice: Future of the nurse practitioner. In L. Aiken & C. Fagin (Eds.), *Charting nursing's future agenda for the 1990s* (pp. 287-297). Philadelphia: J.B. Lippincott Company.

Glass, L.K. (1989). The historic origins of nursing centers. In A. Arvonio (Ed.), *Nursing Centers: Meeting the demand for quality health care* (NLN Pub. No. 21-2311). New York: National League for Nursing.

Goodman, K.W. (2003). *Foundations and history of evidence-based practice in ethics and evidence-based medicine: Fallibility and responsibility in clinical science.* Cambridge: Cambridge University Press.

Hathaway, D., Stegbauer, C., & Graff, C. (2006). The practice doctorate: Perspectives of early adopters. *The Journal of Nursing Education, 45*(12), 487-496.

Havinghurst, C. (1986). The changing locus of decision making in the health care sector. *Journal of Health Politics, Policy and Law, 11*(4), 697-735.

Hayes, E. (1985). The nurse practitioner: History, current conflicts, and future survival. *Journal of Community Health, 34,* 144-147.

Henderson, V. (1960). *Basic principles of nursing.* Geneva: International Council of Nurses.

Horn, B.J. & Swain, M.A. (1978). *Criterion measures of nursing care.* Hyattsville, MD: National Center for Health Services Research. (DHEW Pub. No. HS78-3187.)

International Council of Nurses. (2002, October). Press Release. ICN Announces Position on Advanced Nursing Roles. Retrieved August 22, 2009 from www.icn.ch/PR19_02.htm.

International Council of Nurses. (2008). Press release. Collaborative partnership formed to improve the health of health care workers. Retrieved April 2, 2009, from www.icn.ch/PR21_08.htm.

Johnson & Johnson. (2002). The campaign for nursing's future. Retrieved December 8, 2008 from www.nightingaledeclaration.net/news/jj.

Johnson, M. & Maas, M. (1994). Nursing-focused patient outcomes. Challenge for the nineties. In J. McCloskey & H.K. Grace (Eds.), *Current issues in nursing* (4th ed., pp. 136-142). St. Louis: Mosby.

Kalisch, B., Begeny, S., & Neumann, S. (2007). The image of the nurse on the Internet. *Nursing Outlook, 55,* 182-188.

Kim, M. (2000, November). *Evidence-based nursing* [chart]. Available at http://findarticles.com/p/articles/mi_qa3932/is_200011/ai_n8905921/pg_5/?tag=content;col1.

Kurzweil, R. (2005*). The singularity is near: When humans transcend biology.* New York: Penguin Group.

Lindeman, C.A. (1989). Choices within challenges. *Communicating Nursing Research 22*(1), 3.

Lundeen, S.P. (1994). Community nursing centers. Implications for health care reform. In J. McCloskey & H.K. Grace (Eds.), *Current issues in nursing* (4th ed., pp. 382-387). St. Louis: Mosby.

Lundeen, S.P (1993). Comprehensive, collaborative, coordinated, community based care: A community nursing center model. *Family and Community Health, 16,* 57-62.

McCloskey & H.K. Grace (Eds.). *Current issues in nursing* (4th ed.). St. Louis: Mosby.

McCormick, K.A. & Jones, C.J. (1998, September). Is one taxonomy needed for health care vocabularies and classifications? *The Online Journal of Issues in Nursing.* 3(2).

Miller, M. (2009). *The tyranny of dead ideas.* New York: Henry Holt and Company.

Moore, G.E. (2003). No angels here. The closing of the Pine Street Inn Nurses Clinic, 1972-2003. In S. Sered, *Symposium on religious healing in Boston: Body, spirit, community* (pp. 35-38). Cambridge, MA: Harvard Divinity School.

National League for Nursing. (1985, December 5). Legislative update, *The League,* 1.

National Nursing Center Consortium. (2009). *Nurse-managed health centers are changing the face of health care.* Retrieved April 1, 2009 from http://nncc.us.

Patterson, C. & Haddad, B. (1992). The advanced nurse practitioner common attributes. *Canadian Journal of Nursing Administration, 5*(4), 18-22.

Rogers, M. (1975). Nursing is coming of age…through the practitioner movement. *American Journal of Nursing, 75*(10), 1834-1843.

Sackett, D.L., Rosenberg, W.M.C., Gray, J.A.M., Haynes, R.B., & Richardson, W.S. (1996). Evidence-based medicine: What it is and what it isn't. *British Medical Journal, 312*(7023), 71-72.

Schober, J. (2004). Global perspective on advanced practice. In L.A. Joel (Ed.), *Advanced practice nursing: Essentials for role development,* (pp. 73-96). Philadelphia: F.A. Davis Co.

Sered, S., ed. (2003*). Religious healing in Boston: Body, spirit, community.* Cambridge: Center for the Study of World Religions.

Sered, S., ed. (2004). *Religious healing in Boston: Body, spirit, community.* Cambridge: Center for the Study of World Religions.

Simms, L.M. (1991). The professional practice of nursing administration, *Journal of Nursing Administration, 21*(5), 37-46.

Sowell, R.L. & Meadows, T.M. (1994). An integrated case management model: Developing standards, evaluation, and outcome criteria. *Nursing Administration Quarterly, 18*(2), 53-64.

Stanley, D.J. (2008). Celluloid angels: a research study of nurses in feature films 1900-2007. *Journal of Advanced Nursing.* 64(1), 84-95.

Stewart, I.M. (1943). *The education of nurses.* New York: The Macmillan Company.

Styles, M.M. (1992). Specialization and credentialing. In L. Aiken & C. Fagin: *Charting nursing's future agenda for the 1990s* (pp. 29-39). Philadelphia: J.B. Lippincott Company.

Sussman, D. (2000, October 23). Image overhaul. Media still are off-target portraying nurses. *NurseWeek.* Available at http://www.nurseweek.com/news/features/00-10/tv.asp.

Thede, L.Q. (2006). *ANA recognized standardized terminologies for use in computerizing nursing documentation.* Retrieved May 5, 2009 from http://dlthede.net/Informatics/Chap13/RecognizedDatasets.html.

Toffler, A. & Toffler, H. (1970). *Future shock.* New York: Random House.

Toffler, A. & Toffler, H. (1980). *The third wave.* New York: Morrow.

Toffler, A. & Toffler, H. (1995). *Creating a new civilization. Politics of the third wave.* Atlanta: Turner Publishing, Inc.

Warren, J.J. (1994). Nursing diagnosis taxonomy development. Overview and issues. In J. McCloskey & H.K. Grace (Eds.), *Current issues in nursing* (4th ed., pp. 122-128). St. Louis: Mosby.

Werley, H., Zorn, C.R., & Devine, E.C. (1994). Why the nursing minimum data set (NMDS)? In H. Werley & N.M. Lang (Eds.). (1988). *Identification of the nursing minimum data set.* New York: Springer.

Youso, K. (2009, February 21). Approaching singularity. *The Minneapolis Star Tribune,* pp. E1, E3.

UNIT EIGHT

Allen, I.E. & Seaman, J. (2006). *Making the grade: Online education in the United States.* Needham, MA: Sloan-C™.

American Holistic Nurses Association. (2007). *Holistic nursing: Scope and standards of practice.* Silver Spring, MD: Nursebooks.org: The Publishing Program of ANA.

American Nurses Association. (2008). *Nursing informatics: Scope and standards of practice.* Silver Spring, MD: American Nurses Publishing.

Carnegie, M.E. (1986). *The path we tread: Blacks in nursing, 1854-1984.* Philadelphia: J. B. Lippincot.

Center for Spirituality and Healing. (2009). Retrieved May 13, 2009 at www.csh.umn.edu/about/home.html

Cooper, J.B. & Taqueti, V.R. (2004). A brief history of the development of mannequin simulators for clinical education and training. *Quality and Safety in Health Care.* 13, 11-18.

Decker, S., Sportsman, S., Puetz, L., & Billings, L. (2008). The evolution of simulation and its contribution to competence. *The Journal of Continuing Education in Nursing, 39*(2), 74-80.

Donahue, M.P. (1996). *Nursing: The finest art: An illustrated history* (2nd ed.). St. Louis: Mosby.

Donahue, M.P. (2004). Turning points in nursing history. In L. Haynes, T. Boese, & H. Butcher, *Nursing in contemporary society* (pp. 2-34). Upper Saddle River, NJ: Pearson Prentice Hall.

Dossey, B.M., Keegan, L., Guzzetta, C.E., & Kolkmeier, L.G. (Eds.). (1995). *Holistic nursing: A handbook for practice* (2nd ed.), Gaithersburg, MD: Aspen.

Farella, C. (2001, March 19). Frustration, perspiration, and innovation: Nurse-inventors create in the name of patient care. *Nurseweek.*

Gaba, D.M. (2004). The future vision of simulation in health care. *Quality and Safety in Health Care,* 12, 2-10.

Gadow, S. (1977, March). *Humanistic issues at the interface of nursing and the community*. Unpublished manuscript presented at the Conference of Humanists and Nursing. Hartford, CT.

Goodrich, A.W. (1932). *The social and ethical significance of nursing*. New York: The Maxmillan Company.

Graves, J.R. & Corcoran S. (1989). The study of nursing informatics. *Image: The Journal of Nursing Scholarship*, 21(4), 227-231.

Greene, L.J., Saunders, G.A., & Wilson, J. (2005). *Clinical documentation panel: HIMSS Nursing Informatics*, HIMSS. Retrieved from www.HIMSS.org/content/files/2005proceedings/nursing004.pdf.

Hamilton, D. (1994). Constructing the mind of nursing. *Nursing History Review, 2*, 3-28.

Heller, B., Romano C., Moray I., & Gassert, C. (1989). The implementation of the first graduate program in nursing informatics. *Computers in Nursing*, 7(5), 209-213.

Herrmann, E. (1981). Mrs. Chase: A noble and enduring figure. *American Journal of Nursing*, 81(10), 1836.

Herrmann, E.K. (2000, March-May). Connecticut nursing history vignettes. *Connecticut Nursing News*. Available at http://findarticles.com/p/articles/mi_qa3902/is_200003/ai_n8887739/?tag=content;col1.

Institute of Medicine, Committee on Quality of Health Care in America. (2000). *To err is human: Building a safer health system*. Washington, DC: National Academy Press.

International Council of Nurses. (2004). *Guidelines on the nurse entre/intrapreneur providing nursing service*. Geneva, Switzerland: International Council of Nurses.

Internet Trends. (2009, April-May). Retrieved May 14, 2009 from www.internettrends.org.

Johnson, V.Y. & Walsh, E.G. (2005). Nurses making a difference: the process of technology transfer. *Journal of Neuroscience Nursing*, 37(5), 279-282.

Kalisch, P.A. & Kalisch, B.J. (1982). *The politics of nursing*. Philadelphia: J.B. Lippincott Company.

Kingma, M. (1998). Marketing and nursing in a competitive environment. *International Nursing Review*, 45(2), 45-50.

Koerner, J.G. (2007). *Healing presence: The essence of nursing*. New York: Springer Publishing Co.

Lasseter, F. (1999). A nursing legacy—political activities at the turn of the century. *Association of periOerative Registered Nurses Journal*, 70(5), 902.

Lesse, S. (1981). *The future of the health sciences*. New York: Irvington.

Lewenson, S.B. (1998). Historical overview: Policy, politics, and nursing. In D.J. Mason & J.K. Leavitt (Eds.). *Policy and politics in nursing and health care* (3rd ed.). Philadelphia: W.B. Saunders Co.

Lewenson, S.B. (2002). Pride in our past: Nursing's political roots. In D.J. Mason, J.K. Leavitt, & M.W. Chaffee (Eds), *Policy and politics in nursing and health care* (4th ed.). St. Louis: Elsevier Health Sciences.

Mason, D.J. (1990). Nursing and politics: A profession comes of age. *Orthopaedic Nursing*, 9(5), 11-17.

McBride, A.B. (2006). Informatics and the future of nursing practice. In C.A. Weaver, C.W. Delaney, P. Weber, & R.L. Carr, *Nursing and informatics for the 21st century* (pp. 5-12). Chicago: Healthcare Information and Management Systems Society.

McCormick, K.A. & Jones, C.J. (1998, September 30). Is one taxonomy needed for health care vocabularies and classifications? *The Online Journal of Issues in Nursing*, 3(2).

Metier, R. (2005, November). Sophisticated apparel: A collection by nurse inventors. Presentation at Sigma Theta Tau International Convention, Atlanta, GA.

Mikhailov, A.I., Chernyl, A.I., & Gilyarevskii, R.S. (1967). Informatics—new name for the theory of scientific information. *FID News Bull.*, 17(2), 70-74. In M. Forman (2002), *Informatics*. (Informatics Research Report EDI-INF-RR-0139). Division of Informatics. Retrieved May 17, 2009 from www.informatics.ed.ac.uk.

Naisbitt, J., Naisbitt, N., & Philips, D. (1999). *High tech/high touch: Technology and our search for meaning*. New York: Broadway Books.

National Institutes of Health National Center for Research Resources. (2006). *Electronic health records overview*. McLean, Virginia: The MITRE Corporation.

Nightingale, F. (1863). *Notes on hospitals* (3rd ed., enlarged and for the most part rewritten) (pp. 175-176). London: Longman, Green, Longman, Roberts, & Green.

Ozbolt, J.G. & Saba, V.K. (2008, September/October). A brief history of nursing informatics in the United States of America. *Nursing Outlook*, 56(5), 199-205.

Peteani, L. (2004). Enhancing clinical practice and education with high-fidelity human patient simulators. *Nurse Educator*, 29(1), 24-30.

Riesch, S. (1992). Nursing centres: An analysis of the anecdotal literature. *Journal of Professional Nursing* 8(1), 16-25.

Robson, B. (1993). Independence in nursing: Reclaiming the past. *AARN Newsletter*, 49(9), 25-27.

Saba, V.K. (2001). Nursing informatics: yesterday, today and tomorrow. *International Nursing Review, 48*, 177-187.

Sandelowski, M. (2000). *Devices & desires: Gender, technology, and American nursing*. Chapel Hill, NC: The University of North Carolina Press.

Scholes, M., Bryant, Y., & Barber B. (Eds.). (1983). *The impact of computers in nursing: An International Review*. Amsterdam, The Netherlands: Elsevier Science.

Weaver, C.A., Delaney, C.W., Weber, P., & Carr, R.L. (2006). *Nursing and informatics for the 21st century: An international look at practice, trends and the future*. Chicago: Healthcare Information and Management Systems Society.

Zielstoff, R.D. (Ed.). (1980). *Computers in nursing*. Rockville, MD: Aspen Systems.

Zytkowski, M.E. (2003). Nursing informatics. The key to unlocking contemporary nursing practice. *AACN Critical Issue, 14*(3), 271-281.

UNIT NINE

Anderson, G., Read, C.V., & Monsen, R. (2000). Genetics, nursing, and public policy: Setting an international agenda. *Policy, Politics, and Nursing Practice*, 1(4), 245-255.

Andrews, M.M. (1988). Education preparation for international nursing. *Journal of Professional Nursing*, 4, 430-435.

Aroskar, M.A. (1987). The interface of ethics and politics in nursing, *Nursing Outlook*, 35(6), 268.

Buchan, J. (1993). The same but different. *Nursing Standard*, 7, 21.

Buchan, J. & Calman, L. (2005). *Summary. The global shortage of registered nurses*. Geneva, Switzerland: International Council of Nurses. Retrieved June 29, 2009 from www.icn.ch/global/summary.pdf.

Crigger, N.J. (2008). Towards a viable and just global nursing ethics. *Nursing Ethics*, 15(1), 17-27.

Donahue, M.P. (1978). The nurse: A patient advocate? *Nursing Forum*, 17(2), 143-151.

Donahue, M.P. (1985). Advocacy. In G.M. Bulechek & J.C. McCloskey (Eds.), *Nursing interventions: Treatments for nursing diagnoses* (pp. 338-351). Philadelphia: W.B. Saunders Company.

Ebersole, P.R. (2006, November-December). NCGNP pioneers. *Geriatric Nursing, 27*(6), 343-344.

ESTIA-Net. (2003). *ESTIA-Net Partner Details*. Retrieved June 19, 2009 from www.estiatn.net/year1/partnerdetails.php?code=FI1.

Feder, D. (2008, March 5). Demographic Winter. *MercatorNet*. Retrieved June 15, 2009 from www.mercatornet.com/articles/demographic_winter.

Federal Emergency Management Agency. (2009). *Annual major disaster declarations total*. Retrieved June 15, 2009 from www.fema.gov/news/disaster_totals_annual.fema.

Fenton, M.V. (1994). Development of models of international exchange to upgrade nursing education. In J. McCloskey & H.K. Grace (Eds.), *Current issues in nursing* (4th ed., pp. 202-206). St. Louis: Mosby.

Ferguson, M. (1980). *The Aquarian conspiracy*. Los Angeles and New York: J.P. Tarcher, Inc. & St. Martin's Press.

Greco, K.E. & Mahon, S.M. (2003). Genetics nursing practice enters a new era with credentialing. *Internet Journal of Advanced Nursing Practice*, 5(2), 1-23.

Holloran, C.A. (1994). What are the ethical issues from a worldwide viewpoint? In J. McCloskey & H.K. Grace (Eds.), *Current Issues in Nursing* (4th ed., pp. 763-770). St. Louis: Mosby.

Human Genome Program (2008). *Human Genome Project information*. Retrieved June 14, 2009 from www.ornl.gov/sci/techresources/Human_Genome/home.shtml.

International Council of Nurses. (2001). *Ethical nurse recruitment.* Retrieved June 14, 2009 from http://www.icn.ch/psrecruit01.htm.

International Council of Nurses. (2001) *Nurses and disaster preparedness.* Retrieved June 15, 2009 from www.icn.ch/PS_A11_NursesDisaster-Prep.pdf.

International Council of Nurses. (2003). *International nurse mobility: Trends and policy implications.* Retrieved June 14, 2009 from http://www.icn.ch/Int_Nurse_mobility%20final.pdf.

International Council of Nurses. (2009). ICN Congress results: ICN to look different in the future [press release]. Available at www.icn.ch/PR19_01.htm.

International Council of Nurses (nd). *Genetics and nursing fact sheet.* Retrieved July 22, 2009 from www.icn.ch/matters_genetics.htm.

Johnson, S. (2006). *The ghost map: The story of London's most terrifying epidemic—and how it changed science, cities, and the modern world.* New York: Riverhead Books.

Lindquist, G.J. (1984). A cross-cultural experience: Comparative study in nursing and health care. *Journal of Nursing Education,* 23, 212-214.

Lindquist, G.J. (1990). Integration of international and transcultural content in nursing curricula: A process for change. *Journal of Professional Nursing,* 6(5), 272-279.

Longman, P. (2004). *The empty cradle: How falling birthrates threaten world prosperity and what to do about it.* New York: The Perseus Books Group.

Maglacas, A.M. (1988). Health for all: Nursing's role. *Nursing Outlook,* 36, 66-71.

Maglacas, A.M. (1989). Close encounters in international nursing: Impact on health policy and research. *Journal of Professional Nursing,* 5(6), 304-314.

Marek, K.D. & Rantz, M.J. (2000). Aging in place: A new model for long-term care. *Nursing Administration,* 24(3), 1-11.

May, K.A. & Meleis, A.I. (1987). International nursing: Guidelines for core content. *Nurse Educator,* 12(5), 36-40.

Newmann, M.E. (2008). *Transforming presence: The difference that nursing makes.* Philadephia: F.A. Davis Company.

Olson, V.M. & Styles, M.M. (1994). International nursing. The role of the International Council of Nurses and the World Health Organization. In J. McCloskey & H.K. Grace (Eds.), *Current issues in nursing* (4th ed., pp. 407-415). St. Louis: Mosby.

Rapp, M.P. (2006, November, 27). Should the Gerontological Nurse Practitioner exam be offered as a certificate of added qualifications? *Geriatric Nursing,* 6, 344-345.

Redfield, J. (1993). *The celestine prophecy.* New York: Warner Books.

Salmon, M., Talashek, M., & Tichy, A. (1988). Health for all: A transnational model for nursing. *International Nursing Review,* 35(4), 107-109.

Styles, M.M. (1993). Macrotrends in nursing practice: What's in the pipeline? *Journal of Continuing Education in Nursing,* 24 (1), 7-12.

American Nurses Association. (1991, April). ANA starts center for international nursing. *The American Nurse,* 23, 5.

United Nations Chronicle. (1992).

University of Alabama School of Nursing. (2009). W.H.O. Collaborating Center. Retrieved June 14, 2009 from http://main.uab.edu/Sites/nursing/IntPrograms/WhoCenter.

University of Ulster. (1997, November). *Teaching nurses to cope with disaster* [news release]. Available at http://news.ulster.ac.uk/releases/1997/8.html

University of Ulster. (2002, September). *World's leading disaster relief nurses graduate at UU* [news release]. Available at http://news.ulster.ac.uk/releases/2002/581.html.

Weiner, E. (2006, November). Preparing nurses internationally for emergency planning and response. *Online Journal of Issues in Nursing,* 11(3). Available at www.ncbi.nlm.nih.gov/pubmed/17279859.

World Health Organization (1985). *Nurses lead the way.* Geneva: World Health Organization.

World Health Organization. (2008). *World malaria report 2008.* Retrieved August 3, 2009 from http://apps.who.int/malaria/wmr2008.

World Health Organization. (2009). *Global tuberculosis control report 2009.* Retrieved August 3, 2009 from www.who.int/tb/publications/global_report/2009/en/index.html.

UNIT TEN

Koerner, J.G. (2007). *Healing presence: The essence of nursing.* New York: Springer Publishing Co., xii.

Stewart, I.M. (1929). The science and art of nursing, editorial. *Nursing Education Bulletin,* 2, 1.

Tarnas, R. (2002). Is the modern psyche undergoing a rite of passage? *ReVision,* 24(3), 2-10.

Selected Bibliography

Abdellah, F.G., Beland, I.L., Martin, A., & Matheney, R.V. (1960). *Patient centered approaches to nursing*. New York: Macmillan Publishing Co., Inc.

Abdellah, F.G. & Levine, E. (1979). *Better patient care through nursing research*. New York: Macmillan Publishing Co., Inc.

Adams, F. (1939). *The genuine words of Hippocrates*. Baltimore: Williams & Wilkins Co.

Addams, J. (1935). *Forty years at Hull House*. New York, NY: The Macmillan Co.

Aiken, L.H. & Fagin, C.M. (1992). *Charting nursing's future: Agenda for the 1990s*. Philadelphia: J.B. Lippincott Co.

Albert, J. (1953). Air evacuation from Korea—A typical flight. *Military Surgeon*, 112(4), 256-259.

Alcott, L.M. (1863). *Hospital sketches, camp and fireside stories*. Boston: James Redpath.

Alcott, L.M. (1885). *Hospital sketches*. Boston: Roberts Brothers.

Alexander, G. (2006, August). Ensuring history does not repeat itself. *Kai Tiaki: Nursing New Zealand (Wellington, N.Z.: 1995)*, 12(7), 25.

Alexander, W. (1782).*The history of women from earliest antiquity to the present time*. London: C Dilly.

Alger, R.A. (1901). *The Spanish-American War*. New York: Harper & Brothers.

Allen, I.E. & Seaman, J. (2006). *Making the grade: Online education in the United States*. Needham, MA: Sloan-C™.

Allen ,T.B., Berry, F.C., & Polmar, N.(1991). *CNN: War in the Gulf*. Atlanta: Turner Publishing, Inc.

American Foundation for Mental Hygiene. (1938). *The mental hygiene movement: Origin, objects and work of the National Committee and of the American Foundation for Mental Hygiene*. New York: American Foundation for Mental Hygiene.

American Journal of Nursing. (1950). *The story of the journal*. New York: American Journal of Nursing.

American Medical Association, House of Delegates. (1930). *Proceedings of the eighty-first annual session of the House of Delegates* (pp. 35-41). Chicago: American Medical Association.

American Nurses Association. (1941). *The A.N.A. and you*. New York: American Nurses Association.

American Nurses Association. (1950). *Proceedings of the 37th Biennial Convention of the American Nurses' Association*. New York: American Nurses Association.

American Nurses Association (1965). First position paper on education for nurses. *American Journal of Nursing*, 65(12), 106-107.

American Nurses Association. (1980). *Nursing: A social policy statement*. Kansas City, MO: American Nurses Association.

American Nurses Association. (1986). *The nursing center: Concept and design*. Kansas City, MO: American Nurses Association.

American Nurses Association. (1988). *Nursing case management*. Kansas City, MO: American Nurses Association.

American Nurses Association. (1991, April). ANA starts center for international nursing. *The American Nurse*, 23, 5.

Anderson, G., Read, C.V, & Monsen, R. (2000). Genetics, nursing, and public policy: Setting an international agenda. *Policy, Politics, and Nursing Practice*, 1(4), 245-255.

Andrews, C. (1921). *The fathers of New England*: The chronicles of America (vol. 6). New Haven, CT: Yale University Press.

Andrews, M.M. (1988). Education preparation for international nursing. *Journal of Professional Nursing*, 4, 430-435.

Armstrong, G. (1856). *The summer of pestilence: A history of yellow fever*. Philadelphia: J.B. Lippincott & Co.

Aroskar, M.A. (1987). The interface of ethics and politics in nursing, *Nursing Outlook*, 35(6), 268.

Ashley, J. (1975). Nursing and early feminism. *American Journal of Nursing*, 75, 1465-1467.

Ashley, J. (1976). *Hospitals, paternalism, and the role of the nurse*. New York: Teachers College Press.

Association of Collegiate Schools of Nursing. (1943). *Proceedings of the tenth annual meeting*. New York: Association of Collegiate Schools of Nursing.

Auel, J.M. (1980). *The clan of the cave bear*. New York: Bantam Books, Inc.

Austin, A.L. (1957). *History of nursing source book*. New York: GP Putnam's Sons.

Austin, A.L. (1971). *The Woolsey sisters of New York: 1860-1900*. Philadelphia: American Philosophical Society.

Aynes, E.A. (1973). *From Nightingale to eagle*. Englewood Cliffs, NJ: Prentice-Hall, Inc.

Bache, D. (1899). The place of the female nurse in the Army. *Journal of the Military Service Institution*, 25, 307.

Bacon, F. (1895). Founding of the Connecticut training school for nurses. *Trained Nurse*, 15, 187-189.

Bargagliotti, L. (2007, May). President's message: Gathering wisdom in the global nursing village. *Nursing Education Perspectives*, 28(3), 114. Retrieved June 10, 2008 from CINAHL Plus with Full Text database.

Baker, N.B. (1952). *Cyclone in calico: The story of Mary Ann Bickerdyke*. Boston: Little, Brown & Co.

Baker, R. (1944). *The first woman doctor: The story of Elizabeth Blackwell, M.D.* New York: Julian Messner.

Baker, R. (1959). *America's first trained nurse, Linda Richards*. New York: Julian Messner.

Bamford, J. (1983). *Puzzle palace: AA report on America's most secret agency*. New York: Penguin Group (USA) Incorporated.

Bamford, J. (2005). *Pretext for war: 9/11, Iraq, and the abuse of America's intelligence agencies*. New York, New York: Random House.

Barrus, C. (1908). *Nursing the insane*. New York: The Macmillan Co.

Bartels, J. (2005, December). Educating nurses for the 21st century. *Nursing & Health Sciences*, 7(4), 221-225.

Barton, G. (1897). *Angels of the battlefield: A history of the labors of the Catholic sisterhoods in the late Civil War*. Philadelphia: Catholic Publishing Co.

Barton, W.E. (1922). *Life of Clara Barton*. Boston: Houghton-Mifflin Co.

Bauknecht VL. (1986). Congress overrides veto, nursing gets center for research. *The American Nurse*, 18(1), 1, 24.

Beard, R.O. (1923, February). The report of the Rockefeller Foundation on Nursing Education: A review and critique. *American Journal of Nursing*, 23(5), 358-365.

Beckett, B. (1985). *The illustrated history of the Vietnam War*. Poole, Dorset: Blandford Press.

Bedford, W.K.R. & Holbeche, R. (1902). *The order of the Hospital of St. John of Jerusalem*. London: FE Robinson & Co.

Beeber, L.S. (1990). To be one of the boys: Aftershocks of the World War I nursing experience. *Advances in Nursing Science*, 12(4), 32-43.

Berdoe, E. (1893). *The origin and growth of the healing art.* London: Swan, Sonnenschein & Co.

Bessey, M. (1966). *Magic and the supernatural.* London: Spring Books.

Bhishagratna, K.K.L. (1907). *The sushruta samhita* [The father of surgery]. Calcutta: J.N. Bose.

Billings, J.S. & Hurd, H.M. (Eds.). (1894). *Hospitals, dispensaries, and nursing, International Congress of Charities, Correction and Philanthropy* (sec. 3). Baltimore: Johns Hopkins Press.

Blackwell, E. (1895). *Pioneer work in opening the medical profession to women: Autobiographical sketches.* New York: Longmans, Green & Co.

Blair, A.H. (1992). *At war in the Gulf.* College Station, TX: Texas A&M University Press.

Boardman, M.T. (1915). *Under the Red Cross flag at home and abroad.* Philadelphia: J.B. Lippincott Co.

Bodansky, Y. (2004). *The secret history of the Iraq War.* New York: Harper Collins Publishers.

Bonds, R. (Ed.). (1979). *The Vietnam War: The illustrated history of the conflict in Southeast Asia.* New York: Crown Publishers, Inc.

Bower, K. (1988). Managed care: Controlling costs, guaranteeing outcomes. *Definition, 3,* 14.

Boyd, L.C. (1915). *State registration for nurses* (2nd ed.). Philadelphia: W.B. Saunders Co.

Bradford, S. (1961). *Harriet Tubman: The Moses of her people.* New York: Corinth Books.

Brainard, A.M. (1922). *The evolution of public health nursing.* Philadelphia: W.B. Saunders Co.

Breasted, J.H. (1938). *The conquest of civilization.* New York: Harper & Brothers.

Breay, M. & Fenwick, E.G. (1931). *The history of the International Council of Nurses, 1899-1925.* Geneva: The International Council of Nurses.

Breckinridge, M. (1952). *Wide neighborhoods.* New York: Harper & Brothers.

Bridges, D.C. (1967). *A history of the International Council of Nurses, 1899-1964.* Philadelphia: J.B. Lippincott Co.

Bridgman, M. (1953). *Collegiate education for nursing.* New York: Russell Sage Foundation.

Brown, A.F. (1958). *Research in nursing.* Philadelphia: W.B. Saunders Co.

Brown, B. (2004). Global nursing exchange. *Nursing Administration Quarterly, 28*(1), 1-2.

Brown, E.L. (1936). *Nursing as a profession.* New York: Russell Sage Foundation.

Brown, E.L. (1948). *Nursing for the future.* New York: Russell Sage Foundation.

Brown, E.L. (1970). *Nursing reconsidered: A. study of change* (pt. 1): The professional role in institutional nursing. Philadelphia: J.B. Lippincott Co.

Brown, E.L. (1971). *Nursing reconsidered: A study of change* (pt. 2): The professional role in community nursing. Philadelphia: J.B. Lippincott Co.

Buchan, J. (1993). The same but different. *Nursing Standard, 7,* 21.

Bulechek, G.M. & McCloskey, J. (1994). Nursing interventions classification (NIC): Defining nursing care. In J. McCloskey, H.K. Grace (Eds.), *Current issues in nursing.* (4th ed., pp. 129-135). St. Louis: Mosby.

Bulger, R.J. (1988). *Technology, bureaucracy, and healing in America: A postmodern paradigm.* Iowa City: The University of Iowa Press.

Bullough, B. (1992). Alternative models for specialty nursing practice, *Nursing and Health Care, 13,* 254-259.

Bullough, B. & Bullough, V.L. (Eds.). (1994). *Nursing issues for the nineties and beyond,* New York: Springer Publishing Company.

Bullough, V.L. & Bullough, B. (1984). *History, trends, and politics of nursing,* Norwalk, CT: Appleton-Century-Crofts.

Bullough, V.L., Bullough, B., & Stanton, M.P. (Eds.). (1990). *Florence Nightingale and her era: A collection of new scholarship,* New York: Garland.

Bulwer-Lytton, E. (1834). *The last days of Pompeii,* New York: Dodd, Mead, & Co.

Burgess, M.A. (1928). *Nurses, patients and pocketbooks.* New York: National League of Nursing Education.

Burgess, M.A. (1934). *Nursing schools today and tomorrow.* New York: National League of Nursing Education.

Bush, H. & Mettler, M. (1994). NPs as entrepreneurs: Three case histories. *American Journal of Nursing, 94*(12), 16A.

Bush, L.P. (1890). Reminiscences of the Philadelphia Hospital and remarks on old time doctors and medicine. *Philadelphia General Hospitals Reports, 1,* 68-77.

Butler, A. (1934). *The lives of the saints.* (12 vols.). H. Thurston & A. Attwater (rev. ed.).London: Burns, Oates & Wasbourne, Ltd.

Caldwell, T. (1959). *Dear and glorious physician.* New York: Doubleday & Co.

Carlisle, R. (1893). *An account of Bellevue Hospital.* New York: Society of Alumni of Bellevue Hospital.

Carnegie, M. (2005). Educational preparation of black nurses: A historical perspective. *The ABNF Journal: Official Journal of the Association of Black Nursing Faculty in Higher Education, Inc, 16*(1), 6-7.

Carnegie, M.E. (1976). *Historical perspectives of nursing research.* Boston: Nursing Archive of Boston University.

Carnegie, M.E. (1986). *The path we tread: Blacks in nursing, 1854-1984.* Philadelphia: J.B. Lippincott.

Carnegie, M.E. (1991). *The path we tread: Blacks in nursing, 1854-1990* (2nd ed.). New York: National League for Nursing.

Carnegie, M.E. (1995). *The path we tread: Blacks in nursing worldwide, 1854-1994* (3rd ed.). New York: National League for Nursing Press.

Carpenter, R., et al. (Gilbert Grosvenor, editor in chief.). (1951). *Everyday life in ancient times: Highlights of the beginnings of Western Civilization in Mesopotamia, Egypt, Greece, and Rome.* Washington, DC: National Geographic Society.

Carty, R. (2004). Views of global nursing leadership: A tribute to Florence Nightingale. © Florence Nightingale Service, Washington National Cathedral, May 9, 2004. *Virginia Nurses Today, 12*(3), 29-29.

Castiglioni, A. (1947). *A history of medicine* (2nd ed.). (E.B. Krumbhaar, trans.). New York: Alfred A. Knopf.

Catlin, G. (1926). *North American Indians* (vol. 1). Edinburgh: John Grant.

Caulfield, E. (1931). *The infant welfare movement in the eighteenth century.* New York: Paul B Hoeber.

Central Finland College of Health and Lancashire College of Nursing and Health Studies. (1994). *Preliminary plan for joint curriculum.* Central Finland College of Health and Lancashire College of Nursing and Health Studies. Retrieved August 1, 2009 from www.estiatn.net/year1/partnerdetails, pHp?code-FI1.

Cheney, E.D. (Ed.). (1889). *Louisa May Alcott: Her life, letters, and journals.* Boston: Little, Brown & Co.

Chesterton, G.K. (1924). *St. Francis of Assisi.* New York: George H Doran Co.

Chow, R.K., Hope, G.S., Nelson, E.A., Sokoloski, J.L., & Wilson, R.A. (1978). Historical perspectives of the U.S. Air Force, Army, Navy, Public Health Service, and Veterans Administration Nursing Services, *Military Medicine, 143*(7), 457-463.

Christensen, C., Bohmer, R., & Kenagy, J. (2000). Will disruptive innovations cure health care? *Harvard Business Review, 78*(5), 102.

Christy, T.E. (1969). *Cornerstone for nursing education: A history of division of nursing education of Teachers College, Columbia University, 1899-1947.* New York: Teachers College Press.

Christy, T.E. (1969, January). Portrait of a leader: M. Adelaide Nutting. *Nursing Outlook, 17*(1), 20-24.

Christy, T.E. (1969, March). Portrait of a leader: Isabel Hampton Robb. *Nursing Outlook, 17*(3), 26-29.

Christy, T.E. (1969, June). Portrait of a leader: Lavinia Lloyd Dock. *Nursing Outlook, 17,* 72-75.

Christy, T.E. (1969, October). Portrait of a leader: Isabel Maitland Stewart. *Nursing Outlook, 17*(10), 44-48.

Christy, T.E. (1970, March). Portrait of a leader: Lillian D. Wald. *Nursing Outlook, 18*(3), 50-54.

Christy, T.E. (1970, August). Portrait of a leader: Annie Warburton Goodrich. *Nursing Outlook. 18*(8), 46-50.

Christy, T.E. (1971, February). Equal rights for women: Voices from the past. *American Journal of Nursing, 71*(2), 288-293.

Christy, T.E. (1975, July). The fateful decade, 1890-1900. *American Journal of Nursing, 75*(7), 1163-1165.

Christy, T.E. (1976). Historical perspectives on accountability. In J.A. Williamson (Ed.), *Current perspectives in nursing education.* St. Louis: The CV Mosby Co.

Christy, T.E. (1980). Clinical practice as a function of nursing education: A historical analysis. *Nursing Outlook, 28*(8), 493-497.

Churchill, F. (1851). *On the theory and practice of midwifery.* Philadelphia: Blanchard & Lea.

Clark, J. (1994). The international classification of nursing. In J. McCloskey & H.K. Grace (Eds.), *Current issues in nursing* (4th ed., pp. 143-147). St. Louis: Mosby.

Clay, R.M. (1909). *Medieval hospitals of England.* London: Methuen & Co.

Cohen, I.B. (1984). Florence Nightingale. *Scientific American, 250,* 128-137.

Commission on Nursing Research, American Nurses Association. (1976). *Priorities for research in nursing.* Kansas City, MO: Commission on Nursing Research.

Committee on the Grading of Nursing Schools. (1928). *Nurses, patients, and pocketbooks.* New York: Committee on the Grading of Nursing Schools.

Committee on Nursing and Nursing Education in the United States. (1923). *Nursing and nursing education in the United States.* New York: The Macmillan Co.

Committee on the Structure of National Nursing Organizations. (1950). *New horizons in nursing.* New York: The Macmillan Co.

Cook, Sir Edward (1914). *The life of Florence Nightingale* (vols.1-2). London: The Macmillan Co.

Cooper, P. (1946). *Navy nurse.* New York: McGraw-Hill Book Co.

Cope, Z. (1958). *Florence Nightingale and the doctors.* Philadelphia: J.B. Lippincott Co.

Cox, E. & Briggs, S. (2004). Disaster nursing: New frontiers for critical care. *Critical Care Nurse, 24*(3), 16.

Coyle, G., Sapnas, K., & Ward-Presson, K. (2007, July). Dealing with disaster. *Nursing Management, 38*(7), 24-29.

Crawford, R. (1914). *The plague and pestilence in literature and art.* New York: Oxford University Press.

Crigger, N. (2008). Towards a viable and just global nursing ethics. *Nursing Ethics, 15*(1), 17-27.

Croutier, A.L. (1992). *Taking the waters. Spirit, art, sensuality.* New York: Abbeville Press.

Cunningham, J.T. (1976). *Clara Maass—A nurse—A hospital—A spirit.* Belleville, NJ: Rae Publishing Co.

Curran, C., Sheets, D., Kirkpatrick, B., & Bauldoff, G. (2007). Virtual patients support point-of-care nursing education. *Nursing Management, 38*(12), 27-33.

Curtayne, A. (1935). *St. Catherine of Siena,* New York: Sheed & Ward.

Curtis, D. (1902). Early history of the Boston Training School. *American Journal of Nursing, 2*(5), 331-335.

D'Antonio, P. Baer, E.D., Rinker, S.D., & Lynaugh, J.E. (Eds.). (2007). *Nurses' work: Issues across time and place.* New York, NY: Springer Publishing Company, LLC.

Damel-Rops, H. (1961). *Monsieur Vincent.* New York: Hawthorn Books.

David, P. (1991). *Triumph in the desert: The challenge, the fight, the legacy.* New York: Random House.

Davis, M.B. (1886). *The woman who battled for the boys in blue—Mother Bickerdyke.* San Francisco: Pacific Press Publishing House.

Davison, W.C. (1943, April). Nursing as the foundation of medicine. *North Carolina Medical Journal,* 141.

De Back, V. (2001). What would Florence do? *International Nursing Review, 48*(3), 131.

Defoe, D. (1966). *A journal of the plague year (1721).* New York: Penguin Books.

Delano, J.A. (1918). Nursing as it relates to the war. *American Journal of Nursing.* 18, 1064.

Delano, J.A. (1919). How American nurses helped win the war. *Modern Hospital,* 12, 7.

Dennison, C. (1942). Nursing service in the emergency room, *American Journal of Nursing, 42*(7), 774-784.

Deutsch, A. (1937). *Mentally ill in America: A history of their care and treatment from colonial times.* New York: Doubleday.

Deutsch, A. (1946). *The mentally ill in America.* (2nd ed.). New York: Columbia University Press.

Devane, R.S. (1948). *The failure of individualism.* Dublin: Browne & Nolan, Ltd.

Dewar, M. & the Press Association. (1992). *The Gulf War: A photographic history.* London: Robert Hale.

Dick, R.S. & Stein, E.B. (Eds.). (1991). *The computer-based patient record: An essential technology for health care.* Washington, DC: National Academy Press.

Dickens, C. (1859). *A tale of two cities.* New York: E.P. Dutton & Co.

Dickens, C. (1910). *Martin Chuzzlewit.* New York: The Macmillan Co.

Dock, L.L. (1890). *Textbook of materia medica for nurses,* New York: G.P. Putnam's Sons.

Dock, L.L. (1901). History of the reform in nursing in Bellevue Hospital. *American Journal of Nursing, 2*(2), 89-98.

Dock, L.L. (1901). Secretary's report of the meeting of the International Council of Nurses, Buffalo, New York (Official Reports of Societies). *American Journal of Nursing, 2*(1), 51-53.

Dock, L.L. (1912). *Hygiene and morality.* New York: G.P. Putnam's Sons.

Dock, L.L. & Cottle J. (1901). Letters to the editor. *American Journal of Nursing, 2*(3), 231-232.

Dock, L.L. & National Red Cross Nursing Service. (1922). *History of American Red Cross nursing.* New York: The Macmillan Co.

Dock, L.L. & Stewart, I.M. (1925). *A short history of nursing* (2nd ed.). New York: G.P. Putnam's Sons.

Dock, L.L. & Stewart, I.M. (1938). *A short history of nursing* (4th ed.). New York: G.P. Putnam's Sons.

Dolan, J.A., Fitzpatrick, M.L., & Hermann, E.K. (1983). *Nursing in society: A historical perspective* (15th ed.). Philadelphia: W.B. Saunders Co.

Donahue, M.P. (1978). The nurse: A patient advocate? *Nursing Forum, 17*(2), 143-151.

Donahue, M.P (1981). *Isabel Maitland Stewart's philosophy of education* (doctoral dissertation, The University of Iowa). *Dissertation Abstracts International, 42*(5), 2018A. (University Microfilms No. 8123310).

Donahue, M.P. (1983). Isabel Maitland Stewart's philosophy of education. *Nursing Research, 32*(4), 140-146.

Donahue, M.P. (1985). Advocacy. In G.M. Bulechek & J.C. McCloskey (Eds.), *Nursing interventions: Treatments for nursing diagnoses* (pp. 338-351). Philadelphia: W.B. Saunders Company.

Donahue, M.P. (1985). *Nursing: The finest art. An illustrated history.* St. Louis: Mosby.

Donahue, M.P. (1996). *Nursing: The finest art. An illustrated history* (2nd ed.). St. Louis: Mosby.

Donahue, M.P. (2004). Turning points in nursing history. In L. Haynes, T. Boese, & H. Butcher, *Nursing in contemporary society* (pp. 2-34). Upper Saddle River, NJ: Pearson Prentice Hall.

Dossey, B.M., Selanders L.C., Beck, D., & Attewell, A. (2005). *Florence Nightingale today: Healing leadership global action.* Silver Spring, MD: American Nurses Association.

Douglas, M. (Ed.). (1970). *Witchcraft: Confessions and accusations.* London: Tavistock Publications.

Dreves, K.D. (1975). Nurses in American history: Vassar Training Camp for nurses. *American Journal of Nursing, 75*(11), 2000-2002.

Duffield. C. (1988). Nursing in the 1980s and 1990s: A challenge for managers. *International Journal of Nursing Studies, 25*(2), 125-134.

Duffus, R.L. (1938). *Lillian Wald, neighbor and crusader.* New York: The Macmillan Co.

Dunn, L. (1997). A literature review of advanced clinical nursing practice in the United States of America. *Journal of Advanced Nursing, 25*(4), 814-819.

Eckenstein, L. (1896). *Women under monasticism.* Cambridge: Cambridge University Press.

Edwards, A.B. (1892). *Pharaohs, fellahs, and explorers.* New York: Harper & Brothers.

Ehrenreich, B. & English, D. (1973). *Witches, midwives, and nurses: A history of women healers.* New York: The Feminist Press.

Ehrhart, W.D. (Ed.). (1989). *Carrying the darkness: The poetry of the Vietnam War.* Lubbock, TX: Texas Tech University Press.

Elgood, C. (1951). *A medical history of Persia.* London: Cambridge University Press.

Elmore, J.A. (1976, March). Black nurses: Their service and their struggle. *American Journal of Nursing, 76*(3), 435-437.

Erickson, J. & Ditomassi, M. (2005). The clinical nurse leader: New in name only. *The Journal of Nursing Education, 44*(3), 99-100.

Evans, A.D. & Howard, L.G.R. (1930). *The romance of the British voluntary hospital movement.* London: Hutchinson & Co. Ltd.

Faddis, M.O. (1973). *A school of nursing comes of age.* Cleveland: The Alumni Association of The Frances Payne Bolton School of Nursing.

Fairman, J. & Lynaugh, J.E.(1998). *Critical care nursing: A history.* Philadelphia: University of Pennsylvania Press.

Faulkner, H.V. (1931). *The quest for social justice, 1899-1914.* New York: The Macmillan Co.

Faxon, N.W. (1949). *The hospital in contemporary life.* Cambridge: Harvard University Press.

Felton, G. (1989). Nursing: A profession to celebrate. *Journal of Professional Nursing,* 5(5), 273-278.

Fenton, M.V. (1994). Development of models of international exchange to upgrade nursing education. In J. McCloskey & H.K. Grace (Eds.). *Current issues in nursing* (4th ed., pp. 202-206). St. Louis: Mosby.

Ferguson, M. (1980). *The Aquarian conspiracy.* Los Angeles and New York: J.P. Tarcher, Inc. & St. Martin's Press.

Fischer, J. & Stone, R (1986). *Images of war.* Boston: Boston Publishing Company.

Fiske, A. (1911). *Structure and functions of the body: A handbook of anatomy and physiology for nurses and others desiring a practical knowledge of the subject.* Philadelphia: W.B. Saunders Co.

Fitzpatrick, J.J. & Zanotti, R.(1995). Where are we now? Nursing diagnosis internationally. *Nursing Diagnosis,* 6(1), 42-47.

Fitzpatrick, M.L. (1975). *The National Organization for Public Health Nursing, 1912-1952: Development of a practice field.* New York: National League for Nursing.

Fitzpatrick, M.L. (1983). *Prologue to professionalism.* Bowie, MD: Robert J Brady Co.

Flanagan, L.C. (1976). *One strong voice: The story of the American Nurses Association.* Kansas City, MO: American Nurses Association.

Flesner, M. (2004). Care of the elderly as a global nursing issue. *Nursing Administration Quarterly,* 28(1), 67-72.

Flikke, J.O. (1943). *Nurses in action: The story of the Army Nurse Corps.* Philadelphia: J.B. Lippincott Co.

Foran, J.K. & Morrissey, S.H. (1931). *Jeanne Mance; or, the angel of the colony.* Montreal: Sisters of the Hôtel Dieu.

Ford, L.C. (1992). Advanced nursing practice: Future of the nurse practitioner. In L. Aiken & C. Fagin (Eds.). *Charting nursing's future agenda for the 1990s* (pp. 287-297). Philadelphia: J.B. Lippincott Company.

Frank, Sister C.M. (1953). *The historical development of nursing.* Philadelphia: W.B. Saunders Co.

Freedman, D. & Rhoads, J. (Eds.). (1987). *Nurses in Vietnam: The forgotten veterans.* Austin, TX: Texas Monthly Press.

Friedrich, O. (1991). *Desert Storm: The war in the Persian Gulf.* Boston: Little, Brown and Company.

Fuller, J. (1968). *The days of St. Anthony's fire.* New York: Macmillan Publishing Co., Inc.

Fullerton, J., Schuiling, K., & Sipe, T. (2005). Presidential priorities: 50 years of wisdom as the basis of an action agenda for the next half-century. *Journal of Midwifery & Women's Health,* 50(2), 91-101.

Furlong, E., & Smith, R. (2005). Advanced nursing practice: policy, education and role development. *Journal of Clinical Nursing,* 14(9), 1059-1066.

Gadon, E.W. (1989). *The once and future goddess.* San Francisco: Harper.

Garrison, F.H. (1913). *An introduction to the history of medicine.* Philadelphia: W.B. Saunders Co.

Gelinas, A. (1946). *Nursing and nursing education.* New York: The Commonwealth Fund.

Gibbon, E. (1900). *The decline and fall of the Roman Empire.* New York: Viking Press.

Gibbon, J.M. & Mathewson, M.S. (1947). *Three centuries of Canadian nursing.* Toronto: The Macmillian Co. of Canada Ltd.

Ginzberg, E. (1949). *A pattern of hospital care.* New York: Columbia University Press.

Giordani, I. (1959). *Catherine of Siena.* Milwaukee: Bruce Publishing Co.

Glass, L.K. (1989). The historic origins of nursing centers. In A. Arvonio (Ed.), *Nursing centers: Meeting the demand for quality health care* (NLN Pub. No. 21-2311). New York: National League for Nursing.

Glittenberg, J. (2003). The tragedy of torture: A global concern for mental health nursing. *Issues in Mental Health Nursing,* 24(6-7), 627-638.

Goertz Koerner, J. (2007). *Healing presence: The essence of nursing.* New York: Springer Publishing Company.

Goldsmith, M. (1937). *Florence Nightingale: The woman and the legend.* London: Hodder & Stoughton.

Goodnow, M. (1942). *Nursing history,* Philadelphia: W.B. Saunders Co.

Goodrich, A.W. (1932). The school of nursing and the future, *Proceedings of the thirty-eighth annual convention of the National League of Nursing Education.* New York: National Headquarters.

Goodrich, A.W. (1932). *The social and ethical significance of nursing.* New York: The Macmilliam Co.

Goodstray, S. (1954). Isabel Maitland Stewart, *American Journal of Nursing,* 54(3), 302-306.

Grace, H.K. (1978). The development of doctoral education in nursing: A historical perspective. In N.L. Chaska (Ed.), *The nursing profession: Views through the mist,* New York: McGraw-Hill Book Co.

Grattan, J.H.G. & Singer, C. (1952). *Anglo-Saxon magic and medicine.* New York: Oxford University Press.

Griffin, G.J. & Griffin, H.J. (1973). *History and trends of professional nursing.* St. Louis: The CV Mosby Co.

Grindel, C. (2005). AACN presents the clinical nurse leader and the doctor in nursing practice roles: A benefit or a misfortune? *Medsurg Nursing: Official Journal of the Academy of Medical-Surgical Nurses,* 14(4), 209-210.

Grippando, G.M. (1977). *Nursing perspectives and issues.* Albany: Delmar Publishers, Inc.

Haeser, H. (1857). *Geschichte christlicher krankenpflege und pflegerschaften.* Berlin: Anmerkungen.

Haggard, H.W. (1929). *Devils, drugs, and doctors.* New York: Harper & Brothers.

Haggard, H.W. (1933). *Mystery, magic and medicine.* New York: Doubleday, Doran & Co., Inc.

Hahn, R.E. (1927). A history of nursing scrapbook, *American Journal of Nursing,* 27(4), 279-280.

Hakesley-Brown, R. (2005). The global nursing workforce: Liberating the skills of refugee nurses. *International Nursing Review,* 52(4), 241-242.

Haldeman, J.C. & Abdellah, F.G. (1959, May). Concepts of progressive patient care. *Hospitals,* 33(10), 38-42.

Hale, S. (1871). Lady nurses. *Godey's Lady's Book and Magazine.* 82,188.

Hall, L. (1963). A center for nursing. *Nursing Outlook,* 11, 805-806.

Hathaway, D., Jacob, S., Stegbauer, C., Thompson, C., & Graff, C. (2006). The practice doctorate: Perspectives of early adopters. *The Journal of Nursing Education,* 45(12), 487-496.

Hampton, I.A. (1893). *Nursing: Its principles and practice for hospital and private use.* Philadelphia: W.B. Saunders Co.

Hampton, I.A., et al. (1949). *Nursing of the sick 1893.* New York: McGraw-Hill Book Company, Inc.

Hanaford, P. (1882). *Daughters of America, or women of the century.* Augusta, ME: True & Co.

Hardaway, R.M. (1988). *Care of the wounded in Vietnam.* Manhattan, KS: Sunflower University Press.

Harnack, A. (1909). *Luke, the physician.* New York: G.P. Putnam's Sons.

Haynes, L., Boese, T., & Butcher H. (2004). *Nursing in contemporary society. Issues, trends and transition to practice.* Upper Saddle River, NJ: Pearson Education Inc.

Henderson, V. (1966). *The nature of nursing.* New York: Macmillan Publishing Co., Inc.

Henrietta, Sister (1939). A famous New Orleans hospital. *American Journal of Nursing,* 39(3), 249-256.

Hermann, P. (1954). *Conquest by man.* New York: Harper & Brothers.

Hill, D. (1968). *Magic and superstition.* London: Hamlyn Publishing Group.

Himali, U. (1955). Managed care: Does the promise meet the potential? *The American Nurse,* 27(4), 1, 14-16.

Himali, U. (1995). More than 25,000 RNs march on Washington, issuing a wake-up call to consumers and lawmakers. *The American Nurse,* 27, 1, 20-21.

Hine, D.C. (1985). *Black women in the nursing profession: A documentary history,* New York: Garland.

Hine, D.C. (1989). *Black women in white: Racial conflict and cooperation in the nursing profession, 1890-1950*. Bloomington: Indiana University Press.

Hiro, D. (1992). *Desert shield to desert storm*. New York: Routledge.

Hobson, W. (1963). *World health and history*. Bristol: John Wright & Sons.

Holland, M.A. (1895). *Our Army nurses*. Boston: B. Wilkins & Co.

Holloran, C.A.(1994). What are the ethical issues from a worldwide viewpoint? In J. McCloskey, H.K. Grace (Eds.), *Current issues in nursing* (4th ed., pp. 763-770). St. Louis: Mosby.

Holm, J.M., Wells, S.P. (1993, November). Air Force women in the Vietnam War. In *Celebration of Patriotism and Courage: Dedication of the Vietnam Women's Memorial*. Washington, DC: Vietnam Women's Memorial Project.

Horn, B.J. & Swain, M.A. (1978). *Criterion measures of nursing care*. Hyattsville, MD: National Center for Health Services Research. (DHEW Pub. No. HS78-3187).

Hovis, B. (1991). *Station hospital Saigon: A navy nurse in Vietnam, 1963-1964*, Annapolis, MD: Naval Institute Press.

Howard, J. (1791). *An account of the principal lazarettos in Europe*. London: Johnson, Dilly & Cadel.

Hughes, E.C., Hughes, H.M., & Deutscher, I. (1958). *Twenty thousand nurses tell their story*, Philadelphia: J.B. Lippincott Co.

Hunt, L. (1889). *Essays—The monthly nurse*. London: Frederick Warne & Co.

International Congress of Charities, Correction and Philanthropy. (1893 Chicago). (1949). *Nursing of the sick, 1893*. New York: McGraw-Hill Book Co.

International Labour Office. (1994). *The remuneration of nursing personnel. An international perspective*. Geneva: International Labour Office.

International Nursing Foundation of Japan (1977). *Nursing in the world: The needs of individual countries, and their programmes*. Tokyo, Japan: International Nursing Foundation of Japan.

International perspectives: Global nursing profession loses a renowned leader, educator and scholar...Dr Margretta Madden Styles. (2006). *International Nursing Review*, 53(1), 4-7.

Ireland, M. (1998). The nurse entrepreneur redefined. Are you one? *Revolution (Staten Island, N.Y.)*, 8(3-4), 110-111.

Jacobs, J.B. (1921). Elizabeth Fry, Pastor Fliedner and Florence Nightingale. *Annals of Medical History*, 3(1), 17-25.

Jacobs, S. (2007). The pivotal role of politics in advancing nursing practice. *Nursing New Zealand (Wellington, N.Z.: 1995)*, 13(11), 14-16.

Jamieson, E.M. & Sewall, M.F. (1950). *Trends in nursing history*. Philadelphia: W.B. Saunders Co.

Jaret, P. (2008). *Nurse: A world of care*. Atlanta, Georgia: Emory University.

Jennings, C. (2001). The evolution of U.S. health policy and the impact of future trends on nursing practice, research, and education. *Policy, Politics, & Nursing Practice*, 2(3), 218-227.

Johns, E. & Pfefferkorn, B. (1934). *An activity analysis of nursing*. New York: New York Committee on the Grading of Nursing Schools.

Johns, E. & Pfefferkorn, B. (1954). *The Johns Hopkins Hospital School of Nursing, 1889-1949*, Baltimore: Johns Hopkins University Press.

Johnson, M. & Maas, M. (1994). Nursing-focused patient outcomes: Challenge for the nineties. In J. McCloskey & H.K. Grace (Eds.), *Current issues in nursing* (4th ed., pp. 136-142). St. Louis: Mosby.

Johnson, S. (2006). *The ghost map. The story of London's most terrifying epidemic and how it changed science, cities and the modern world*. New York, NY: Riverhead Books.

Joint Committee on Nursing in National Security. (1951). Mobilization of nurses for national security. *American Journal of Nursing*, 51(2), 78-79.

Jolly, E.R. (1927). *Nuns of the battlefield*. Providence, RI: Providence Visitor Press.

Jones, P. (1996). Humans, information and science. *Journal of Advanced Nursing*, 24(3), 591-598.

Jones, W.H.S. (1909). *Malaria and Greek history*. Manchester: Manchester University Press.

Judson, H. (1941). *Edith Cavell*. New York: The Macmillan Co.

Kalisch, P.A. & Kalisch, B.J. (1978). *The advance of American nursing*. Boston: Little, Brown & Co.

Kalisch, P.A. & Kalisch, B.J. (1982). *The politics of nursing*. Philadelphia: Lippincott.

Kalisch, P.A. & Kalisch, B.J. (1987). *The changing image of the nurse*. Menlo Park, CA: Addison-Wesley Publishing Company.

Kalisch, P.A. & Kalisch, B.J. (1995). *The advance of American nursing* (3rd ed.). Philadelphia: J.B. Lippincott Company.

Kalisch, P.A. & Kalisch, B.J. (2004). *American Nursing: A history* (4th ed.). Philadelphia: Lippincott Williams & Wilkins, A Wolters Kluwer Company.

Kane, J.N. (1934). *Famous first facts*. New York: The H.W. Wilson Co.

Kansas State Nurses' Association. (1942). *Lamps on the prairie: A history of nursing in Kansas*. Emporia, KS: Emporia Gazette Press.

Kavanagh, J. (1852). *Women of Christianity*. New York: D. Appleton Co.

Kellogg, F.S. (1907). *Mother Bickerdyke as I knew her*. Chicago: Unity Publishing.

Kelly, H.A. (1923). *Walter Reed and yellow fever*. New York: G.P. Putnam's Sons.

Kenton, E. (Ed.). (1925). *The Jesuit relations and allied documents (1610-1791)*. New York: A & C Boni.

Kernodle, P.B. (1949). *Red Cross nurse in action: 1882-1948*. New York: Harper & Brothers.

Ketter, J. (1994, October). Nurses worldwide speak the same language. *The American Nurse*, 26(9), 8-9.

Kimber, D.C. & Gray, C.E. (1893). *Anatomy and physiology for nurses*. New York: The Macmillam Co.

King, I.M. (1971). *Toward a theory of nursing*. New York: John Wiley & Sons, Inc.

King, L.S. (1958). *The medical world of the eighteenth century*. Chicago: University of Chicago Press.

Kingma, M. (2006). *Nurses on the move: Migration and the global health care economoy*. Ithaca, NY: Cornell University Press.

Kingsley, C. (nd). *Hypatia*. New York: Lovell, Coryell & Co.

Kramer, M. (1974). *Reality shock: Why nurses leave nursing*. St. Louis: The CV Mosby Co.

Krampitz, S.D. (1981). Clinical specialization: Historical antecedents of today's issues. In J.C. McCloskey & H.K. Grace, *Current issues in nursing*. Boston: Blackwell Scientific Publications, Inc.

Lamb, H. (1930). *The crusades: Iron men and saints*. New York: Doubleday, Doran & Co.

Lambertsen, E.C. (1953). *Nursing team organization and functioning*. New York: Teachers College, Columbia University.

Lambertsen, E.C. (1958). *Education for nursing leadership*. Philadelphia: J.B. Lippincott Co.

Lardner, J. & Marcus, M. (2008, March 7). For nurses, a barrier broken. It's a test insurers are backing: Can primary care work without doctors? *U.S. News & World Report, L.P.* Retrieved March 7, 2008 from http://health.usnews.com.

Lasseter, F. (1999). A nursing legacy—political activities at the turn of the century. *AORN Journal*, 70(5), 902-907.

Lavin, M., Avant, K., Craft-Rosenberg, M., Herdman, T., & Gebbie, K. (2004). Contexts for the study of the economic influence of nursing diagnoses on patient outcomes. *International Journal of Nursing Terminologies & Classifications*, 15(2), 39-47.

Lazaro, A.R. (1949). The role of the flight nurse in air evacuation. *Military Surgeon*, 105(1), 60-64.

Leake, C.D. (1952). *The old Egyptian medical papyri*. Lawrence, KS: University of Kansas Press.

Lear, L.E. (1989*). Coping of nurses who served in the Vietnam conflict*. Unpublished thesis, The University of Iowa. Iowa City, IA.

Lee, E. (1942). *History of the School of Nursing of the Presbyterian Hospital, 1892-1942*. New York: G.P. Putnam's Sons.

Lesnik, M.J. & Anderson, B.L. (1947). *Legal aspects of nursing*. Philadelphia: J.B. Lippincott Co.

Lesse, S. (1981). *The future of the health sciences*. New York: Irvington.

Lewis, E.P. (1980). *A collection of editorials from Nursing Outlook 1971-1980*. New York: American Journal of Nursing Company.

Lewis, F. (1983, November 13). Quantum mechanics of politics—And life. *Des Moines Sunday Register*, 1C.

Lin, Y. (1942). *The wisdom of China and India*. New York: Random House.

Lindeman, C.A. (1989). Choices within challenges. Western Institute for Nursing Research Communicating Nursing Research Conference Proceedings, 22(1), 3.

Lindquist, G.J. (1984). A cross-cultural experience: Comparative study in nursing and health care. *Journal of Nursing Education*, 23, 212-214.

Lindquist, G.J. (1990). Integration of international and transcultural content in nursing curricula: A process for change. *Journal of Professional Nursing*, 6(5), 272-279.

Link, E.P. (1971). Elizabeth Blackwell, citizen and humanitarian. *Woman Physician*, 26, 451-458.

Lippard, L.R. (1990). *A different war*. Whatcom Museum of History & Art, Bellingham & Seattle, WA: The Real Comet Press.

Lippmann, W. (1944, December, 19). American women and our wounded men, *Washington Post*. (Reprinted in the *Congressional Record* as an extension of the remarks of Hon. Edith Nourse Rogers, December 19, 1944.)

Longmore, T. (1883). *The sanitary contrasts of the British and French armies during the Crimean War*. London: C. Griffin & Co.

Loomis, J., Willard, B., & Cohen, J. (2007, December 22). Difficult professional choices: Deciding between the PhD and the DNP in nursing. *Online Journal of Issues in Nursing*, 12(1), 6. Retrieved June 9, 2008 from MEDLINE with Full Text database.

Lord, J. (1885). *Beacon lights of history* (vol. 5, *Great women*). New York: Fords, Howard & Hulbert.

Loshak, D. (1994). *Munch*. New York: Smithmark Publishers, Inc.

Lowenfels, W. (1961). *Walt Whitman's Civil War*. New York: Alfred A Knopf, Inc.

Lundeen, S.P (1993). Comprehensive, collaborative, coordinated, community based care: A community nursing center model. *Family and Community Health*, 16, 57-62.

Lundeen, S.P. (1994). Community nursing centers. Implications for health care reform. In J. McCloskey & H.K. Grace (Eds.), *Current issues in nursing* (4th ed., pp. 382-387). St. Louis: Mosby.

Lyons, A.S. (1978). Ancient China. In A.S. Lyons & R.J. Petrucelli, *Medicine: An illustrated history*. New York: Harry N. Abrams, Inc.

Lyons, A.S. (1978). Ancient Hebrew medicine. In A.S. Lyons & R.J. Petrucelli, *Medicine: An illustrated history*. New York: Harry N. Abrams, Inc.

Lyons, A.S. (1978). Hippocrates. In A.S. Lyons & R.J. Petrucelli, *Medicine: An illustrated history*. New York: Harry N. Abrams, Inc.

Lyons, A.S. (1978). Medicine in Roman times. In A.S. Lyons & R.J. Petrucelli, *Medicine: An illustrated history*. New York: Harry N. Abrams, Inc.

Lyons, A.S. (1978). Medicine under Islam (Arabic medicine). In A.S. Lyons & R.J. Petrucelli, *Medicine: An illustrated history*. New York: Harry N. Abrams, Inc.

Lyons, A.S. (1978). The nineteenth century (the beginnings of modern medicine). In A.S. Lyons & R.J. Petrucelli: *Medicine: An illustrated history*. New York: Harry N. Abrams, Inc.

Lyons, A.S. & Petrucelli, R.J. (1978). *Medicine: An illustrated history*. New York: Harry N Abrams, Inc.

Maglacas, A.M. (1988). Health for all: Nursing's role. *Nursing Outlook*, 36, 66-71.

Maglacas, A.M. (1989). Close encounters in international nursing: Impact on health policy and research. *Journal of Professional Nursing*, 5(6), 304-314.

Mannino, A.J. (1951). Men in nursing. *American Journal of Nursing*, 51(3), 198-199.

Marram, G., Barrett, M. & Bevis, E. (1979). *Primary nursing: A model for individualized care* (2nd ed.). St. Louis: The C.V. Mosby Co.

Marshall, H.E. (1937). *Dorothea Dix, forgotten Samaritan*. Chapel Hill, NC: University of North Carolina Press.

Marshall, H.E. (1972). *Mary Adelaide Nutting*. Baltimore: Johns Hopkins University Press.

Marshall, K. (1987). *In the combat zone: An oral history of American women in Vietnam, 1966-1975*. Boston: Little, Brown and Company.

Martin, K.S. & Scheet, N.J (1992). *The Omaha System: Applications for community health nursing*. Philadelphia: W.B. Saunders.

Mason, D. (1990). Nursing and politics: a profession comes of age. *Orthopaedic Nursing*, 9(5), 11-17.

Mason, O.T. (1894). *Woman's share in primitive culture*. New York: D. Appleton & Co.

May, K.A. & Meleis, A.I. (1987). International nursing: Guidelines for core content. *Nurse Educator*, 12(5), 36-40.

Maynard, T. (1939). *Apostle of charity: The life of St. Vincent de Paul*. New York: Dial Press.

Maynard, T. (1956). *St. Benedict and his monks*. London: Staples Press.

McCartney, P. (2000). Information technology in maternal/child nursing: past, present, and future. *MCN: The American Journal of Maternal Child Nursing*, 25(6), 336-339.

McCrary, L. (1995, March 31). Nurses to protest in D.C., saying job cuts erode care. *The Philadelphia Inquirer*, pp. A1, A20.

McIsaac, I. (1909). *Bacteriology for nurses*. New York: The Macmillan Co.

McJunkin, J.N. & Crace, M.D. (1983). *Visions of Vietnam*. Novato, CA: Presidio Press.

McKenzie, J.L. & Chrisman, N.L. (1977). Healing herbs, gods and magic. *Nursing Outlook*, 25(3), 326-329.

McMahon, N. (1959). *The story of the Hospitallers of St. John of God*. Westminster, MD: Newman Press.

McManus, R.L. (1962). Isabel M. Stewart—Foremost researcher. *Nursing Research* 11(1), 4.

Mead, K.C. (1938). *History of women in medicine*. New York: Haddam Press.

Merejkowski, D. (1902). *The romance of Leonardo da Vinci*. New York: Random House.

Merton, R.K. (1958). *Issues on the growth of a profession*. New York: American Nurses Association.

Metarazzo, J.D. & Abdellah, F.G. (1971). Doctoral education for nurses in the United States. *Nursing Research*, 20, 404-414.

Middleton, J. (Ed.). (1967). *Magic, witchcraft and curing*. New York: The Natural History Press.

Military nurses rally for Operation Desert Shield [headline news]. (1990). *The American Journal of Nursing*, 90(10), 7 & 11.

Miller, H.S. (1968). *The history of Chi Eta Phi Sorority, Inc., 1932-1967*. Washington, DC: Negro Life and History, Inc.

Miller, M. (2009). *The tyranny of dead ideas: Letting go of the old ways of thinking to unleash a new prosperity*. New York: Times Books, Henry and Company, LLC.

Millett, A.R. (Ed.). (1978). *A short history of the Vietnam War*. Bloomington & London: Indiana University Press.

Mollett, W. (1888). On the necessity of legal registration for nurses. *Nursing Record*. London.

Moloney, T.W. & Rogers, D.E. (1979). Medical technology—A different view of the contentious argument over costs. *New England Journal of Medicine*, 301, 1413-1419.

Montag, M.L. (1951). *The education of nursing technicians*. New York: G.P. Putnam's Sons.

Montag, M.L. (1959). *Community college education for nursing: An experiment in technical education for nursing*. New York: McGraw-Hill Book Co.

Morison, S.E. (1965). *The Oxford history of the American people*. New York: Oxford University Press.

Morison, S.E. & Commager, H.S. (1942). *The growth of the American republic* (vols. 1-2). New York: Oxford University Press.

Morten, H. (1894). *Nurse's dictionary of medical terms and nursing treatment*. Philadelphia: W.B. Saunders Co.

Morton, T.G. (1897). *The history of the Pennsylvania Hospital, 1751-1895*. Philadelphia: Times Printing House.

Mumey, H. (1918). *Hygiene for nurses*. St. Louis: The C.V. Mosby Co.

Munson, H.W. (1948). Linda Richards. *American Journal of Nursing*, 48(9), 551-555.

Munson, H.W. & Stevens, K. (1934). *Story of the National League of Nursing Education*. Philadelphia: W.B. Saunders Co.

Murphy-Ende, K. (2002). Advanced practice nursing: Reflections on the past, issues for the future. *Oncology Nursing Forum*, 29(1), 106-112.

Murray, J. (2005). President's message: Working collaboratively to provide leadership for global nursing education. *Nursing Education Perspectives*, 26(3), 138.

NACGN—Four decades of service. (1945). New York: The National Association of Colored Graduate Nurses.

National Commission for the Study of Nursing and Nursing Education. (1970). *An abstract for action*. New York: McGraw-Hill Book Co.

National Federation for Specialty Nursing Organizations Public Relations Committee (1984). *NFSNO: The first ten years*. Washington, DC: The Federation.

National League for Nursing. (1985, December 5). *Legislative update*. New York: National League for Nursing.

National League of Nursing Education. (1917). *Standard curriculum for schools of nursing*. New York: National League of Nursing Education.

National League of Nursing Education. (1937). *A curriculum for schools of nursing*. New York: National League of Nursing Education.

Navy Nurse Corps observes forty-fifth anniversary [release]. *Military Surgeon*, 113(1), 45-47.

Nelson, S. & Gordan, S. (Eds.) (2006). *The complexities of care: Nursing reconsidered*. Ithaca, NY: Cornell University Press.

Neuman, L. (2006). Creating new futures in nursing education: Envisioning the evolution of e-nursing education. *Nursing Education Perspectives*, 27(1), 12-15.

Newman, M. (2008). *Transforming presence: The difference that nursing makes*. Philadelphia: F.A. Davis Company.

Newcomb, C. (1958). *St. John of God*. New York: Dodd, Mead & Co.

Newman, M.A. (1979). *Theory development in nursing*. Philadelphia: F.A. Davis Co.

Newton, M.E. (1949). *Florence Nightingale's philosophy of life and education*. Unpublished dissertation of Leland Stanford Junior University.

Nightingale, F. (1860). *Notes on nursing*. New York: D. Appleton & Co.

Nightingale, F. (1867). *Notes on hospitals* (3rd ed.). London: Longmans.

Nightingale, F. (1883). Nurses, training of. In R. Quain (Ed.), *A dictionary of medicine*. New York: Apppleton and Co.

Noble, D.L. (1992). *Forgotten warriors: Combat art from Vietnam*. Westport, CT: Praeger.

Norman, E.M. (1990). *Women at war: The story of fifty military nurses who served in Vietnam*. Philadelphia: University of Pennsylvania Press.

Nutting, M.A. (1905, June). Some results of preparatory courses for nurses. *American Journal of Nursing*, 5, 654.

Nutting, M.A. (1912). Educational status of nursing. *U.S. Bureau of Education Bulletin* (no. 7, no. 475). Washington, DC: U.S. Government Printing Office.

Nutting, M.A. (1925, October 27-29). Greeting at the New York State League for Nursing. In *Souvenir programme of the annual convention of the New York State Nurses' Association*. Albany, NY: The New York Organization for Public Health Nursing.

Nutting, M.A. (1926). *A sound economic basis for schools of nursing*. New York: G.P. Putnam's Sons.

Nutting, M.A. & Dock, L.L. (1907 & 1912). *A history of nursing: The evolution of nursing systems from earliest times to the foundations of the first English and American training schools for nurses* (vols.1-4). New York: G.P. Putnam's Sons.

Ogden, Brother Daniel (1957). *Of valiant men: A chronicle of the congregation of Alexian Brothers*. Gresham, WI: The Novitiate Press.

Ohlson, V.M. & Styles, M.M. (1994). International nursing. The role of the International Council of Nurses and the World Health Organization. In J. McCloskey & H.K. Grace (Eds.), *Current issues in nursing* (4th ed., pp. 407-415). St. Louis: Mosby.

O'Malley, I.B. (1931). *Florence Nightingale, 1820-1856*. London: Thornton Butterworth.

On the genius and character of Hogarth. (1818). In *The works of Charles Lamb*. London: Printed for C. and J. Ollier.

Orem, D. (1971). *Nursing: Concepts of practice*. New York: McGraw-Hill Book Co.

Orlando, I.J. (1961). *The dynamic nurse-patient relationship: Function, process, and principles*. New York: G.P. Putnam's Sons.

Osler, W. (1932). *Aequanimitas*. Philadelphia: Blakiston Co.

O'Sullivan, A., Carter, M., Marion, L., Pohl, J., & Werner, K. (2005, September 30). Moving forward together: The practice doctorate in nursing. *Online Journal of Issues in Nursing*, 10(3), 5-5. Retrieved June 9, 2008, from MEDLINE with Full Text database.

Oursler, F. (1949). *The greatest story ever told*. New York: Doubleday & Co., Inc.

Oursler, F. (1951). *The greatest book ever written*. New York: Doubleday & Co., Inc.

Pachter, H. (1961). *Paracelsus: Magic into science*. New York: Collier Books.

Paget, S. (1897). *Ambroise Paré and his times*. New York: G.P. Putnam's Sons.

Parker, W.W. (1892). Woman's place in the Christian world: Superior morally, inferior mentally to man: Not qualified for medicine or law; the contrariety and harmony of the sexes, *Transactions of the Medical Society of Virginia*, 23, 86-107.

Partin, B. (2005). The doctorate of nursing practice: A natural evolution. *The Nurse Practitioner*, 30(11), 23.

Patron, J., Greely, H., Higginson, T.W., Abbott, J.S.C., Hoppin, J., Winter, W., et al. (1868). *Eminent women of the age being narratives of the lives and deeds of the most prominent women of the present generation*. Hartford, CT: S. M. Betts & company; Chicago. IL: Gibbs & Nichols.

Payne, G.H. (1916). *The child in human progress*. New York: G.P. Putnam's Sons.

Pennock, M. (Ed.). (1940). *Makers of nursing history*. New York: Lakeside Publishing Co.

Peplau, H. (1952). *Interpersonal relations in nursing*. New York: G.P. Putnam's Sons.

Peters, M. (2007). Clinical nurse leader: A go to person. *The Pennsylvania Nurse*, 62(3), 17.

Petrucelli, R.J. (1978). Art and science. In A.S. Lyons & R.J. Petrucelli, *Medicine: An illustrated history*. New York: Harry N. Abrams, Inc.

Petrucelli, R.J. (1978). The dark ages. In A.S. Lyons & R.J. Petrucelli, *Medicine: An illustrated history*. New York: Harry N. Abrams, Inc.

Pilcher, J.E. (1907). The Red Cross. *Military Surgery*, 20, 230.

Pimlott, J. & Badsey, S. (Eds.). (1992). *The Gulf War assessed*. London: Arms and Armour Press.

Poole, E. (1935). *Nurses on horseback*. New York: The Macmillian Co.

Porter-O'Grady, T. (1997, Fall). The private practice of nursing: The gift of entrepreneurialism. *Nursing Administration Quarterly*, 22(1), 23-29.

Porter-O'Grady, T. (1998). The making of a nurse entrepreneur. *Seminars for Nurse Managers*, 6(1), 34-40.

Power, E. (1924). *Medieval people*. New York: Barnes & Noble.

Powers, E.J. (1866). *Hospital pencilings*. Boston: Edward L Mitchell.

Preston, A. (1863). *Nursing the sick and the training of nurses*. Philadelphia: King & Baird.

Pugh, G.F. & Fisher, A.J.B. (1970). *Ethics and health in late Victorian society*. London: Arundel.

Punam, E.J. (1921). *The lady*. New York: G.P. Putnam's Sons.

Quinn, N.K. & Somers, A.R. (1974). The patient's bill of rights: A significant aspect of the consumer revolution. *Nursing Outlook*, 22(4), 240-244.

Rathbone, W. (1890). *History and progress of district nursing*. New York: The Macmillam Co.

Rathbone, W. (1890). *Sketch of the history and progress of district nursing from its commencement in the year 1859 to the present date*. New York: The Macmilliam Co.

Ravenel, M.R. (Ed.). (1912). *Half century of public health*. New York: American Public Health Association.

Rayfield. S., Stimson, M., & Tattershall, L.M. (1930, October). A study of Negro public health nursing. *Public Health Nursing*, 22, 525.

Ream, A.C. (1982, October 25). Our undertrained nurses. *Newsweek*, 17.

Redfield, J. (1993). *The celestine prophecy*. New York: Warner Books.

Reeder, S.J. (1978). The social context of nursing. In N.L. Chaska (Ed.), *The nursing profession: Views through the mist*, New York: McGraw-Hill Book Co.

Reinach, S. (1930). *Orpheus: A history of religions*. New York: Liveright, Inc.

Riesman, D. (1936). *The story of medicine in the Middle Ages*. New York: Harper & Brothers.

Robb, I.H. (1898-1899). Some of the lessons of the late war and their bearing upon trained nursing, *Cleveland Medical Gazette*, 14, 463.

Robb, I.H. (1900). Nursing as a profession. *Albany Medical Annals*, 21, 491.

Robb, I.H. (1900). *Nursing ethics: For hospital and private use*. Cleveland: Koeckert.

Robb, I.H. (1905). The affiliation of training schools for nurses for educational purposes, *American Journal of Nursing*, 5, 666-679.

Robb, I.H. (1907). *Educational standards for nurses, with other addresses on nursing subjects*. Cleveland: Koeckert.

Robb, W. (2005). PhD, DNSc, ND: The ABCs of nursing doctoral degrees. *Dimensions of Critical Care Nursing: DCCN*, 24(2), 89-96.

Robeck, N. de (1953). *Saint Elizabeth of Hungary*. Milwaukee: Bruce Publishing Co.

Roberts, M.M. (1954). *American nursing: History and interpretation*. New York: The Macmillan Co.

Roberts, M.M. (1956). Lavinia Lloyd Dock: Nurse, feminist, internationalist. *American Journal of Nursing, 56*(2), 176-179.

Robinson, V. (1946). *White caps: The story of nursing.* Philadelphia: J.B. Lippincott Co.

Rockefeller Foundation, Division of Medical Education. (1932). *Nursing education and schools of nursing.* New York: The Foundation.

Rodabaugh, J.H. & Rodabaugh, M.J. (1951). *Nursing in Ohio: A history.* Columbus: The Ohio State Nurses Association.

Roddis, L.H. (1935). The U.S. hospital ship *Red Rover* (1862-1865). *Military Surgeon, 77,* 92.

Rogers, M.E. (1970). *An introduction to the theoretical basis of nursing.* Philadelphia: F.A. Davis Co.

Rosen, G. (1958). *A history of public health.* New York: MD Publications, Inc.

Rosenberg, C. (1962). *The cholera years.* Chicago: The University of Chicago Press.

Rosenberg, C.E. (1987). *The care of strangers.* New York: Basic Books, Inc.

Rosenthal, M.M. & Frenkel, M (1992). *Health care systems and their patients. An international perspective.* Boulder, San Francisco, Oxford: Westview Press.

Roy, C. (1967). *Introduction to nursing: An adaptation model.* Englewood Cliffs, NJ: Prentice-Hall, Inc.

Rushforth, H. & Glasper, E. (1999). Implications of nursing role expansion for professional practice. *British Journal of Nursing (Mark Allen Publishing), 8*(22), 1507-1513.

Saba, V. (1992). The classification of home health care nursing: Diagnoses and interventions. *Caring Magazine, 11*(3), 50-56.

Saba, V. (2001). Nursing informatics: Yesterday, today and tomorrow. *International Nursing Review, 48*(3), 177-187.

Saint Jerome. (1893). Letters. In *Nicene and post-Nicene fathers of the Christian church* (vol. 6). New York: The Christian Literature Co.

Saint Thomas Aquinas. (1945). *Basic writings.* New York: Random House.

Salmon, M., Talashek, M., & Tichy, A. (1988). Health for all: A transnational model for nursing. *International Nursing Review, 35*(4), 107-109.

Sandwith, F.M. (1914-1915). The nursing and care of the sick prior to 1850. *Hospitals, 56,* 273.

Sanford, J., Hall, P., & Roussel, L. (2007). The clinical nurse leader: New role in nursing. *Mississippi RN, 69*(1), 17.

Satterly, F. (2004). *Where have all the nurses gone? The impact of nursing shortage on American healthcare.* Amhurst, NY: Prometheus Books.

Schermerhorn, E. (1940). *On the trail of the eight pointed cross: A study of the heritage of the Knights Hospitallers in feudal Europe.* New York: G.P. Putnam's Sons.

Scovil, E.R. (1888). *In the sickroom: The art of nursing.* New York: Montgomery.

Seaman, V. (1800). *The midwives monitor, and mothers mirror, being three concluding lectures of a course of instruction on midwifery; containing directions for pregnant women; rules for the management of natural births, and for early discovering when the aid of a physician is necessary; and cautions for nurses, respecting both the mother and child. To which is prefixed, a syllabus of lectures on that subject.* New York: Issac Collins.

Seelye, Rev L.C. (1874). *The need of a collegiate education for women.* North Adams, MA: American Institute of Instruction.

Sellew, G. & Nuesse, C.J. (1946). *The history of nursing.* St. Louis: The C.V. Mosby Co.

Seymer, L.R. (1932). *A general history of nursing.* London: Faber & Faber Ltd.

Seymer, L.R. (1940). *Florence Nightingale.* London: Faber & Faber Ltd.

Shames, K. (1996). Financial empowerment: the holistic nurse entrepreneur. *Beginnings, 16*(7), 10.

Shaw, E. (1973). *The black nurse—Then, now, and?* Paper presented for continuing education, Nashville, TN: Meharry Medical College.

Shields, E.A. (Ed.). (1981). *Highlights in the history of the Army Nurse Corps.* Washington, DC: U.S. Army Center of Military History.

Shryock, R.H. (1959). *The history of nursing: An interpretation of the social and medical factors involved.* Philadelphia: W.B. Saunders Co.

Sigerist, H.E. (1934). *American medicine.* New York: W.W. Norton & Co., Inc.

Simmons, L.W. (1945). *The role of the aged in the primitive society.* New Haven, CT: Yale University Press.

Simms, L.M. (1991). The professional practice of nursing administration, *Journal of Nursing Administration, 21*(5), 37-46.

Simpson, R. (2004). The softer side of technology: How IT helps nursing care. *Nursing Administration Quarterly, 28*(4), 302-305.

Smith, F.B. (1982). *Florence Nightingale: Reputation and power.* London: Croom Helm.

Smith, G.R. (1975). From invisibility to blackness: The story of the National Black Nurses' Association. *Nursing Outlook, 23,* 225-229.

Smith, L. (1991). The history of nursing and politics in the United States. *Advancing Clinical Care: Official Journal of NOAADN, 6*(4), 6-7.

Smith, W. (1992). *American daughter gone to war: On the front lines with an Army nurse in Vietnam.* New York: William Morrow & Company, Inc.

Smith-Rosenberg, C. & Rosenberg, C. (1973). The female animal: Medical and biological views of woman and her role in nineteenth century America. *Journal of American History, 60*(2), 332-356.

Smolan, R., Moffitt, P.H., & Nathons, M. (1990). *The power to heal: Ancient arts and modern medicine.* New York: Prentice Hall Press.

Sowell, R.L. & Meadows, T.M. (1994). An integrated case management model: Developing standards, evaluation, and outcome criteria. *Nursing Administration Quarterly, 18*(2), 53-64.

Spalding, H.S. (1920). *Talks to nurses: The ethics of nursing.* New York: Benziger.

Spelts, D. (1986). Nurses who served—And who did not return. *American Journal of Nursing, 86*(9), 1037-1039.

Stafford, B.M. (1993). *Body Criticism. Imaging the unseen in enlightenment art and medicine.* Cambridge, MA: The MIT Press.

Stanton, S.L. (1986). *Vietnam order of battle.* New York: Galahad Books.

Staupers, M.K. (1961). *No time for prejudice.* New York: Macmillan Publishing Co., Inc.

Steuer, R.O., Saunders, J.B. de C.M. (1959). *Ancient Egyptian and Cnidian medicine.* Berkeley: University of California Press.

Stevens, E.F. (1928). *American hospital of the twentieth century: A treatise on the development of medical institutions, both in Europe and in America, since the beginning of the present century* (2nd ed.). New York: Architectural Record Co.

Stevens, R. (1971). *American medicine and the public interest.* New Haven, CT: Yale University Press.

Stewart, H.R. (1919). The value of the public health nurse to the community. *Modern Medicine, 1,* 429.

Stewart, I.M. (1909). *The hospital economics course from the students' standpoint.* Paper presented before the Maryland Nurses' Association.

Stewart, I.M. (1918). How can we help to improve our teaching in nursing schools? *Canadian Nurse 22,* 1593.

Stewart, I.M. (1921, November). Popular fallacies about nursing education. *The Modern Hospital, 18,* 1-2.

Stewart, I.M. (1929): The science and art of nursing [editorial]. *Nursing Education Bulletin, 2,* 1.

Stewart, I.M. (1939). Florence Nightingale—Educator. *Teachers College Record, 41*(3), 208-223.

Stewart, I.M. (1943). *The education of nurses.* New York: The Macmillan Co.

Stewart, I.M. (1961). *Reminiscences of Isabel M. Stewart.* New York: Oral History Research Office, Columbia University.

Stewart, I.M. & Austin, A.L. (1962). *A history of nursing* (5th ed.). New York: G.P. Putnam's Sons.

Stimson, J.C. (1925). Earliest known connection of nurses with Army hospitals in the United States, *American Journal of Nursing, 25*(1), 18.

Stimson, J.C. (1937). *History and manual of the Army Nurse Corps.* Carlisle, PA: Army Medical School.

Stirling, M. & National Geographic Society (U.S.). (1955). *National Geographic on Indians of the Americas: A color illustrated record.* Washington, DC: National Geographic Society.

Stobart, J.C. (1934). *The glory that was Greece* (rev. ed.). Boston: Beacon Press.

Storer, H. (1868). *Nurses and nursing.* Boston: Lee & Shepard.

Strachey, G.L. (1918). Florence Nightingale. In *Eminent Victorians.* London: G.P. Putnam's Sons.

Strachey, R. (1928). *The cause: A short history of the women's movement in Great Britain.* London: G. Bell & Sons.

Streef, M.B. (1994). Third-party reimbursement issues for advanced practice nurses in the '90s. In J. McCloskey & H.K. Grace (Eds.), *Current issues in nursing* (4th ed., pp. 437-449). St. Louis: Mosby.

Struthers, L.R. (1917). *The school nurse.* New York: G.P. Putnam's Sons.

Styles, M.M. (1977). Doctoral education in nursing: The current situation in historical perspective. In *National Conference on Doctoral Education in Nursing.* Philadelphia: University of Pennsylvania.

Styles, M.M. (1982). *On nursing: Toward a new endowment.* St. Louis: The CV Mosby Co.

Styles, M.M. (1992). Specialization and credentialing. In L. Aiken & C. Fagin, *Charting nursing's future agenda for the 1990s* (pp. 29-39). Philadelphia: J.B. Lippincott Company.

Styles, M.M. (1993). Macrotrends in nursing practice: What's in the pipeline? *Journal of Continuing Education in Nursing,* 24(1), 7-12.

Summers, S. & Summers H.J. (2009). *Saving lives: Why the media's portrayal of nurses puts us all at risk.* New York: Kaplan Publishing.

Sutton, F. & Smith, C. (1995). Advanced nursing practice: New ideas and new perspectives. *Journal of Advanced Nursing,* 21(6), 1037-1043.

Swenson, M., Salmon, M., Wold, J., & Sibley, L. (2005). Addressing the challenges of the global nursing community. *International Nursing Review,* 52(3), 173-179.

Taft, W.H. (1917, September). A distinct call to women. *Ladies Home Journal,* 34, 5.

Talley, C. (1925). *Ethics: A textbook for nurses.* New York: G.P. Putnam's Sons.

Taylor, E.J. (1925). The school of nursing at the Yale University. *American Journal of Nursing,* 25, 9-14.

Taylor, H.O. (1922). *Greek biology and medicine.* Boston: Marshall Jones Co.

Thatcher, V.S. (1953). *History of anesthesia with emphasis on the nurse specialist,* Philadelphia: J.B. Lippincott Co.

The American Society of Superintendents of Training Schools for Nursing. (1912). *Proceedings of the eighteenth annual convention of the American Society of Superintendents of Training Schools for Nursing.* New York: The American Society of Superintendents of Training Schools for Nursing.

The nurses have not lagged behind. (1945, April 28). Editorial. *The Saturday Evening Post.*

The State Board Test Pool Examination. (1952). *American Journal of Nursing,* 52(5), 613-615.

Thibodeau, J.A. (1983). *Nursing models: Analysis and evaluation.* Belmont, CA: Wadsworth Health Sciences.

Thompson, J. (1972). *The ANA in Washington.* Kansas City, MO: American Nurses Association.

Thompson, M. (1954). *The cry and the covenant.* New York: Doubleday & Co.

Thoms, A.B. (1929). *Pathfinders: A history of the progress of colored graduate nurses.* New York: Kay Printing House.

Thoms, A.B. & Bullock, C.E. (1928). Developing of facilities for colored nurse education, *Trained Nurse and Hospital Review,* 80, 722.

Thorwald, J. (1963). *Science and secrets of early medicine,* New York: Harcourt, Brace, & World, Inc.

Tiffany, F. (1937). *Life of Dorothea Lynde Dix.* Boston: Houghton.

Tinkham, C. & Voorhees, E. (1972). *Community health nursing—Evolution and process,* New York: Appleton-Century-Crofts.

Toffler, A. & Toffler, H. (1970). *Future shock.* New York: Random House.

Toffler, A. & Toffler, H. (1980). *The third wave.* New York: Morrow.

Toffler, A. & Toffler, H. (1995). *Creating a new civilization. Politics of the third wave,* Atlanta: Turner Publishing, Inc.

Tucker-Allen, S. (1998). Entrepreneurship in nursing practice: A vision for the future? *ABNF Journal,* 9(2), 27.

Tuker, M.A. & Malleson, H. (1900). *Handbook to Christian and ecclesiastical Rome.* New York: The Macmillan Co.

Tuttle, G.T. (1906, October). The male nurse. *American Journal of Insanity,* 63, 191-204.

Uhlhorn, G. (1883). *Christian charity in the ancient church.* New York: Charles Scribner.

U.S. Council of National Defense. (1971). *First annual report of the Council of National Defense [fiscal year 1917].* Washington, DC: U.S. Government Printing Office.

Vallery-Radot, D. (1923). *Life of Pasteur.* Garden City, NY: Doubleday.

Van Doren, M. (1945). *Walt Whitman.* New York: Viking Press.

Van Loon, H.W. (1931). *RVR: The life and times of Rembrandt.* New York: Liveright Publishing Co.

van Maanen, H.M.T. (1990). Nursing in transition: An analysis of the state of the art in relation to the conditions of practice and society's expectation. *Journal of Advanced Nursing,* 15, 914-924.

Vietnam Veterans' Association. (1984, October). Women vets profiled in new VA study, *Veteran,* 5.

Vreeland, E.M. (1950). Fifty years of nursing in the federal government nursing services. *American Journal of Nursing* (anniversary issue), 50(10), 626-631.

Wakeford, C. (1917). *The wounded soldiers' friends: The story of Florence Nightingale, Clara Barton, and others.* London: Headley-Brothers.

Wald, L. (1934). *Windows on Henry Street.* Boston: Little, Brown & Co.

Wald, L.D. (1915). *The house on Henry Street.* New York: Henry Holt & Co.

Walsh, J. & Aulich, J. (Eds.). (1989). *Vietnam images: War and representation.* Houndmills, Basingstoke, Hampshire, England: Macmillam Press Ltd.

Walsh, J.J. (1929). *The history of nursing.* New York: P.J. Kenedy & Sons.

Waltari, M. (1949). *The Egyptian.* New York: G.P. Putnam's Sons.

Warren, J.J. (1994). Nursing diagnosis taxonomy development: Overview and issues. In J. McCloskey & H.K. Grace (Eds.), *Current issues in nursing* (4th ed., pp. 122-128). St. Louis: Mosby.

Waters, Y. (1909). *Visiting nursing in the United States.* New York: Charities Publication Committee.

Weaver, C.A., Delaney, C.W., Weber, P., & Carr, R.L. (Eds.) (2006). *Nursing and Informatics for the 21st century. An international look at practice, trends and the future.* Chicago: Healthcare Information and Management Systems Society.

Weeks-Shaw, C.S. (1885). *A textbook of nursing for the use of training schools, families, and private students.* New York: Appleton.

Weinberg, D.B. (2003). *Codegreen: Money-driven hospitals and the dismantling of nursing.* Ithaca, NY: Cornell University Press.

Weinreb, N. (1953). *The Babylonians.* New York: Doubleday & Co.

Weinstein, S.M. & Brooks A.T. (2007). *Nursing without borders: Values, wisdom, success makers.* Indianapolis: Sigma Theta Tau International.

Wells, C. (1964). *Bones, bodies, and disease.* New York: Frederick A Praeger.

Werley, H., Ryan, P., Zorn, C.R., & Devine, E.C. (1994). Why the nursing minimum data set (NMDS)? In J. McCloskey & H.K. Grace (Eds.), *Current issues in nursing* (4th ed., pp. 113-122). St. Louis: Mosby.

West, M. & Hawkins, C. (1950). *Nursing schools at the mid-century.* New York: National Committee for the Improvement of Nursing Services.

Wheeler, H. (1889). *Deaconesses, ancient and modern.* New York: Hunt & Eaton.

Whitehead, A.N. (1929). *The aims of education and other essays.* New York: The Macmillan Co.

Whitman, W. (1898). *The wound-dresser: A series of letters written from the hospitals in Washington during the war of the rebellion.* Boston: Small, Maynard.

Whitman, W. (1961). *Leaves of grass* [selections]. New York: Crown Publishers.

Whitman, W. (1968). *The works of Walt Whitman.* New York: Funk & Wagnall's, Inc.

Whitney, J. (1936). *Elizabeth Fry.* Boston: Brown & Co.

Wilson, F. (1941). *Crusader in crinoline: The life of Harriet Beecher Stowe.* Philadelphia: J.B. Lippincott Co.

With the Army Nurse Corps in Korea. (1951, June). *American Journal of Nursing,* 51(6), 387.

Woelful, N. (1933). *Molders of the American mind.* New York: Columbia University Press.

Wong, K.C. & Wu, Lieu-The (1936). *History of Chinese medicine.* Shanghai: National Quarantine Service.

Woodham-Smith, C. (1951). *Florence Nightingale.* New York: McGraw-Hill Book Co.

Woody, T. (1929). *A history of women's education in the United States* (vol. 2). New York: The Science Press.

Woolf, S.J. (1937, March 7). Miss Wald at 70 sees her dreams realized. *New York Times.* 22.

Woolley, L. (1963). *History unearthed.* London: Ernest Benn Ltd.

Woolsey, J.S. (1868). *Hospital days,* New York: Van Nostrand.

World Health Organization. (1985). *Nurses lead the way.* Geneva: World Health Organization.

Wylie, W.G. (1877). *Hospitals: Their history, organization and construction.* New York: Appleton.

Zander, K. (1994). Nurses and case management. To control or to collaborate? In J. McCloskey & H.K. Grace (Eds.) *Current issues in nursing* (4th ed., pp. 254-260). St. Louis: Mosby.

Zaret, H. (1944). *Song of the Army Nurse Corps* [music by Lou Singer]. MCA Music, a division of MCA Inc., 445 Park Avenue, New York, New York 10022.

Zarnitz, P., & Malone, E. (2006). Surgical nurse practitioners as registered nurse first assists: The role, historical perspectives, and educational training. *Military Medicine*, 171(9), 875-878.

Zielger, P. (1969). *The black death.* New York: John Day Co.

Zimmermann, A. (1976). ANA: Its record on social issues. *American Journal of Nursing,* 76(4), 588-590.

Zinsser, H. (1934). *Rats, lice and history.* New York: Blue Ribbon Books, Inc.

Zytkowski, M. (2003). Nursing informatics: the key to unlocking contemporary nursing practice. *AACN Clinical Issues: Advanced Practice in Acute & Critical Care*, 14(3), 271-281.

Index

Page numbers followed by *f* and *t* indicate figures and tables, respectively.

375